Joseph Mertes
August 1989

THE RETARDATION OF
AGING AND DISEASE
BY DIETARY RESTRICTION

THE RETARDATION OF AGING AND DISEASE BY DIETARY RESTRICTION

By

RICHARD WEINDRUCH, PH.D.

Biomedical Research and Clinical Medicine Program
National Institute on Aging
National Institutes of Health
Bethesda, Maryland

and

ROY L. WALFORD, M.D.

Department of Pathology
University of California
Los Angeles, California

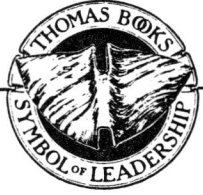

CHARLES C THOMAS • PUBLISHER
Springfield • Illinois • U.S.A.

Published and Distributed Throughout the World by
CHARLES C THOMAS • PUBLISHER
2600 South First Street
Springfield, Illinois 62794-9265

This book is protected by copyright. No part of
it may be reproduced in any manner without
written permission from the publisher.

© *1988 by* CHARLES C THOMAS • PUBLISHER
ISBN 0-398-05496-7
Library of Congress Catalog Card Number: 88-12288

With **THOMAS BOOKS** *careful attention is given to all details of manufacturing and design. It is the Publisher's desire to present books that are satisfactory as to their physical qualities and artistic possibilities and appropriate for their particular use.* **THOMAS BOOKS** *will be true to those laws of quality that assure a good name and good will.*

Printed in the United States of America
Q-R-3

Library of Congress Cataloging in Publication Data
Weindruch, Richard.
    The retardation of aging and disease by dietary restriction / by Richard Weindruch and Roy L. Walford.
      p. cm.
    Bibliography: p.
    Includes index.
    ISBN 0-398-05496-7
    1. Aging—Nutritional aspects. 2. Low-calorie diet. 3. Rats—Physiology. 4. Mice—Physiology. 5. Diet in disease. I. Walford, Roy L. II. Title.
    [DNLM: 1. Aging. 2. Diet. 3. Diet Therapy. 4. Life Expectancy. WT 104 W423r]
QP86.W45   1988
612'.67—dc19
DNLM/DLC
for Library of Congress   88-12288
                                                                                       CIP

To . . .
>   *Clive McCay*
>   *Albert Tannenbaum*
>   *Morris Ross*
>   *. . . for starting all this.*

PREFACE

IT HAS BEEN known for slightly over fifty years that dietary restriction (DR), if properly executed, will greatly extend the maximum life span of rodents and decrease the incidence of cancer and other late-life diseases. For most of that time, however, the phenomenon has been regarded more as an interesting curiosity than as a unique model system for investigating not only aging and cancer but a variety of physiologic processes.

Our own interest in the model began in the late 1960s when we sought to use a DR regimen in mice as a necessary albeit insufficient test of the immunologic theory of aging. If immune dysfunction were involved in aging, we reasoned, this life span (LS)-extending procedure should delay the onset of age-related immune functional changes. Indeed this proved to be the case.

Interest in DR-induced phenomena increased substantially in the 1970s and even more in the 80s, due in part to the increased focus on the aging process in the United States and other developed countries, and in part to the gathering realization of the magnitude and consistency of the changes provoked by appropriate DR regimens. This growing interest in DR encompasses not only LS alteration but disease parameters and a wide variety of other biologic parameters. Dietary restriction has emerged over competitor methodologies as the only procedure that can actually and strikingly retard aging in homeothermic vertebrates.

A reflection of the developing interest in DR is the fact that the National Institute on Aging (NIA) has recently established a colony numbering about 30,000 rodents (rats and mice), of various inbred and hybrid strains, including animals fed ad libitum and others subjected to DR. These are scheduled for study by NIA-supported grantee laboratories to seek to establish the validity and usefulness of a variety of different potential so-called "biomarkers of aging." The rodents are being maintained at the National Center for Toxicological Research at Jefferson, Arkansas. In early 1987, the NIA also set up a primate colony to determine whether DR will affect primates as it does other vertebrates.

In its recent report, "Aging in Today's Environment," the National Research Council's Committee on Chemical Toxicity and Aging identifies the DR model as potentially one of the most fruitful areas for modern gerontologic research.

In view of the above and our own long-term preoccupation with DR, it seems timely and appropriate to undertake a critical review of the field to date, to present our own interpretations of many of the phenomena involved, and to suggest future avenues of research. Such is the purpose of this book. It should be noted that to facilitate ease of reading we have rounded off most figures dealing with ages, weights, disease incidences, and certain other parameters.

In Chapter 1 the DR model is introduced, key issues are raised, and a wide-ranging overview is presented, according to five historical and conceptual subdivisions. The remainder of the book expands on these introductory topics. Chapter 2 considers effects of DR on LS, Chapter 3 its effects on susceptibility to, and incidence of various (mostly late-life) diseases, and Chapter 4 the effect of DR on other biological parameters which include the so-called "biomarkers of aging." Chapter 5 then discusses the central question: How does DR retard the aging process or processes? What is the mechanism, or the mechanisms, whereby it exerts its wide-ranging multi-system, multi-process effects? The search for mechanisms is becoming a more active aspect of the DR field. Chapter 6 examines the human side of DR. Will it retard aging in humans? How can this question be approached short of a life-time experiment? Long-term preventive health measures in humans may require a different orientation towards evidence than has been customary in the largely therapeutic medicine practiced up to the present time. We conclude our book with suggested research needs, particularly in terms of human application.

On points of controversy we have not hesitated to argue our own position, and moreover have freely speculated on various issues throughout the book, believing that these insertions may serve a useful function in stimulating thought and research, and hopefully make the book more than a dry coverage of what is now a massive, rapidly expanding data base on the manifold aspects of the DR paradigm.

ACKNOWLEDGMENTS

MANY COLLEAGUES have contributed greatly to our studies on DR and we are especially indebted to Doctors Maria Gerbase-DeLima, Robert K. Liu, Meg Mathies, George Smith, Ted Konen, R. Mickey, K.E. Cheney, S.R.S. Gottesman, P.J. Meredith, A. Koizumi, S.S. Ball, T.W. Bruice, S.B. Harris, R.B. Effros, F. Licastro, J. Davis, P.J. Leveille, J. Horwitz, M.K. Cheung, M.A. Verity, D.K. Ingram, S. Fligiel, D. Hollander, D. Guthrie, B. Devens and H.V. Raff. We appeciate the skilled and good spirited technical assistance of James Kristie, Glenda MeFeeters, Paula Wilhelmi, Edith Zeller, Mel Harris, Augusto Tayag, and Beagle Mullen, and the care extended to our mice by the UCLA Division of Laboratory Animal Medicine. The administrative assistance of Larry Weber and Helga Bradish is gratefully acknowledged, as is the word processing of Susan Halleman. We appreciate the support of our work given by the several Chairmen of the Department of Pathology, UCLA Medical Center, Doctors Sidney Madden, Julien Van Lancker, and P.A. Cancilla. We sincerely thank Doctors Huber Warner and Steve Harris for their comments on the manuscript, and Doctor Evan Hadley for his encouragement. The patience and drawings of Robin Weindruch are much appreciated, as are the additional drawings of Kirsty Iredale and the photography of Carol Appleton. Our research on DR has been supported by the National Institute on Aging, the National Cancer Institute, the Life Extension Foundation, and the Paul Glenn Foundation.

CONTENTS

                                                                                       Page

Dedication v
Preface vii
Acknowledgments ix

Chapter 1
AN OVERVIEW

A. INTRODUCTION.. 3
    1. The Goals of Gerontology.................................... 3
    2. Approaches to the Study of Aging 3
    3. Strategies for Increasing LS 4
    4. Maximum LS in Developed Societies Today 5
B. FIVE HISTORICAL PHASES OF DR RESEARCH.................. 6
    1. LS Extension 7
        a. *Invertebrates and Poikilothermic Vertebrates* 7
        b. *Rodents* 8
    2. Disease Incidence... 15
    3. Physiologic Changes: The "Biomarkers of Aging" 16
        a. *Criteria for a Biomarker* 17
        b. *Division of Biomarkers into Sets* 19
        c. *Genetic Complication to Biomarker Utility*................ 19
        d. *Some Biomarkers Are Not Influenced by DR* 20
    4. Mechanisms 21
        a. *Dietary Restriction and the "Theories of Aging"* 21
        b. *Uni- and Multi-Factorial Aging*.......................... 24
        c. *Dietary Restriction and Between-Species/Within-Species*
           Comparisons 26

	Page
5. Human Application	28
C. STATISTICAL TREATMENT OF DATA	28
D. SUMMARY	29

Chapter 2
DIETARY RESTRICTION: EFFECTS ON SURVIVORSHIP

A. INTRODUCTION	31
B. ANALYSIS OF SURVIVORSHIP	31
C. STUDIES IN INVERTEBRATES	36
D. STUDIES IN VERTEBRATES	39
1. Studies of DR in Non-Rodent Vertebrates	39
2. Studies of DR in Rodents	40
a. *Types of Diets*	40
b. *Feeding Strategies for DR*	41
i. *Restricted Feeding of an Adequate Diet*	42
ii. *Low Protein Diets*	43
c. *Fasting*	44
d. *Early-Onset Dietary Restriction (EDR)*	45
i. *Growth, Puberty Onset and Health*	45
ii. *Longevity*	48
e. *Adulthood-Onset Dietary Restriction (ADR)*	60
f. *Growth Rate, Body Weight and Life Span*	68
E. SUMMARY	71

Chapter 3
DIETARY RESTRICTION: EFFECTS ON DISEASE

A. INTRODUCTION	73
B. SPONTANEOUS DISEASES	76
1. Dietary Restriction Started Early in Life (EDR)	76
a. *Studies with Rats*	76
b. *Studies with Mice*	84
i. *Short-Lived Strains*	85
ii. *Long-Lived Strains*	89
2. Dietary Restriction Started in Adulthood (ADR)	95
a. *Studies with Rats*	95

	Page
b. *Studies with Mice*	97
C. INDUCED DISEASES	101
1. Studies with Mice	102
a. *What is the Relationship Between the Severity of DR and Induced Tumor Incidence and Time of Onset?*	102
b. *Does DR Affect Tumor Initiation and/or Promotion?*	104
c. *Must DR be Started Early in Life to Retard Induced Tumors?*	104
d. *How Does the Quality of the DR Regimen Affect Induction of Tumors?*	105
2. Studies with Rats	108
a. *Importance of Restriction of Dietary Energy vs. Fat in Inhibiting Chemical Tumorigenesis*	108
b. *Intestinal Tumorigenesis by Chemicals*	112
c. *Radiation-Induced Tumors*	113
d. *Hormones and Cancer*	114
e. *Diabetes*	114
D. SUMMARY	114

Chapter 4
DIETARY RESTRICTION: EFFECTS ON BIOLOGICAL PARAMETERS

A. INTRODUCTION	117
B. MOLECULAR PARAMETERS	118
1. Collagen	118
2. Enzymes and Metabolites	120
a. *Long-Term DR*	120
b. *Short-Term DR*	135
3. Neuroendocrine	137
a. *Reproductive Aspects*	138
b. *Non-Reproductive Aspects*	143
i. *Thyroid Axis*	143
ii. *Growth Hormone (GH) and Somatomedins*	147
iii. *ACTH and Corticosterone*	148
iv. *Insulin and Glucagon*	149
v. *Catecholamines*	155

      vi. *Parathyroid Hormone (PTH) and Calcitonin*.................156
      vii. *Brain Receptors*.................156
   c. *Synopsis*.................159
4. Nucleic Acid Content, Expression and Repair.................159
   a. *Content*.................160
   b. *Expression*.................166
   c. *Repair*.................167
5. Protein Content, Synthesis and Turnover.................167
   a. *Content*.................168
   b. *Synthesis and Turnover*.................171
6. Lipid Content and Peroxidation.................173
   a. *Lipid Content*.................174
   b. *Lipid Peroxidation and Lipofuscin*.................176
7. Other Serum Components.................178

C. IMMUNOLOGIC PARAMETERS.................179
1. Thymus.................179
2. Cell Numbers, Proportions and Subpopulations.................183
3. Immune Response Capacities.................186
4. Autoimmunity.................196
5. Lymphoid Biochemistry.................197

D. PHYSIOLOGIC PARAMETERS.................197
1. Metabolic Rate.................197
   a. *Lifetime Energy Intake*.................198
   b. *O_2 Consumption and Heat Production*.................201
   c. *Mitochondria*.................203
2. Body Temperature.................209
3. Body Composition.................213
4. Muscle.................215
5. Adipose Tissue.................218
6. Bone.................221
7. Reproductive Senescence.................223
8. Other Physiologic Parameters.................226

E. LEARNING AND BEHAVIORAL PARAMETERS.................227
F. SUMMARY.................229

Chapter 5
MECHANISMS: HOW DOES DIETARY RESTRICTION RETARD AGING?

- A. INTRODUCTION...231
- B. EVOLUTIONARY PERSPECTIVE 234
  1. Totter's Hypothesis 234
  2. Sacher's Equations..235
- C. ENERGY METABOLISM 237
  1. Background 237
     a. Age Changes in Normal Metabolism 237
        i. Metabolic Rate...237
        ii. Mitochondria..239
     b. Free Radicals and Aging..................................241
        i. Energy Coupling in Mitochondria..................243
        ii. Free Radical Production in Mitochondria.........245
        iii. Free Radical Neutralization........................246
     c. Metabolic Efficiency.....................................248
  2. Dietary Restriction and Energy Metabolism 251
     a. Dietary Restriction and Metabolic Rate 252
     b. Metabolic Efficiency and Energy Intake................253
     c. Decreased Free Radical Production by DR.............256
     d. Increased Free Radical Neutralization by DR 256
     e. Other Possibilities.......................................260
- D. BODY TEMPERATURE 260
  1. Poikilotherms 260
  2. Homeotherms...261
- E. PROTEIN SYNTHESIS, DNA, CHROMATIN, GENE EXPRESSION, DNA REPAIR 263
  1. Protein Synthesis 265
  2. DNA and Chromatin 267
  3. Gene Expression 268
  4. DNA Repair..270
- F. NEUROENDOCRINE INTERPRETATION 272
  1. Hypothalamic-Pituitary Axis................................273

			Page
	2. Reproductive Senescence and the Hypothalamus	276
	3. Glucocorticoid and Neuroendocrine Cascades	278
	4. Neuroendocrine-Immune Interactions	279
	5. Conclusion	280
G.	IMMUNOLOGIC INTERPRETATION	281
	1. Aging, Immune Function, and MHC-Related Functions	281
	2. Dietary Restriction, Immune Function, and the MHC	282
	a. *Long-Lived Strains*	283
	b. *Short-Lived Strains*	284
	c. *MHC-Influenced but Non-Immune Functions*	285
	3. Conclusion	286
H.	THE BASAL/INDUCED ACTIVITY HYPOTHESIS	286
I.	SYSTEMS ANALYSIS	289
J.	CONCLUSION AND INTERPRETATION	293

Chapter 6
PROSPECTS FOR RETARDING HUMAN AGING BY DIETARY RESTRICTION

A.	INTRODUCTION	295
B.	PROOF AND PROBABILITY IN MEDICAL PRACTICE	296
C.	PROFESSIONAL "AGEISM"	299
D.	EVIDENCE AND CONJECTURE IN FAVOR OF THE PROPOSITION	300
	1. Are the Animal Data Translatable to Humans?	300
	2. Human Studies	301
	a. *The Okinawan Population Isolate*	301
	b. *Vallejo's Experiment*	303
	c. *Anorexia Nervosa*	303
	d. *Long-Term Dietary Studies*	304
	e. *Other Dietary Studies*	305
	f. *Comment on Human Studies*	306
E.	EVIDENCE AND CONJECTURE AGAINST THE PROPOSITION	306
	1. Actuarial Analyses	306
	2. Masoro's Objections	311

| 3. Other Arguments..314
F. LEVEL OF RESTRICTION AND METHODOLOGY
   APPROPRIATE FOR A HUMAN STUDY.....................316
        1. When to Begin...316
        2. Rapidity of Weight Loss...................................317
        3. How Much Weight Loss....................................317
        4. Energy Requirements......................................319
        5. Essential Nutrients.......................................321
        6. Summary of Dietary Recommendations......................322
G. POTENTIAL DANGERS AND/OR DISADVANTAGES OF
   DR FOR HUMANS...323
H. POTENTIAL BENEFITS OF DR BESIDES LS EXTENSION....326
I. SOCIAL EFFECTS OF LS EXTENSION......................328
J. RESEARCH NEEDS AND RECOMMENDATIONS FOR
   HUMAN STUDIES..330
        1. Biomarkers of Aging.......................................330
        2. Primate Populations.......................................335
        3. Testing of Human Cohorts................................335
        4. Social Planning..336
K. SUMMARY..336

Bibliography..339
Abbreviations...399
Author Index..401
Subject Index...425

THE RETARDATION OF
AGING AND DISEASE
BY DIETARY RESTRICTION

CHAPTER 1

AN OVERVIEW

INTRODUCTION

WHILE THE extension of life span (LS) has been one of humankind's oldest preoccupations, indeed one of the great dreams of our species (Walford, 1983), biogerontology, whose classic goal has been to realize this dream, remained what may be labeled a "fringe science" until relatively recent times. This attitude has been changing. The establishment of the National Institute on Aging (NIA) in 1974 was a milestone event for American aging research. Biogerontology is now attracting new investigators from diverse backgrounds, in part because of increased funding availability, but perhaps mainly because, as Smith-Sonneborn (1988) has so aptly put it, "The feasibility threshold has been reached."

The Goals of Gerontology

The goals of modern biogerontology (hereafter referred to simply as "gerontology") include: (1) a better understanding of the biologic cause(s) of aging, (2) extending the maximum LS of humans, which goal includes the retention of functional vigor (i.e., not simply adding "old years onto old"), and (3) improving the quality of the later years of life (more properly the domain of geriatrics than of fundamental aging studies).

Approaches to the Study of Aging

The approaches used to date to study the fundamental biology of aging fall into five categories, as outlined in Table 1.1. Each category is now occupied by a sizeable body of research studies, but there has been some tendency for research to remain confined within the categories. For example, while interesting biochemical and other differences exist *between* species which seem to relate to the great differences in LSs between species, the data have rarely been integrated or reflected upon with respect to biochemical changes that take place with normal aging *within* a species. Also, non-gerontologists working with diseases which show features of accelerated aging (e.g. systemic lupus erythematosus [Barnett et al., 1981], or diabetes mellitus [Walford et al., 1981b]), have rarely considered the gerontologic aspects of those maladies, i.e., have not looked for interactive relationships between categories 3 and 4 (Table 1.1). Dietary restriction (DR), the subject of the present treatise, is a subdivision of category 5. One emphasis maintained throughout our book will be to inquire how DR integrates with and sheds light upon other approaches to the study of aging.

TABLE 1.1

Ways to Investigate the Biology of Aging

1. Differences in LSs between species
2. Differences in LSs between strains, races or individuals
3. Changes with normal aging in morphology and function
4. Models of accelerated aging (e.g. Down's syndrome, autoimmune diseases, thymectomy)
5. Models of decelerated aging (e.g. dietary restriction)

Strategies for Increasing LS

A number of strategies have been employed in the attempt to increase the LSs of different species (i.e., Category 5, Table 1.1), either as a device that might be applicable to humans on an empirical basis, or as a model system for the study of aging. These strategies are listed in Table 1.2 (see page 9), with selected references for those reporting actual survival data.

Among the strategies, a lowering of core body temperature has been found to retard aging and extend LS in invertebrates and poikilothermic vertebrates (reviewed in Sohol, 1981, and in Liu & Walford, 1972), as has antioxidant administration in certain invertebrates (Balin, 1982);

but only DR has been shown to extend the species-characteristic maximum LS in nearly all species so far tested, including a number of invertebrates (*Amoeba* and honeybees may be exceptions, but for specialized reasons: see "STUDIES IN INVERTEBRATES," Chapter 2), fish, and homeothermic vertebrates such as mammals. The effect of controlled DR on primate longevity, including the longevity of humans, has never been adequately tested. But epidemiologic observations as well as inferential data derived from physiologic alterations during long-term weight loss regimens for obesity, suggest that humans would respond to DR in a manner similar to other animals.

Maximum LS in Developed Societies Today

A look at survival curves for USA females in 1900, 1960 and 1980 (Figure 1.1) may be instructive.[1] We see that the *average* LS has increased from about 60 years in 1900 to 80 years in 1980. Despite this 30 percent increase in average LS during the 1900s, the *maximum* LS has increased far less, if at all. A slight increase in maximum human LS in the USA does appear to have occurred quite recently (Schneider & Brody, 1983; Myers & Manton, 1984), with the oldest segment of the population showing the greatest increase in life expectancy. That the USA mortality rate over age 85 is decreasing for both sexes at a proprotionately greater rate than for under 85 age-groups can be interpreted to suggest that neither sex is near its biological maximum LS limit, or else that the limits are being increased (Schneider & Brody, 1983). This depends on how one defines maximum LS. Accepting the average age of the longest lived 10 percent of the population (the 10th decile of survivorship) as a good index of maximum LS, then maximum LS seems to be increasing in modern Western societies. However, if maximum LS is defined either as the average age of the very longest lived 0.0005 percent of the population, or the age of the longest lived individual, then it is not clearly increasing. Despite important advances in medicine and public health which have allowed for better prevention and treatment of diseases, and for an increase in average LS, the maximum LS barrier for humans (as defined by the latter criterion) has not been breached. Nor has the maximum LS barrier been breached for other mammals, except for the DR model, which is the subject of this book.

---

[1]It should be noted that to facilitate ease of reading we have rounded off most figures dealing with ages, weights, disease incidences, and certain other parameters.

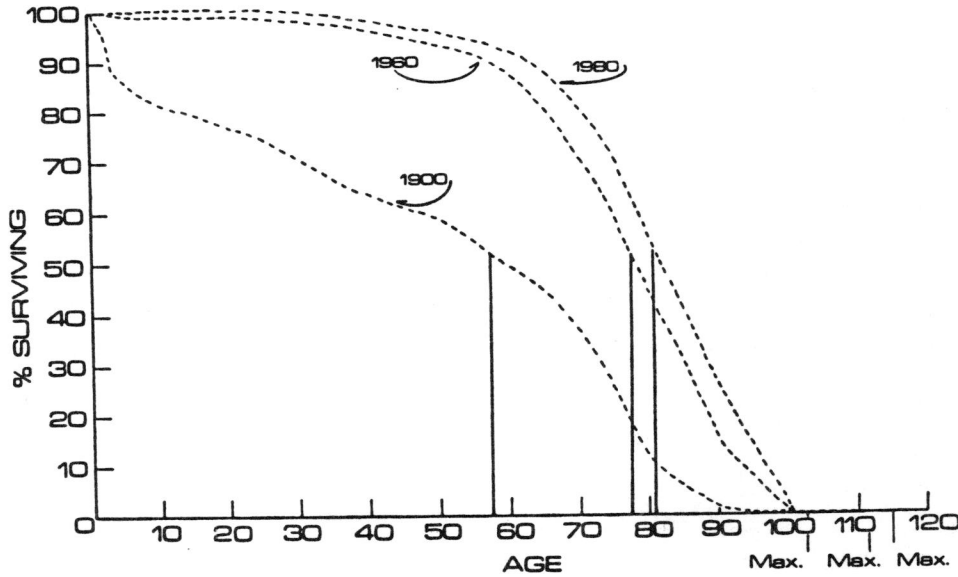

Figure 1.1. Survival curves for U.S. females in 1900, 1960, 1980. Vertical lines indicate 50 percent survivals subject to the mortality risks of 1900, 1960, and 1980 respectively. The "Max." points indicate "life endurancy," or the age to which one in 100,000 persons could expect to survive based on the mortality risks of 1900, 1960 or 1980. Adapted from Meyers and Manton (1984).

FIVE HISTORICAL PHASES OF DR RESEARCH

Energy intake restriction without essential nutrient deficiency, also labeled by the catch-phrase "*under*nutrition without *mal*nutrition" and here called "DR" (dietary restriction), retards aging and extends LS in nearly all species so far tested, and across wide phylogenetic differences. Historical phases of this model system for studying aging have included: (1) modulation of the survival curve along with lowering the mortality rate, (2) effects on disease incidence and ages of onset, (3) effects on the physiological changes that occur normally with aging, (4) a new phase that is focused on possible mechanisms whereby DR influences such widely diverse phenomena, (5) and the phase of human application which is still at an early stage. While we shall use such a framework in both this introductory chapter and throughout the book, it should be underscored that the various phases are perhaps more conceptual than chronologic. All the above are still going on, although current emphasis is on physiological changes and how studying them may uncover basic mechanisms.

For example, while LS extension represents the first phase, investigators are still improving dietary methodology to obtain even further extension, and are perhaps at the step of adding additional techniques, including even non-DR techniques, to a basic restriction regimen in order to further increase LS. Ambient temperature control might be such an example. Within limits, external temperature makes little difference to LS in fully fed homeotherms. However, the effect of ambient temperature on survival of rats which have been severely energy restricted to the point of starvation, as shown in Figure 1.2, suggests that a similar survival effect might obtain in DR animals, which might be able to be maintained on an even lower energy intake at an appropriately higher temperature, as opposed to normal laboratory temperature. (Other evidence to be presented later, for example on correlations between LS and body weight (BW) within a DR population, support the idea that one cannot necessarily predict the behavior of DR animals from that of a fully fed population.) Recently, Harrison and Archer (1987a) added a new twist to the DR methodology by finding that some additional increase in the LS of DR mice was achieved by relaxing the degree of energy restriction at the end stage of the animals' lives. Thus, the "first phase" in the history of DR research is in fact still viable.

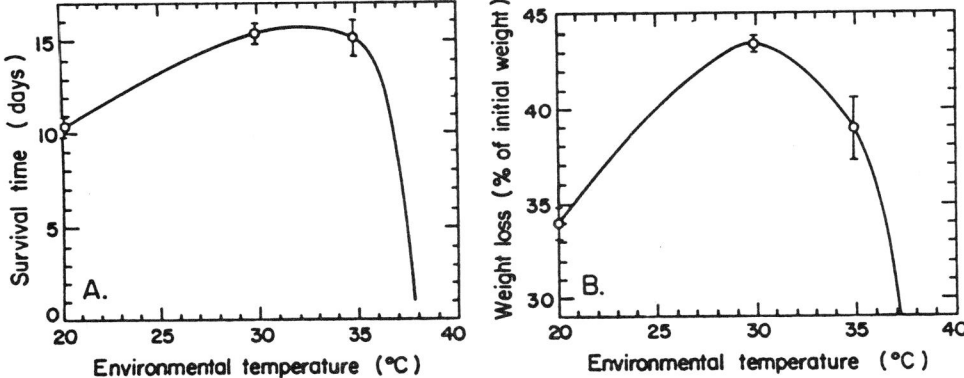

Figure 1.2. The effect of environmental temperature on survival and weight loss by time of death of fasting (water only) rats. Adapted from Kleiber (1975).

LS Extension

Invertebrates and Poikilothermic Vertebrates

Various types of restricted feeding regimens extend LS in lower animals, including the protozoan *Tokophyra* (Rudzinska, 1952), rotifers

(Fanestil & Barrows, 1965), *Daphnia* (Ingle et al., 1937), *Drosophila* (Loeb & Northrop, 1917), spiders (Austad, 1988), and fish (Comfort, 1963; Walford, 1983). These and related findings are discussed at greater length in Chapter 2.

Rodents

Almost all DR work with homeothermic vertebrates has been with rats and mice. Among many putative anti-aging interventions tested (Table 1.2), DR is the sole strategy which retards a broad spectrum of age-related biologic changes, convincingly reduces the mortality rates (Sacher, 1977), and extends maximum LS (Ross, 1978; Cutler, 1981; Schneider & Reed, 1985a and 1985b).

The extension of maximum rodent LS via DR was first clearly shown more than 50 years ago by McCay and coworkers (1935). An earlier report of Osborne et al. (1917) is sometimes credited as being first but the data therein do not actually show DR (called "stunting" in that report) to increase the maximum LS in the test animals (rats). The work of Ross (for review see Ross, 1978) from the 1950s until his death in 1984 provided extensive information on DR's influence on LS, as well as on diseases and biochemical parameters in obesity-prone male Sprague-Dawley rats. Over the last decade or so, other research groups have studied aging in rodents on DR. These include Masoro's group at the University of Texas, San Antonio (reviewed in Masoro, 1984), Barrows (reviewed by Barrows & Kokkonen, 1984) and Goodrick, Ingram and colleagues at the NIA's facility at Baltimore, the group of Good, Fernandes, and Yunis, all originally at the University of Minnesota (reviewed by Fernandes, 1984 and Good & Gajjar, 1986), Merry and colleagues at the University of Hull, England (see Holehan & Merry, 1986), our own group at UCLA (reviewed by Weindruch, 1984), and others.

Successful DR regimens do *not* lead to *mal*nutrition, but instead provide the essential nutrients in adequate amounts while restricting calorie intake to a range 30-70 percent below the ad lib level. The LS extending effects seem to depend quite specifically on energy (calorie) restriction alone, since restriction of fat (French et al., 1953; Birt et al., 1982a), protein (Nakagawa et al., 1974; Birt et al., 1982b; Feldman et al., 1982) or carbohydrate (Dalderup & Visser, 1969) *without* energy restriction does not increase the maximum species-specific LS of rodents. Maximum LS is also not increased by pre-weaning DR (Widdowson & Kennedy, 1962; Cheney et al., 1983), overall vitamin supplementation

TABLE 1.2

Strategies Tested in Rodents for Lifespan Extension[a]

	Reference(s)[b]
Nutritional:	
Dietary Restriction	(1)
Protein Level	(2,3)
Fat Level	(4,5)
Carbohydrate Level	(6)
Source of Protein, Fat or Carbohydrate	(7,8,9)
Vitamin Level (overall)	(10)
Vitamin E and other nutrient antioxidant supplementation	(11,12)
Mineral Level	(13)
Self-Selection of Diet	(14)
Drugs, Hormones & Metabolic Factors:	
Antioxidants (non-nutrient ones = 2-MEA, BHT, ethoxyquin)	(15,16)
Centrophenoxine	(17)
L-DOPA	(18)
Gerovital-H_3	(19)
Beta-aminopropionitrile (BAPN)	(20)
Anterior Pituitary	(21)
Prednisolone	(22)
Surgery:	
Hypophysectomy	(23)
Immunologic Reconstitution	(24)
Parabiosis	(25)
Castration (males)	(26)
Exercise:	(27)
Ambient Temperature:	(28)

[a]This lists some, but not all, of the strategies tested. The complete names for the two abbreviated antioxidants are 2-mercaptoethylamine and butylated hydroxytoluene.

[b]References: (1) Chapter 2, this volume; (2) Nakagawa et al. (1974); (3) Feldman et al. (1982); (4) French et al. (1953); (5) Birt et al. (1982a); (6) Dalderup and Visser, (1969); (7) Iwasaki et al. (1988a); (8) Kaunitz and Johnson (1975); (9) Durand et al. (1968); (10) Kokkonen and Barrows (1985); (11) Blackett and Hall (1981); (12) Schroeder and Mitchener (1971); (13) Iwasaki et al. (1988b); (14) Ross et al. (1976); (15) Harman (1968); (16) Kohn (1971); (17) Hochschild (1973); (18) Cotzias et al. (1977); (19) Verzar (1959); (20) LaBella and Vivian (1975); (21) Robertson and Ray (1919); (22) Bellamy (1968); (23) Everitt et al. (1980); (24) Walford et al. (1977); (25) Ludwig and Elashoff (1972); (26) Drori and Folman (1976); (27) Holloszy et al. (1985); (28) Kibler and Johnson (1966).

(Kokkonen & Barrows, 1985), or supplementation with vitamin E (Tappel et al., 1973; Ledvina & Hodanova, 1980; Porta et al., 1980; Blackett & Hall, 1981) or other antioxidants (Harman, 1968; Comfort et al., 1971; Kohn, 1971; Clapp et al., 1979; Heidrick et al., 1984) (for review of survival curves from antioxidant-treated populations, see Walford, 1986a, page 389). Nor does variation in the type of dietary fat (Morin, 1967; Kaunitz & Johnson, 1975; Horn et al., 1979) or carbohydrate (Durand et al., 1968) or type of protein (Iwasaki et al., 1988a) extend maximum LS. We refer here to maximum species-specific LS, not merely strain-specific LS. The LS of various short-lived strains can be influenced by dietary manipulations other than energy restriction, probably by influencing disease susceptibility or progression rather than basic aging. However, even here calorie restriction gives by far the most impressive results (Good & Gajjar, 1986).

Loss of body weight (BW) or slow growth can occur with antioxidant feeding (for review see Schneider & Reed, 1985b) and after adding other potential anti-aging substances (e.g. L-DOPA [Cotzias et al., 1977; Papavasaliou et al., 1981]; centrophenoxine [Hochschild, 1973]; dehydroepiandrosterone (DHEA) [Nyce et al., 1984; Weindruch et al., 1984]) to the diet. Thus any positive findings in experimental animals which weigh less than controls cannot be attributed with certainty to a particular test substance because inadvertent DR may have been ongoing. For studies where rodents are fed a potential anti-aging substance, it is crucial to: (1) very carefully monitor the food intake and, (2) if differences obtain between treated and control groups, include a pair-fed group eating the control diet at the same energy intake as the test animals. Only thereby can one separate influences of the test substance from those of DR.

In a recent study (Weindruch et al., 1986) we fed control and DR mice the purified diets shown in Table 1.3. Note that the mice on DR received on an intermittent basis a diet enriched in protein (casein), vitamins, and minerals such that per week intakes of these nutrients were quite similar for DR and control mice. The DR mice received substantially less carbohydrate (cornstarch and sucrose) and somewhat less fat and fiber per week than the controls. In our experience, best results occur when only calorie intake, as opposed to essential nutrient intake, differ between test and control populations.

The vast majority of DR studies have tested early-onset DR (henceforth abbreviated EDR) and not adult-onset DR (abbreviated ADR). Typically, EDR is started on 3-6 week old, rapidly growing animals. In

TABLE 1.3
Composition of Diets

Ingredient	Diet 1[a]		Diet 2[b]	
	g/kg of diet	(g/mouse)·wk	g/kg of diet	(g/mouse)·wk
Casein	200.0	4.3	350.0	4.3
Cornstarch	260.8	5.7	157.6	2.0
Sucrose	260.8	5.7	157.6	2.0
Corn oil	135.0	2.9	135.0	1.7
Mineral mixture	60.0	1.3	110.0	1.4
Fiber	56.4	1.2	40.0	0.5
Vitamin mixture	23.0	0.50	42.2	0.52
Brewer's yeast	4.0	0.09	7.4	0.09
Zinc oxide	0.05	1.1×10^{-3}	0.1	1.2×10^{-3}

[a]Diet 1: Diet fed to control mice as seven 3.0 to 3.2 g feedings per week providing 85 kcal per week. Composition is given as g ingredient/kg diet. The per week intake of each ingredient for each mouse is also given. For details, see Weindruch et al. (1986).

[b]Diet 2: Diet fed to restricted mice. A purified diet enriched in casein, mineral and vitamin mixtures, brewer's yeast and zinc oxide. Fed as four 2.4 to 3.2 g feedings per week providing 40 to 50 kcal per week to the various DR groups.

this book we shall take 3 months of age as the youngest age for onset of ADR in rodents, and consider onset of restriction before 3 months as EDR. As will be detailed, both EDR and ADR extend maximum LS.

Our own DR studies have mostly dealt with mice from naturally long-lived strains. We were the first to show in such strains that gradual institution of ADR (onset at 12 months) would increase maximum LS (Weindruch & Walford, 1982) and retard immunologic aging (Weindruch et al., 1982a & b). We view ADR as an extremely important (and understudied) area because ADR might be applicable to humans.

Figure 1.3 presents data from our recent study (Weindruch et al., 1986) showing how EDR strongly influences LS and late-life tumor incidence in mice from a long-lived hybrid strain. It compares mice fed the diets shown in Table 1.3: "Normal" calorie diet (85 kcal/week, which is actually about 25 percent less than the average ad libitum intake, so that the "normal" or control mice eat all the food but do not become obese) or the EDR diet (40 kcal/week). Early-onset DR increased the average LS to 45.1 ± 0.9 months (SEM) from 32.7 ± 0.7 months (a 38% increase), and increased by 34 percent the maximum (10th decile) LS to

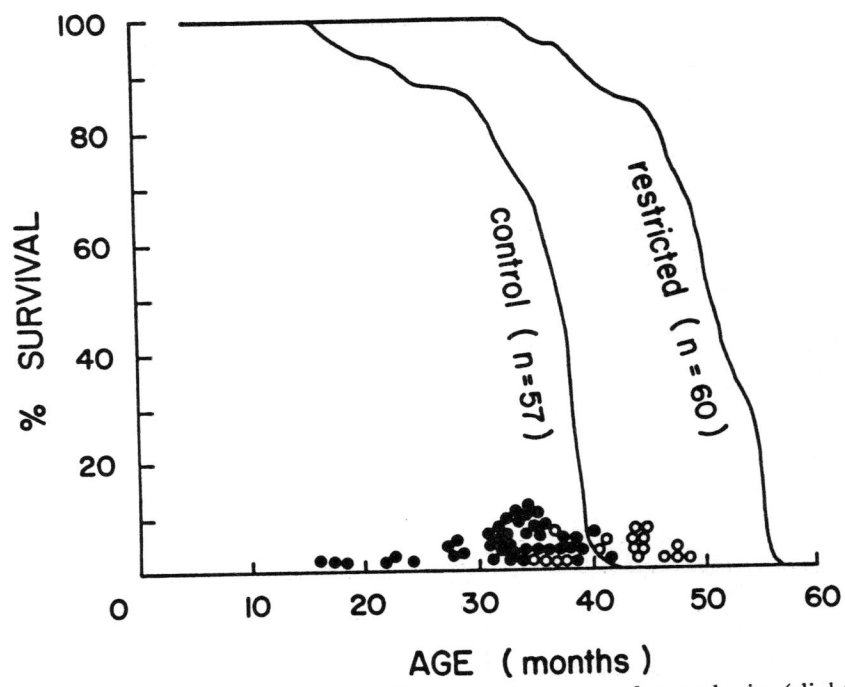

Figure 1.3. Survival curves and age-specific tumor incidence of control mice (slightly restricted, ●) and test mice (severely restricted, ○) with restriction initiated at time of weaning. Symbols show age of death for tumor-bearing mice. Adapted from Weindruch et al. (1986).

53.0 ± 0.3 from 39.7 ± 0.6 months. To our knowledge, this 53 month maximum decile exceeds reported values for mice of any strain.

Not all gerontologists share our view that DR really retards aging in rodents. We have discussed these and other contrarian views elsewhere (Weindruch, 1984; Walford, 1985). Three of the main arguments and our responses thereto follow.

Argument #1: Cherkin (1979) proposed that experimental evidence from DR studies "equally supports an opposite interpretation, namely, that dietary excesses cause reduced life span." He points toward "the unstated assumption that an ad libitum diet is 'normal' or 'optimal' as the source of this problem." **Response:** The caged, ad lib fed rodent does indeed age at a more rapid rate than rodents fed less food. In our recent study (Weindruch et al., 1986), the average LS for ad lib fed mice was 27 months, vs. 33 months for what we in fact consider our "control" mice (fed 25% less than the ad lib level), vs. 45 months for "test" mice fed about 65 percent less than ad lib or 40 percent less than "control" mice.

Up to the point where energy restriction approaches an actual starvation level, the greater the DR the greater the LS. Cherkin's argument thus becomes irrelevant. There is no necessary assumption in DR studies that the ad lib rodent is the "normal" rodent.

Argument #2: Cutler (1982) believes that DR returns "the animal back to the aging rate it would normally have in its natural ecological niche" and does not extend LS beyond the "normal genetic potential for the animal." **Response:** These are in fact two arguments. The first argument is clearly wrong. Wild mice show greatly accelerated mortality compared to laboratory mice, due largely perhaps to the hazards of existence in the wild (Berry et al., 1973). Fifty percent mortality occurs in field mice at about 6 months of age. Only a rare mouse survives longer than 9 months. Now laboratory rats on DR show delayed sexual maturation (albeit a striking prolongation of reproductive LS) (Merry & Holehan, 1979), and female mice on DR regimens tend to become acyclic (see "Neuroendocrine" section, Chap. 4), although upon refeeding even at a late age they may bear litters (Carr et al., 1949). Despite the potential prolongation of reproductive LS, the total progeny output is decreased in DR animals, and there may be an increased degree of cannibalism of the young. The high environmentally-related early and continued mortality rate of wild rodents coupled with the delayed and/or decreased reproductive fitness known to be associated with a fullblown DR regimen would mitigate strongly against survival of a wild rodent population on DR. Thus, DR, at least to the extent used to achieve the longest LS, cannot be the "natural state" of most wild rodents. Cutler's view may hold however for certain rodents having a natural habitat in a hot, arid environment, for example the spiny mouse, which has adapted to living under conditions of severely restricted food supplies (Wise, 1977a & b).

Interestingly, rapid growth in wild populations of Columbian ground squirrels during times of abundant natural food resources resulted in earlier maturation and shorter LSs (Zammuto & Millar, 1985). Also, within mammalian species living in the wild, the age at which females first reproduce is strongly positively correlated with life expectancy, after correction for the effects of body size (Harvey & Zammuto, 1985). Thus, slow growth and diminished food supply correlate with longer lives in both research colony and wild environs. Like Cherkin's argument, the thesis about an animal's "aging rate . . . in its natural ecologic niche" becomes meaningless. Dietary restriction retards aging in both laboratory and wild populations.

The "normal genetic potential" argument becomes in fact two, having an evolutionary and a purely genetic component. If what is "normal" in evolutionary terms equates to what is best for *species* survival, as opposed to *individual* survival, then DR cannot be considered a "normal" state for wild populations, for the reasons given above. In evolutionary terms, greatest species survival usually correlates with rapid growth rate, large body size (for the particular species), and high fecundity. Dietary restriction mitigates against all of these.

The "genetic component" aspect of the argument becomes a sort of word game. A genetic influence on rate of aging would be most manifest where environmental factors that might accelerate aging are minimized, or where the environment was "optimized" to allow maximum survival under the genetic potential of the species. Calorie intake is certainly an environmental factor, therefore DR becomes a necessary part of an "optimized environment" in terms of assessing genetic components of aging. Williams et al. (1987) have touched upon this issue, as discussed in the next chapter. And Totter (1985) proposed that energy for maintaining temperature and reproduction are the main sources of oxygen radical flux, which he assumes causes aging, but that energy diverted to food gathering, i.e., work energy, is not so involved. He suggests that in times of food shortage in the wild (or of DR in the laboratory) diversion of energy to muscular work (to search for food) and away from basal metabolism and reproduction might therefore lead to a relatively slower rate of aging (see also "EVOLUTIONARY PERSPECTIVE," Chapter 5). In this sense then, or in the sense of optimized environment for individual survival, DR might be considered as a "natural" state.

A good example of the confusion of the "natural state" argument when comparing survival of wild with laboratory populations is illustrated by Figure 1.4, from Austad (1988). Maximum LS of spiders of the family *Linyphiidae* was 30 days for wild spiders (who usually consume the equivalent of 8 flies per week), 99 days for laboratory spiders fed 5 flies per week, and 139 days for spiders fed 1 to 3 flies per week. Indeed the use of the words "normal" and "natural" in interpreting the DR paradigm is about as meaningless as when they appear on the labels of cans of processed food.

Argument #3: It has been stated that rodents on EDR experience more deaths early in life than do normally fed controls and that ". . . we are finally looking at the longevity of a group highly selected by a destructive failure test" (Morrison, 1983). **Response:** Even when this argument was written it did not accord with much of the published literature.

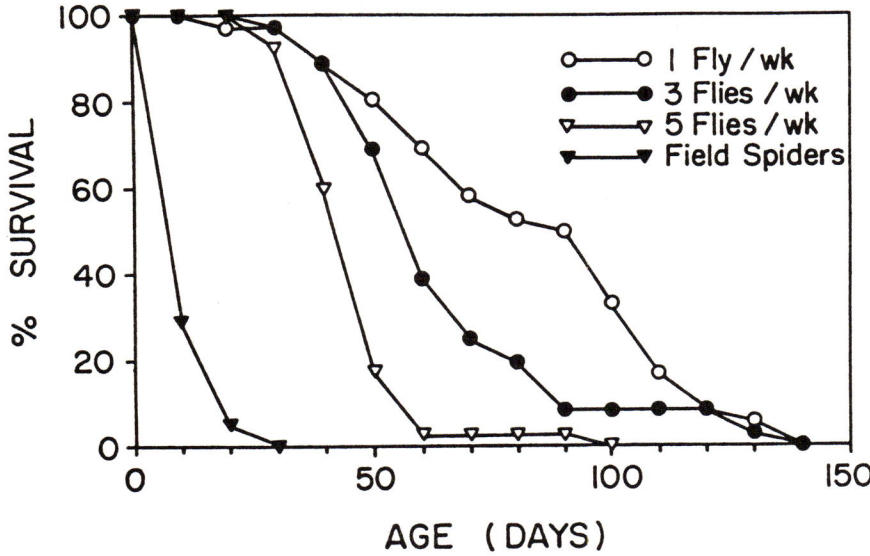

Figure 1.4. Survival curves for the bowl and doily spider (family *Linyphiidae*) in the field and in the laboratory in relation to food intake. Field spiders usually consume the equivalent of about 8 flies per week. Adapted from Austad (1988).

That early deaths need not accompany LS-prolonging EDR has been clearly confirmed by work of Yu et al. (1985) and Weindruch et al. (1986).

Disease Incidence

The original studies of McCay and coworkers (1935) showed that, besides increasing LS, DR lowers the incidences of tumors and certain other diseases. In the 1940s and early 1950s, the studies of Tannenbaum (reviewed in Tannenbaum & Silverstone, 1953) showed clearly that DR reduced the incidence of both spontaneous and induced tumors in mice. Ross (1978) published abundant data on the effect of DR on diseases of rats. Not only is total tumor incidence decreased by DR, but the age of death from tumors is delayed, as illustrated in mice by Figure 1.3. In general, DR both decreases incidence and delays the age of onset of late-life diseases.

DR strikingly prolongs LS of genetically short-lived rodent strains which develop a particular disease at (in terms of species longevity) an early age (typically well before 20 months). All of the following genetically ill rodent strains have their late-life health problems delayed or even cured by DR: the systemic lupus erythematosus-like syndrome of

(NZB × NZW) F_1 female mice (abbreviated B/WF$_1$) (Fernandes et al., 1976c, 1978a; Gajjar et al., 1987), genetically obese C57BL/6J ob/ob mice (Harrison et al., 1984), the lymphoproliferative disease of the MRL/lpr mouse (Fernandes & Good, 1984), the hydronephrosis of the kd/kd mouse (Fernandes et al., 1978b), the spontaneous hypertension of a susceptible rat strain (Lloyd, 1984), and maladies of the "senescence accelerated mouse" (Kohno et al., 1985). It is not always clear whether the increased LSs caused by DR in some of the above animal strains (which can be as much as 2 or 3 times that of their ad lib counterparts) are due to prevention of the specific disease, or retardation of basic aging; but probably both are involved. The long list of DR-prevented or -ameliorated diseases suggests the possibility that DR merits consideration as a preventive regimen for certain human diseases having a clear-cut genetic propensity.

Physiologic Changes: The "Biomarkers" of Aging

The third phase in the history of DR, ushered in by studies of the effects of DR on collagen (Everitt, 1971) and on immune responses (Walford & Tittor, 1973; Walford et al., 1973/74), concerns the demonstration that many not-clearly-disease-related parameters which are altered by age, are altered at a slower rate in DR animals. These investigations have also dealt with liver enzymes, response to hormones, neuroendocrine parameters, eye lens proteins, protein turnover, age pigment, and behavioral and psychomotor indexes, plus others (Bertrand, 1983; Weindruch, 1984; Masoro, 1985a & b; Holehan & Merry, 1986), and will be treated individually and at some length in Chapter 4.

There is no clearcut distinction between physiological changes that occur with age and what may be labeled "biomarkers of aging." However, the term "biomarkers of aging" implies parameters which hopefully allow one to arrive at a reliable estimate of biological or "functional" age, as opposed merely to chronologic age, for any subject. A good biomarker or set of biomarkers might also be expected to offer predictive information on the future longevity of an individual. It is obviously not sufficient merely to follow a parameter that undergoes a change with age and treat that as a biomarker. For example, even though average caloric consumption declines linearly with age in man, the caloric intake of an individual would clearly not make a good assessment of that person's "functional" age.

Criteria for a Good Biomarker

The development of good biomarkers, if such can be done, is much needed. In animals with a relatively short LS (such as rodents), average and maximum LS data can serve as indicators whether intervention into aging by a particular method has been successful. In longer lived species, such as humans, this is not practical, and methods to determine over a relatively short space of time whether the *rate* of aging is being influenced are required. The NIA has wisely supported development of this controversial area (controversial because gerontologists do not agree on what a biomarker is or whether any really exist), including 1981 and 1986 conferences to evaluate biomarkers for rodents and humans (Reff & Schneider, 1982a). According to the 1981 conference organizers (Reff & Schneider, 1982b), desirable features for a good biomarker include that: (1) it be measurable without harming the subject, (2) it be highly reproducible and reflect physiologic ("functional") age, (3) it show significant age changes within a relatively brief time period (in relation to the LS of the organism), and (4) the clinical functions should be crucial to the health of the species.

Harrison (1982) and Harrison and Archer (1984) list four criteria for a biomarker assay based on physiological changes: (1) the results must change significantly with age (2) changes should be repeatable in the same individual, (3) assays for independent physiological parameters should give similar estimates for age for the same individual, and (4) the "age" indicated by the biomarker should correlate with subsequent LS, i.e., it should be *predictive* of how long the animal has yet to live (Harrison et al., 1988).

It is worth emphasizing that while predictive value of subsequent LS represents an important criterion, it could be quite misleading if it relates primarily to disease susceptibility. Hypercholesterolemia predicts on the average a shorter LS, but due to the risk of an early cardiac death, not necessarily from accelerated aging. Ingram (1984) discussed what criteria to use in selecting biomarkers, especially behavioral ones. These include *content* validity (The test must be appropriate to the cohort: do not use a too sophisticated intellectual test for children.), *construct* validity (Does the change really have meaning? [Gray hair correlates with chronologic age but does not correlate at all with the rate of aging.]), and *predictive* validity (Does it predict LS, health and/or rate of aging?).

Because much of modern experimental gerontology employs rodents, it is worth a cautionary note that the use of an inbred strain can be misleading in terms of biomarker studies, because inbreeding forces fixation of all loci, those relevant and those not relevant to the phenotype being studied. A case can be made that future biomarker research in rodents should concentrate either on congenic strains (single locus variable) or include or be checked against fully outbred strains.

In our view a good biomarker should reflect, as much as possible, intrinsic changes which are little influenced by extraneous environmental factors. One cannot say "all" environmental factors because the intervention itself (e.g., DR or antioxidants) may be considered an environmental factor. Exercise resulting in enhanced muscular, cardiovascular, or skeletal fitness is an environmental factor which doubtless influences average LS but has not been shown to raise maximum species-specific LS. Those age-sensitive parameters which are greatly influenced by physical fitness (e.g., glucose tolerance, serum lipids) may not be reliable biomarkers except for what may be termed "segmental" aging (Schneider et al., 1982). Or they may be satisfactory if all individuals in the study are equally physically fit, or equally sedentary; or if in a longitudinal study the degree of physical fitness of the individual(s) is kept constant. Maximum oxygen consumption (VO_2max) is a good example of such an interaction of variables (Suominen et al., 1980; Bruce, 1984) as illustrated in Figure 1.5, which also shows that vital capacity falls with age in humans but is *not* influenced by the degree of fitness.

Age-related changes may occur within organisms which have nothing to do with any of the above, which are time-dependent but do not necessarily act upon physiologic processes. An example is the increasing racemization of aspartic acid with age (Helfman & Bada,

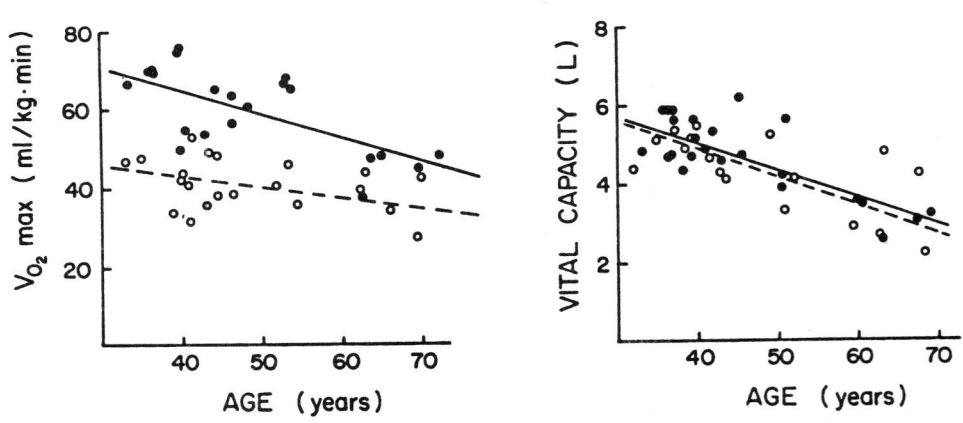

Figure 1.5. Maximum oxygen consumption and pulmonary vital capacity in relation to age in physically fit (●, ———) and sedentary (○, ---) individuals. From Suominen et al. (1980).

1976), which likely reflects merely the passage of time analogous to inherent radioactive decay of an isotope.

Division of Biomarkers into Sets

Biomarkers can be divided into sets, and each set into categories. One set includes those biomarkers which hopefully reflect increases in maximum LS (i.e., a true retardation of the aging process); those which reflect a change in average LS only (i.e., usually by squaring the survival curve via a decrease in disease susceptibility but probably not via a decrease in the rate of basic aging); and those which reflect alterations in segmental aging such as calcium loss from bone. Any biomarker fitting into the first category would also fit into the 2nd and 3rd. Borkan (1983, 1986) lists 24 age-related variables used to estimate biological age profiles in humans from the Baltimore Longitudinal Study of Aging.

Genetic Complication to Biomarker Utility

A major potential complication (and a rather intractable one at present for human studies) is that of genetic influences on a particular biomarker. Our concept here can be illustrated by the influence of the major histocompatibility complex (MHC) on the age-related decline in the response to the T-lymphocyte mitogen phytohemagglutinin (PHA), as in the studies of Meredith and Walford (1977) in mice and Batory et al. (1983) in humans. It is clear from the curves of Figure 1.6, for example, that for B10.AKM ($H-2^m$) mice the response to PHA would be a poor biomarker beyond 14 months of age, whereas for B10 ($H-2^b$) and B10.RIII ($H-2^r$) it would be suitable up to about 38 months of age. These strains are inbred and differ only at the MHC, i.e., at one relatively small genetic region. In an outbred colony, a low PHA response for an individual mouse might indicate great age if the mouse were genetically like the B10.RIII, but not necessarily for a mouse with the $H-2^m$ allele. In line with this, Covelli et al. (1984) found that in an outbred mouse strain selection for antibody responsiveness did not always appear to influence LS.

Humans are on the whole a highly outbred population, and we presently have no good way to assess whether a biomarker parameter in one human reflects predominantly a genetic or an aging influence. This genetic situation greatly complicates the biomarker field, and failure to realize it and deal with it may be the chief reason why this field (particularly in humans) remains less useful than one would hope.

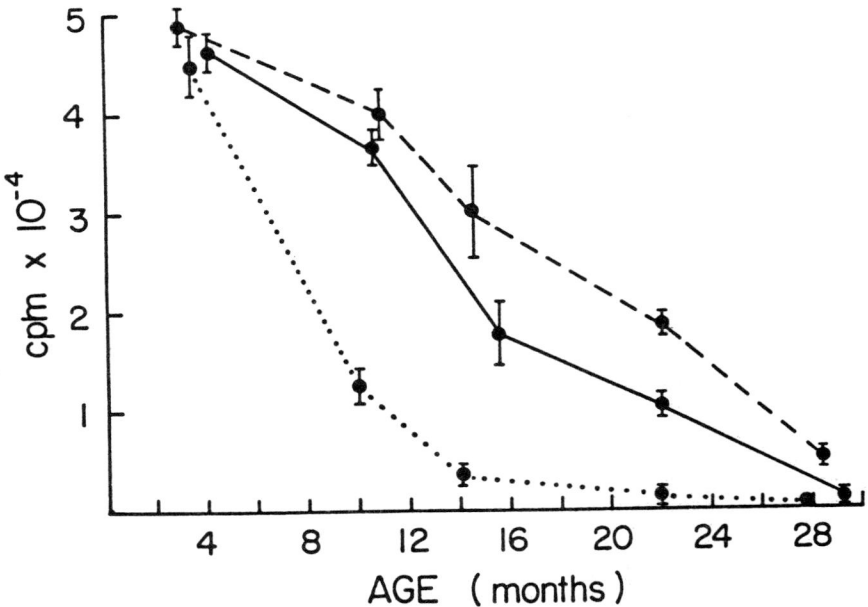

Figure 1.6. Age-related decline in responses of splenocytes from three strains of mice congenic at the major histocompatibility complex (the H-2 locus) to stimulation by the mitogen, phytohemagglutinin (PHA). B10.RIII (H-2^r) (●-----●); C57BL/10 (H-2^b) (●———●); B10.AKM (H-2^m) (● · · · · · ●). From Meredith and Walford (1977).

Some Biomarkers Are Not Influenced by DR

As will become clear in Chapter 4, DR in rodents leads to retarded rates of age-related change for most *but not all* age-sensitive biologic parameters. Certain of the potential biomarkers which are not much influenced by DR may be particularly important in understanding aging processes, and may reflect a *multi*factorial as opposed to a *uni*factorial mechanism of aging (see following section for discussion of these terms). Those biomarkers not influenced by DR would appear to be either irrelevant to aging, or on the contrary may help explain why rodents on DR do not live even longer.

The vast majority of age-related variables tested to date do stay "younger longer" in DR rodents. Representing a broad array of age-sensitive biologic phenomena, these provide additional evidence that DR is the best available method for studying the biology of decelerated aging. This deceleration probably comes about by direct retardation of processes which cause aging and/or by improving the efficacy of processes which oppose senescence.

Mechanisms

The fourth historical phase in DR research—and the one now attracting much interest—is the search for mechanisms. How does simple energy intake restriction exert its multiple profound effects? Studies to this end have been fueled by the assumption that a treatment like DR, whose LS prolonging effects have been demonstrated in diverse animals, must operate at a very fundamental level, perhaps by manipulating a single root mechanism of aging. Thus, the implication is, at least until recently, that there is a *uni*factorial causality. Accordingly, DR has been considered experimentally in relation to many of the major existing theories of aging, including those concerned with immunology, cellular proliferation, rate-of-living, DNA repair, free radical damage, protein synthesis, and others.

Dietary Restriction and the "Theories of Aging"

Many theories of aging have been proposed (reviewed by Martin, 1980; Sacher, 1980; Hart & Turturro, 1983, 1985; see also the book edited by Warner et al., 1987), as well as classification schemes for the main theories. Table 1.4 presents our modification of a classification scheme originally set forth by Hart and Turturro (1983). This provides a framework for thinking about the biology of aging, and the role DR may potentially play in unraveling this enigma. While we shall not undertake here to review all the major theories of aging, and while the closely related subject of "mechanisms of the DR effect" will be considered at length in Chapter 5, certain comments on these subjects may be useful of themselves, and serve as background for the chapters to come.

The immune system may be involved in the etiopathogenesis of aging, or as a "pacemaker" of aging (Walford, 1969, 1987). Dietary restriction slows down and in some circumstances reverses the immune decline, and inhibits the upswing in autoimmune phenomena that occur with aging (Weindruch, 1984; Weindruch et al., 1982b).

Dietary restriction may act in part by retarding the basal turnover rate of proliferative cell populations, or what may be termed the "idling" rate of all cell populations, but at the same time potentiate for an increased response when such is called for (Walford et al., 1987). The metaphor here would be with a well-tuned automobile which idles quietly at the intersection but responds promptly and well when the light changes. Such a condition would have the dual benefits of retarding programmatic or deteriorative aging, while increasing adaptability to

TABLE 1.4
A Classification of Theories of Aging[a]

1. **Cellular-Based Theories**
   - Free radical damage
   - Glycosylation and other cross-links
   - Changes in DNA or chromatin
   - Decreases in the accuracy or quantity of protein synthesis
   - Limited cell division capacity ("Hayflick limit")
   - Decrease in DNA repair capacity

2. **Organ System(s)-Based Theories**
   - Role of immune phenomena
   - Role of neuroendocrine phenomena

3. **Population-Based Theories**
   - Theories associating aging with differentiation or growth cessation
   - Rate of living
   - Theories based on the evolution of LS in mammals
     - e.g. Sacher's equations on relations between metabolism, brain and body weight, and LS
     - e.g. Cutler's work on repair and protective processes

4. **Integrative Theories** (=combination of 2 or more of the above)
   - e.g. free radicals → DNA damage → neuroendocrine aging
   - e.g. neuroendocrine aging → immunologic aging

5. **Systems Analysis and Other Mathematical Theories of Aging**

[a]Adapted from the classification of Hart & Turturro (1983). This is not a complete listing.

environmental stimuli, and would accord with the observation that DR animals are both long-lived and show increased resistance to disease. We have shown that while, compared to controls, splenic natural killer cell (NK) activity is low in unstimulated DR animals, the response after stimulation (by an interferon inducer) rises to a higher level in DR animals than in controls (Weindruch et al., 1983).

The potential influence of long-term DR on specific metabolic rate and energy metabolism was analyzed by Sacher (1977), who supported a rate-of-living theory of aging by concluding on the basis of data from the literature that DR decreases energy use per unit BW per day, with life-time energy use on a per BW basis remaining constant. However, findings by Masoro and co-workers (see Masoro, 1985b) did not accord with this analysis, and these workers rejected metabolic rate reduction as DR's mode of action.

In our view metabolic rate effects still have a candidacy. To begin with, it is quite clear from studies in a number of laboratories (Ross & Bras, 1973; Weindruch et al., 1986), including Masoro's (Yu et al., 1985), that restriction of energy intake, i.e., simply of calories, as opposed to variation in any other dietary factor, is by far the most crucial variable in the age-retardation induced by DR. At an admittedly naive level, a phenomenon tied entirely to energy ought to translate into some kind of metabolic rate effect. And a reduced basal rate of cell turnover or "idling rate" in DR animals would also imply, although it would not prove, a metabolic alteration. There is a well-known relationship between species' maximum LSs and the metabolic rates of the different species, as illustrated in Figure 1.7, which shows a curve where lifetime energy intake, for each species shown (except man), is about 200 calories per gram BW (Man is about 800.). While comparing between-species (LS and metabolic rate) variables with effects observed within a species (DR on LS and metabolic rate) can be quite hazardous (see below), we are for the reasons given above and for several others reluctant to exclude a metabolic rate effect at some level or locale as DR's mode of action (see "ENERGY METABOLISM," Chapter 5).

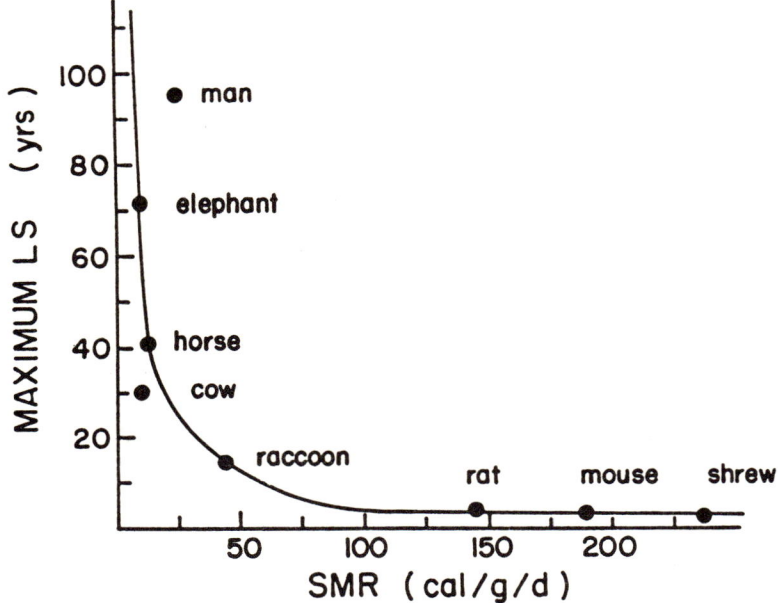

Figure 1.7. Life spans and specific metabolic rates (SMR) for eight different species of mammals. Adapted from Cutler (1978).

Capacity to repair DNA may be related to aging (for review see Tice & Setlow, 1985). Cells from longer-lived species have proportionately greater capacity to repair UV-induced damage to DNA. In this regard, studies in our laboratory in mice point towards DR's slowing the decline in DNA repair capacity that occurs with aging (Licastro et al., 1986 & 1988).

DR may extend LS by affecting the generation or persistence of free radicals (reviewed by Harman, 1986). It is reasonable to suppose that a decreased energy intake would generate fewer free radicals, although reduction might be relevant only to certain critical organ systems. As for the effect of DR on free radicals, experimental evidence is limited. Lipid peroxidation is lower and catalase activity (but not the activities of superoxide dismutase and glutathione peroxidase) higher in the livers of DR than in control mice (Koizumi et al., 1987a). Thus the total "peroxide tone" (Ball et al., 1986) might be expected to be *decreased* in DR animals. This would, according to the free-radical theory of aging, increase LS.

Free radical scavengers are characteristically increased as a response to the generation of free radicals, and DNA repair mechanisms are increased following either injury to DNA or a proliferative stimulus. In DR, the situation may be different. We have suggested that DR leads to a *selective* upregulation of certain DNA repair and certain antioxidant defense systems, by mechanisms *other than* feedback-response to DNA damage or to free radical production (Walford et al., 1987). This could point to a fundamental process, probably involving gene expression, whereby DR influences aging.

Uni- and Multi-Factorial Aging

The above possibilities all clearly share the idea that aging can be traced to a few causes or a single cause. However, DR may be useful in analyzing an alternate possibility to such a unifactorial approach. The "multifactorial" concept (Harrison & Archer, 1984; Schneider & Reed, 1985b; Walford et al., 1987) posits that the physiologic systems of an animal go awry with age, but not from a single cause. Aging is then the summation of this gathering disarray.

Figure 1.8 illustrates how DR might impinge upon such a multifactorial concept. We have selected thymic hormone levels, DNA repair, and protection against free radical injury as functions whose alterations might contribute to multifactorial aging. Panel A (Figure 1.8) illustrates

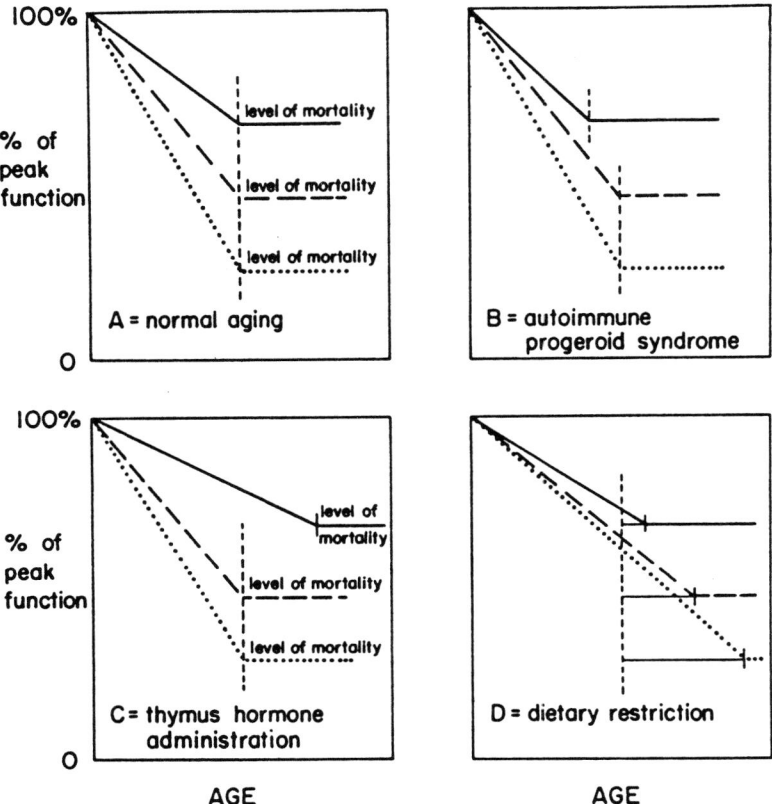

Figure 1.8. Dietary restriction and multifactorial aging: a heuristic model showing (A) decline in multifactors in a long-lived strain, (B) accelerated decline in one factor in an autoimmune, progeroid syndrome, (C) behavior of multifactors following thymus hormone administration in a long-lived strain, (D) effect of dietary restriction. Thymic hormone levels (———); DNA repair (— — —); protection against free radical damage (· · · · ·). From Walford et al. (1987).

the proposition that in a long-lived strain these and other multifactors, while perhaps declining at different rates, nevertheless all reach their respective levels of mortality at about the same time in life. If this were *not* the case, then those which reached the lethal level substantially later than others would not be directly involved in mortality, and we would be reduced to a less-than-multifactorial causality.

Certain disease states exist where one or a few age-related factors decline at an accelerated rate, as illustrated for thymic hormone levels (Fig. 1.8B). These accelerated aging syndromes (Martin, 1978), such as Down's syndrome, insulin-dependent diabetes, or the autoimmunity of

B/WF$_1$ mice (for review see Gottesmann & Walford, 1982) never show *all* the features of aging. Furthermore, in the mouse autoimmune syndromes, the shortened LS can be substantially prolonged by specific therapy (= segmental intervention) (Gabrielsen & Olson, 1977). The B/WF$_1$ and other mouse strains, in which immune function as a single factor selectively changes at an accelerated rate (Fig. 1.8B), can thus be regarded as subgroups of normal aging (Gottesman & Walford, 1982). By contrast, in long-lived mouse strains attempts at specific therapy, such as administration of thymic hormone or free radical scavengers, have not convincingly prolonged maximum LS (Walford, 1986a; Hiramoto et al., 1987). Inducing a change in (for example) only one factor (as Fig. 1.8A → C for thymic hormone administration) may be insufficient to prolong survival, if, as in a long-lived strain, many factors are involved in aging.

We have suggested (Walford et al., 1987) that in long-lived rodent strains the rates of change of the multifactors involved in aging may be differentially altered by DR, so that now the factors tend to reach their lethal levels at different times relative to one another, as illustrated in Figure 1.8D. Thus, DR creates a new pattern which, although seen on a longer time scale, somewhat resembles an expansion of that observed for accelerated aging syndromes. Dietary restriction leads to a broad but ultimately "segmental juvenescence." In the heuristic example shown in Figure 1.8D, DR has significantly retarded the progression of those multifactors represented by DNA repair and free radical damage, but to a lesser degree the fall-off in thymic hormone levels. In fact, taken together, studies by Licastro et al. (1986), Koizumi et al. (1987a), and Weindruch et al. (1988) do present evidence, as yet inconclusive, for such a sequence of events in DR mice.

It follows from the above that some of the factors which are *not* (or only marginally) altered by DR but seem for other reasons to be possibly important in aging may be responsible for the fact that DR animals do not live even longer. Hence, a further extension might be obtained by manipulation of these DR insensitive factors within a cohort already rendered long-lived by the DR regimen.

Dietary Restriction and Between-Species/Within-Species Comparisons

As hinted at in our discussion above of between-species metabolic rate differences in relation to species' LSs, it is a convenient assumption that what correlates with maximum LS differences between species ought to be involved in some way in the aging process. DNA repair as an example was cited above. Mice have low repair capacity and short LSs, humans high capacity and long life, and data for other mammals are proportionate in both categories.

Table 1.5 assembles representative data on certain liver biochemical parameters related to antioxidant defense mechanisms as these may be affected by age *within* rodent species (mice and/or rats), plus the effects, where known, of DR thereon. How these same parameters vary *between* species in relation to the maximum LSs differences of the species is also indicated. One might anticipate that parameters which correlate directly or inversely with species maximum LSs would, if they are truly fundamental to aging, be similarly influenced by DR, and in both cases in a direction opposite to the changes found in normal aging. However, the data do not entirely support this simple, albeit attractive surmise. From the table it is clearly *not* possible (although tempting) to infer directly from comparisons *between* species of differing maximum LSs how a particular parameter might change when the LS is altered by DR *within* a single species. Catalase activity may be lower in longer-lived species (Cutler, 1985a), but is increased by DR. Superoxide dismutase (SOD) activity is higher in longer-lived species but not always influenced by DR, according to existing data. Internal body temperature, incidentally, is an additional example that such inferences can be hazardous. Between species, an increase in maximum LS goes with higher core body teperatures (Sacher, 1977), but within a (poikilothermic) vertebrate the reverse obtains (Liu & Walford, 1966, 1972). Other examples where between-species correlations do not conform to within-species comparisons are given by Storer (1967).

Despite the above (and clearly such comparisons need much further exploration), we think it possible that comparison of the effects of DR on physiologic and/or biomarker parameters *within* a species, with the same parameters in relation to LS differences *between* species, may help identify those variables which are best candidates to be involved in the pathogenesis of aging. For example, both DR and between-species comparative studies seem to agree that increased DNA repair capacity correlates with an increased maximum LS, thus making DNA repair of continued interest in designing future studies of aging—for example, to find out precisely which among the repair pathways or repair of what kinds of damage show this tripartite relationship.

TABLE 1.5

Liver Enzymes and Substrates Involved with Antioxidant Defense: Correlations with Differences in LS Between Mammalian Species, Effects of Increasing Age, and of Long-Term DR in Rodents[a]

Liver Enzyme or Substrate	Between-species change with increase in LS	Within-species change with aging	Within-species change with long-term DR
1. Catalase	↓	↓ mouse & rat	↑ mouse & rat
2. Superoxide dismutase total activity	↑	↓, ↔ rat	↔ mouse
MnSOD		↓ mouse	
CuZnSOD		↓ rat	
		↓, ↔ rat, mouse	↔ mouse
3. Glutathione peroxidase	↓	↓ mouse	↔ mouse
4. Glutathione	↓	↓, ↔ mouse	
5. Reduced glutathione		↓, ↔ mouse	
6. P450 activity	↓	↓ rodents	↔ mouse
			↑ rat

[a]For example, First column: liver catalase activity is less in longer lived mammals, such as man, than in short-lived mammals such as mice, with other mammals such as rhesus monkeys being proportionately intermediate for both LS and catalase activities. Second column: in rodents, liver catalase activity declines with age. Third column: DR animals show increased liver catalase activities compared to controls. "↔" indicates no effect. Blank spaces indicate that data are unavailable. Adapted from Walford et al. (1987): see for references.

Human Application

The final and fifth historical phase in DR research concerns the possibility of human application (Walford, 1986a). We think there is a very high order of probability that the animal data are translatable to humans, in terms of retardation of aging and LS extension as well as disease prevention. Furthermore, what epidemiologic, experimental, and inferential data are available (not many exist but in fact more than is commonly thought) point also in the direction of human applicability. Chapter 6 will be devoted to this important subject.

STATISTICAL TREATMENT OF DATA

In the above we have not touched upon an extremely important factor in evaluating overall mortality and survival curves and physiologic changes in relation to aging and the DR model, particularly to the extent that the physiologic changes qualify as biomarkers. That factor is the statistical handling of the data. Such handling is much influenced, for example, by whether one views aging as uni- or multi-factorial.

Mortality and survival statistics in DR studies will be outlined in Chapter 2.

Regression analysis of biomarker data obtained on randomly selected individuals usually reveals a great deal of scatter. For most physiologic functions the coefficient of variation about the mean increases with age (Bafitis & Sargent, 1977). When results for a number of biomarkers are combined, rather high correlation coefficients for chronologic age can be obtained (Holingsworth et al., 1965; Conard et al., 1966; Suominen et al., 1980; Borkan, 1983; Harrison & Archer, 1987b). Yet, it can be argued that if aging is multifactorial and multi-process, and proceeds at different rates in different organs, efforts to produce biologically meaningful composite scores may be futile (Costa & McCrae, 1980b). But even this inversion can be reinverted: if aging is multifactorial, a diversified battery ought to be selected on the basis of the relative independence of the parameters, on the basis of their internal consistency being relatively low (Ingram, 1984). A more detailed consideration of the treatment of physiologic/biomarker data will be given later (see "Biomarkers of Aging in Humans," Chap. 6).

SUMMARY

The classic goal of gerontology is to understand the basic biology of aging, and of applied gerontology to retard aging and increase healthful LS. Dietary caloric restriction is the only method which accomplishes the latter in nearly all species so far tested, from protozoans to mammals. The progress of DR research can be divided to some extent historically and certainly conceptually into five areas: effects on survival, on diseases (e.g. cancer, renal disease, diabetes, autoimmune disease), effects on the physiologic changes that occur with aging and the evaluation of biomarker data, the search for the mechanism(s) whereby DR exerts these diverse effects, and potential human application of the DR paradigm. Additionally, DR is useful in exploring other facets of aging, for example in determining whether aging is uni- or multi-factorial in causality, and the significance of certain physiologic variables in relation to LS differences between species. Dietary restriction is emerging as a major methodology in the study of aging.

CHAPTER 2

DIETARY RESTRICTION: EFFECTS ON SURVIVORSHIP

INTRODUCTION

THE EFFECTS of DR on average and maximum LSs and the mortality rate parameters strongly support the view that DR slows fundamental aging processes. Survival curves from DR studies in four widely diverse species (*Tokophyra* [a protozoan], *Daphnia* [the water flea], *Rattus* [the rat], *Lebistes* [the guppy]) are shown in Figure 2.1. Maximum LSs were increased by DR by 40-85 percent in the first three species and by 5 percent in *Lebistes* (the guppies were on DR only for the first third of life).

Following a discussion of ways to analyze survivorship, the present chapter focuses upon the main published experiments about DR and LS. All species tested will be evaluated, but only the rodent work tabulated. Early-onset (before 3 months of age) and adult-onset DR will be treated separately. We will also consider in this chapter the effects of DR on the onset of puberty and general health and appearance of the animals. Longevity data indicate that DR regimens can be made to work even though differing in the severity of caloric restriction, the relative intakes of the three energy-furnishing food types (proteins, carbohydrates and fats), sources of nutrients, length of the fasting interval and the age at which DR is started. However, all DR regimens which extend maximum LS do share one feature: *caloric restriction.*

ANALYSIS OF SURVIVORSHIP

There are several ways to express longevity data. The commonest of these is the survival curve as shown in Figures 1.3 and 2.1. Two other

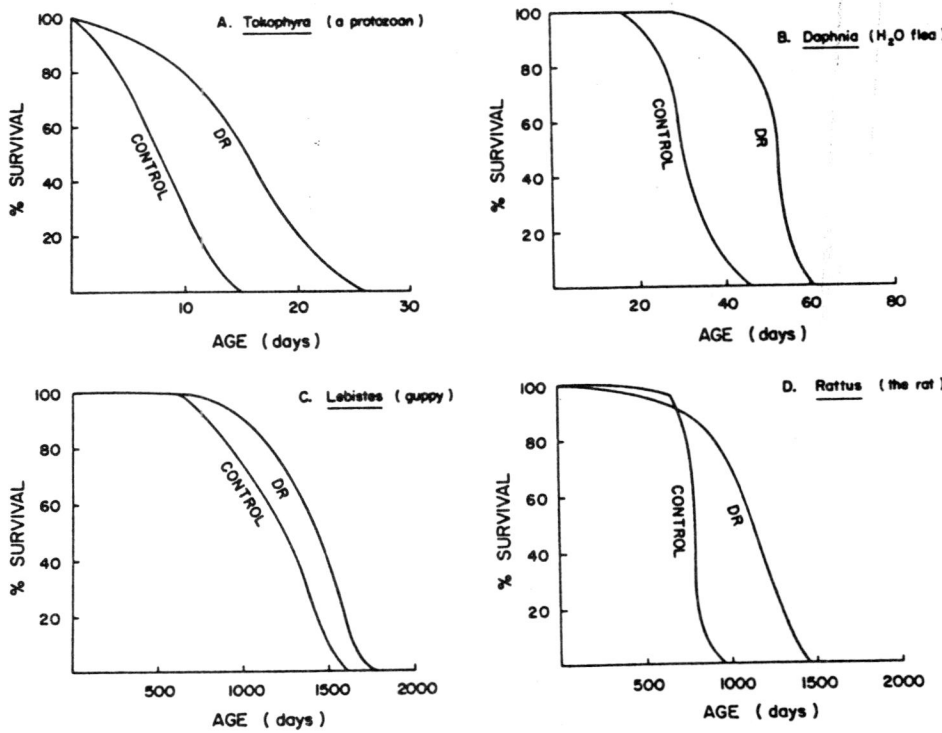

Figure 2.1. Survival curves for DR and control populations from four species. *Panel A* gives curves approximated from data of Rudzinska (1952) for *Tokophyra*. *Panel B* shows survival of *Daphnia* using the data of Ingle et al. (1937). *Panel C* is the survival of guppies fed as described by Comfort (1963). *Panel D* was drawn from data reported for rats by Yu et al. (1982).

ways are graphed in Figure 2.2, using published data from DR rodents. According to Mos and Hollander (1987) cohort sizes larger than 80 animals do not much further improve confidence limits for 50 and 10 percent survivals.

Figure 1.3 shows percent survival vs. age for female $C3B10RF_1$ mice from our colony of control and DR animals. The onset of DR was 3 weeks of age. The curves reveal that: (1) deaths soon after weaning were not observed in either group; (2) the onset of age-dependent increases in mortality began at about 30 months for controls vs. 40 months for DR mice; (3) the respective median LSs were about 35 and 50 months; (4) the maximum (10th decile) LSs were 40 months for controls and 53 months for DR mice; (5) the slopes of the survival curves appear similar, although the DR curve may decline slightly more gradually for the population's longest-lived one-half.

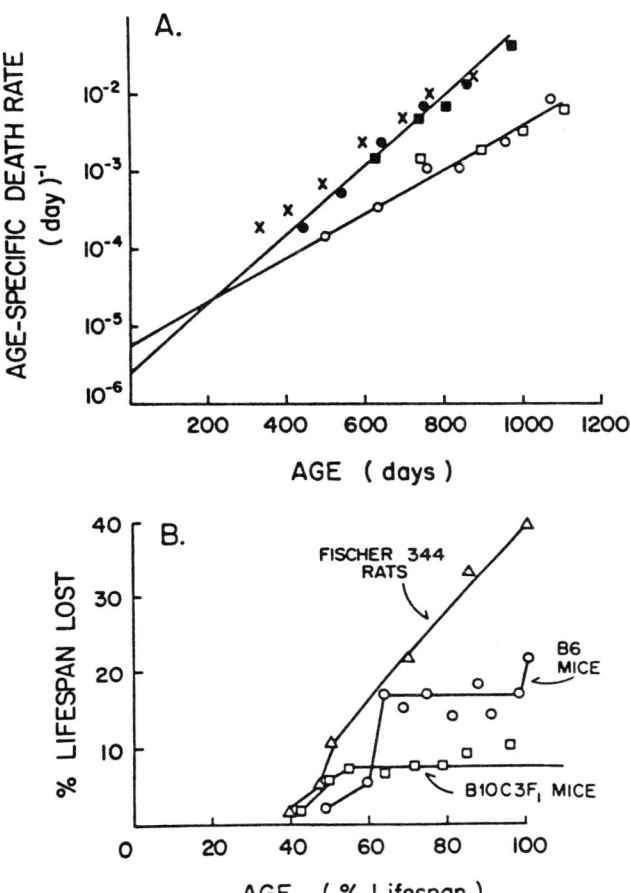

Figure 2.2. *Panel A:* Gompertz diagram for DR and control rats. Open symbols are for DR rats, closed symbols are for corresponding ad lib fed animals. Squares are from data reported by Berg and Simms (1960); circles are from Ross (1961). The 'x's represent a control population cited by and redrawn from Sacher (1977). *Panel B:* Reduction in remaining life expectancy associated with ad lib feeding compared to EDR and ADR. The DR was initiated either at 6 weeks of age on Fischer 344 rats (data of Yu et al., 1982) or at 12 months of age on B6 and B10C3F$_1$ mice (data of Weindruch & Walford, 1982). △ = Fischer 344 rats; ○ = B6 mice; □ = B10C3F$_1$ mice. Adapted from Williams et al. (1987).

Gompertz analysis (Figure 2.2A) provides another view of survival data. Perhaps the most informative discussion of this type of analysis was provided by Sacher (1977). Survival curves for mammals in favorable environments are sigmoidal in shape, and the age-specific death rate increases exponentially with age according to the Gompertz equation,

$$\left[\frac{1}{N_{(t)}} \frac{dN}{dt}\right] = q_0 e^{\alpha t}$$

where the term

$$\left[\frac{1}{N_{(t)}} \frac{dN}{dt}\right]$$

is the fractional death rate at time t, $N_{(t)}$ is the number in the population at time t, and q_0 is the initial vulnerability parameter. The slope term, α, is a rate term which Sacher calls the *actuarial aging rate*. It describes the exponential rate of increase of mortality with age. The equation may be made linear:

$$\ln\left[\frac{1}{N_{(t)}} \frac{dN}{dt}\right] = \ln q_0 + \alpha t$$

The term $\ln q_0$ is the log of the initial rate of mortality and is calculable by extrapolating the linear form of the Gompertz equation back to age zero.

The mortality rate is perhaps most understandably expressed by the *doubling time*, $T_d = \ln 2/\alpha = 0.69/\alpha$, or the time needed for the fractional death rate to double. This is constant for a population obeying the Gompertz equation. The term q_0 is the *basal vulnerability* parameter, and extrapolates the population's fractional mortality rate to age zero. Sacher hypothesized that q_0 is determined by genotype. A sampling of values for these mortality parameters in several mammals is shown in Table 2.1. Longer-lived species have longer T_d's and lower q_0 and α values. Sacher envisioned two main actuarial ways to increase LS: increase T_d (i.e. decrease α), and decrease q_0. How does DR affect these parameters?

Panel A (Figure 2.2) shows a Gompertz plot (log of fractional death rate vs. age) of published data for rats fed control and DR regimens. The T_d values of 105-130 days for DR rats were about 2 times that for controls (66 days). The q_0 value for the DR rats was 8×10^{-6}, almost three times that of the controls (2.7×10^{-6}). Thus, the early actuarial effects of DR were negative here; however, newer DR studies do not show higher early mortality. A main conclusion of Sacher's was that *DR is the only strategy proven to retard the actuarial rate of aging (i.e. decrease α) in homeotherms*. He attributed this to a slowdown in the rate of energy metabolism, a notion which has been challenged (Masoro et al., 1982), and is discussed at length in Chapter 5.

TABLE 2.1
Gompertz Mortality Parameters in Mammalian Species[a]

Species	Life Expec.(d)	$q_o(d^{-1})$	$T_d(d)$	α
Mus musculus (house mouse)	600	3.0×10^{-4}	220	.0032
Peromyscus leucopus (white-footed mouse)	1,500	1.2×10^{-4}	450	.0015
Canis familiaris (beagle dog)	3,600	2.7×10^{-5}	800	.0009
Equus caballus (horse)	6,300	6.0×10^{-6}	1330	.0005
Homo sapiens (USA, 1969)	27,700	1.5×10^{-7}	3100	.0002

[a]Data adapted from Sacher, 1977. d = days. The term q_o is the initial vulnerability parameter. T_d is the doubling time of the mortality rate. The rate term, α, is the age-specific death rate per day.

Similar reductions in mortality rate have been reported for DR mice from our colony (Cheney et al., 1980 & 1983). But in later cohorts of DR mice with great increases in LS, α was not always decreased compared to controls (Figure 1.3 plus Harris et al., in preparation).

Panel B (Figure 2.2) gives a toxicologist's analysis of DR data, as presented by Williams et al. (1987). The relative loss of longevity produced by a "toxic stress" is plotted on an age-specific basis (expressed as % of LS). Two types of toxic agents are considered: (1) those accelerating the aging rate and, (2) those lowering the age when the mortality rate starts to increase. This type of analysis looks at the life-shortening effects of "toxins" via principles expressed by the two main Gompertz terms (α, q_0). For DR studies, the percent of LS lost due to a "toxic stress" (i.e. ad lib eating) is plotted against age as illustrated in Panel B using Yu and co-workers' (1982) data for rats on DR since they were 6 weeks old, and our data for mice on DR since 12 months of age (Weindruch & Walford, 1982). Williams et al. (1987) conclude that the pattern of LS lost for the ad lib-fed rats resembled that produced by an agent which accelerated aging rate uniformly per unit time, whereas the pattern for our ad lib-fed mice suggested a reduced threshold to mortality's onset. It would seem worthwhile to conduct this type of analysis on more DR longevity data. Notice that real time (months or days) is nowhere seen in Panel B. One must be careful not to ignore absolute LSs when using the "Williams plot" because a LS prolonging effect in a short-lived strain may not resemble that in a hardier one.

STUDIES IN INVERTEBRATES

For background on aging in invertebrates, see Comfort (1979) and Barrows and Kokkonen (1982). Most of the work on DR in invertebrates was carried out between 1915-1965. These studies clearly show that LS extension by DR can be seen in diverse species, and is not simply an improved diet for overfed, inactive, caged rodents.

The amoeba is an exception to the rule that DR extends LS in invertebrates. But it is also a special case in that on an unlimited diet amoeba show no aging at all, but form an immortal clone. Working with *A. proteus* and *A. discoides*, Muggleton and Danielli (1958) noted that if immortal clones were fed a reduced food supply to the extent that growth and cell division were inhibited for some weeks, and then returned to unlimited feeding, the clones survived only another 6 to 9 months. Further study of these "alternative states" of amoeba by Kaufman and Rao (1980) showed that prolonged arrest of amoeba cells by reduced culture conditions resulted in altered nuclear functions including markedly reduced DNA and RNA synthesis.

Another possible exception, the honey bee, is also a special case. The summer honey bee has an average LS of 25 to 35 days; the winter honey bee, 7 to 8 months. If a bee born in spring or summer is overfed on protein-rich pollen during its first 10 to 14 days, it becomes a "winter bee" with the characteristic extended LS (Maurizio, 1961).

Rudzinska (1952) found that the protozoan *Tokophyra infusionum* lives longer when fed less. She fed young *Tokophyra* in 3 ways: (1) abundant food (= 8-15 *Tetrahymena*/organism/day), (2) abundant food every 2nd day and, (3) a small amount of food (1-3 *Tetrahymena* every 2nd or 3rd day). The average LSs for these groups were 7, 10 and 13 days, respectively. Of the 60 individuals in each diet group, the number living beyond 9 days was 11, 32 and 46. Only the severely restricted Group 3 animals lived beyond 17 days. Chronologically old but underfed *Tokophyra* showed morphologic features of youth, including less accumulation of age pigment and diminished age-related loss of mitochondria compared to more fully fed controls (Rudzinska, 1962).

A species of rotifer *(Philodina acuticornis)* lived longer when underfed starting early in life (Fanestil & Barrows, 1965; Barrows & Kokkonen, 1982). Three diet groups (n = 30) were followed: group 1, abundant food (fresh pond water daily with added algae); group 2, fresh pond water daily but without algae and, group 3, fresh algae-less pond water on Mondays, Wednesdays and Fridays. Life spans averaged about 35, 45 and 55 days, respectively. Food restriction also raised the age at which egg production ceased: from 12 days for the control group 1, to about 25 days for group 2 and 30 days for group 3. Thus, the survival time after cessation of egg production was uninfluenced by diet. Rotifers underfed in the same fashion as those in group 2, but starting when egg production ceased, lived a total of 42 ± 3 (SEM) days, vs. 33 ± 1 days for controls. Thus, rotifer LS was increased by ADR.

Another rotifer *(Asplanchna brightwelli)* showed average and maximum LSs about 15 percent longer than those of controls if the diet was either restricted or vitamin E-supplemented (Sawada & Carlson, 1987). DR was carried out by offering a medium with one-ninth the concentration of *Paramecium* (the food source), but actual intakes were not known. Lipid peroxidation rose with age and was retarded by both LS-extending regimens.

The nematode *Caenorhabditis elegans* lives longer when food is restricted. In one study, the average LS for worms cultured with 10^8 *E. coli*/ml was 26 days, vs. 15-16 days with 10^9-10^{10} *E. coli*/ml (Klass, 1977). Fecundity was less for the restricted worms. Early-onset DR in *C. elegans* increased average LS by 52 percent, whereas ADR beginning on days 6 or 8 after the reproductive period led to 19 and 12 percent increases. Johnson et al. (1984) reported a 66 day average LS for *C. elegans* subjected to DR under axenic conditions (i.e., no other organism present in the media). Both larval and adult periods were extended. Russell and Jacobson (1985) reviewed studies of nematode aging. They argued against the view that worms grown monoxenically (i.e., with one additional organism present, usually *E. coli*) suffer pathological damage from eating the accompanying organism. They considered the results of nematode DR studies as complementing those in rodents, and supporting the relevance of this animal model. Under harsh conditions such as starvation or crowding, *C. elegans* as well as the related *C. briggsae* and *T. aceti* may form dauerlarvae (an arrested developmental form). These can live a long time, up to 60 days. They do not appear to undergo aging, since when reactivated by return to a normal environment, they display a normal LS. Thus the dauer state appears to represent a "time out" from aging as well as from larval development (Johnson, 1984).

Daphnia longispina also lives longer when underfed. Ingle et al. (1937) imposed DR on *Daphnia* by diluting (1:36) the growth medium (Figure 2.1B). The average and maximum LSs for controls were 30 and 46 days, vs. 40 and 48 days for those on DR for their entire lives. Animals underfed until the 15th to 18th instar (quite late in the LS) and then normally fed lived even longer (average LS of 45-50 days, maximum LS 60 days). Underfeeding lowered the heart rate.

Dunham (1938) confirmed that lifelong underfeeding of *Daphnia* extended average and maximum LSs. Adult-onset DR was also tested and average LSs ranked: DR for the entire life (46 days) > DR from 3rd or 6th instar (40 days) > no DR (37 days) > DR from 9th or 12th instar (29 days). The author notes that animals not underfed until either the 9th or 12th instars were 60 percent larger than age-matched animals which had always been underfed. Thus the *Daphnia* subjected to ADR were comparatively more severely restricted than those animals always on DR. Concerned that the ADR might have been too severe, Dunham attempted to impose it gradually (e.g. 1:10 medium at the 9th instar, 1:20 at the 10th, 1:30 at the 11th, and 1:40 thereafter). This failed to improve survival.

Studies of the development (egg → larva → pupa → imago [= adult]) and aging of underfed *Drosophila* were reported by Northrup (1917) and Loeb and Northrup (1917). The development of *Drosophila* could be retarded by maintaining larvae on an inadequate food source. When yeast was added, pupae would form and flies emerge. If yeast was added to the larvae on day 0, pupae formed on day 4, flies emerged on day 8, and average overall LS was about 19 days. In contrast, larvae first given yeast on day 10 formed pupae 3 days later, became adults on day 17, and showed an average LS of 29 days. Thus, any increase in LS was due to lengthening the egg → larval → pupal period, and DR had no effect on the next stage, that of the imago.

Another study (David et al., 1971) carried out ADR on *Drosophila* by diluting an axenic medium (8% Brewer's yeast, 8% cornflour) with an agar solution to produce a final concentration of foodstuff from 16 percent (no dilution) down to 1 percent (16× diluted). Longevity for flies fed these media ranked 4-16 > 2 > 1 percent, suggesting that very severe ADR adversely affected LS. It is also possible that in some circumstances axenic media are nutritionally inadequate. Holmes and Holmes (1987) observed shorter LSs and greater accumulation of DNA damage in *Paramecium tetraurelia* in axenic compared to nonaxenic media, although neither population was restricted from feeding.

Two other early reports on DR in insects are relevant. Kellogg and Bell (1903) observed that the mulberry silkworm *(Bombyx mori)* responds to severe DR by increasing the time required to moult and by increasing the number of larval moults (from 4 to 5). Kopec (1924) reported that intermittent starvation of young caterpillars (*Lymantria dispar*) would prolong larval life, while not influencing the duration of the adult portion of the LS.

As indicated in Chapter 1 (Fig. 1.4), the bowl and doily spider responds to DR by living longer (Austad, 1988). In the field, this spider ate about 8 *Drosophila* per week and died by 30 days of age. In the laboratory, limiting the number of *Drosophila* from 5 to 3 to 1 progressively increased longevity and decreased fecundity.

Fischer-Piette (1939) reported that when food is abundant, the mollusc *Patella vulgata* only lives 2.5 years, whereas in waters poor in organic material its survival may reach 16 years.

While confirming biomarker data are only available for *Tokophyra* and nematodes, the above findings strongly suggest that an appropriate DR regimen will retard aging in a variety of invertebrate species. Furthermore, DR does not have to be imposed during the phase of active growth in order to increase LS in several of these species, although there is some question whether it will do so in holometabolous insects once the imago (post-mitotic) stage is reached (Comfort, 1960). The far more extensive studies of DR in rodents, which we next discuss, tell a similar, albeit more definitive story.

STUDIES IN VERTEBRATES

Vertebrates have been used for the majority of DR longevity studies, chiefly mice and rats, plus a few studies of fish and cows. A major knowledge gap in the DR field concerns primates. The effect of DR on aging in primates has not yet been directly tested although such a study was recently started by investigators at the NIA's Gerontology Research Center.

Studies of DR in Non-Rodent Vertebrates

Comfort (1963) reported that underfeeding sufficient to inhibit the growth of fish (female guppies [*Lebistes*]) increased the LS (Figure 2.1C). The guppies were fed *Tubifex* worms weekly or biweekly from early in life until 600 days of age, after which they were switched to full feeding. These realimented guppies showed an average gain in life expectancy of about 200 days (a 20% increase). A three-fold increase in the LS of the annual fish *Cynolebias adloffi* maintained on reduced food intake was noted by Walford (1982).

Another "fish story" involved brook trout experimentally stocked in a small, remote lake in the High Sierra. Reimers (1979) describes this 1951-1975 study, in which some trout lived well into their 24th year of life. This period, amounting to at least a *doubling* of the previous maximum LS for the species, was attributed to a combination of food scarcity, low temperature, and a remote environment (with few anglers). That these fish reached an *extremely* great age is suggested by the fact that only 1 of 14 previously studied brook trout populations reported fish reaching 7 years of age. This study argues pointedly against the idea that DR findings are not applicable to wild populations.

A small amount of evidence exists for longer LSs in range beef cows given less food in the winter (Pinney et al., 1972). Effects on BW were minor. Average LS in one restricted group was 14.7 vs. 10.9 years for those not restricted. The maximum LS was not determined.

Studies of DR in Rodents

Types of Diets

Greenfield and Briggs (1971) critically reviewed nutritional methods used in rat research. They found that of the 100 rat studies reported in the 1969 *Journal of Nutrition* only 24 employed diets adequate in both vitamin and mineral contents! Mineral deficiencies were most common. This situation is now thought to be improved with the increasing use of the AIN-76™ diet (AIN is the American Institute of Nutrition; this diet is described below).

Of course, statements of "adequacy" or "deficiency" should be viewed realizing that little is known about what comprises optimal rodent nutrition. The nutrient requirements for laboratory mice were the subject of a National Research Council report (1978) which wisely brings to the fore a recurring question to anyone contemplating nutrient requirements: Requirements for what? We seek optimal intakes for a healthful increase in LS brought on by a deceleration of biologic aging. Others may seek maximum growth rate, body size, or fecundity. Optimum nutrition is demonstrably not the same for these different goals.

Most longevity studies in rodents have used either commercially available nonpurified diets (NPDs) or defined purified diets (PDs). Both diet types were thoroughly discussed in the 1977 report of the AIN's

Committee on Standards for Nutritional Studies. (This report and the aforementioned National Research Council [1978] publication, are essential reading for workers in rodent nutrition.) Two types of NPDs exist: *open* formula (which has a defined, fixed composition [e.g. NIH-7 Open Formula Diet]) and *closed* formula (in which the commercial manufacturer does not disclose exact composition [e.g. Purina Laboratory Chow™]).

The PDs differ from NPDs in being made of commercially refined proteins (casein is most commonly used), carbohydrate (e.g. sucrose, cornstarch) and fat (usually corn oil), with added vitamin and mineral mixtures. The compositions of a much used open formula NPD (NIH-7) and a PD (AIN-76™) are given in Table 2.2. A potential disadvantage of NPDs is that nonnutritive substances can contaminate NPDs more readily than for the PDs. Thus, PDs are better defined nutritionally as well as affording the investigator the power to manipulate diet content. A third type of diet is the "chemically defined diet" which differs in supplying protein as purified amino acids, carbohydrate from refined mono- or disaccharides, and fat from purified fatty acids or triglycerides. Chemically-defined diets are generally too expensive for long-term, gerontological testing.

The 1977 AIN report suggested that AIN-76™ be the standard PD for rodent studies. Its use appears to be widespread and increasing. The general use of a single diet is positive in allowing meaningful comparison of data but is negative in discouraging new attempts to optimize diet composition. This may be especially pertinent here since the AIN Committee ". . . decided that the diet should not contain quantities of vitamins and minerals highly in excess of the requirements for rats and mice as set forth by the Committee on Animal Nutrition, National Research Council (1978)." Despite the obvious appeal of using a completely defined diet for many nutritional studies, the AIN diet itself must be shown to yield maximum LSs as great as less defined or less widely used diets, in order to be considered adequate for longevity studies.

Feeding Strategies for DR

Two basic methods of DR are known to increase LS. These are either to restrict the intake of an adequate diet or to allow animals to eat a protein deficient diet ad libitum. Because animals eat less of a poor diet than a good one, low protein diets commonly lead to caloric restriction.

TABLE 2.2

Compositions of a Nonpurified and Purified Rodent Diet[a]

NIH-7 Open Formula[b] Ingredient	%	AIN-76™ Purified Diet[c] Ingredient	%
Dried skim milk	5.0	Casein	20.0
Fish meal (60% protein)	10.0	DL-Methionine	0.3
Soybean meal (49% protein)	12.0	Cornstarch	15.0
Alfalfa meal (17% protein)	4.0	Sucrose	50.0
Corn gluten meal (60% protein)	3.0	Fiber	5.0
Ground shelled corn	24.5	Corn oil	5.0
Ground hard winter wheat	23.0	AIN mineral mix	3.5
Wheat middlings	10.0	AIN vitamin mix	1.0
Brewers dried yeast	2.0	Choline bitartrate	0.2
Dry molasses	1.5		100.0
Soybean oil	2.5		
Sodium chloride	0.5		
Dicalcium phosphate	1.2		
Ground limestone	0.5		
Pre-mixes	0.3		
	100.0		

[a]Adapted from the "Report of the American Institute of Nutrition Ad Hoc Committee on Standards for Nutritional Studies" (American Institute of Nutrition, 1977) wherein details (e.g. composition of vitamin and mineral mixes, comparison of actual nutrient intakes to recommended levels) about these diets are reported.
[b]The calculated composition is crude protein=23.5%, crude fat=5%, crude fiber=4.5%, and ash=7.0%.
[c]The AIN committee commented that the 50% sucrose content of this diet may have adverse long-term effects. They note that substituting other carbohydrates may introduce other variables (e.g. starch contains unsaturated lipid, commercial glucose has about 10% moisture).

Restricted Feeding of an Adequate Diet. By far, the most solidly established and effective way to prolong life in rodents is to feed PDs in limited amounts. This is best done by feeding the animal a known reduced amount of food, but has also been accomplished by allowing ad lib access for a fixed period of time (e.g. for 12 hours every other day). In most studies the DR animals consumed 40-70 percent of the number of calories eaten by adult controls. The diets fed in restricted amounts are sometimes (but not always) enriched in certain essentials to guard against malnutrition. Diets which provide identical intakes of all known essential nutrients even though differing in calories may be referred to as "isonutrient diets."

The DR and control regimens used in our laboratory were detailed in Table 1.3. The diet we feed to restricted mice is richer in proteins, vitamins and minerals than the control diet. Our DR mice are fed only on Mondays, Wednesdays and Fridays. However, impressive LS extension can also follow a reduction in total food intake for animals fed every day (e.g. Ross, 1961; Merry & Holehan, 1981; Yu et al., 1982).

As will be detailed, NPDs and PDs not further enriched in essential nutrients have also increased average and maximum LSs when fed on a low calorie basis. Presumably, all these rations are adequate to avoid malnutrition and provide a healthful, low calorie diet. This presumption is supported by the finding that rats on EDR (50% of ad lib intake of an AIN-76™-like diet not enriched in minerals) did not differ from controls in concentrations of zinc, copper and manganese in several tissues at 1 year of age (Burch & Hahn, 1982).

Low Protein Diets. The longevity of rodents freely eating diets providing amounts of protein insufficient for normal growth has been studied (Leto et al., 1976a; Stoltzner, 1977; Goodrick, 1978). Life span is far more impressively increased by nutrient-adequate DR than by these low protein (typically 4-10% casein) diets. Low dietary protein levels can reduce the food intake and BW of animals compared to normally fed controls. Payne (1975) observed that low protein diets may lead to an anorexia that is more severe for 30 day old than for 70 day old rats. Thus, these regimens likely cause a complex pattern of protein malnutrition and calorie restriction during the growth period. Table 2.3 presents certain observations made in rodents fed low protein diets (LS data are considered separately below). The data suggest that a reduced calorie intake may accompany ad lib feeding of low protein diets.

Labelling either of these restriction protocols *"caloric restriction"* or *"protein restriction"* may be misleading. The restricted feeding of an adequate diet leads to lower intakes of all ingredients which have not been proportionately enriched in the restricted diet. Thus, fat and protein restriction accompany most published work using DR regimens, thereby making the label "caloric restriction" imprecise in these instances. With regard to the term "protein restriction," young rodents given free access to low protein diets eat less than do controls fed normal diets. Thus, intakes of calories and all non-enriched ingredients are less for the "protein restricted" animals than for controls. It is also possible that restricted feeding of even an isonutrient diet might result in relative protein restriction, if protein must be used for catabolic and not anabolic

TABLE 2.3
Findings in Rodents Fed Low Protein Diets Ad Lib Since Weaning

Study[a]	Animal	Diets[b]	Effect of Low Protein Diet
1.	Mouse, Balb/c	4% vs. 24%	Adult BW for 4% pro = 23 g vs. 32 g for controls. ↓ Organ wts.
2.	Mouse (3 strains)	4% vs. 26%	4% pro → BW at 6 mo of 16-23 g (vs. 28-37 g), ↓ rectal temp., ↑ O_2 consump.
3,4.	Mouse, B6	4% vs. 26%	4% pro → ↓ BW (35%), ↓ rectal temp., ↑ O_2 consump., ↓ activs. of liver & kidney enzymes.
5.	Rat, albino	9% vs. 27%	At 3 mo, the BW of rats fed 9% pro. was 50% that of controls. Many restr. rats were sick.
6.	Rat, Wistar	5% vs. 21%	5% pro. → ↓ BW, ↓ RNA and free amino acids in skeletal muscle.

[a](1) Stoltzner (1977); (2) Goodrick (1973); (3) Leto et al. (1976a); (4) Leto et al. (1976b); (5) Boyd (1972); (6) Giovannetti and Strothers (1975).
[b]Values give the protein content of the diets.

purposes. For these reasons, we favor use of the term "dietary restriction" as a general label applicable to most of the literature in this field; however, it is clear that the restricted feeding of an adequate diet retards aging far more convincingly than the ad lib feeding of low protein diets.

Fasting

The duration of the fasting interval varies among studies which restrict food intake. Some workers provide daily feedings of small portions while others may offer larger rations on alternating days. In either case, DR rodents may go several hours or even a day or two without food.

The literature which describes the biology of fasting in rodents has therefore some pertinence to DR studies. Noteworthy outcomes of acute fasting (discussed variously in Chapters 4, 5 and 6; see also Table 6.1) include decreases in body temperature, O_2 consumption, and thyroid activity. Several other endocrine parameters besides thyroid activity may also be depressed. Levels of and synthesis rates for several fats decline. Heart rate and rate of cardiac protein degradation fall.

It is not unreasonable to expect that rodents on those DR regimens involving fasts exceeding one day may share common biologic alterations with acutely fasted animals. While this seems to be the case, and while certain of the phenomena of fasting may provide hints as to the actions of DR in retarding aging, one must keep in mind that significant differences exist between acute starvation or total fasting, and long-term hypocaloric diets.

Coprophagy can influence the length of fasting as well as the actual numbers of calories ingested. A recent report (Williams & Senior, 1985) described a 20-30 percent loss of BW by rats subjected to ADR. However, the digestibility of the food offered in restricted amounts was higher than for the food fed ad lib, and this higher digestibility vanished if coprophagy by the ADR animals was prevented. The preclusion of coprophagy did not influence digestibility of food fed ad libitum. To precisely quantitate actual caloric intakes and energy balance for DR rodents requires that coprophagy be considered as a potential variable.

Early-Onset Dietary Restriction (EDR)

Growth, Puberty Onset and Health. The growth rates and adult BWs of young rodents subjected to DR approximate the levels of caloric intake. Growth curves for female $C3B10RF_1$ mice studied in our laboratory are shown in Figure 2.3. The heaviest mice were allowed free access to Purina Lab Chow™. The other diet groups were fed nutritionally adequate PDs (Table 1.3) at about 85, 50 or 40 kcal per week. Mice fed 85 kcal per week of Diet 1 served as controls for the EDR mice but were themselves diet restricted by about 25 percent when compared to the intake for mice freely fed the Lab Chow™.

Early-onset DR delays the onset of puberty in female rodents. This was described in rats long ago by Evans and Bishop (1922). McCay's colleagues, Asdell and Crowell (1935), observed first estrus for ad lib fed rats at about 2 months of age (BW, 140 g), vs. 12 months (BW, 85 g) for DR rats. The time interval separating vaginal opening and first estrus was increased by DR.

Studying female Wistar rats, Glass et al. (1976) found a highly significant inverse linear relation between age of onset of puberty (as judged by vaginal opening and first estrus) and growth rate (which was caused to vary either by restricted feeding of a defined amino acid diet, or by giving a valine deficient ration). Body weights at puberty were not constant, and the growth rate seemed more important than arrival at a particular BW in affecting the timing of puberty.

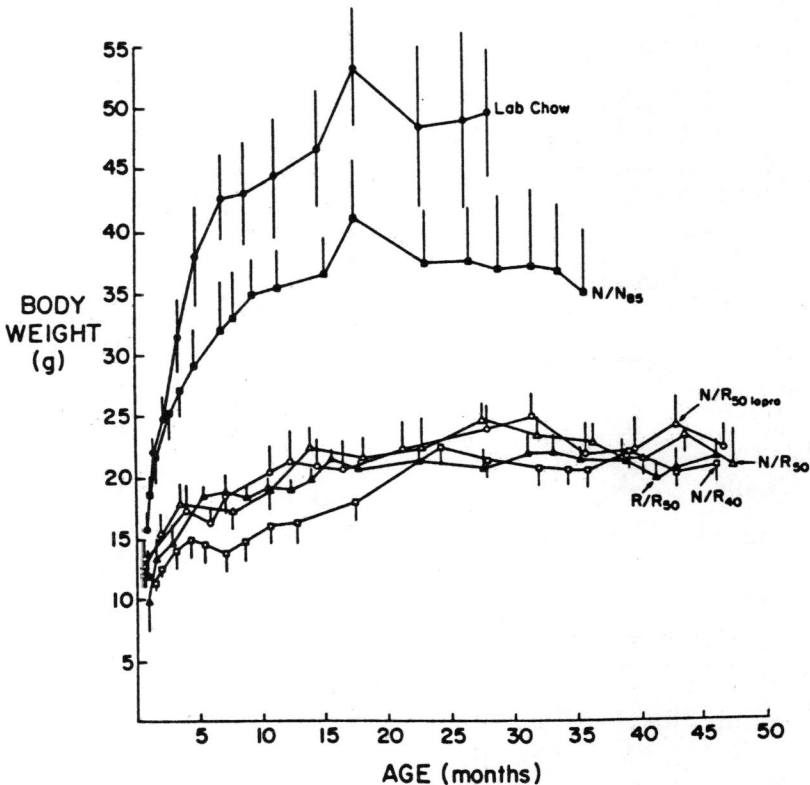

Figure 2.3. Influences of diet on BW of female C3B10RF$_1$ mice. Values represent mean ± SD. Diet groups: Lab Chow, Purina Lab Chow™ ad libitum; N/N$_{85}$, fed normally before and after weaning, postweaning diet fed at 85 kcal/week (25% less than ad libitum); N/R$_{50}$, fed normally before weaning, restricted postweaning to 50 kcal/week; R/R$_{50}$, restricted in feeding level both before and after weaning; N/R$_{50lopro}$ restricted after weaning to 50 kcal/week with a decrease with age in the protein content of the diet; N/R$_{40}$, restricted after weaning to 40 kcal/week. Diet compositions are shown in Table 1.3. From Weindruch et al. (1986).

Female Sprague-Dawley rats subjected to about 25 percent reductions in the intake of NPDs at weaning were older and leaner at first estrus than were ad lib fed controls; however, DR and control rats did not differ in BW or body length at time of puberty (Willen & Naftolin, 1978; Bronson, 1987). Furthermore, within DR and control groups at first estrus, later maturers were larger in length and BW, were fatter, and had consumed less food per BW than had early maturers (Willen & Naftolin, 1978).

Additional information about the influences of EDR on onset of puberty in rats comes from the studies of Merry and Holehan from the

Wolfson Institute, University of Hull, England. (They have also studied several age-sensitive biologic parameters in DR rats [Chapter 4].) Vaginal opening and first estrus in Sprague-Dawley rats on DR (50% of ad lib) was delayed (Merry & Holehan, 1979). All controls were mature by 45 days of age (range = 36-45 days) whereas only about 50 percent of the DR animals were mature by 160 days. All DR rats (n = 100) had reached maturity by 227 days. Thus, DR delayed but did not prevent sexual maturation in female rats. Later work (Holehan & Merry, 1985a) indicated that the onset of puberty occurred at the same BW in DR and control rats.

A 25 percent food restriction imposed on weanling mice from a randomly bred strain delayed vaginal opening by only about 5 days (from 35 to 40 days of age) (Hansen et al., 1983). As will be discussed (Chapter 4), female mice subjected to more severe DR usually do not display estrus cycles and thereby differ from restricted rats which continue to cycle.

Findings on the onset of sexual maturity in underfed male rats were reviewed by Glass and Swerdloff (1980). Several types of undernutrition cause hypoandrogenism attributable to a hypothalamic-pituitary defect. Despite this, spermatogenesis is usually preserved in DR male rats and the testicular weight: BW ratio increases. Merry and Holehan (1981) observed that male Sprague-Dawley rats fed half of an ad lib intake showed 10 to 20 day delays in the pubertal peak of serum testosterone. Reduced fertility was observed in these EDR rats when tested at 63-84 days of age but not at the next ages (107-128 days) tested. Hamilton and Bronson (1986) reported that reproductive development is less sensitive to inhibition by DR in male than in female mice. Yet, earlier observers (Lee et al., 1951) saw reduced fertility with DR in male C3H mice. Severe DR (30% of ad lib) more readily disrupted spermatogenesis in deer mice *(Peromyscus)* than in house mice (Blank & Desjardins, 1983).

A few comments are in order on the general health of DR rodents. Early studies reported high infant mortality rates, but this no longer obtains, and was very likely due to essential nutrient deficiency rather than a simple decrease in caloric intake. Generally, we find that less than 2 percent of a large group of weanling mice will die prior to 6 months of age and that this figure is the same for DR and control groups. Our DR mice, fed regimens isonutrient to those fed to controls, appear quite healthy and very active. Other current workers are finding these same outcomes. The coats and appearances of DR rodents have long been reported to be better maintained to older ages than for controls (McCay et al., 1935; Berg & Simms, 1960), which accords with our observations for mice restricted either early or much later in life.

The excellent health of underfed rodents is attested to by a study of exercise capacity in Sprague-Dawley rats (Hansen-Smith et al., 1977a). Young males (125 g, no age given) were assigned to one of five PD groups and fed for 8-10 weeks. Group 1 ate a 27 percent casein diet ad lib (16 g/day → BWs of 350 g), group 2 a 15 percent casein diet ad lib (16 g/day → BWs of 315 g), groups 3-5 were restricted (final BWs 190 g). Group 3 was fed an 8 percent casein diet ad lib (9 g/day), group 4 was fed the 27 percent casein diet but was restricted to 6.5 g per day, and group 5 was fed 6.5 g per day of the 15 percent casein diet. Swimming endurance times were determined. Restricted groups 3-5 could swim for as long or longer than controls. Group 3 showed the greatest endurance.

The remarkable life history of Emperor penguins provides a stunning example of functionality and fitness during long-term fasting which occurs during the rigors of the Antarctic winter (Dewasmes et al., 1980). Only able to feed at sea, these birds must fast when they leave the ocean to migrate to breeding rookeries (located on sea ice and as far as 120 km from open water). The birds court, copulate, and after about 45 days, each female lays one egg and leaves this with the mate for incubation (65 days). She returns to sea (maternity leave?) and reappears near the time of hatching, at which time the fasted male walks back to sea. Thus, the male's fast approaches 4 months. Males have lost about 50 percent of their BW by the time they return to the sea to feed. Dewasmes and colleagues have measured metabolic rates at rest and during treadmill walking in emperors after 63-118 days of fasting. Resting rates (not adjusted to BW) decrease linearly with BW throughout the fast. When normalized to BW, neither type of metabolic rate differed through most of the fast.

Longevity. Before evaluating the abundant rodent data on DR and LS, it is appropriate to ask: How long have laboratory rodents (rats and mice) been observed to live? To our knowledge, the oldest rat or mouse described in a regular scientific report (Schroeder & Mitchener, 1971) was a female Long-Evans rat who lived to be 60 months of age. This rat was given extra-selenate in the drinking water and its LS was *double* the average LS for the treatment group. Reports of exceptional or atypical LSs for isolated animals must, however, remain suspect in view of the possibilities of mislabelling, mutation, or other untoward events.

Exceptionally long-lived rodents were described in a letter to the editor of *Thymus* written by the Polish scientists Czaplicki and Blonska

(1981). They injected mice, rats and guinea pigs with "early fetal thymic pig extracts (ETPE) or early fetal thymic calf extracts (ETCE)" and observed: (1) two male mice from the R3 strain injected IP thrice weekly for 2.5 months (age of treatment not stated) lived 66-67 months; (2) an ETPE-treated guinea pig lived 12 years; and (3) young (6 month old) Wistar rats treated with ETCE (45 injections) showed brief LSs on the average (most dead by 29 months) but a few lived to 54 months before all succumbing to a laboratory heating system failure. These spectacular results (heating failure excluded) resemble nothing in the modern gerontological literature. The injections were also accompanied by immunologic alterations. These we have been unable to confirm in mice, although LS data are not yet in (S. Harris & R.L. Walford, unpublished observations).

A report by Osborne et al. (1917) is often cited as providing the first evidence that diets which stunt growth can increase LS. Growth of rats was slowed by either food restriction, low protein diets, or qualitatively inadequate protein sources. Four females were described which were stunted since about 6 weeks of age. They were then given adequate food and allowed to resume growth respectively at 6, 12, 13 or 18 months of age (when weighing only 100 g). These rats produced litters at ages (16-29 months) when normally fed rats could not. They died of lung disease between 26-33 months of age, which is long for both the colony (where about 2 of 3 controls do not reach 24 months) and for the era. But maximal LS for controls was 34 months meaning that this report did not in fact provide evidence of extended maximum LS.

Tables 2.4 and 2.5 summarize LS studies respectively of rats and mice subjected to EDR. Reports were excluded from this analysis if less than 10 individuals were included per treatment group. Also, we have made no attempt to catalog every diet group of every report. We do seek to indicate: (1) how the severity of EDR influences LS, (2) which DR regimens appear qualitatively superior, and (3) any relation between length of the fasting interval and LS in DR rodents.

Inspection of Table 2.4 reveals that diverse DR regimens can produce extremely old rats. The greatest maximal LSs, expressed as 10th decile of survivorship, for males all occurred in the Sprague-Dawley strain and were reported by Ross (1961: Grp 7g = 49 months, Grp 7c = 46 months), Merry and Holehan (1981: Grp 15a = 47 months) and Ross and Bras (1973: Grp 9e = 45 months). Ross used PDs, and Merry and Holehan a NPD. Body weights varied considerably (from 170-400 g) among these various DR groups.

TABLE 2.4
Longevity Studies Using Rats Fed Restricted Diets Starting Early in Life[a]

Study[b]	Strain	Diet Groups[c]	Peak BW[d]		Ave. LS[e]	Max. LS[f]
1.	"white"	1a. R (23F,13M), PD, ↑cas, ↑vit, DF[c]	210	(59%)	25,27	45,43
		1b. C (22F,14M), PD, ad lib	355		26,16	38,27
2.	"white"	2a. R until 900d (10F,10M), PD + nat'l foods, DF	195	(71%)	37,36	41,39
		2b. C (19F,19M), as above + ad lib NPD	275		24,20	37,30
3.	Wistar	3a. R (15F,15M), NPD ad lib one day, fast the next	235[d]	(86%)	24,22	34,31
		3b. C (19F,14M), NPD ad lib	275		23,20	31,26
4.	Sprague-Dawley	4a. R (20[c]), PD, DF (28 kcal)	180[d]	(47%)	12/20 alive@24 mo[f]	
		4b. C (20[c]), PD+sucrose, DF (52 kcal)	380		4/20 alive@24 mo[f]	
5.	Wistar	5a. R (27), NPD, DF (5-7g/d)	265	(55%)	28	5/27@36 mo
		5b. C (586), NPD ad lib	485		24	0/586@36 mo
6.	Sprague-Dawley	6a[c]. R (39F,79M), NPD, DF (54% of ad lib)	170	(61%)	41,33	>40[f],35
		6b. C (79F,89M), NPD, ad lib	280		30,25	33,28
7.	Sprague-Dawley	7a. R (210M), PD, 30% cas, 61% suc, DF (41 kcal)	450		30	42
		7b. C (25M), PD, 30% cas, 61% suc, ad lib (71 kcal)	NR		10	11
		7c. R (120M), PD, 51% cas, 34% suc, DF (25 kcal)	250		31	46
		7d. C (25M), PD, 51% cas, 34% suc, ad lib (78 kcal)	NR		20	26
		7e. R (210M), PD, 8% cas, 83% suc, DF (41 kcal)	400		27	38
		7f. C (25M), PD, 8% cas, 83% suc, ad lib (61 kcal)	NR		27	39
		7g[c].R (195M), PD, 21% cas, 54% suc, DF (16 kcal)	170		31	49
		7h[c].C (25M), PD, 21% cas, 54% suc, DF (83 kcal)	NR		20	28
		7i. C (210M), NPD, ad lib (83 kcal)	600		24	32
8.	Chas. River	8a. R (250M), PD, DF (25 kcal)	200	(29%)	27	43
		8b. R to 70d→C (150M), PD, ad lib	680		19	30
		8c. C (250M), PD, ad lib (80 kcal)	720		20	27
9.	Chas. River	9a. R. (352M), PD, 10% cas, 70% suc, DF (25 kcal)	185	(29%)	25	38
		9b. C (250M), PD, 10% cas, 70% suc, ad lib	650		20	29
		9c. R (250M), PD, 22% cas, 59% suc, DF (25 kcal)	200	(27%)	28	43
		9d. C (250M), PD, 22% cas, 59% suc, ad lib	750		20	27
		9e. R (250M), PD, 51% cas, 30% suc, DF (25 kcal)	200	(31%)	32	45
		9f. C (250M), PD, 51% cas, 30% suc, ad lib	650		21	28

TABLE 2.4
(Continued)

Study[b]	Strain	Diet Groups[c]	Peak BW[d]		Ave. LS[e]	Max. LS[f]
10.	Holtzman	10a. R (20M), NPD, DF	400	(72%)	24	28
		10b. C (40M), NPD, ad lib	550		20	24
11.	Sprague-Dawley	11a. R (60M), NPD, ad lib for 2 hours/day	450	(82%)	23	30
		11b. C (60M), NPD, ad lib	550		19	25
12.	Long-Evans	12a. R (24F), PD, tryptophane deficient, ad lib	150	(43%)	33% alive@23 mo[f]	
		12b. C (14F), NPD, ad lib	350		86% alive@23 mo[f]	
13.	Albino	13a. R (49M), NPD, ad lib for 6 hours/day	400	(80%)	29	39
		13b. C (49M), NPD, ad lib	500		24	33
14.	Sprague-Dawley	14a. R (45F), NPD, DF (50% of ad lib)	300	(50%)	36	43
		14b. C (200F), NPD, ad lib	600		23	33
15.	Sprague-Dawley	15a. R (100M), NPD, DF (50% of ad lib)	400	(42%)	33	47
		15b. C (397M), NPD, ad lib	950		23	33
16.	Wistar	16a. R (25M), NPD, DF (40% of ad lib)	170	(34%)	28	42
		16b. C (25M), NPD, ad lib	500		26	33
17.	Wistar	17a. R (20M), NPD, DF (12.5 kcal/d)	NR		10	19
		17b. R (25M), NPD, DF (25 kcal/d)	125	(42%)	28	39
		17c. R (25M), NPD, DF (50 kcal/d)	185	(62%)	31	39
		17d. C (20M), NPD, ad lib (75 kcal/d)	300		24	33
18.	Wistar	18a. R (20M), NPD, DF (7g/d)	180	(36%)	29	36
		18b. R (15M), NPD, DF (15g/d)	350	(70%)	30	38
		18c. C (20M), NPD, ad lib (19g/d)	500		25	35
19.	Wistar	19a. R (25M), NPD, DF (7g/d)	180	(36%)	29	41
		19b. C (25M), NPD, ad lib (~20g/d)	500		24	33
20.	Fischer 344	20a. R (115M), PD, ↑vit, DF (60% of ad lib)	300	(55%)	32	43
		20b. C (115M), PD, ad lib	550		23	29
21.	Fischer 344	21a[c]. R (40M), PD, ↑vit, ↑min, DF (60% of ad lib)	290	(53%)	35	41
		21b[c]. C→R (40M), as above but onset of DR = 6 mo	300	(55%)	31	39
		21c[c]. R→C (40M), switched from R→C @6 mo	500	(91%)	27	30
		21d. C (40M), PD, ad lib	550		23	27
22.	Wistar	22a. R (24M), NPD, ad lib but every other day	400	(62%)	32	39
		22b. C (28M), NPD, ad lib	650		18	22
23.	Wistar	23a. R (24M), NPD, ad lib but every other day	420	(81%)	29	35
		23b. C (52M), NPD, ad lib	520		24	28
24.	Wistar	24a. R (36M), PD (18% cas), DF (66% of ad lib)	400	(70%)	23	NR[f]
		24b. R (36M), PD (30% cas), DF (66% of ad lib)	400	(67%)	>24[e]	NR[f]

TABLE 2.4
(Continued)

Study[b]	Strain	Diet Groups[c]	Peak BW[d]		Ave. LS[e]	Max. LS[f]
		24c. R (36M), PD (42% cas), DF (66% of ad lib)	400	(70%)	>24[e]	NR[f]
		24d. C (36M), PD (12% cas), ad lib	570		20	NR[f]
		24e. C (36M), PD (20% cas), ad lib	600		22	NR[f]
		24f. C (36M), PD (28% cas), ad lib	570		23	NR[f]
25.	Wistar	25a[c]. R (45M), NPD, IF (ad lib every other day)	330	(63%)	38	46
		25b[c]. C→R (45M), NPD, Diet C to 12 mo, then IF	410	(77%)	35	41
		25c[c]. R→C (45M), NPD, IF until 12 mo, then diet C	465	(88%)	34	42
		25d. C (45M), NPD, ad lib	550		31	39
26.	Sprague-Dawley	26a. R (829), NPD, DF (66% of ad lib)	320	(62%)	15	28
		26b. C (969), NPD, ad lib	520		14	25

[a]DR started in most studies at 3-5 weeks of age. Starting later were studies #3, 19-21 (onset=6-7 wk) and #11, 16, and 18 (10 wk). This table includes two studies (#21, 25) each testing both EDR and ADR.

[b]References (listed chronologically for the most part): (1) McCay et al. (1935); (2) McCay et al. (1943); (3) Carlson and Hoelzel (1946); (4) Riesen et al. (1947); (5) Gilbert et al. (1958); (6) Berg and Simms (1961); (7) Ross (1961); (8) Ross and Bras (1971); (9) Ross and Bras (1973); (10) Kibler and Johnson (1966); (11) Leveille (1972); (12) Segall and Timaris (1976); (13) Drori and Folman (1976); (14) Merry and Holehan (1979); (15) Merry and Holehan (1981); (16) Everitt et al. (1980); (17) Everitt et al. (1982); (18) Everitt et al. (1983); (19) Wyndham et al. (1983); (20) Yu et al. (1982); (21) Yu et al. (1985); (22) Goodrick et al. (1982); (23) Goodrick et al. (1983a); (24) Davis et al. (1983); (25) Beauchene et al. (1986); (26) Zamenhof and van Marthens (1982).

[c]Abbreviations used: R=restricted diet group; C=control diet group; F=female; M=male; NPD=nonpurified diet, which includes both commercially available pelleted diets and natural product diets; PD=purified diet; cas=casein (the usual sole protein source in PDs); suc=sucrose; vit=vitamins; min=minerals; ↑=diet enriched in that ingredient (e.g. ↑ cas. =diet enriched in casein); DF=daily feeding; IF=intermittent feeding. When gender of animal is not shown next to the number of animals studied, this indicates that both sexes were studied but not separately reported. For group 1a, a "stairstep" method was used to retard growth rate. The amount of food given allowed a growth of ~10 g per 2-3 month interval. In study #4, each group consisted of 10 F and 10 M. For groups 6a & 6b, the building housing the rats was "demolished" when the rats were ~800 days old. Some of the R survivors (37 F & 64 M) were killed leaving 20 F and 26 M for LS study. All surviving controls (58 F, 31 M) were killed at that time. Mortality data are for controls which had previously completed their LSs. Groups 7g & 7h ate diets enriched in vitamins and minerals relative to the other groups in the study. Studies #21 and 25 tested both EDR and ADR. In #21, grp. 21a was started on DR at 6 weeks of age and maintained this way until death; 21b was switched to ADR at 6 months of age; 21c was returned to ad lib feeding at 6 months. In study #25, grp. 25a was started on DR at 30 days of age. Grp. 25b was switched from ad lib to DR at 12 months. Grp. 25c was switched from DR to ad lib at 12 months.

[d]Largest average BW (g) attained. NR=not reported. Values for females in those studies of both sexes. Value in parentheses next to R value gives peak BW of R/peak BW of C, an index of the severity of the DR. For study #3, the BW values are for 300 days of age (peak BW not stated). For study #4, rats were not separated by sex for reporting of BW and LS data.

[e]Average LS of cohort in months. A few reports do not give this value and an estimate is shown here. Study #24 was terminated at 24 months. When LSs of both sexes were separately described in a report, values for females preceed those for males.

[f]Average LS of the cohort's longest lived decile in months. Usually, this value was not reported and was estimated here. Again, LSs of females preceed those of males. The rats of study #4 were observed for 24 months. For group 6a, 73% of the R females were alive at 40 months which is the oldest age for which data are given. For study #12, all 7 restricted rats alive at 23 months were living at 30 months. In contrast, 6 of 12 rats in group 12b died during that period. Study #24 ended at 24 months.

It is perhaps noteworthy that specific pathogen free housing conditions as used by Masoro's group (studies #20 and 21) did not increase the maximum LS of rats: 10th decile of 29 months for controls and 43 months for DR rats. This is in keeping with the thesis, that, except for calorie restriction itself, *maximum* LS (as opposed to *average* LS) for the species seems independent of environment. And evidence from Holloszy's laboratory suggests that even exercise is no exception (Holloszy et al., 1985). Also illustrating this point is the finding that the median LS of ad lib-fed Wistar rats is 32 months if raised in conventional quarters as opposed to 35 months in germ-free environs; however, median LSs for rats on DR (70% of ad lib) are about 40 months in either environment (Snyder & Pollard, 1987).

Data for female rats are also given in Table 2.4. Females have not been studied as extensively as males. The greatest 10th decile LSs were reported by McCay et al. (1935: #1a = 45 months), Berg and Simms (1961: #6a = 73% of the population alive at 40 months when observation ceased) and Merry and Holehan (1979: #14a = 43 months). Again, the studies differed widely in the DR regimen used as reflected in BWs of 170-300 grams. Also, we note that what are classified as "Sprague-Dawley rats" appear to be a heterogeneous group, since Berg and Simms' ad lib fed controls at 280 g weighed less than Merry and Holehan's DR group (300 g)! Merry and Holehan (1979) discuss vast differences in growth potentials of Sprague-Dawley rats.

Clearly there are more ways than one to underfeed a rat, and several types of diets work well at LS extension. Most studies in rats have utilized daily feeding of fixed amounts of adequate but not necessarily isonutrient diets. The relative severity of DR as judged by the ratio of peak BWs of EDR:control varied from 0.31-0.61 in the studies just identified as being most successful. Of course, such percentages can be misleading due to variable degrees of obesity in the control groups. And daily fed DR animals who eat their entire ration quickly (as several of our DR mice do) experience 20-23 hour fast each day of their lives. Intermittent fasting (one day in two) was imposed by Carlson and Hoelzel (study #3) but they did not limit food intake on eating days, resulting in the opportunistic EDR rats weighing nearly as much (86%) as ad lib controls, and maximum LSs of less than 35 months. Certain other studies listed in Table 2.4 (#11, 13, 22, 23) also carried out DR by giving rats free access to food for a limited period of time, and none of these produced maximum LSs exceeding 39 months of age.

Ross' studies offer much information on how the makeup of restricted diets influences LS. Ross (1961) constructed restricted diets (Table 2.4, Diets 7a, 7c, 7e, 7g) to respectively provide 41, 25, 41, and 16 kcal/day while giving equal daily amounts of fat, vitamins and minerals. These four diets differed in casein and sucrose levels. Casein intakes for rats fed diets 7a and 7c were balanced (3.0 g/rat·day) as were the casein intakes of rats fed diets 7e and 7g (0.8 g/rat·day). These combinations could therefore be considered isonutrient. Sucrose intakes for rats in groups 7c and 7g were equal (2.0 g/rat·day) and those of the other two DR groups nearly so (6.1-8.3 g/rat·day). Groups 7c and 7g ate the fewest kcal per day and lived the longest. Rats eating diet 7g, the most severely underfed, showed the greatest early mortality and also extremely long LSs. The low protein diet (7e, 8% casein) fed on a restricted basis was least beneficial.

In a later study, Ross and Bras (1973: Table 2.4, #9) balanced the calorie intakes (25 kcal/day) of rats subjected to EDR but varied the casein:sucrose ratio of the three diets tested. The average LS of rats on DR increased as the amount of protein in the diet increased suggesting that effects of DR on LS may be enhanced by diets high in protein content. A later report (Davis et al., 1983) supports this view.

Segall and Timaris (1976) studied the effects of a tryptophan deficient diet on survival in rats (Table 2.4, #12). Only one-third of the deficient rats lived until 23 months, but increased longevity of post-23-months survivors was observed. The regimen caused the rats to eat little food (despite ad lib presentation) producing BWs less than 50 percent those of controls fed a normal diet. Several other rat studies have tested the effects of low protein diets on LS but these involved ADR intervention (see "*Adulthood-Onset Dietary Restriction (ADR),*" this Chapter).

Everitt and co-workers studied the effects of hypophysectomy (Hx) and DR on aging in male Wistar rats (Table 2.4, studies #16-19). Because hypophysectomized (Hxed) rats eat only about 40 percent as much food as intact rats, and DR groups were required to serve as pair-fed, intact controls. In these studies LS was fairly equally increased by Hx and DR, but the maximum LSs reached were unimpressive (usually < 40 months). It is difficult to separate the effects of Hx and DR in these experiments.

The average LSs of normotensive and hypertensive rats were increased by EDR, from 19 and 25 months (respectively) to 30 and 32 months (Lloyd, 1984). The rats were genetically prone to develop hypertension, but on DR showed pathologies more typical of old age than of hypertension (see Chapter 3).

Longevity studies in mice from both short-lived and long-lived strains subjected to EDR are outlined in Table 2.5. Judging by the peak BW index, the degree of DR imposed is often less for mice than for rats. Note (Table 2.5) the very short LSs (irrespective of diet) of mice in the early studies. Maximal LSs of more than 40 months have been observed less often in mice than in rats and only by Harrison's group (#18, 19) and Nelson and Halberg (#21), and in our colony (studies #6, 15-17). Most of our mice were intermittently fed limited amounts of vitamin-, mineral- and protein-enriched diets. Feeding low protein diets ad lib to mice from long- and medium-lived strains (studies #11-13) did not yield such extreme LSs despite some peak BW ratios of about 0.6. These results seem to accord with the finding of Ross and Bras (1973) that high protein diets accentuate DR-induced gains in the LS of rats.

An impressive body of literature describes striking benefits of early-onset DR in inbred mouse strains predetermined to develop a fatal disease at an early age. Much of this work was pioneered by experiments carried out at the University of Minnesota and Sloan-Kettering by Robert Good, Gabriel Fernandes, Edmund Yunis and their colleagues who studied four strains.

(1) NZB mice (which develop autoimmune hemolytic anemia during the first year of life) eating a 6 percent casein diet such that fat and calorie intakes were the same as for controls eating a 22 percent casein diet, showed lower BWs but nonsignificant increases in LS (Table 2.5, study #7).

(2) C3H/Umc females (which have a very high incidence of fatal mammary adenocarcinomas starting at 10 months) showed *no* mammary cancer when underfed; however, LS extension was not reported in study #8 (but the 3 longest lived mice were restricted).

(3) When B/WF$_1$ mice (the lupus model) were fed one of a variety of diets (study #9), LS increased dramatically with DR. Although this study ended at 23 months, one can surmise which DR regimens were most promising for LS extension by ranking survivorship at this age (females and males considered together). Sixteen of 25 mice in restricted group 9a (22% casein, 5% fat) were alive, and a similar number in restricted group 9g (6% casein, 20% corn oil). Mice eating 6 percent casein/5 percent corn oil or 22 percent casein/20 percent corn oil did less well, with only about one-third of each group alive at 23 months.

TABLE 2.5
Longevity Studies Using Mice Fed Restricted Diets Starting Early in Life[a]

Study[b]	Strain	Diet Groups[c]	Peak BW[d]		Ave. LS[e]	Max. LS[f]
1.	"white"	1a. R (24F,24M), NPD, ad lib for 5d, fast for 2d	28	(100%)	27,25	34,33
		1b. C (24F,24M), NPD, ad lib.	28		25,23	31,33
2.	AK	2a. R (47F,47M), NPD, DF (1.5 g/d)	17	(68%)	12[e]	23[e]
		2b. C (52F,52M), NPD, ad lib.	28		8[e]	13[e]
3.	A	3a. R (46F), NPD, ↑cas, ↑vit, ↑min, DF (1.5 g/d)	17	(61%)	14	23
		3b. C (72F), NPD, DF (2g/d)	28		11	15
4.	C3H	4a. R (~18M), NPD, ↑cas, ↑vit, ↑min, DF (2g/d)	20	(50%)	23	31
		4b. C (~18M), NPD, ad lib	40		15	17
5.	A	5a. R (30F), NPD, IF (24 kcal/2d)	NR		18	30
		5b. C (35F), NPD, ad lib	NR		17	26
6.	B6	6a. R (100F), PD, ↑vit, ↑min, IF (14 kcal/2d)	21	(84%)	>34[e]	>40[e]
		6b. C (100F), PD, DF (14 kcal/d)	25		30	38
7.	NZB	7a. R (22F,27M), PD, 6% cas, DF (20 kcal/d)	23	(55%)	17,16	25,20
		7b. C (26F,36M), PD, 22% cas, DF (20 kcal/d)	42		15,15	20,20
8.	C3H	8a. R (18F), PD, DF (10 kcal/d)	23[d]	(72%)	13	18
		8b. C (17F), PD, DF (16 kcal/d)	32[d]		14	16
9.	B/WF$_1$	9a. R (12F,12M), PD, 22% cas, 5% fat, ↑vit, ↑min, 10 kcal/d	30	(67%)	>19,>22[e]	>23,>23[e]
		9b. C (12F,12M), PD, 22% cas, 5% fat, 20 kcal/d	45		11,12	14,14
		9c. R (12F,12M), PD, 6% cas, 5% fat, ↑vit, ↑min, 10 kcal/d	28	(70%)	15,>22[e]	18,>23[e]
		9d. C (12F,12M), PD, 6% cas, 5% fat, 20 kcal/d	40		11,16	17,21
		9e. R (12F,12M), PD, 22% cas, 20% fat, ↑vit, ↑min, 12 kcal/d	37	(93%)	>16,>19[e]	>23,>23[e]
		9f. C (12F,12M), PD, 22% cas, 20% fat, 24 kcal/d	40		12,15	19,20
		9g. R (12F,12M), PD, 6% cas, 20% fat, ↑vit, ↑min, 12 kcal/d	30	(100%)	>19,>21[e]	>23,>23[e]
		9h. C (12F,12M), PD, 6% cas, 20% fat, 24 kcal/d	30		12,14	13,19
	DBA/2f	9i. R (12F,12M), PD, 22% cas, 5% fat, ↑vit, ↑min, 10 kcal/d	NR		14,12	18,16
		9j. C (12F,12M), PD, 22% cas, 5% fat, 20 kcal/d	NR		>14[e],14	>21[e],18
		9k. R (12F,12M), PD, 6% cas, 5% fat, ↑vit, ↑min, 10 kcal/d	NR		14,>17[e]	18,>21[e]
		9l. C (12F,12M), PD, 6% cas, 5% fat, 20 kcal/d	NR		>17[e],>21[e]	>21,>21[e]

TABLE 2.5
(Continued)

Study[b]	Strain	Diet Groups[c]	Peak BW[d]		Ave. LS[e]	Max. LS[f]
10.	kd/kd	10a. R (9), PD, 22% cas, ↑vit, ↑min, 8 kcal/d	NR		>16[e]	>16[e]
		10b. C (20), PD, 22% cas, 16 kcal/d	NR		<8	<8
		10c. C (20), PD, 6% cas, 16 kcal/d	NR		<8	<8
		10d. R→C (9), PD, as 10a until 8 mo, then as 10b	NR		9	9
11.	B6	11a. R (70F), PD, 4% cas, ad lib	24	(63%)	28	38
		11b. C (70F), PD, 26% cas, ad lib	38		23	27
12.	Balb/c	12a. R (200M), PD, 4% cas, ad lib	23	(72%)	22	30
		12b. R (200M), PD, 8% cas, ad lib	29	(91%)	21	30
		12c. C (200M), PD, 24% cas, ad lib	32		20	28
13.	A/J	13a. R (50M), PD, 4% cas, ad lib	23	(72%)	23	30
		13b. C (50M), PD, 26% cas, ad lib	32		21	27
	B6	13c. R (50M), PD, 4% cas, ad lib	28	(62%)	24	32
		13d. C (50M), PD, 26% cas, ad lib	45		21	27
	(A/J × B6)F$_1$	13e. R (50M), PD, 4% cas, ad lib	29	(57%)	28	37
		13f. C (50M), PD, 26% cas, ad lib	51		24	32
14.	Swiss albino	14a. R (50F,50M), NPD, DF (4 g/d)	32	(73%)	28,28	35,36
		14b. C (50F,50M), NPD, DF (5 g/d)	44		23,24	31,30
15.	B6	15a. R (41F), PD, ↑vit, ↑min, IF (60 kcal/wk)	20	(61%)	28	44
		15b. C (34F), PD, DF (105 kcal/wk)	33		29	39
		15c. C (63F), NPD, ad lib	33		29	35
16.	B10C3F$_1$	16a[c]. R (37F), PD, ↑vit, ↑min, IF (60 kcal/wk)	21	(64%)	40	NR[f]
		16b[c]. R (33F), as for 16a, but also on DR before weaning	21	(64%)	43	50
		16c[c]. R (30F), switched from C→R at 14 mo	20	(61%)	39	45
		16d. C (36F), PD, DF (105 kcal/wk)	33		36	41
17.	C3B10RF$_1$	17a. R (60F), PD, ↑cas, ↑vit, ↑min, IF (40 kcal/wk)	21	(42%)[d]	45	53
		17b. R (71F), PD, ↑cas, ↑vit, ↑min, IF (50 kcal/wk)	22	(44%)[d]	42	51
		17c. R (56F), PD, ↓ingcas.[c], ↑vit, ↑min, IF (50 kcal/wk)	23	(46%)[d]	40	49
		17d. C (57F), PD, IF (85 kcal/wk)	36	(72%)[d]	33	40
		17e. C (49F), NPD, ad lib (115 kcal/wk)	50		27	35
18.	B6	18a. R (39F, ob/ob[c]), NPD, DF (7 kcal/d)	30	(40%)	27	41
		18b. C (29F, ob/ob[c]), NPD, ad lib (15 kcal/d)	75		17	27
		18c. R (38F, +/+[c]), NPD, DF (7 kcal/d)	20	(67%)	27	39
		18d. C (32F, +/+[c]), NPD, ad lib (11 kcal/d)	30		25	32
19.	B6	19a. R (48M, ob/ob), NPD, DF (40% of ad lib)	30	(37%)	27	38

TABLE 2.5
(Continued)

Study[b]	Strain	Diet Groups[c]	Peak BW[d]		Ave. LS[e]	Max. LS[f]
		19b. C (53M, ob/ob), NPD, ad lib	82		16	25
		19c. R (48M, +/+), NPD, DF (66% of ad lib)	24	(66%)	20	36
		19d. C (45M, +/+), NPD, ad lib	36		28	36
	B6CBAF$_1$	19e. R (34M), NPD, DF (66% of ad lib)	25	(63%)	39	~50[f]
		19f. C (35M), NPD, ad lib	40		31	40
20.	Han: NMRI	20a. R (150F, "fat"[c]), NPD, DF (12 kcal/d)	38	(73%)	24	37
		20b. C (150F, "fat"[c]), NPD, ad lib (15 kcal/d)	52		20	30
		20c. R (150F, "lean"[c]), NPD, DF (12 kcal/d)	35	(85%)	22	39
		20d. C (150F, "lean"[c]), NPD, ad lib (15 kcal/d)	41		19	30
		20e. R (150F, "non-selected"[c]), NPD, DF (12 kcal/d)	38	(79%)	26	39
		20f. C (150F, "non-selected"[c]), NPD, ad lib, (15 kcal/d)	48		22	30
21.	CD2F$_1$	21a. R (92F), NPD, DF (75% of ad lib)	26	(84%)	31	43
		21b. (168F), NPD, ad lib (3.8 g/d)	31		27	35

[a]DR started at 3-6 weeks of age in all studies except for #5 and #19 (onset @ 8 wks) and #10 (onset @ 8-10 wks). This table also includes one report (#16) which compared both EDR and ADR.

[b]References: (1) Robertson et al. (1934); (2) Saxton et al. (1944); (3) Ball et al. (1947); (4) Lee et al. (1956); (5) Silberberg et al. (1962); (6) Gerbase-DeLima et al. (1975); (7) Fernandes et al. (1976a); (8) Fernandes et al. (1976b); (9) Fernandes et al. (1976c); (10) Fernandes et al. (1978b); (11) Leto et al. (1976a); (12) Stoltzner (1977); (13) Goodrick (1978); (14) Tucker (1979); (15) Cheney et al. (1980); (16) Cheney et al. (1983); (17) Weindruch et al. (1986); (18) Harrison et al. (1984); (19) Harrison and Archer (1987a); (20) Rehm et al. (1985a); (21) Nelson and Halberg (1986).

[c]See footnote [c], Table 2.4 for abbreviations. Group 16b was also restricted prior to weaning (i.e. taken from large litters and separated from mothers every other day from 1 wk of age until weaned). Grp. 16c was put on DR at 14 months of age. Group 17c was fed progressively less casein as they aged. Study #18 examined both genetically obese (ob/ob) and non-obese (+/+) B6 mice. Study #20 involved three sublines of outbred Han:NMRI mice: "fat"=selected for high BW at 4 weeks, "lean"=selected for low body fat content, and "non-selected."

[d]Largest average BW (g) attained. NR=not reported. Values for females are given for those studies of both sexes. Value in parentheses next to R value is peak BW of group R/peak BW of C (an index of the severity of the DR). For study #8, values were reported for 3 month old mice and probably are not peak BW. In study #20, relative BWs for restricted mice are calculated as % of ad lib fed controls (group 20e).

[e]Average LS of cohort in months. A few reports do not give this value and an estimate is shown here. In study #2, survivorship of females and males were not separately reported. In study #6, observation ceased at 40 months of age. Study #9 was written when the B/WF$_1$ mice were 23 months old and the DBA mice were 21 months of age. Study #10 covers the short-lived kd/kd mice up to 16 months of age.

[f]Average LS of the cohort's longest lived decile in months. Usually, this value was not reported and an estimate is shown here. In some cases (i.e. reports written before all mice died [see note "[e]"]) a good estimate is not possible. In group 16a, the last survivors died accidentally. In group 19e, the longest-lived mouse was switched from DR to ad lib feeding at 51 months of age and died at 57 months.

(4) In kd/kd mutant mice (which develop another type of renal disease), LS was prolonged by calorie but not by protein restriction (study #10).

Recently, Good's group varied the fat and protein contents of the diets fed to energy-restricted B/WF$_1$ female mice. Kubo et al. (1987a) found that LSs were most strikingly prolonged by DR when moderate fat intakes (38% of energy as fat) and not very high fat intakes (69% of energy as fat) were used. Variation of protein level in DR mice did not alter longevity (Gajjar et al., 1987).

Tucker (#14) and Rehm et al. (#20) each observed that mild DR (80% of ad lib) resulted in 20 to 30 percent gains in average and maximum LSs over those of ad lib fed, obese (50 g) controls.

Harrison et al. (1984) conducted an important study (#18) on genetically obese (ob/ob) and normal B6 mice. Extending an earlier study by Lane and Dickie (1958), they found that the longevity of ob/ob mice increased markedly with DR! The restricted ob/ob were still fatter (48% body fat) than +/+ mice fed normal (22% body fat) or restricted (13% body fat) diets, but had less body fat than ob/ob mice fed the control diet (67% fat). These data suggest that DR may be quite beneficial for metabolically thrifty, fat-prone individuals. Favorable effects of DR on the LS of genetically obese mice were also described by Goodrick et al. (1983c).

Harrison and Archer (1987a, #19) next reported that DR was very effective in prolonging life in both genetically obese (ob/ob) B6 mice and normal BW B6CBAF$_1$ mice but not in genetically normal B6 male mice. However, this lack of effect of DR contrasts with prior findings of a DR-induced increase in maximum LS for males of this same strain. The study by Harrison and Archer (1987a) is notable in having produced the longest-lived individual mouse on record (57 months, named "Freddy" by the Jackson Laboratory caretakers) who was switched from DR to ad lib feeding at 51 months of age.

Nelson and Halberg (1986) found that meal-timing did not significantly influence LS in CD2F$_1$ mice subjected to DR. Food was presented as a single meal during either early lightness or darkness or as six very small meals at 2 hour intervals. All DR groups showed maximum decile LSs of 41-43 months.

The other very longest lived DR mice in Table 2.5 are from two studies (#16, 17) from our laboratory. Both involved female mice from already long-lived hybrid strains fed enriched PDs. These studies showed that: (1) DR mice can live beyond 50 months and, (2) pre-weaning DR has no major impact on LS. A main diet difference was that of protein enrichment in study #17, amounting therefore (with the vitamin and mineral enrichment) to a nearly isonutrient diet (The fat intake of DR mice was less than that of controls.). The longest lived group of DR mice yet reported is #17a and this regimen approximated as severe a restriction as can be well tolerated by weanling female mice of this hybrid strain. Study #17 also showed no improvement of survival if the protein intake for DR mice was started off high (35% casein) and reduced over the LS (to 25% at 4 months, 20% at 12 months, and 15% from 24 months to death). Figure 2.4 gives survival curves for the 6 diet groups of study #17. Comparing this with the growth curves for these groups (Figure 2.3), one sees that the heaviest mice (NPD ad lib) died earliest. The next heaviest group (N/N$_{85}$) were the next to die, followed by the various DR groups.

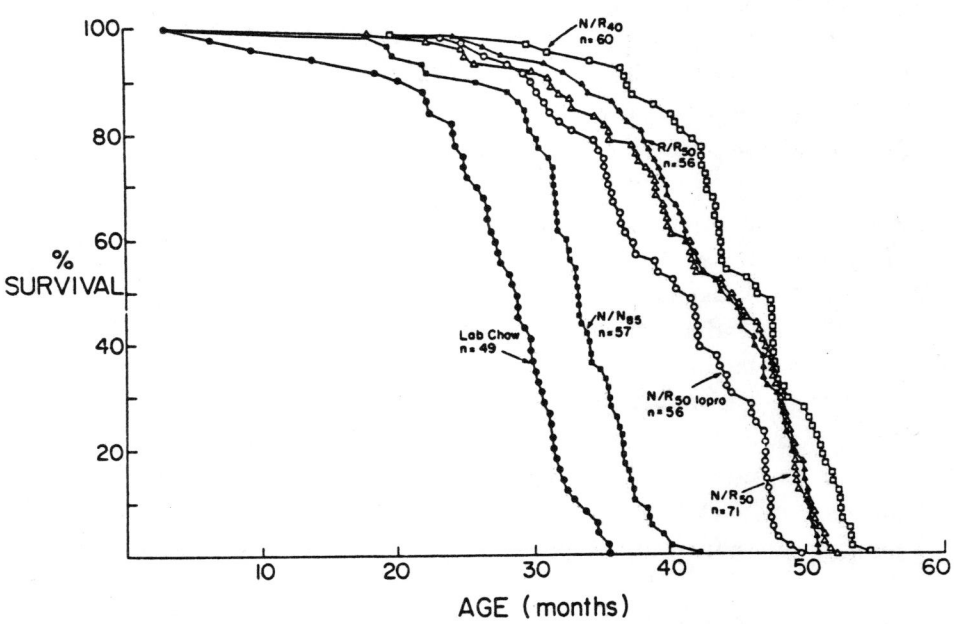

Figure 2.4. Influences of EDR on survival of C3B10RF$_1$ female mice. Each symbol represents an individual mouse. See Figure 2.3 for diet groups. From Weindruch et al. (1986).

Adult-Onset Dietary Restriction (ADR)

Table 2.6 summarizes the principal LS studies limited to rodents restricted beginning in adulthood, at 3 to 25 months of age. Three additional reports (studies #21 & 25 in Table 2.4 and #16 in Table 2.5) compare both EDR and ADR groups. Average LSs of ADR rodents exceeded those of controls in all but 2 of the 15 studies. Maximum LSs were not usually reported in the 1960s and 1970s, but good evidence for extension by ADR now exists and is mounting. A prominent knowledge gap concerns the LS of rodents first restricted quite late in life (say over 20 months old). The one study (#12) starting at 25 months showed that a very mild ADR regimen (BW of ADR 80-90% that of control) did not influence average LS. We are now studying longevity of male B6 mice first restricted at 23-25 months of age.

TABLE 2.6
Longevity Studies Using Rodents Fed Restricted Diets Starting in Adulthood

Study[a]	Animal	Onset[b]	Diet Groups[c]	Peak BW[d]		Ave. LS[e]	Max. LS[f]
1.	"white" rat	7-15[b]	1a. R (17M), PD, DF (10% < ad lib)	224	(93%)	22	31
			1b. C (17M), PD, ad lib	240		20	29
2.	Wistar rat	13-19[b]	2a. R (89M), NPD, DF (50% of ad lib)	275	(55%)	21	NR
			2b. C (83M), NPD, ad lib	500		22	NR
3.	rat (NR)	10	3a. R (10M), PD, ↑vit, ↑min, DF (52% of ad lib)	350	(50%)	26	NR
			3b. C (10M), PD, ad lib	700		20	NR
			3c. R (10M), NPD, DF (60% of ad lib)	400	(67%)	25	NR
			3d. C (10M), NPD, ad lib	600		23	NR
4.	Chas. River rat	12	4a. R (NR[c]), PD, DF (10 g/d)	350	(38%)	27	NR
			4b. C (NR[c]), PD, ad lib	915		22	NR
5.	"hooded" rat	4	5a. R (10F), NPD, low pro. (4% of kcals), ad lib	380	(69%)	32	38
			5b. C (10F), NPD, normal pro. (12% of kcals), ad lib	550		25	33
6.	Sprague-Dawley rat	3	6a. R (35F,35M), PD, DF (60% of ad lib)	480	(55%)	31,31	NR[f]
			6b. R (35F,35M), PD, DF (80% of ad lib)	620	(70%)	29,26	NR[f]
			6c. C (35F,35M), PD, ad lib	880		25,23	NR[f]
7.	Wistar rat	12	7a. R (25M), 50% of ad lib[c]	550	(85%)	26	>30[f]
			7b. C (25M), ad lib[c]	650		18	30
	mouse (NR)	12	7c. R (100M), 50% of ad lib[c]	NR		26	30
			7d. C (100M), ad lib[c]	NR		21	26
	hamster (NR)	12	7e. R (100M), 50% of ad lib[c]	NR		30	33
			7f. C (100M), ad lib	NR		23	28
8.	Wistar rat	12	8a. R (25-30), NPD, IF (ad lib every other night)	NR		35	NR

TABLE 2.6
(Continued)

Study[a]	Animal	Onset[b]	Diet Groups[c]	Peak BW[d]		Ave. LS[e]	Max. LS[f]
9.	B10C3F$_1$ mouse	12	8b. C (25-30), NPD, ad lib	NR		31	NR
			9a. R (67M), PD, ↑cas, ↑vit, ↑min, IF (90 kcal/wk)	30	(71%)	37	45
			9b. C (68M), PD, DF (160 kcal/wk)	42		33	41
	B6 mouse	12	9c. R (29M), same as 9a but 80 kcal/wk	26	(77%)	30	38
			9d. C (24M), same as 9b but 110 kcal/wk	34		25	32
10.	Wistar rat	10.5	10a. R (12M), NPD, IF (ad lib every other day)	400	(67%)	26	32
			10b. C (24M), NPD, ad lib	600		20	23
		18	10c. R (24M), NPD, IF (ad lib every other day)	450	(75%)	25	31
			10d. C (24M), NPD, ad lib	600		23	25
11.	B6 mouse	6	11a. R (24M), NPD, IF (ad lib every other day)	29	(91%)	29	37
			11b. C (24M), NPD, ad lib	32		26	31
12.	B6 mouse	25	12a. R (56M), PD, IF (ad lib for a total = 56 h/wk)[c]	29	(81%)	29	NR
			12b. R (57M), PD, IF (ad lib for a total = 80 h/wk)	32	(89%)	30	NR
			12c. C (55M), PD, ad lib	36		29	NR
13.	Long-Evans rat	6	13a. R (36M), NPD, 18 g/d	420	(70%)	37	43
			13b. C—exercised (32M), NPD, 23 g/d	420	(70%)	33	40
			13c. C—sedentary (54M), NPD, 26 g/d	600		30	40

[a]This table does not include three reports which tested both EDR and ADR (these reports in Tables 2.3, 2.4 & 2.7). References: (1) McCay et al. (1941); (2) Barrows and Roeder (1965); (3) Ross (1966); (4) Ross (1972); (5) Miller and Payne (1968); (6) Nolen (1972); (7) Stuchlikova et al. (1975); (8) Beauchene et al. (1979); (9) Weindruch and Walford (1982); (10) Goodrick et al. (1983b); (11) Talan and Ingram (1985); (12) Kokkonen and Barrows (1985); (13) Holloszy et al. (1985).

[b]Onset of the ADR in months. In study #1, the specific ages of the 7-15 month old rats studied in each diet group were not made clear. In #2, the LS data for rats started on ADR at 13 or 19 months were combined.

[c]For abbreviations, see Table 2.3. In study #4, Ross states that >1300 rats were used in the several experiments reported. In study #7, diet composition and feeding strategy were not described. Study #12 also tested feeding low protein diets (4,6,8,10 or 12% casein) ad lib to 25 month old mice. The result (not in table) was that average LS was not thereby influenced.

[d]Value for controls is the largest average BW (g) attained. Values for ADR rodents is the stable BW arrived at in response to ADR. Values for females given in those studies of both sexes. Value in parenthesis next to R value is peak BW for R group/peak BW for C group (an index of the severity of ADR).

[e]Average LS of cohort in months. In studies of both sexes, the value for females preceeds that for males.

[f]Average LS of the cohort's longest lived decile in months. Often this was not reported and unestimable from what was reported. Study #6 was (unfortunately) terminated when the rats reached 36 months at which time survivorship was 6a = 36% of females, 24% of males; 6b = 24% of F, 8% of M; 6c = 4% of F, 0% of M. In group #7a, 10% of the cohort was alive when reported at 30 months of age.

The history of rodent ADR longevity studies is as follows. McCay and colleagues reported in 1941 on LSs of rats underfed or exercised starting at 7-15 months of age (Table 2.6, study #1). Several diet groups (in addition to those tabulated herein) were studied. The ADR regimen was very mild, producing only a 10 percent fall in peak BW. Rats kept thinner than normal in this way showed a mild boost in average and maximum LSs. Neither exercise nor the level or source of dietary protein strongly affected LS. No rat lived longer than 38 months (not very old for rats). The authors did state that chronic lung disease of uncertain etiology was a major late life disease in their colony. Such lung disease of unclear (but probable infectious) origin appears as a major pathology in several of the earlier rat reports. Apparently, the rats in this first ADR study did not reach old age but were eliminated earlier by diseases. Ingram and Reynolds (1983) subjected the data of McCay et al. (1941) to statistical analysis and found that most of his observation-based conclusions were statistically sound.

A negative impact of ADR (50% of ad lib intake of Purina Lab Chow™) on LS in male Wistar rats was reported (study #2) by Barrows and Roeder (1965). Adult DR was started at 13 or 19 months of age. Both ADR groups and the controls had similar average LSs (21-22 months). Again, these are unimpressive LSs.

Ross investigated the ability of ADR to modify LS in rats. A 1966 report (study #3) described 10 month old males switched to ADR after previously being fed ad lib. Only one of four PDs fed on a restricted basis increased average LS (diet 3a is the successful regimen [other 3 diets not listed]). Continued feeding of the commercial diet in restricted amounts also raised average LS. Maximum LSs were not reported. In 1972, Ross described male Charles River rats subjected to ADR (study #4). Rats fed a PD became quite large (900 g) when allowed an ad lib intake (20 g/day). Rats restricted at 10-12 months to 8-10 g per day showed lower mortality ratios and greater life expectancies than ad lib fed rats. More severe ADR (6 g/day) imposed at 10-12 months of age was poorly tolerated and reduced survival below that of ad lib controls. With increasing age, the severity of the restriction must be less, to achieve optimum LS extension.

In two other studies (#5, 6) DR was started on 3 to 4 month old rats. Miller and Payne (#5) fed three diets ad lib that differed in protein content. They accomplished this by using a NPD (which all rats ate until 4 months old) and diluting it with starch. Rats switched to the lowest protein diet (group 5a = 4% of kcals as protein) weighed about 70 percent as much as controls (group 5b = 12% of kcals as protein), and lived longer. But rats fed this same diet since weaning failed to thrive, and died young (before 500 days). Thus, the same low protein diet may benefit adults but harm young rats. The other study (Nolen, 1972; #6) began with both 3 week and 3 month old Sprague-Dawley rats of both sexes, and found that rats subjected to DR at either age lived equally longer than controls. As shown in Table 2.5, rats fed 60 or 80 percent of control (ad lib) intake levels were outliving controls at the experiment's premature cessation.

Stuchlikova and co-workers (study #7) imposed ADR on 12 month old male mice (strain unstated), golden hamsters and Wistar rats. Three other diet groups were also tested: (1) ad lib since weaning, (2) EDR, or (3) EDR switched to ad lib at 12 months of age. Adult-onset DR raised average LSs above those of controls but did not increase maximum LSs. In all three species the regimen producing the greatest average LS was for animals switched from EDR to an ad lib intake. Note that average LSs in this study were *very* short (18-23 months) and of 400 mice studied, none lived beyond 36 months! It is both difficult and risky to draw conclusions about dietary effects on *aging* from this often cited but, we believe, over-rated study.

Beauchene and co-workers (study #8) reported (in abstract form) an experiment of very similar design which tested the same four diet groups (always ad lib, EDR, ad lib switched to ADR [at 12 months], and EDR switched to ad lib [at 12 months]) in male Wistar rats. Dietary restriction was achieved by allowing the animals free access to food, but only on every other evening. Average LSs ranked: EDR > EDR switched to ad lib = ad lib switched to ADR > always ad lib. The average LSs were impressive with ADR rats averaging 35 months. Indeed, the average LS of the ad lib controls here was 31 months, exceeding that for all control rats in Table 2.6.

Survey of the ADR longevity data through 1976 left us with the strong feeling that it was still unclear whether or not the careful restriction of middle-aged or older rodents can produce survival benefits in terms of species-specific maximum LSs. The literature also left us with the strong impression that older, full grown rodents should be *gradually* restricted. A 1977 pilot study of ours encouraged us further: a 4.5 month course of ADR started on 12 month old mice led to higher splenic T lymphocyte proliferative responses than for controls (Weindruch et al.,

1979). Next, we began a large study (#9 in Table 2.6) on LS and spontaneous tumor incidence in male mice started on ADR at 12 months of age. Two long-lived strains (B10C3F$_1$ and B6) were investigated. Adult-onset DR was gradually imposed on mice previously fed a NPD ad lib. The ADR mice were fed an isonutrient diet (except for fat which was at the same percentage in both diets so that less of it was eaten by the ADR mice), consuming 60 percent of the number of the calories eaten by controls. Body weights and survival are shown in Figure 2.5. The ADR mice averaged 10-20 percent increases in average and maximum LSs compared to control mice. The restricted B10C3F$_1$ mice attained particularly long LSs (Table 2.6).

Each of three reports published between 1983 and 1986 tested both EDR and ADR. These reports were summarized in the EDR tables (2.4 and 2.5). They offer the best information on the comparative impact each type of DR exerts on LS. As shown in Table 2.7, in all three studies

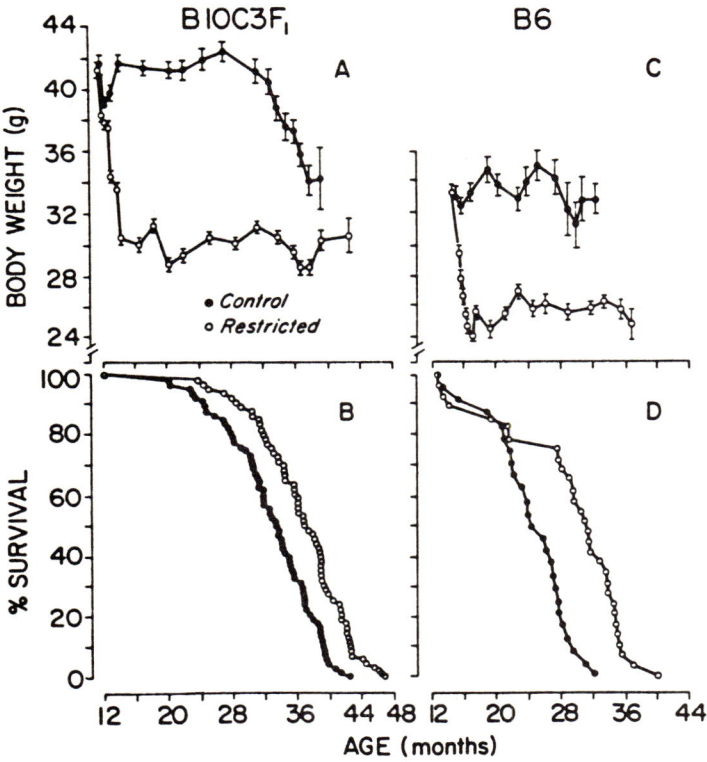

Figure 2.5. Body weights and survival curves of B10C3F$_1$ mice (A and B) and B6 mice (C and D) fed control or ADR diets. The ADR started at 12 months of age. Each point in the survival curves represents one male mouse. From Weindruch and Walford (1982).

DR starting in young adulthood or midadulthood extended average and maximum LSs 89 to 95 percent as much as that started in early life. This consistency is of interest in view of the short age gap (4.5 months) separating early and later onset DR in the study of Yu et al. (1985) and the longer period (11-13 months) in the other studies. Clearly, DR first started in midadulthood is nearly as effective as that started much earlier in life in extending survival. Within these ranges, most of the retardation of aging by DR is independent of slow growth and the onset of puberty.

Two reports (Table 2.6, #10, 11) from the NIA's Gerontology Research Center also suggest that ADR increases longevity. In study #10, 10.5 and 18 month old Wistar rats were subjected either to ADR (EOD feeding) or to the opportunity to exercise (voluntary wheel running) or both. The LSs of these rats were compared to those of exercised and non-exercised ad lib fed controls. Survival for the 18 month onset group, as shown in Figure 2.6, revealed that: (1) this colony was not exceptionally long-lived (None of 156 rats studied lived beyond 37 months.) and, (2) EOD feeding exerted stronger prolongevity and anti-obesity effects than did voluntary exercise. The other NIA study (#11) found that a small (10%) reduction in BW caused by the EOD feeding of 6 month old B6 mice increased longevity slightly. On the basis of resultant BWs and LSs, EOD ad lib feeding regimens do not appear severe enough to increase LS strongly.

TABLE 2.7
Three Longevity Studies Testing Both Early- and Late-Onset DR

Study[a]	Animal	Onsets[b]	Average LS[c]				Max. LS[d]			
			Cont.	EDR	ADR	A:E	Cont.	EDR	ADR	A:E
1.	mouse, B10C3F$_1$	1, 14	36	43	39	0.91	41	50	45	0.90
2.	rat, Fischer 344	1.5, 6	23	35	31	0.89	27	41	39	0.95
3.	rat, Wistar	1, 12	31	38	35	0.92	39	46	41	0.89

[a] (1) Cheney et al. (1983); (2) Yu et al. (1985); (3) Beauchene et al. (1986).
[b] The onsets (in mo) for EDR and ADR.
[c] Values are in months. "Cont." gives values for controls. A:E gives the ratio for the LS of ADR:EDR groups.
[d] The value given is the average LS in months for each group's longest-lived 10%. Other abbreviations as in "c" (above).

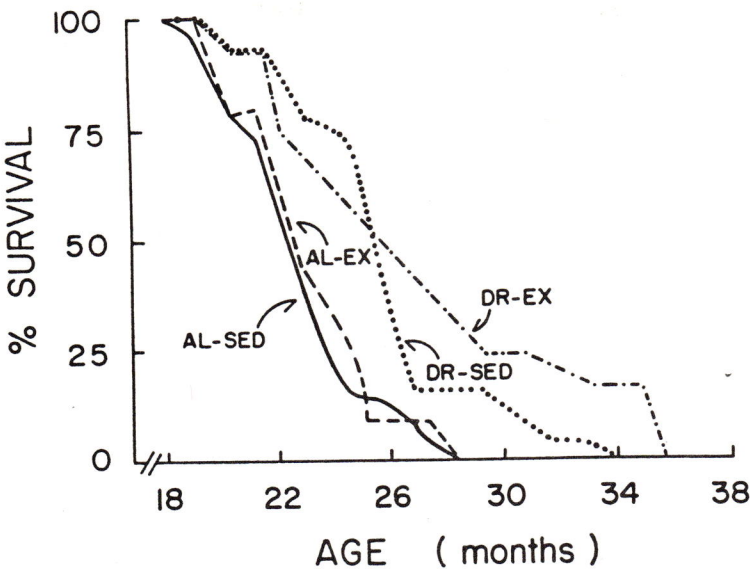

Figure 2.6. Influences of DR and/or exercise on survival of 18 month old male Wistar rats. The DR was via EOD feeding. Each group consisted of 18-24 rats. Abbreviations: AL, ad libitum; EX, exercised; SED, sedentary. Adapted from Goodrick et al. (1983b).

The longevity studies of Holloszy and co-workers (Table 2.6, #13) tested exercise (voluntary wheel activity) or ADR imposed on 6 month old Long Evans rats. The ADR was gauged to yield BWs like those of the running rats. Adult DR led to increases in average and maximum LSs of 23 and 8 percent respectively, whereas only average LS rose (by 10%) with exercise. Indeed, Holloszy and Smith (1986) suggest that exercise may have a detrimental effect on primary aging, which is obscured by its health benefits in decreasing susceptibility to certain diseases.

It is noteworthy indeed that ADR has also been observed to benefit short-lived, disease-prone mouse strains with *ongoing* disease, i.e. to exert not only a preventive but a therapeutic effect. Friend et al. (1978) restricted B/WF$_1$ mice at either weaning or 4 to 5 months of age (at which time their lupus-like syndrome was clinically manifest). At about 9 months of age, mice on early or later onset DR showed far less autoimmune nephropathy than controls (LS was not determined). Later studies in the MRL/lpr mouse strain (which develop an autoimmune lymphoproliferative condition very early in life) revealed a strong impact of ADR on this syndrome and on LS. Mark and colleagues reported (1984a) that 5 to 6 month old mice previously fed a NPD ad lib, and then restricted, showed a dramatically improved appearance 4-6 weeks thereafter. The mice were more active than fully fed controls and greatly outlived them (all controls were dead by 11 months of age vs. 40% of the ADR group still alive at 13 months). Kubo et al. (1984a) subjected MRL/lpr mice to ADR at about 3 months of age. The median LS for was 15 months vs. 7 months for controls. These results suggest that ADR might well slow the advance of certain diseases in humans (see "POTENTIAL BENEFITS OF DR BESIDES LS EXTENSION," Chapter 6).

Recently completed but not yet published studies from our laboratory provide additional information on the survival advantages which follow ADR in mice. A.CA/Sn mice (a non-obese strain which develops a variety of late-life tumors) were restricted at either 1, 5 or 10 months of age, or not at all. Average LSs were 26 months for controls vs. 31-33 months for the DR groups. Maximum LSs were 34 months for controls vs. 38-41 months for the DR mice. The group restricted at 1 month of age displayed only a slightly higher maximum LS than the ADR groups. Again, this constitutes evidence that DR at any pre-middle age extends LS.

Growth Rate, Body Weight and Life Span

The foregoing material suggests that both EDR (which reduces growth rates and peak BW) and ADR (which, if started sufficiently late in life, affects neither growth rate nor peak BW) may increase LS. Are there associations between LS and growth rate or between LS and peek BW which are evident in normally fed and DR rodents?

Robertson and Ray (1920) reported a tendency for longer LSs for fast growing mice; however, in our view, their data remain unconvincing. Fifteen years thereafter, Sherman and Campbell (1935) did not report any LS differences between fast and slow growing ad lib fed rats. Carlson and Hoelzel (1946) found that rats which were heaviest at 6 weeks of age (the study's onset) tended to live longest. In ad lib fed male Wistar rats, Everitt and Webb (1957) observed that rats destined to be short-lived grew more slowly between 200-400 days of age than the longer-lived rats. And peak BWs of long-lived rats were higher.

These various results would seem at odds with DR studies. However, McCay (1952) did offer an intriguing explanation as to why results from his and other laboratories did not accord with those reported by Robertson and Ray (1920). He suggested that the test mice, being a heterogeneous group, included sick animals which grew at a slower rate and died prematurely. He concluded that relationships between growth rate and LS are very difficult to determine in a heterogeneous lot of animals permitted to grow at maximum rates.

Goodrick studied possible interrelationships between growth rate, BW and LS. He reported (Goodrick, 1977) an inverse relationship between growth rate and LS in B6 mice fed ad lib, but that the duration of growth was longer for longer-lived mice. Among the inbred mice described in Table 2.5 (study #13) fed low protein or control diets, a slow growth rate for individual mice was associated with greater longevity. Wistar rats (both sexes, ad lib fed, some exercised) also showed an inverse correlation between LS and growth rate, and a direct correlation between LS and growth duration (Goodrick, 1980). Goodrick's repeated finding that slow growth associates with longevity agrees with expectations based on the EDR results. However, in all three of Goodrick's reports, a sporadic tendency existed for individual animals with the highest BWs to live longest.

Goodrick's work was continued (following his death in 1981) by Ingram and colleagues. The data in Goodrick's 1980 report were reanalyzed using a multivariate correlational approach (Ingram et al., 1982). For ad lib fed rats the rates of early BW gain were found to be unrelated to LS in either control or exercised rats. After 9 months of age, rates of BW gain were positively related to LS. In another study, Ingram et al. (1983) examined relationships of genotype, sex, BWs and growth rate to LS in 9 inbred and 6 hybrid mouse strains. Several growth parameters were significantly related to LS but the directions of the correlations were sex-dependent. For male mice, BW and growth rate were positively correlated with LS, while among females the relationships were weak or negative. After reviewing the tangled literature on BW and LS relationships in rodents, Ingram and Reynolds (1987) found ". . . little support for the hypothesis that leanness per se confers long life in laboratory rodents."

Still other observations reveal longer LSs for slower growing, low peak BW individual rodents. In a study by Yu et al. (1982), those male Fischer 344 rats fed ad lib which grew slowly and weighed less tended to live longest. Other workers (Lesser et al., 1973) found that in a population of male Sprague-Dawley rats, the longest-lived individuals had the lowest BWs and fat-free BWs and maintained a stable body composition in old age. Likewise, Sprague-Dawley rats of both sexes with high BWs developed diseases (tumors, nephropathy) more frequently, and died sooner than did the low BW rats (Turnbull et al., 1985). In mice, a hyperphagic strain with about twice the usual growth rate was developed from a randomly bred strain, by selection for BW gain from 21-24 days of age over many generations (Eklund & Bradford, 1977). The rapid growing and ultimately fat mice (peak BW of 70 g!) showed an average LS of 12 months (males) and 20 months (females), vs. 26 months for normally growing controls (BW 40 g). Results of this last study likely reflect the health consequences of extreme obesity, and tell little about BWs which might be optimal for longevity.

Ross and colleagues allowed ad lib fed Sprague-Dawley rats to choose among three diets (10, 22 and 51% casein) listed in Table 2.4, #9). Body weights and intakes of each diet were recorded for each rat until death. Food intake from 2 through 12 months of age was very strongly and negatively correlated with LS ($r = -.40$) (Ross & Bras, 1975). Twenty rats eating a daily average of 18 g of food between 100 and 199 days of age displayed an average LS of 24 months, vs. 18 months for 21 rats eating 24 g per day. Body weight variables correlated more closely with LS than did the dietary variables (Ross et al., 1976). The strongest direct correlations found with ultimate LS ($r = .46-.49$) were the times to reach specific BWs whereas peak BW was not strongly related to LS.

In Ross' last published report (Ross et al., 1985 [He died on April 30, 1984.]) the same self-selection model was studied. A multivariate statistical model to predict LS on the basis of pre-adult diet habits and growth responses was evaluated prospectively. Four variables (age at 250 g BW, average daily food intake from 99 to 147 days, average gross food efficiency from 148 to 196 days, and mature BW) produced an average error between individually predicted and observed LSs of only 11 percent! Again, a short LS was associated with a large food intake before adulthood, especially when combined with a highly efficient conversion of food to BW, with rapid growth rate, and with early attainment of peak BW.

Evidence from two studies suggests a positive correlation exists between adiposity and LS as well as BW and LS for early-onset DR rodents. Bertrand et al. (1980a) found that DR in Fischer 344 rats resulted in significant positive correlations between LS and peak absolute fat mass ($r = 0.63$, $p < 0.001$), and between LS and maximum percent body fat ($r = 0.63$, $p < 0.001$). These associations were not observed in the ad lib fed group. (This rat population was later fully described by Yu et al. [1982].). Our recently reported results (Weindruch et al., 1986) for BW-LS correlations in C3B10RF$_1$ mice are shown in Table 2.8. They tell a similar story: heavier DR mice tended to live longer than lighter ones. Like the rat study of Bertrand et al. (1980a), such correlations were not found among controls. Apparently, the thrifty, energy-efficient members of DR cohorts experience the greatest longevity. The fact that this is less often seen in ad lib fed animals may simply reflect too much noise in such populations and/or the negative consequences of obesity.

TABLE 2.8

Correlations Between Body Weight (BW) and Lifespan (LS)[a]

Group	BW_w–LS	BW_5–LS	BW_{10}–LS	BW_{15}–LS	BW_{22}–LS
NPD	0.115	0.026	−0.020	−0.053	0.224
N/N$_{85}$	0.192	0.053	0.050	−0.014	−0.014
N/R$_{50}$	−0.016	−0.063	0.045	0.257*	0.223^t
R/R$_{50}$	−0.002	−0.216	−0.003	0.066	0.264*
N/R$_{50lopro}$	−0.208	0.005	0.313*	0.355**	0.211
N/R$_{40}$	0.174	0.058	−0.078	0.210	0.140

[a]Adapted from Weindruch et al. (1986). Abbreviations BW_w = body weight at weaning (3 wks of age), BW_5 = BW at 5 months of age, BW_{10} = BW at 10 months, BW_{15} = BW at 15 months, BW_{22} = BW at 22 months. All mice studied for longevity were used for this analysis. Pearson product-moment correlations were used. Statistical significance indicated by: ^{t}, $p<0.10$; *, $p<0.05$; **, $p<0.01$.

SUMMARY

The growing body of data suggesting that DR increases LS in diverse species is long-standing, extensive, and convincing. In rodents, DR slows the actuarial aging rate and/or decreases the population's initial vulnerability to mortality. Many DR regimens act to strikingly prolong survivorship and all of these share the common variable of *caloric* restriction. The most impressive results have been obtained by feeding isonutrient diets, or diets nutritionally adequate but in restricted amounts such that the peak BWs of DR animals are only 30 to 60 percent those of control animals. Within DR groups, but not notably within ad lib groups, the heavier and fatter animals appear to live longest. Both EDR and ADR can increase longevity, and oftentimes the results of ADR approach those of its early-onset counterpart. Although EDR can delay puberty, it appears that LS extension via DR does not in fact depend on interrupting maturation for much of its effect. Studies in short-lived, disease-prone mouse strains show that ADR can retard the course of pre-existing disease. Rodents subjected to DR are not only long-lived, but healthy, sleek and active as well.

CHAPTER 3

DIETARY RESTRICTION: EFFECTS ON DISEASE

INTRODUCTION

THE SPONTANEOUS diseases which occur predominately in late life reflect in part an increased susceptibility secondary to basic aging processes. In humans, certain diseases of aging are the main causes of death (e.g. cardio- and cerebrovascular diseases, cancer, diabetes) while others (e.g. arthritis, osteoporosis, dementia, cataracts) increase the likelihood of accidents and limit life's enjoyment. Undoubtedly, these diseases also influence other age-related phenomena, and the student of aging must sort out how much of an observed age-related change might stem from disease(s) and not from aging *per se*. Likewise, the geriatrician must differentiate diseases from aging processes.

Studies in rodents clearly reveal that DR both forestalls the onset of the major late-life diseases and alters their incidences. On the other hand, very little is known about the influences of DR on late-life diseases in non-rodent species. One rare example is the trout study of Reimers (1978) who observed few signs of overt disease in very old (12-18 years) fish whose great LSs are attributed to food scarcity, low temperature, and a remote environment. In "lower non-rodents" (e.g. protozoans, *Caenorhabditis elegans*) it is not even clear if "diseases" occur in old age. And in "higher non-rodents" (e.g. primates) nothing is known about influences of DR on diseases, with the possible exception of certain human data (see Chapter 6).

The appreciation that DR retards spontaneous diseases in rodents was predated by evidence that severe underfeeding slows the growth of implanted or induced tumors. Moreschi (1909) found that mouse sarcoma grafts grew less frequently and more slowly in malnourished mice.

Rous (1914) reported that mice fed a nutritionally inadequate diet showed slower growth of certain transplanted tumors (Figure 3.1). He also surgically disseminated spontaneous mammary carcinomas in individual mice, then fed them either a normal or inadequate diet. Mice losing BW on the poor diet showed a delay or stoppage in the growth of the tumor grafts.

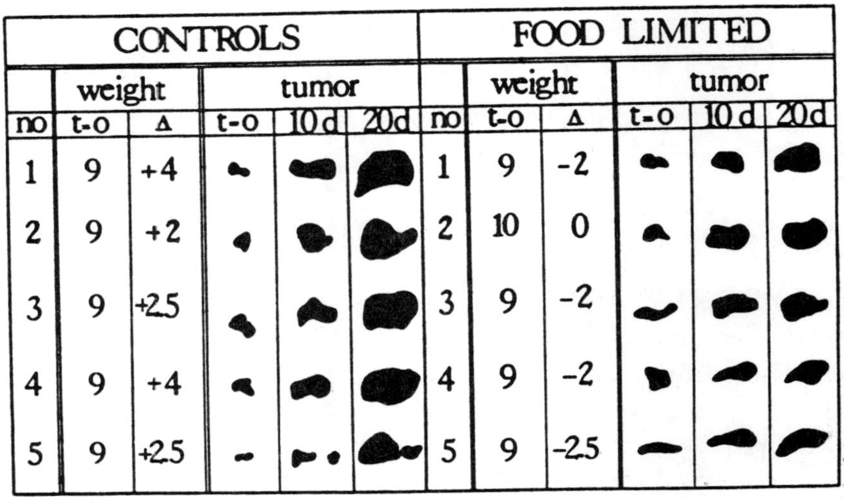

CONTROLS						FOOD LIMITED					
	weight		tumor				weight		tumor		
no	t-0	Δ	t-0	10d	20d	no	t-0	Δ	t-0	10d	20d
1	9	+4				1	9	-2			
2	9	+2				2	10	0			
3	9	+2.5				3	9	-2			
4	9	+4				4	9	-2			
5	9	+2.5				5	9	-2.5			

Figure 3.1. Influence of severe DR on growth of a transplantable adenocarcinoma in mice. "no" is mouse number, t = 0 is BW (in g) at start of the experiment, "Δ" is gain or loss of BW over the 20 day experiment. Tumor sizes at 0, 10 and 20 days are illustrated. Note that the tumors were of a substantial size when the diet was started. Redrawn from Rous (1914).

What are the main diseases of aging in selected mouse and rat strains whose long LSs render these suitable for gerontologic research? Table 3.1 summarizes disease patterns in large populations of ad lib-fed BALB/c mice (Cosgrove et al., 1978), B6/Icrfa mice (Rowlatt et al., 1976), Lewis rats (Feldman & Woda, 1980), and Fischer 344 rats (Maeda et al., 1985). Of course, the number and types of pathologies reported are strongly influenced by genotype, colony conditions, how many tissues the investigator scrutinized, and how close the scrutiny. Also, even though a number of pathologic lesions are quite well-defined for rodents, it is not always possible (as is the case for humans) to confidently establish a cause of death for rodents from long-lived strains. By contrast, most short-lived strains die of an overt disease afflicting nearly all individuals. The subject of diseases of aging in mammals is well reviewed in *Mammalian Models for Research on Aging* (1981), where the important point is made that, especially for mouse work, the study of neoplasias has far overshadowed that of non-neoplastic lesions, and the contributions of the latter to mortality have rarely been examined.

TABLE 3.1
Representative Disease Incidences in Mice and Rats Fed Ad Libitum[a]

Disease	Incidence (%)			
	Mouse Strain		Rat Strain	
	BALB/c	B6/Icrfa	Lewis	Fischer
Neoplasms:				
Total neoplasms	94	40	37	53[b]
Leukemia/Lymphoma	67[b]	16	5	3
Mammary gland	13	---	6	---
Lung	32	6	0	0
Adrenal cortex	29	0	1	0
Pituitary	8	NR	17	7
Ovarian carcinoma	<1	---	30	---
Non-neoplasms:				
Glomerulosclerosis	74	NR	5	99
Lung lesions[c]	0	51	81	NR
Adrenal cort. atrophy	70	0	7	NR
Myocardial degen.	0	NR	16	89
Amyloidosis	<1	37	NR	NR
Ovarian cyst	8	---	11	---
Bile duct hyperplasia	NR	NR	NR	78

[a]Data adapted from Cosgrove et al. (1978) for female BALB/c mice (n=331, ave. LS=25 mo), Rowlatt et al. (1976) for B6/Icrfa mice (n=497 males for neoplasms and n=43 [total] mice of both sexes for non-neoplasms; ave. LS=27 mo for 464 males), Feldman and Woda (1980) for female Lewis rats (n=165, ave. LS=24 mo), and from Maeda et al. (1985) for male Fischer 344 rats (n=71, ave. LS of similarly fed rats=23 mo). Only the most common pathologies are tabulated. NR, not reported.

[b]For BALB/c mice, almost all of these were reticulum cell sarcomas. For Fischer 344 rats, the overall tumor incidence does not include testicular interstitial cell tumors (83% incidence) which were not viewed as a major cause of death.

[c]Several non-neoplastic lung lesions have been observed. The B6/Icrfa mice showed inflammatory infiltrates and crystals in air spaces. Lewis rats developed emphysema-atelectasis and consolidation as result of the colony being infected with a chronic murine pneumonia. Lung lesions of Fischer rats were not quantified although it was stated that pulmonary edema and congestion were commonly seen in animals expiring spontaneously but not among sacrificed rats.

We shall here review studies where diseases were investigated in rodents fed restricted diets. Such work has overwhelmingly concerned effects of DR on spontaneous or induced tumors. Useful reviews of the early studies are those of Albanes (1987a), Keys et al. (1950), Tannenbaum (1947), and Tannenbaum and Silverstone (1957).

SPONTANEOUS DISEASES

Dietary Restriction Started Early in Life (EDR)

Studies with Rats

Twelve studies on the incidence of spontaneous diseases in rats subjected to EDR are summarized in Table 3.2. (Many of these are the same reports cited for LS data in Table 2.4.) As detailed in footnote "c", in some experiments rats were allowed to die naturally while in others the rats were sacrificed and autopsied. The table gives the incidences of the most commonly reported neoplastic and non-neoplastic diseases. Overall incidence values do not provide information about the age of onset of disease. Also, incidence values for certain diseases may be misleading. For example, rats on DR occasionally show a high incidence of a disease which was uncommon in controls. However, this usually occurs for diseases afflicting quite long-lived animals, i.e., those reaching ages not normally obtained by controls, which die earlier of diseases prevented by DR. In some instances, for example, disease may relate mainly to length of time of exposure to a noxious agent, so that longer living DR animals may simply be exposed for a longer time. One must take into account both incidences and age-specific onsets when thinking about the effects of DR on disease.

An early report of DR retarding diseases in rats was that of Saxton (1945), who studied rats from McCay's colony, where the commonest affliction was chronic pneumonia with bronchiectasis. The pulmonary disease was retarded by DR (Table 3.2, study #1, footnote "e") but not prevented. Pituitary chromophobe adenomas, lung lymphosarcomas, and glomerulonephritis afflicted about half of the control group, but were rarely observed in DR rats. Myocardial fibrosis occurred later in DR rats, but final incidence was not influenced.

Carlson and Hoelzel (1946) reported that Wistar rats subjected to the very mild restriction of intermittent fasting showed five-fold fewer mammary tumors than controls (Table 3.2, study #2). Also, tumor weights were higher for fully fed rats.

TABLE 3.2
Disease Incidence in Rats Fed Restricted Diets Starting in Early Life[a]

Study	Strain[b]	Diet Groups[c]	Neoplasms[d]							Non-Neoplasms[e]						
			Pit	Adr	Lym	Mam	Lng	Fib	Pnc	Glm	Myo	Skl	Per	Rad	Lng	Bdh
1.	"white"	1a. R (=2a, Tbl. 2.4), 71%[c]	1	-	-	-	6[d]	-	-	0	58	-	1	-	76[e]	-
		1b. C (=2b, Tbl. 2.4)	51	-	-	-	46[d]	-	-	50	37	-	10	-	82[e]	-
2.	Wistar	2a. R (=3a, Tbl. 2.4), 86%	-	-	-	7	-	-	-	-	-	-	-	-	-	-
		2b. C (=3b, Tbl. 2.4)	-	-	-	37	-	-	-	-	-	-	-	-	-	-
3.	Wistar	3a. R (=5a), Tbl. 2.4), 55%	7	52	0	0	0	0	0	-	-	-	-	-	-	-
		3b. C (=5b, Tbl. 2.4)	11	54	6	18	0	1	2	-	-	-	-	-	-	-
4.	S-D	4a. R (=6a, Tbl. 2.4), 61%[c]	[d]overall inc. =12% for F, 26% for M.							0	16	4	2	100[e]	-	-
		4b. C (=6b, Tbl. 2.4)[c]	[d]overall inc. =41% for F, 58% for M.							72	47	6	43	93[e]	-	-
5.	S-D	5a. R (=7a, Tbl. 2.4), 75%	-	0	7	-	2	6	4	-	-	-	-	-	-	-
		5b. R (=7c, Tbl. 2.4), 42%	-	2	2	-	0	2	3	-	-	-	-	-	-	-
		5c. R (=7e, Tbl. 2.4), 67%	-	0	2	-	0	9	1	-	-	-	-	-	-	-
		5d. R (=7g, Tbl. 2.4), 28%	-	1	1	-	0	3	1	-	-	-	-	-	-	-
		5e. C (=7i, Tbl. 2.4)	-	0	5	-	0	5	2	-	-	-	-	-	-	-
6.	S-D	6a. R (=8a, Tbl. 2.4), 29%	1	2	2	0	2	2	2	-	-	-	-	-	-	-
		6b. R to 70d→C (=8b)	4	<1	3	<1	6	0	5	-	-	-	-	-	-	-
		6c. C (=8c, Tbl. 2.4)	10	<1	2	<1	6	2	6	-	-	-	-	-	-	-
7.	S-D	7a. R (=9a, Tbl. 2.4), 29%	1	1	2	0	2	1	2	-	-	-	-	-	-	-
		7b. C (=9b, Tbl. 2.4)	6	1	7	0	3	3	4	-	-	-	-	-	-	-
		7c. R (=9c, Tbl. 2.4), 27%	1	2	3	0	2	3	2	-	-	-	-	-	-	-
		7d. C (=9d, Tbl. 2.4)	10	<1	2	<1	6	2	6	-	-	-	-	-	-	-
		7e. R (=9e, Tbl. 2.4), 31%	2	1	3	0	1	1	1	-	-	-	-	-	-	-
		7f. C (=9f, Tbl. 2.4)	8	1	3	<1	5	3	7	-	-	-	-	-	-	-
8.	Norway	8a. R (=13a, Tbl. 2.4), 80%	14	overall inc. (non-pit.) =11%						22	-	-	-	-	64[e]	-
		8b. C (=13b, Tbl. 2.4)	8	overall inc. (non-pit.) =10%						25	-	-	-	-	65[e]	-
9.	Wistar	9a. R (=18a, Tbl. 2.4), 36%[c]	overall inc. =6%							-[e]	-	-	-	-	56	-
		9b. R (=18b, Tbl. 2.4), 70%	overall inc. =8%							-[e]	-	-	-	-	77	-
		9c. C (=18c, Tbl. 2.4)	overall inc. =33%							-[e]	-	-	-	-	80	-
10.	Wistar	10a. R (=19a), Tbl. 2.4), 36%[c]	overall inc. =40%							-[e]	-	-	-	-	45	-
		10b. C (=19b, Tbl. 2.4)	overall inc. =65%							-[e]	-	-	-	-	60	-

Table 3.2 (continued)

Study	Strain[b]	Diet Groups[c]	Neoplasms[d]							Non-Neoplasms[e]						
			Pit	Adr	Lym	Mam	Lng	Fib	Pnc	Glm	Myo	Skl	Per	Rad	Lng	Bdh
11.	F344	11a. R (=20a, Tbl. 2.4), 55%[c]	-	-	-	-	-	-	-	3	-[e]	-	0[e]	-[e]	-[e]	13
		11b. C (=20b, Tbl. 2.4)	-	-	-	-	-	-	-	95	-[e]	-	18	-	-	36
12.	F344	12a. R (=21a, Tbl. 2.4), 53%[c]	7	0	21	-	-	0	0	5	7	<8[e]	2[e]	-	-[e]	43
		12b. C→R (=21b, Tbl. 2.4), 55%	8	4	13	-	-	8	4	4	19	<8[e]	0	-	-	30
		12c. R→C (=21c, Tbl. 2.4), 91%	12	21	6	-	-	4	8	49	47	25	10	-	-	58
		12d. C (=21d, Tbl. 2.4)	12	5	3	-	-	2	7	69	62	39	14	-	-	60

[a]DR started in most studies at 3-5 weeks of age. Later starting studies were #2 and 10-12 (6-7 wk) and 9 (10 wk). Most studies reported on only one or a few diseases. "-" indicates that incidences were not reported for that disease. In some studies data were collected for animals allowed to die naturally whereas for others old rats were killed and autopsied.

[b]Abbreviations for rat strains: S-D, Sprague Dawley; F344, Fischer 344. References (listed chronologically except for grouping reports from the same laboratory): (1) Saxton (1945); (2) Carlson and Hoelzel (1946); (3) Gilbert et al. (1958); (4) Berg and Simms (1961); Berg et al. (1962) (5) Ross and Bras (1965); (6) Ross and Bras (1971); (7) Ross and Bras (1973); (8) Drori and Folman (1976); (9) Everitt et al. (1983); (10) Wyndham et al. (1983); (11) Yu et al. (1982); (12) Maeda et al. (1985).

[c]Abbreviations used to describe the diet groups are in Table 2.4. For those studies also in Table 2.4, the diet protocol is not redescribed here and reference is made to the group in Table 2.4. "%" is the peak BW of DR rats as a percentage of that of controls. In study #1, rats from McCay's colony were killed at various ages for study. The data presented are for those killed between 19 and 33 months of age. In study #2, few rats were studied: n=30 (Grp. 2b), n=33 (2b). Study #3 involved 27 DR and 586 control rats. In study #4, the data tabulated are for animals killed at 26 months (n=17-58 for each age-sex-diet combination). Data for both sexes are combined for non-neoplasic diseases in #4. In studies #11 and 12, data are for 17-30 month old rats after either sacrifice or spontaneous death. An exception is the tumor data reported in #12 which were obtained from rats which died spontaneously (n=14 for 12a, n=24 for 12b, n=49 for 12c, n=61 for 12d).

[d]Values are incidences in percent. Abbreviations for neoplasms: Pit=pituitary adenoma; Adr=adrenal; Lym=lymphomoreticular and hematopoietic (excludes reticulum cell sarcoma of lung); Mam=mammary; Lng=lung; Fib=fibroma, fibrosarcoma; Pnc=pancreatic islet cell tumor. In study #1, the lung tumors were lymphosarcomas. In study #4, tumors were not classified by type but it was stated that most were benign with the commonest ones being breast fibroadenoma, thyroid adenoma, pituitary chromophobe adenoma, pheochromocytoma of the adrenal, and islet cell adenoma of the pancreas. In study #11, cancer was not a main focus. However, it was reported that interstitial cell tumors of the testis were quite common in both diet groups but were delayed to an older age by DR.

[e]Values are incidences in percent. Abbreviations for non-neoplasms: Glm=glomerulonephritis; Myo=myocardial degeneration; Skl=skeletal muscle degeneration; Per=periarteritis; Rad=radiculoneuropathy; Lng=lung lesions (often 2° to infection); Bdh=bile duct hyperplasia. In study #1 (McCay's rats), the lung disease was chronic pneumonia. This disease was far more common in Grp. 1b than in DR rats early in life (e.g. 50 vs. 4% incidence for 6-13 mo old rats). In study #4, data on radiculoneuropathy (=myelin degeneration of the cauda equina) were for 33 month old rats. For study #8, the lung disease was pneumonia. A condition observed in Everitt's colony (studies #9 & 10) was hind limb paralysis. This occurred in 30% of ad lib fed rats but was not observed in DR rats. In these two studies, evidence was presented on the suppression of glomerulonephritis by DR (e.g. less proteinuria, less abnormal glomeruli, less casts in tubules) based on observations in 3-6 rats per diet-age group. A chronic lung disease occurred in this colony but its nature was not studied. In studies #11 and 12, nephropathy was graded from 0 (no lesions) through end stage with 4 classes of increasing intermediate severities. The incidence values above are for Grade 4 and end stage. The periarteritis was testicular. It was stated that myocardial fibrosis and degeneration started to appear at 18 months for controls and 30 months for DR rats. Lung lesions were not quantified but it was noted that pneumonia was not observed in this barrier-maintained colony. Study #12 evaluated cardiomyopathy and bile duct hyperplasia by a grading system (Grades 0→3). Rats with lesions of grades 2 or 3 were considered as having either of these conditions in the above incidence figures. Skeletal muscle degeneration was observed and its low incidence (<8%) in the DR groups was far less than for controls.

Gilbert and co-workers (1958) included small numbers of DR rats in their study (Table 3.2, #3) of how several diets affected tumor incidence. The DR was at about half of the ad lib level and its strongest effect was to lower the incidence of mammary tumors.

In studying Sprague-Dawley rats on nonisonutrient DR (54% of ad lib, Table 3.2, #4), Berg and colleagues (Berg & Simms, 1961; Berg et al., 1962) emphasized non-neoplastic diseases such as glomerulonephritis, myocardial and skeletal muscle degenerations, and polyarteritis nodosa. The incidences and severities of these four diseases remained lower for DR rats than for fully fed animals. Although the age of tumor onset was delayed and the overall incidences of tumors were reduced by DR, still greater effects were exerted upon the non-neoplastic diseases. An exception was radiculoneuropathy (myelin degeneration of the cauda equina roots), which was *not* influenced by DR. The data from these primary reports were later graphed in a review article (Berg, 1976) so that incidences and onsets are quite clear (Fig. 3.2). The inhibitory effects of DR on diverse late-life pathologies were brought about by a regimen which nevertheless did allow for the rats to grow and become sexually mature.

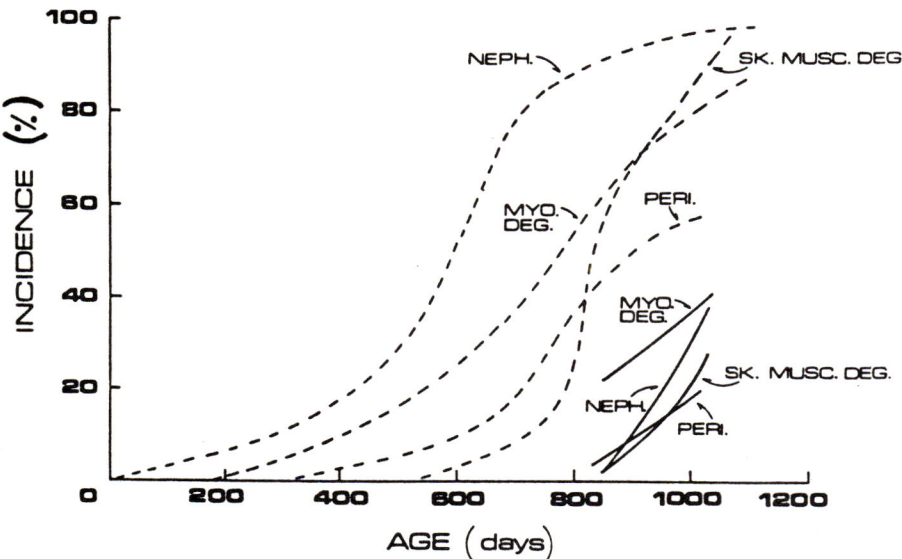

Figure 3.2. Incidence of lesions of 4 major diseases of aging in male Sprague-Dawley rats. Abbreviations: NEPH = nephrosis; MYO DEG. = myocardial degeneration; SK MUSC DEG. = skeletal muscle degeneration; PERI = periarteritis. Control rats, -----; DR rats, ———. Redrawn from Berg (1976).

Much of what is known about DR's influence on spontaneous tumors in rats stems from three reports (#5-7 in Table 3.2) by Ross and Bras. Their work is important for several reasons: routine testing of *many* (200 or so) rats per diet group, well defined diets, and very long LSs of DR animals. Inspection of Table 3.2 reveals that overall incidence values for any tumor did not exceed 10 percent, and indeed only pituitary adenomas reached that level. Other common tumors were fibromas, fibrosarcomas, lymphomas, pulmonary adenomas and carcinomas, reticulum cell sarcomas of lung and lymphoid tissue, and pancreatic islet cell tumors.

In study #5, the two most severely restricted groups (5d, 5b) developed the fewest tumors (overall incidence of 8-16% vs. 22-30% for controls). Group 5d was fed the lowest amount of energy of all groups, lived the longest (see Table 2.4, #7g), and had the lowest tumor incidence and the greatest delay in time of onset of tumors. (Impressed by these results, we formulated our own restricted mouse diets to approximate this diet.) Tumors occurred earliest in life for the ad lib fed group. They were most delayed in group 5d. Tumor incidence was higher for the heavier rats in four of the five diet groups. Diet composition affected tumor patterns. Malignant lymphomas were most common in rats consuming a high protein intake, while fibromas and fibrosarcomas were associated with a low protein intake.

Study #6 compared restricted (#6a, whose diet regimen was similar to that imposed on group 5d) and ad lib fed rats (6c) to a third group restricted only from time of weaning (21 days) until 70 days of age and then switched to ad lib eating (6b, a regimen which did not markedly increase LS [Table 2.4, #8]). Figure 3.3 shows that tumor onset was markedly delayed by long-term uninterrupted DR, but not by the 49 day version. The total incidence of benign tumors declined with DR (lowest for group 6a) while the incidence of malignant tumors was unaltered. The 49 days of DR early in life lowered the risk of benign connective tissue tumors and endocrine adenomas. As in the preceding study, tumor incidence within each group was greater for heavier than for lighter rats.

The third report (study #7) of Ross and Bras tested three diets differing in protein:carbohydrate ratios. Each diet was given both on an ad lib and restricted basis. As noted, longevity of the DR rats in this study was greatest for those fed the high protein (51% casein) diet (group 9e). In a later review, Ross (1976) discussed which tumors were decreased,

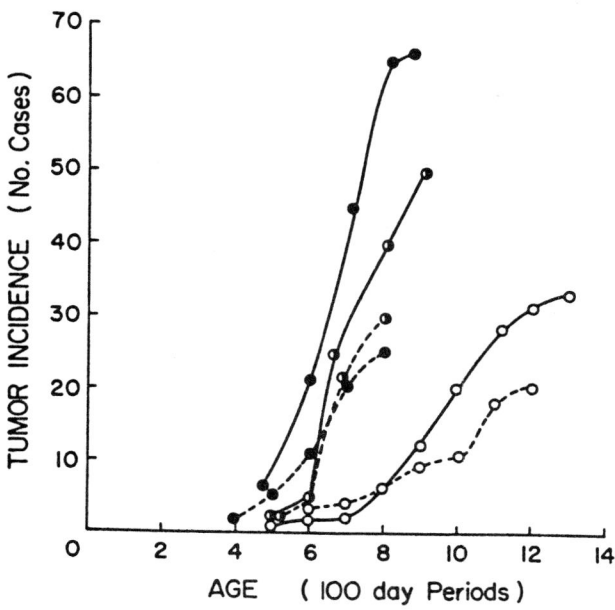

Figure 3.3. Tumor incidence patterns in male Sprague-Dawley rats fed either ad lib (AL, •, n = 250), restricted from weaning to death (DR, o, n = 250), or on DR from weaning to 70 days of age then switched to ad lib feeding (DR → AL, ⊙, n = 150). Benign tumors, ———; Malignant tumors, -----. Redrawn from Ross and Bras (1971).

unaffected or increased by DR in this study. He compared the combined incidences of tumors in the three DR groups to those in the three ad lib groups. As shown in Table 3.3, incidences of the most common neoplasms (pituitary, pancreatic and other adenomas; lymphoreticular and hematopoietic cancers) were decreased by DR. Other, less common tumors were either unaffected or increased by DR. Pituitary chromophobe adenomas were carefully studied in these rats, as detailed in an earlier report (Ross et al., 1970). Early life BWs correlated directly with pituitary adenoma incidence in late life.

Study #7 is important to consider in work aimed at optimizing DR regimens, as it represents one of the few studies comparing different diets fed at the same level of energy restriction. The DR rats fed the high protein diet displayed a lower risk of developing malignant epithelial tumors than DR rats fed the low protein diet. Adrenal and thyroid tumor morbidity were both inversely related to dietary protein among the DR groups. In short, both LS and tumor data suggest that high protein diets accentuated the benefits of DR in Ross' colony.

TABLE 3.3

Effects of DR on Tumor Incidence in Rats[a]

Tumor Type	Decreased[b]	Unaffected[c]	Increased[d]
1. Epithelial (165/197)	Adenoma (122/154)	Papilloma (30/27)	Carcinoma (9/15)
2. Lymphoreticular (63/30)	RCS (lung) (35/8) Thymoma (16/12)		RCS (lymph.) (5/12)
3. Musculoskeletal & Soft Tissue (33/22)	Lipoma (8/0)	Fibroma, Fibrosarcoma (21/15)	
4. Endocrine (121/56)	Pituitary (60/12) Pancreas (40/10)	Thyroid (15/17)	Adrenal (4/10) Parathyroid (1/7)

[a]Values are cases in ad lib group/cases in DR group for the Sprague-Dawley rats described by and adapted from Ross and Bras (1973). Many rats (750/group) were studied. Total tumor incidence was 35% in the ad lib group, vs. 18% in the DR group. The average LSs of ad lib and DR rats (independent of tumor status) were 20 and 30 months, respectively.
[b]The value for adenomas is the sum for all sites. RCS is reticular cell sarcoma. Pituitary tumors were anterior ones. Pancreatic tumors were of islet cell origin.
[c]The papillomas were in the urinary bladder. Values for fibromas and fibrosarcomas are for all sites.
[d]The carcinomas were from all sites. The RCS indicated is for lymphoid organs.

Drori and Folman observed (study #8) that mild DR (ad lib for 6 hours per day, leading to a 20% decrease in adult BW) did not markedly affect disease incidence in random bred male rats.

Two studies (#9 & 10) from Everitt's laboratory showed that DR retarded the development of glomerulonephritis and lowered overall tumor incidence in rats, while not clearly affecting the development of chronic lung disease. Similar results were reported (#9) for hypophysectomized rats consuming the same amount of calories as intact rats on DR. A third study from this group (Wyndham et al., 1983) found that DR started at 50 days of age prevented proteinuria and reduced the incidence of tubular pathology. Electron microscopy showed that foot process retraction and spreading on the glomerular basement membrane were less frequently seen in old DR rats than in controls.

Masoro's group described diseases in Fischer 344 rats maintained under specific pathogen-free conditions (#11 & 12). Chronic nephropathy is the major disease in this colony. In both studies, it occurred at a much earlier age and progressed faster in ad lib fed rats than in DR rats. In study #11, histologic evidence for end-stage real disease was found in 56 of 80 of the ad lib fed rats dying between 18 and 24 months of age, but in none of the DR rats (n = 55) dying between 18 and 48 months. Study #11 also showed that DR prevented or delayed testicular (interstitial cell) tumors, bile duct hyperplasia, and myocardial fibrosis and degeneration.

Study #12 represented an even broader disease survey of rats placed on DR at either 6 weeks (#12a), 6 months (12b), from 6 weeks to 6 months of age (12c), or not at all (12d). Besides nephropathy, neoplasias and cardiomyopathy emerged as the main late-life diseases. Food restriction started at 6 weeks or 6 months was very effective in slowing the development of these three (and other) diseases. Dietary restriction confined to early life (12c) or dietary protein restriction without energy restriction (data in article but not included in Table 3.2) did not profoundly retard diseases. A later ultrastructural study of kidneys from these cohorts showed that continuous DR from 6 weeks or 6 months of age slowed many age changes of this type (e.g. increasing thickness and lesions of the glomerular basement membrane, loss of glomerular epithelial cells) (Hayashida et al., 1986).

Figure 3.4 gives an overview of DR's favorable effects on mortality and tumor incidence in study #12. Deaths (from all causes and from tumors) occurred 6 to 12 months later in DR than in ad lib fed animals. Note (Figure 3.4) that similar effects were rendered by DR started at

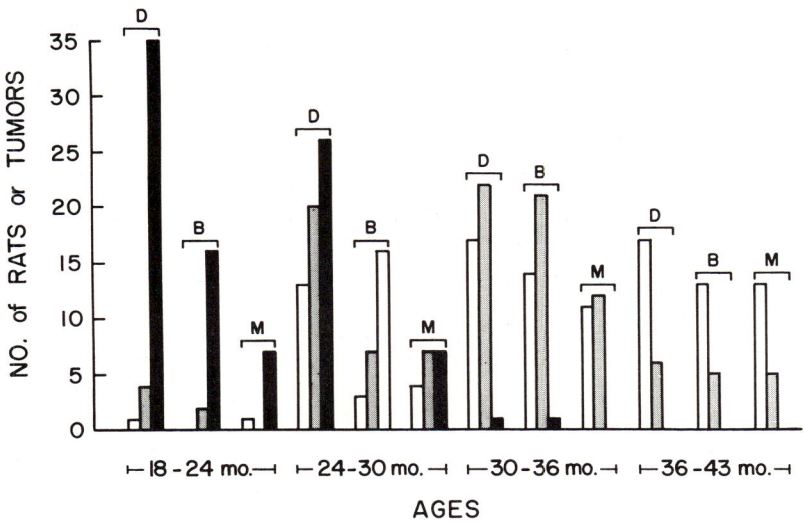

Figure 3.4. Mortality and tumor incidence at four age-periods in male Fischer 344 rats as influenced by EDR and ADR. Open bars = DR from 6 weeks of age (n = 56, average LS of 35 months); stippled bars = DR from 6 months of age (n = 60, average LS of 31 months); solid bars = ad lib (n = 71, average LS of 23 months). "D" denotes the number of deaths from all causes in each age period. "B" gives the number of rats with benign tumors and "M" the number with malignant tumors at each age-period. Drawn from data in Maeda et al. (1985).

either 6 weeks or at 6 months of age. However, the 13 percent increase in the average LS of the 6 week-onset group over that of the 6 month-onset group is appreciable and reflected in tumor onset.

Davis and co-workers (1983) found that the development of renal disease was retarded in male Wistar rats on DR, as judged by para-aminohippuric acid transport (an indicator of the kidney's ability to do osmotic work) and by urinary protein excretion (increased in chronic renal disease). The retardation obtained for the restricted feeding of either low, medium and high protein diets, but not with ad lib feeding over a range of protein intakes.

Tucker (1979) observed that Wistar rats on mild DR (20% less than ad lib intake) developed fewer tumors than controls when studied at 24 months of age. Pituitary and mammary tumors were most common and also most sensitive to inhibition by DR.

As mentioned (Chapters 1 & 2), Lloyd (1984) found that spontaneously hypertensive rats lived longer if on DR. Restricted rats less often displayed histologic changes in heart (edema and fatty infiltration), adrenals (vacuole formation and congestion), and kidneys (interstitial fibrosis) associated with the hypertension of fully fed controls. Instead, the DR rats showed late-life lesions more typical of rat strains not prone to develop hypertension.

Another rat model of illness is the LA/N corpulent strain which is hypercholesterolemic and prone to myocardial infarction. Russell and Amy (1986) found that DR lowered their cholesterol levels. The LA/N rats also respond to DR by showing less DMBA-induced mammary tumors (Klurfeld et al., 1987b).

The self-selection studies of Ross and his colleagues provide yet another example supporting the view that low BWs in rodents are associated with less disease. One recalls that in these studies the rats were allowed to eat ad lib but chose between three diets. The mature BWs of the rats correlated linearly with spontaneous tumor frequency (Ross et al., 1983a). Similarly, those rats which grew rapidly, displaying a high level of conversion of food into BW, more readily developed anterior pituitary tumors (Ross et al., 1983b). Thus a thrifty metabolic phenotype is "bad" for obesity-prone, ad lib fed rats but may be "good" for rodents on DR (see *"Growth Rate, Body Weight and Lifespan,"* Chapter 2).

Studies with Mice

Mice have been used in many underfeeding studies where spontaneous diseases were monitored. Most often the strains selected were relatively short-lived, each with its own characteristic and progressive disease syndrome (e.g. breast cancer, autoimmune nephropathy) affecting nearly all mice in a uniform fashion and with death at ages which would be regarded as merely early middle age for heartier strains. For this discussion, the criterion for classifying a strain as "short-lived" is an average LS for normally fed animals of less than 22 months. In about one-half of the studies, the mice were killed for various analyses and LSs were not determined. The other studies determined diseases present at natural death.

Short-Lived Strains. Table 3.4 summarizes data on disease inhibition in short-lived mice dietarily restricted from early in life. The data are grouped on a disease-by-disease basis and arranged chronologically. The first listed disease, breast cancer, is so placed to reflect it being the subject of the earliest and largest number of studies. Tannenbaum (study #1) reported in 1942 that DR beginning at 10 weeks of age prevented the occurrence of mammary tumors through 20 months of age, whereas controls experienced a 38 percent incidence. Visscher et al. (1942) (study #2) observed no breast tumors at all in severely underfed (14 g peak BW!) C3H mice over 16 months, whereas two of every three ad lib fed mice developed the tumor. This difference cannot be unequivocally attributed to caloric restriction, however, since controls ate a fatty diet (20% lard) and the DR mice were given on a calorie basis 70 percent as much of a diet lower in fat content (15%) lard). At the end of the study, 57 percent of the DR Mice were alive vs. 27 percent of the control group. It was noted incidentally that in A strain mice the same DR regimen yielded 18 g adults, suggesting large strain differences in the metabolic responses to DR.

Study #3 (White & Andervont, 1943) also reported marked inhibition of breast tumors in severely underfed and probably malnourished mice (ad lib access to a 3.9% casein diet, yielding BWs of 12 g at 6 months of age). Restricted and control mice (BW, 25 g) were fed the same diet except that for the controls l-cystine was added (0.5% of the diet, at the expense of corn starch) to eliminate the diet's most serious amino acid deficiency. As with certain other studies, this experimental design does not clarify which nutrients need to be restricted to retard breast tumors.

Tannenbaum published two 1945 reports (#4, 5) showing that DR started at 10 weeks of age prevented breast tumors in DBA mice (breast tumors appear later in life in DBA compared to C3H mice). The NPDs (composed of Fox chow meal, skimmed milk powder and constarch)

TABLE 3.4
Inhibition by EDR of Spontaneous Diseases in Mice from Short-Lived Strains[a]

Disease	Study	Strain	End[b]	Diet Group[c]	Incidence[d]	Onset[e]
Mammary carcinoma	1	DBA	20	1a. R (50F), NPD (2g/d), 66%	0	-
				1b. C (50F), NPD (3g/d)	38	17
	2	C3H	16	2a. R (44F), NPD, ↑vit, ↑min, DF (1.7g/d), 47%	0	-
				2b. C (51F), NPD, ad lib (2.3g/d)	67	9
	3	C3H	22	3a. R (45F), NPD, ↓pro, ad lib, 48%	0	-
				3b. C (42F), NPD, ↓pro+cystine, ad lib	98	6
	4	DBA	23	4a. R (50F), NPD, 7 kcal/d, 67%	0	-
				4b. R (49F), NPD, 8 kcal/d, 73%	12	-
				4c. C (48F), NPD, ad lib (11 kcal/d)	54	17
	5	DBA	31	5a. R (49F), NPD, 9 kcal/d, 73%	47	22
				5b. C (47F), NPD, ad lib (11 kcal/d)	74	18
	6	A	LS	6a. R (=3a, Table 2.5), 61%	0[d]	-
				6b. C (=3b, Table 2.5)	4[d]	-
	7	C3H	LS	7a. R (=8a, Table 2.5), 72%	0	-
				7b. C (=8b, Table 2.5)	71	12
	8	C3H	23	8a. R (=8a, Table 2.5), NR	11	-
				8b. C (=8b, Table 2.5)	60	13
Leukemia	9	AK	LS	9a. R (=2a, Table 2.5), 68%	10	-
				9b. C (=2b, Table 2.5)	65	9
Lung Tumor	10	A	17	10a. R (33F, 24M), NPD, 2g/d, 80%	33	15
				10b. C (17F, 18M), NPD, ad lib	46	11
Hepatoma	11	C3H	15	11a. R (32M), NPD, 8.1 kcal/d	0	-
				11b. R (38M), NPD, 9.2 kcal/d	0	-
				11c. R (46M), NPD, 10.3 kcal/d	11	-
				11d. C (36M), NPD, 14.3 kcal/d	64	NR
Renal disease	12	B/WF$_1$	LS	12a. R (=9a, Table 2.5), 67%	[d]	[e]
				12b. C (=9b, Table 2.5)	100	8
	13	kd/kd	LS	13a. R (=10a, Table 2.5), NR	[d]	[e]
				13b. C (=10b, Table 2.5)	100	5

[a]In seven of these studies, DR commenced at 3 to 5 weeks of age. The later starting ones (#1,3,4,5,11 and 13) began at 8 to 10 weeks of age.

[b]References: (1) Tannenbaum (1942); (2) Visscher et al. (1942); (3) White and Andervont (1943); (4) Tannenbaum (1945a); (5) Tannenbaum (1945b); (6) Ball et al. (1947); (7) Fernandes et al. (1976b); (8) Sarkar et al. (1982); (9) Saxton et al. (1944); (10) Larsen and Heston (1945); (11) Tannenbaum and Silverstone (1949); (12) Fernandes et al. (1976c); (13) Fernandes et al. (1978b). "End" is the age of the mice when the experiment was ended. If mice were allowed to live their full LSs, this is indicated by "LS."

[c]Abbreviations used for diet groups are in Table 2.4. Diet protocols previously summarized in Table 2.5 are not redescribed and references to that table are provided. Figures in first parenthesis give numbers of animals and sex. "%" gives the peak BW of DR as a percentage of control BW. In group 4c, it is noteworthy that the reported ad lib caloric intake (70-84 kcal/wk) is very low for most mouse strains, approximating the caloric intake for *restricted* mice studied by Good's group.

[d]Values are incidences in percent. Note the strong dependency of these values on when each study was terminated. In study #4, values are for virgin females. Breeders in this colony fed the control diet showed a 19% incidence of mammary cancer vs. 0% for DR mice. In study #12, disease incidence was not reported (only LS data were reported); however, as the LS was about doubled, it is quite likely that incidence was lower in #12a than in #12b at most ages when the latter group was afflicted. Incidence was not reported in study #13; however, based on LSs and limited histopathologic data, the disease was clearly suppressed by DR.

[e]Onset values give the age when 25% of the group's mice showed evidence of the disease (e.g. palpable tumor, death). This was usually estimated from each report using various kinds of data. In studies #12 and 13, disease onset was not precisely determined but was inferred for the control group from the survival curves.

were formulated so that DR mice were limited in carbohydrate but not in other essentials. The DR in study #5 was mild, and accordingly, tumor prevention was incomplete.

In study #6 (Table 3.4), the tumor incidence values given were for virgin females and were quite low even in the control group. However, breeders in this colony given the control diet ad lib experienced a 19 percent incidence of mammary tumors (data not shown) vs. 0 percent for DR mice.

Interest in DR's effect on breast cancer in the C3H mouse model reappeared about 30 years later when Fernandes et al. (1976b) (study #7) reported that breast tumors did not occur in DR mice, even though LS was not increased in the small population studied. (The main focus of study #7 was towards immunologic effects of DR [see "IMMUNOLOGIC PARAMETERS" in Chapter 4]). The next study (#8, Sarkar et al., 1982) probed DR's effect on breast tumors using endocrine and virologic approaches aimed at elucidating mechanisms. Again, the incidence of tumors was sharply reduced and the onset delayed by DR, which also led to a reduction of: (1) serum prolactin level (value for DR about half that for control animals, while levels of other hormones [growth hormone, TSH] were not affected), (2) mammary tumor virus production, and (3) the size and number of mammary alveolar lesions. Unlike the case with more severe underfeeding, estrus cycling was not affected by the 70 calorie per week DR regimen employed in these studies.

Saxton's group reported in 1944 (study #9) that AK mice showed lower incidence and later onset of leukemia when underfed with a NPD severe enough to produce 17 g adults. He noted that 10-16 percent of mice died before 6 months of age, either from fighting or pneumonia in the control group or of unknown causes in the DR group. One does not often see early deaths in the more recent studies in which animals usually are singly housed in modern facilities and fed nutritionally adequate diets.

Early-onset DR inhibited the development of pulmonary tumors in A strain mice (Larsen & Heston, 1945: study #10). The restriction regimen was a cystine-supplemented low protein (3.9% casein) diet given at the same intake level as that of mice consuming a cystine-deficient diet ad lib. This latter diet (not in table) produced very small mice (peak BW of 17 g) as well as a lower tumor incidence. The effectiveness of DR even in the presence of an adequate cystine intake suggests that low calorie intake is more important than low cystine intake in retarding lung tumors in A strain mice.

Tannenbaum and Silverstone (1949) observed that hepatoma incidence fell according to the degree of energy restriction in male C3H mice (study #11). Tumors were larger in fully fed than in DR mice. In this study the mice were treated topically with metylcholanthrene to induce skin tumors. This agent did not affect hepatoma patterns.

Lee et al. (1956) observed that DR at a level one-third less than ad lib feeding prolonged LS (Table 2.5) and gave a very low hepatoma incidence. However, as only small numbers of mice were used, we did not include the data in Table 3.4. Also not included are data showing that DR suppresses mammary and liver tumors in C3H/A^{vy} mice (Rowlatt et al., 1973).

An excellent review of dietary effects on hepatic tumors in mice is that of Gellatly (1975). He questioned the term "hepatoma," preferring "hepatic parenchymal nodules" as better reflecting the varied nature of such lesions. Nodules were classified as Type 1 (= nodular hyperplasia), Type 2 (= liver cell adenoma), and Type 3 (= hepatocellular carcinoma). Mice of the B6 strain fed a PD made of 11 percent fat attained mature BWs of 45 g and developed many more nodules than other mice reaching 35 g of BW on an ad lib NPD diet containing 4.5 percent fat.

Additional work by Good and colleagues concerning inhibition of disease by DR in short-lived mouse strains has broadened the array of DR-sensitive pathologies. The renal diseases of B/WF$_1$ (study #12; Izui et al., 1981) and kd/kd (study #13) mice were strongly inhibited by DR. Mice of the B/WF$_1$ hybrid develop an autoimmune, proliferative nephritis associated with xenotropic virus infection, immune complexes and glomerulosclerosis. The diseased kd/kd kidney shows profound mononuclear cell interstitial infiltration with tubular dilatation, atrophy and casts. The pathogenesis of the kd/kd disease (which is said to resemble nephronophthisis in humans) is not clear.

Mechanisms possibly involved in EDR's inhibition of nephropathy in B/WF$_1$ mice were explored. Izui et al. (1981) found that 8 month old mice maintained on DR (10 kcal/day) showed only minimal to mild renal changes, whereas controls (20 kcal/day) displayed severe changes. Further, DR selectively lowered the expression of retroviral envelope glycoprotein (gp70) in serum to a level less than half that seen in controls. This reduction obtained for both free gp70 as well as that complexed to antibody. However, serum levels of the major structural protein of endogenous retroviruses were not affected by DR. Another serum glycoprotein, haptoglobin, was also low in sera from DR mice, whereas albumin levels were not affected. A moderate but significant reduction in serum autoantibodies to single- and double-stranded DNA was observed in the restricted mice.

Mice of the B/WF$_1$ strain are also afflicted with vascular disease. Fernandes et al. (1983) reported that proliferative and fatty-proliferative lesions of the aorta and its branches were reduced by calorie or fat restriction. Ad lib feeding of "lab chow" (= low in fat, high in fiber) retarded the aortic but not the renal pathology.

In a large study (N = 640) attempting "to define certain suitable conditions for the conduct of future carcinogenicity tests," Conybeare (1980) studied the incidence of tumors and other pathologies in 80-member groups of outbred Swiss mice of each sex fed one of two NPDs. Each diet was fed on both an unrestricted and a *mildly* restricted basis (75% of ad lib intake, leading to 30 g females and 40 g males). The experiment terminated at 18 months, at which time about 60 percent of controls and 75 percent of DR mice remained alive. In both sexes and on both diets, DR led to a decrease in neoplasms (overall incidence about 40% for ad lib vs. 15% for DR), the most common tumors being pulmonary (adenomas, adenocarcinomas) and hepatic (graded from proliferative parenchymal foci to metastatic tumors) Pulmonary tumors occurred in 17 percent of control and 8 percent of DR mice. Hepatic tumors occurred chiefly in males, afflicting 31 percent of male controls vs. 8 percent of DR males. The incidences of renal amyloidosis or cataract were not influenced by DR. Conybeare (1980) concluded that, compared to ad lib fed obese animals with a high "background" cancer incidence, the DR rodent represents a better model for carcinogenicity studies. This agrees with the "toxicological perspective" of Williams et al. (1987).

In Conybeare's study and several others food intake was limited to an amount 20-25 percent below the ad lib level. Not surprisingly, the ability of such "mild DR" to prolong LS and forestall diseases is less than that of more severe DR regimens. From the standpoint of human application, however, an effect at 80 percent of ad lib seems relevant because many more adult humans could probably adapt and adhere to this degree of DR than to severer ones.

Long-Lived Strains. We are aware of nine reports on diseases in mice from long-lived strains fed restricted diets since childhood. In six of these mild DR (80% of ad lib level) was imposed on marginally long-lived mouse strains (Tucker, 1979; Rehm et al., 1984; Rehm et al.,

1985a, 1985b, 1985c, and 1987). The three others, all from our laboratory, imposed more severe DR on clearly long-lived strains (Cheney et al., 1980; Cheney et al., 1983; Weindruch et al., 1986). The dissimilarity of the two types of studies can be illustrated by noting that BWs for the restricted mice in the mild DR studies (see Table 2.5, #14a, 20a, c & e) approximated those for certain of the control groups in the severe DR sets (Table 2.5, #15c, 16d, 17d), all being about 35 grams.

The mild DR regimen of Tucker (1979) improved survival (Table 2.5, #14), markedly increased the age for tumor onset, and lowered tumor incidences in both sexes. Tumor onset (as defined in Table 3.4) was 20 months for ad lib fed vs. 30 months for DR mice. Overall tumor incidences were 80 percent for ad lib vs. 50 percent for DR Mice. The most common tumor was pituitary adenoma. In males, 32 percent of controls carried the tumor whereas none were found in DR mice. Incidences were higher in females: 66 percent for ad lib and 38 percent for DR mice. Thirty four percent of fully fed mice developed mammary tumors, but only 6 percent of DR mice.

Recently, Rehm and co-workers have provided much information on the effect of mild DR (20% restriction) on development of diseases. They studied female Han:NMRI mice: 300 individuals from an obese subline, 300 from a lean subline, and 300 controls. Each subline was divided into DR and ad lib groups (see Table 2.5, #20). At death the mice were carefully examined both grossly and microscopically.

Neoplasia was the cause of death in about 50 percent of the mice. The age of development of the tumors was delayed by the DR (Table 3.5). The final incidences of pituitary and mammary tumors were two to four fold lower in the DR group, whereas the incidences of other tumors (ovarian, hematopoietic, pulmonary) were not much influenced. Ovarian and lung tumors only rarely proved fatal, whereas all generalized hematopoietic and some mammary tumors did appear responsible for the death of their hosts. Ovarian tumors, with tubular adenomas, granulosa and Sertoli cell tumors being the most common, were reported separately (Rehm et al., 1984). The authors concluded that for these tumors susceptibility depended most strongly on time of exposure and therefore the longer-living DR mice developed more such tumors, albeit at a later chronologic time in life.

These investigators have also described nonneoplastic lesions of the thyroid (Rehm et al., 1985b), respiratory tract (Rehm et al., 1985c), and stomach (Rehm et al., 1987). The most common thyroid lesion was

TABLE 3.5

Delayed Development of Tumors in Mildly Underfed Mice[a]

Tumor	Incidence (%)		Ave. LS	
	AL	DR	AL	DR
Pituitary	33	8	25	31
Mammary	14	6	25	29
Lymphosarcoma	11	10	20	27
RCA—Type B	7	2	23	26
RCS—Type A	4	3	26	33
Lung—single adenoma	21	13	23	27
Lung—multiple adenoma	6	3	23	29
Lung—adenocarcinoma	11	15	24	28

[a]Data are from Rehm et al. (1985a) using values from the subline not selected for BW. The average LS for the ad lib (AL) fed group was 22 months, vs. 26 months for mice on mild DR (80% of the AL level). RCS is reticulum cell sarcoma. Average LS (mo) of mice bearing that tumor.

a cystic distension of the ultimobranchial bodies, and its occurrence was slightly delayed by mild DR. The main respiratory tract lesions were pulmonary mineralizations and crystal formations and these were largely insensitive to DR. The dominant gastric lesions were ulcers and adenomatous hyperplasia. Ulcers were more common in the DR groups and were a very serious problem for the lean subline, killing 20 percent of the mice (vs. 5% or less in the other lines). The authors suggest that the ulcers may be stress-related and note that housing the DR mice five per cage may have contributed. Adenomatous hyperplasia of the fundus was the most common gastric lesion in ad lib fed mice, and was not apparent clinically.

Our laboratory's three studies on more severely underfed mice from longer-lived strains also showed that DR greatly altered age-specific tumor patterns. The LSs of these mice were discussed in Chapter 2.

The study of Cheney et al. (1980) (Table 2.5, #15) included four cohorts of B6 mice, only one of which ("Cohort IV" of the original report) is in the table. The effects of the DR on tumor patterns were more dramatic than those on LS. The predominant disease was lymphoma, which occurred less frequently and later in life for DR mice.

Cheney et al. (1983) extended this work to the even longer lived B10C3F$_1$ hybrid mouse, studying seven diet groups (four are in Table 2.5, #16). The groups were N/N (i.e. fed "normally" pre- and post-weaning [#16d]), R/N (restricted access to mother before weaning, normal diet thereafter), N/R (#16a), R/R (#16b), N/N/R (switched to DR at 14 months of age [#16c]), N/R/N switched at 14 months to normal diet) and R/R/N. Table 3.6 summarizes tumor incidences for these mice. The two main tumors were lymphoma and hepatoma. Tumor frequency varied with the period in life when DR was imposed. The lowest overall incidences occurred for those three groups restricted during most or all of their adult lives (i.e. R/R, N/R and N/N/R). Lymphoma was less common in mice subjected to any of the five regimens involving post-weaning DR than in groups N/N and R/N. Hepatoma incidence was more complexly affected, with highest incidences occurring in the two groups shifted to normal diets at 14 months of age after being on EDR. Preweaning restriction appeared to raise hepatoma incidence. Figure 3.5 shows the ages of death for tumor bearing mice in this study. The LSs of tumor-bearing mice reflected group LSs.

The third report (Weindruch et al., 1986) was also described earlier in terms of LS effects (Table 2.5, #17). The influences of diet on overall tumor incidence are shown in Table 3.7. The incidence was highest for N/N$_{85}$ mice (78%) and lowest for N/R$_{40}$ mice (38%). Mice on either of the four types of DR did not differ from others freely fed Lab Chow™ in

TABLE 3.6

Tumor Incidence in Seven Diet Groups of B10C3F$_1$ Female Mice[a]

Diet Group	Number	Lymphoma(%)	Hepatoma(%)	Any Tumor(%)
N/N	45	29	20	60
R/N	56	23	27	68
N/R	53	0	15	21
R/R	49	14	35	47
N/N/R	30	10	7	20
N/R/N	29	10	72	79
R/R/N	26	15	54	81

[a]Data are from Cheney et al. (1983). "Number" tells how many mice were studied per group. Other values are the tumor incidences in percent for mice at time of natural death. Values for "Any Tumor" give the group's overall tumor incidence. See text and Table 2.5 (#16) for explanation of the normal ("N") and restricted ("R") diets.

overall tumor incidence. For mice fed Lab Chow™, the average LS of tumor-bearing mice exceeded that of tumor-free mice. Early deaths in mice fed Lab Chow™ occurred largely in tumor-free, obese animals. The LS of tumor-bearing vs. tumor-free mice was not significantly different in the other five groups.

Effects of DR on the incidence of the three most common tumors (lymphoma, hepatoma and soft tissue neoplasms) and on the LS of mice bearing each tumor type are shown in Table 3.8. Lymphoma incidence was highest in the N/N_{85}, Lab Chow™ and $N/R_{50lopro}$ groups. Lymphoma-bearing mice lived by 8-12 months longer in the four DR groups than in the non-DR groups. Hepatoma occurred most frequently

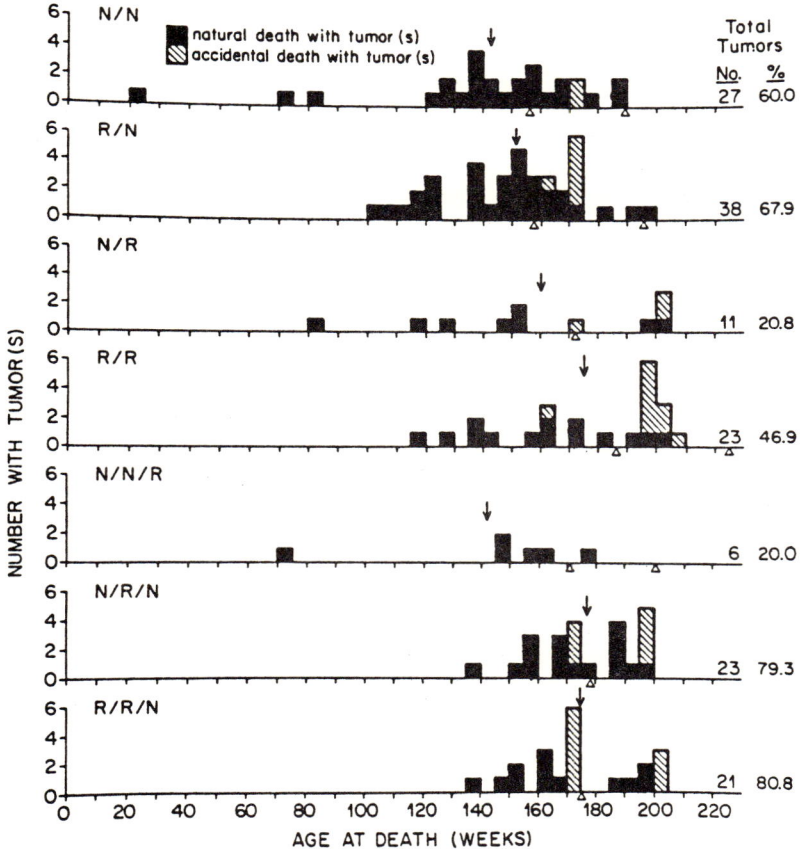

Figure 3.5. Distributions of ages at death for tumor-bearing B10C3F$_1$ mice. Seven diet groups (defined in text) were studied. N = normal diet, R = restricted diet. Arrows (↓) above the distributions give the average LS for tumor-bearing mice. The triangles (△) under the baselines give average and maximum LSs for the whole group (maximum LSs not given for those three groups where the last survivors died accidental deaths). Percentages are of autopsied mice. From Cheney et al. (1983).

TABLE 3.7

Tumor Incidences and Longevity in Six Diet Groups of C3B10RF$_1$ Female Mice[a]

Group[b]	n	Mice with a Tumor		Mice with no Tumor	
		Inc.	Ave. LS	Inc.	Ave. LS
Lab Chow	45	56[ab]	30 ± 1[a]	44[ab]	26 ± 1[a]
N/N$_{85}$	54	78[c]	32 ± 1[a]	22[c]	34 ± 1[b]
N/R$_{50}$	70	51[ab]	42 ± 1[bc]	49[ab]	42 ± 2[cd]
R/R$_{50}$	54	63[bc]	43 ± 1[bc]	37[bc]	44 ± 1[cd]
N/R$_{50lopro}$	55	53[ab]	39 ± 1[b]	47[ab]	40 ± 2[c]
N/R$_{40}$	60	38[a]	44 ± 1[c]	62[a]	46 ± 1[d]

[a]Incidence is the percent of mice in that diet group with or without a tumor at time of natural death. Values for LS are average age (in months) of mice at time of death in each group ± SEM. Values in each column not sharing a common superscript (a–d) were significantly different (p = 0.05). Data adapted from Weindruch et al. (1986).

[b]Diet groups: Lab Chow, Purina Lab Chow™ ad libitum; N/N$_{85}$, fed normally before and after weaning, postweaning diet fed at 85 kcal/week (25% less than ad libitum); N/R$_{50}$, fed normally before weaning, restricted postweaning to 50 kcal/week; R/R$_{50}$, restricted in feeding level both before and after weaning; N/R$_{50lopro}$, restricted after weaning to 50 kcal/week with a decrease with age in the protein content of the diet; N/R$_{40}$, restricted after weaning to 40 kcal/week.

TABLE 3.8

Incidences of Three Types of Tumors in Six Diet Groups of C3B10RF$_1$ Female Mice, and Longevity in Each Diet-Tumor Group[a]

Group	Type of Tumor					
	Lymphoma		Hepatoma		Soft Tissue	
	Inc.	Ave. LS	Inc.	Ave. LS	Inc.	Ave. LS
Lab Chow	31[ab]	30 ± 1[a]	9[a]	29 ± 1[a]	9[ab]	32 ± 1[a]
N/N$_{85}$	46[a]	31 ± 1[a]	20[ab]	34 ± 2[a]	15[a]	34 ± 2[ab]
N/R$_{50}$	23[b]	40 ± 2[b]	21[ab]	45 ± 2[b]	0[c]	-------
R/R$_{50}$	19[bc]	39 ± 3[b]	37[b]	44 ± 1[b]	6[ac]	40 ± 5[ab]
N/R$_{50lopro}$	29[ab]	39 ± 2[b]	18[a]	41 ± 2[b]	4[bc]	33 ± 3[a]
N/R$_{40}$	13[c]	42 ± 2[b]	15[a]	44 ± 2[b]	3[bc]	44 ± 2[b]

[a]Tumor incidence values give the percent of mice in that diet group with that type of tumor. Ave. LS refers to average age of death ± SEM in months for mice with the indicated tumor. Values in each column not sharing a common superscript (a–c) were significantly different (p = 0.05). Data adapted from Weindruch et al. (1986).

in the R/R_{50} cohort and least frequently in mice fed Lab Chow™. Hepatoma-bearing mice from the four most restricted groups displayed average LSs greater by 6-15 months than mice from the other two groups. Soft tissue tumors (mostly sarcomas and breast tumors) and lung tumors (2-7% incidence in the six groups) were far less frequently encountered than were lymphoma and hepatoma, but tended also to be decreased in incidence by DR.

Correlations between BW at 5, 10, 15, or 22 months of age and presence of lymphoma or hepatoma were determined for mice in each of the six groups. Most groups showed several small positive correlations between BW and the eventual development of lymphoma, which were either statistically significant or nearly so. In contrast, the presence of hepatoma appeared unrelated to BW at any age in the six diet groups.

Unlike most rats and short-lived mouse strains which often develop renal disease, mice from long-lived strains usually do not incur such lesions. An exception is documented by Johnson and Barrows (1980) in female B6 mice where intermittent feeding or severe protein restriction opposed the development of glomerular lesions as assessed by scanning electron microscopy.

Dietary Restriction Started in Adulthood (ADR)

One compelling reason to investigate spontaneous disease incidence and progression in rodents subjected to ADR is that such a regimen might plausibly be usable by humans. Could ADR retard the onset of late-life diseases in humans? Could human ADR forestall the progression of, or aid in curing *ongoing* diseases? Although human data are unavailable, results of ADR studies in rodents, although much less extensive than EDR studies, also show favorable effects on late-life disease patterns.

Studies with Rats

Limited but accumulating data indicate that rats introduced to long-term DR at various adult ages stay disease-free to later ages than do their more fully fed counterparts. We have already discussed (Table 3.2, #12; Figure 3.4) the recent study of Maeda et al. (1985), where DR started at 6 months of age in male Fischer 344 rats curbed the development of nephropathy and tumors about as effectively as DR started at 6 weeks of age. We are aware of only five other pertinent studies of diseases in rats subjected to ADR. Ages of onset were 3 to 14 months of age. The earliest-onset ADR studies are of limited value for modelling the human situation.

Nolen (1972; see Table 2.6, #6 for description of 3 of 7 diet groups studied) fed the following regimens to Wistar rats: ad lib, EDR (onset at 3 weeks of age) at 60 percent of ad lib, EDR at 80 percent of ad lib, ADR (3 mo onset) at 60 percent of ad lib, ADR at 80 percent of ad lib, EDR at 60 percent of ad lib switched to ad lib at 3 months, and EDR at 80 percent of ad lib switched to ad lib at 3 months. Disease incidences were not clearly affected by these dietary manipulations; however, disease onsets were delayed by DR, and this effect was most overt in the two groups maintained at 60 percent of ad lib from time of weaning or from 3 months of age (These two groups had many more survivors than any of the others when the experiment was halted in its 36th month.). The leading cause of death among the rats was respiratory disease (suppurative pneumonitis and bronchiectasis). Nephritis, hepatic disease (not detailed), and tumors were also common. These results indicate that it is not critical to restrict rats before 3 months of age to achieve maximum or near-maximum effects on disease parameters.

A genetically obese rat strain afflicted also by renal disease, hyperlipidemia, hypertension, and atherosclerotic vascular disease was studied by Koletsky and Puterman (1977). The syndrome is inherited as a homozygous recessive trait. When fed a NPD ad lib the rats attain BWs of about 700 g by 7 months, show an average LS of 10 months, and are all dead by 14 months of age. Restriction (33% of ad lib intake) begun at 3 months kept BWs below 350 g, eliminated the hypertriglyceridemia and reduced the hypercholesterolemia, and resulted in average and maximum LSs of 23 and 28.5 months. The incidence of atherosclerotic lesions was 48 percent among the obese controls vs. 14 percent for the restricted group. Would DR prove beneficial to members of human families prone to obesity, hyperlipidemia, hypertension and early cardiovascular deaths?

A 6 month course of periodic ADR (3 weeks on, 2 weeks off) imposed on 8 month old obese Zucker rats did not retard their renal disease (glomerulosclerosis) (Kasiske et al., 1986). The rationale for testing this peculiar DR regimen was "to mimic human dietary behavior."

Renal disease as manifested by proteinuria and the electrophoretic profile of excreted proteins was studied in male Wistar rats by Fujita et al. (1984). Adult-onset DR at 50 percent of the ad lib intake of a nutrient non-enriched PD was started at 14 months of age, a time when renal disease was already ongoing. Although leading to a rapid decrease in proteinuria, ADR did not alter the profile of the excreted proteins. Dietary restriction commenced either at weaning or at 14 months improved survivorship in the samll numbers (n = 8 to 12) of rats studied (The ADR experiment was halted at 26 months, and maximum LS was not determined.).

Studies with Mice

Mice have also been examined for the effects of ADR on late-life diseases. Indeed the data are somewhat more plentiful than for the rat. Three phases comprise this work. First, the initial evidence that DR, started at any age, may retard the development of spontaneous tumors derives from studies of short-lived mouse strains reported by Tanenbaum in 1940. Ages of onset in Tannenbaum's Phase I ADR studies ranged from 5 to 14 months. Phase II, comprised of studies on autoimmune mice, also short-lived, began with a report from Good's group (Friend et al., 1978) showing that ADR begun at 4 to 5 months of age largely prevents autoimmune nephropathy in B/WF_1 mice. Beach et al. (1982) also observed that ADR commencing at 6 months of age benefited B/WF_1 mice, and slowed the autoimmune hemolytic anemia of NZB mice (Beach et al., 1981b). Phase III, consisting of our ADR work in long-lived strains, comprised a study of tumor incidence in male $B10C3F_1$ and B6 mice restricted at 12 months of age (Weindruch & Walford, 1982) and a second study on a small group (n = 30) of $B10C3F_1$ females restricted at 14 months of age (Cheney et al., 1983).

The results of Tannenbaum's Phase I studies are shown in Table 3.9. The two reports listed provide evidence for prevention or retardation of mammary carcinoma and pulmonary adenomas by ADR. Starting ADR even as late as 9 months sharply diminished susceptibility to breast cancer. Study #2 quantified relationships between breast cancer incidence and caloric intake. Five intake levels (8.1, 8.9, 9.6, 10.3, and 11.7 kcal/day) were tested (Only three are shown in Table 3.9.). Figure 3.6 reveals that severe caloric restriction was required for a strong reduction in tumor incidence if the experiment was allowed to run until the mice reached 31 months of age. Probably this allowed time for the delayed-onset tumors to manifest. At 18 months of age, less severe DR was effective, probably because the onset of many potential tumors was delayed beyond the time of the experiment. That caloric intake is the key determinant in such results is supported by another report (Tannenbaum &

TABLE 3.9
Tannenbaum's Studies on Spontaneous Tumors in Adult-Restricted Mice

Tumor	Study[a]	Strain	Start[a]	End[a]	Diet Groups[b]	Incidence(%)	Onset[c]
Mammary	1	DBA	5	18	1a. R (50F), NPD, 50% of ad lib, 55%	2	-
					1b. C (50F), NPD, ad lib	40	15
	1	DBA	9	24	1c. R (44F), NPD, 50% of ad lib, 65%	7	-
					1d. C (44F), NPD, ad lib	30	18
	2	DBA	5	31	2a. R (25F), NPD, 8 kcal/d, 80%	36	19
					2b. R (25F), NPD, 9 kcal/d, 82%	68	18
					2c. C (30F), NPD, 12 kcal/d	73	15
Pulmonary	1	ABC[a]	14	23	1e. R (25F, 25M), NPD, 50% of ad lib, 60%	32	NR
					1f. C (25F, 25M), NPD, ad lib	58	NR

[a]References: (1) Tannenbaum (1940); (2) Tannenbaum (1945a). "Start" gives the age (mo) when ADR began. "End" indicates when (in mo) the study was ended. Groups 1e and 1f were treated topically with benzpyrene early in life and studied for induced skin tumors; however, pulmonary tumor incidence and onset were not influenced by applying benzpyrene.

[b]Abbreviations for diet groups are given in Table 2.4. Figures in parentheses give numbers of animals and sex. The final percent figure is the peak BW of R as a percentage of that for C.

[c]Tumor onset values give the age when 25% of the group's mice showed evidence of the tumor.

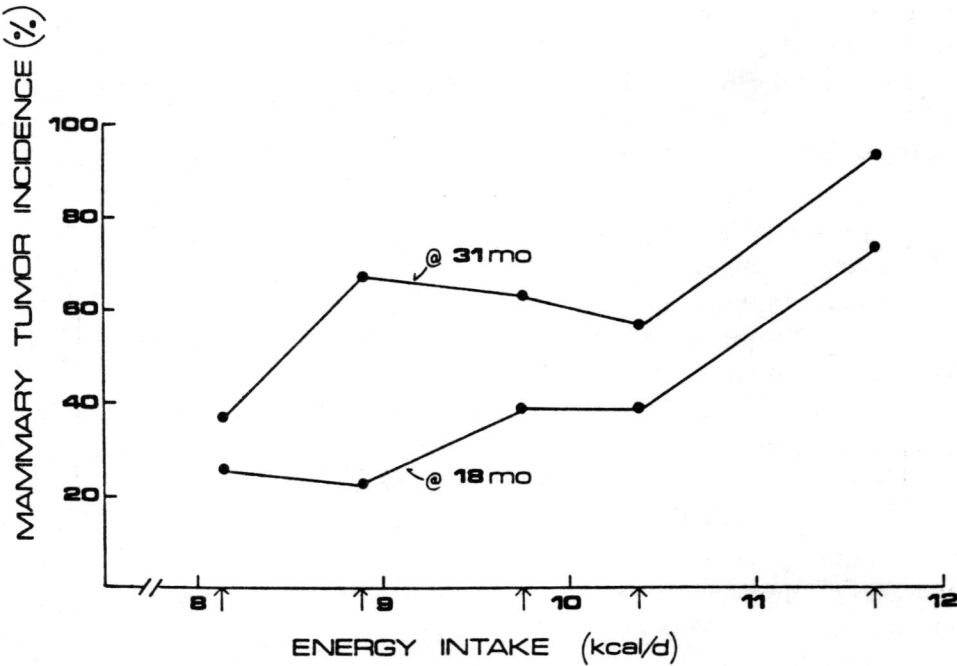

Figure 3.6. Mammary tumor incidence at 18 and 31 months of age in DBA mice fed at one of five levels (all less than ad lib) of energy. Diets were begun at 5 months of age. Redrawn from Tannenbaum (1945a).

Silverstone, 1950) showing that a regimen of intermittent fasting without an actual reduction in total food consumption, started in DBA mice at 8 months of age, failed to retard the development of mammary tumors. Regarding the effect of DR on pulmonary adenomas, not only was the incidence about halved, but the average size of the tumors reached only 70 percent of that found in ad lib fed mice.

The Phase II studies involving autoimmune mouse strains showed that ADR could retard the development of *ongoing* diseases. Mice from the B/WF$_1$ strain were started on DR at 4 to 5 months of age, by which time autoimmune disease is already underway in these strains, and examined at 9 months of age displayed lower levels of serum autoantibodies to DNA (40% of control values) and less severe renal disease as judged by light microscopy (mesangial changes, glomerular proliferation and basement membrane thickening, wire loops, hyalinization) and by immunofluorescent measure of renal immune complex deposition (Friend et al., 1978). Adult-onset DR appeared to ameliorate the course of this disease as well as EDR. In MRL mice, lymphoproliferative disease (Kubo et al., 1984a) and atherosclerosis (intrarenal and aortic branch arteries) (Mark et al., 1984a) were retarded by ADR.

Beach and colleagues' were primarily concerned with testing effects of marginal, moderate or severe dietary zinc deficiency on autoimmune nephropathy (Beach et al., 1981b) and anemia (Beach et al., 1982). Such diets were started at 6 weeks or 6 months of age. However, because "zinc restricted" mice eat only about 3.5 g/day, less than controls allowed a normal diet, additional control populations fed 3.5 g/day of a non-deficient diet were included. The DR was not severe, as BWs for the DR mice in both studies approached 40 g in late life, vs. 30-35 g for moderately and severely zinc deficient mice (Why the pair-fed DR mice outweighed their zinc deficient partners could not be explained.).

For the autoimmune NZB mice, EDR was less effective than early-onset, moderate or severe zinc deficiency in retarding anemia. In contrast, the moderate ADR (5-6 month onset) slowed the progression of anemia to an extent similar to that seen in mice switched to zinc deficient diets in adulthood. A recent report (Vruwink et al., 1987) from this group showed that very mild and late ADR (15% below ad lib intake, 6-8 month onset) imposed on NZB mice did not retard anemia and that zinc deficiency made it worse. Also, for B/WF$_1$ mice, EDR again failed to match the efficacy of early-onset zinc deficiency. Adult-onset DR retarded the development of nephropathy but less strongly than adult-onset zinc deficiency. How zinc deficiency works here is unknown but may have something to do with its essentiality for maintaining thymic-dependent immunocompetence.

Phase III studies included the effects of ADR on tumor development in long-lived mouse strains (for LS comparisons, see Table 2.6, #9). Table 3.10 summarizes tumor data obtained in male B10C3F$_1$ mice. The overall incidence of tumors was 87 percent for controls and 75 percent for ADR mice (p < .06). Lymphoma, pulmonary tumors and multiple tumors were less common in ADR mice but the differences were not statistically significant. Neither hepatoma incidence nor the average age of death for mice with hepatoma was influenced by diet. The average LSs for ADR mice with lymphoma, multiple tumors, or no tumors significantly exceeded those of controls in each category. And ten of the 14 longest lived ADR mice were tumor-free. Tumor status did not impact on the LS of controls.

TABLE 3.10

Tumor Incidence and Longevity in B10C3F$_1$ Mice Subjected to Dietary Restriction at 1 Year of Age[a]

Tumor	Incidence (%)		Average Age of Death (mo)	
	Control	ADR	Control	ADR
Hepatoma	43	40	34 ± 1	35 ± 1[d]
Lymphoma	47[b]	31	32 ± 1[c]	36 ± 1[d]
Lung	12	6	34 ± 2	39 ± 2
Multiple	16[b]	6	34 ± 1[c]	40 ± 2
No Tumor	13[b]	25	34 ± 2[c]	41 ± 1[d]

[a]Data are from 68 control and 67 ADR mice as adapted from Weindruch and Walford (1982). Values following the average age of death are SEM. Mice with multiple tumors bore two or more distinct tumor types at autopsy.

[b]These three comparisons between diet groups failed to attain statistical significance (P < .08) based on testing the significance of difference between two proportions.

[c]Significantly less than the value for mice on ADR (p < .01, two tailed t test).

[d]These comparisons between ADR mice grouped according to type of tumor were significantly different: no tumor > hepatoma (P < .001) and lymphoma (P < .01).

Based on data for mice dying after 22.5 months of age, ADR also lowered tumor incidence in B6 mice (Weindruch & Walford, 1982). Six of 23 ADR mice bore a tumor, compared with 9 of 17 controls. The most common tumor for the controls was lymphoma (8 of 9 tumors) whereas among the ADR group three mice with hepatomas, two with lung tumors, and one with lymphoma were encountered.

The findings of Cheney et al. (1983) on tumor patterns in female $B10C3F_1$ mice were previously examined (Table 3.6, Figure 3.5). The small number of ADR mice tested developed few tumors.

Collectively, these reports indicate that DR started on young adult or even middle-aged mice decreases the total incidence and either delays the age of onset or retards the rate of development of several important diseases associated with aging. The slowed progression obtains even for ongoing autoimmune diseases in short-lived mouse strains. For long-lived mouse strains, DR can be imposed on middle-aged animals and still retard certain tumors. These findings carry major implications for prevention and perhaps even treatment of human diseases.

INDUCED DISEASES

A substantial literature shows that rodents subjected to DR are more resistant to certain experimentally induced diseases than fully fed controls. Almost all studies have involved tumor induction and the control regimen has been ad lib feeding leading to rapid growth and, in some reports, frank obesity. These studies are important not only in modelling diseases but also in providing information on whole animal "toughness"—thereby differing from much of the work to be discussed in Chapter 4, where *in vitro* responses or organ system properties of diet-restricted and control animals are analyzed.

All but one investigation of DR in relation to induced diseases used mice or rats as the experimental animal. The rare exception was a study employing hamsters which found that DR (25% restriction) reduced epithelial thickness and mitotic index, and retarded DMBA carcinogenesis in the cheek pouch (Andreou & Morgan, 1981). Unlike most investigations of the effects of DR on rodent maladies, in the case of induced diseases study of the mouse came before the rat: 15 of the 20 reports on induced diseases in DR mice were published prior to 1950 whereas 15 of the 18 reports involving rats appeared in the 1980s. Except for the early work of Tannenbaum (1940), the effect of ADR on induced diseases has been largely unexplored.

Studies with Mice

Work originating with Moreschi (1909) and continued by Rous (1914) showed that severe underfeeding can retard the growth of transplanted tumors. Extending these observations, Bischoff et al. (1935) showed that mice subjected to 50 percent restriction of a "calf meal" diet supported slower growth of "sarcoma 180" transplants over a 15 day period. Twenty percent restriction was ineffective. It was next shown that the slower growth reflected caloric restriction *per se* rather than deficiency of other nutrients (Bischoff et al., 1938). In very short term studies (usual duration less than 1 month), it was also demonstrated that severely underfed mice outlive controls after inoculation with various mouse leukemias (Flory et al., 1943). Rare DR studies of that era not concerned with tumors were those of Foster et al. (1944a & b): DR at about half of ad lib intake increased the resistance of mice against developing paralysis and dying after polio virus injection.

We know of ten reports published during the 1940's on induced tumors in mice on EDR. These are summarized in Table 3.11. Most of the work involved benzpyrene-induced skin tumors. The Table's main message is clear: *every* study found that tumor incidence was reduced and/or the onset delayed by DR. More specific information can be set forth in the form of four questions.

What is the Relationship Between the Severity of DR and Induced Tumor Incidence and Time of Onset?

Two studies (#5 & 9) addressed this question, each testing several levels of DR. (For each study the table only gives data for the most severely underfed cohort plus the fully fed controls.) In both studies, increasing food intake was associated with earlier occurrence and higher incidence of skin tumors. Figure 3.7 presents data from study #5, plotting tumor incidence against daily energy intake. A rapid ascent to earlier onsets and higher incidences occurred for intakes greater than 9.6 kcal/day. Mice fed 8.1 kcal/day did not differ in tumor patterns from those fed 8.9 kcal/day but both groups were clearly more resistant than ice fed 9.6 kcal/day. A comparison of Figures 3.6 and 3.7 reveals similar overall quantitative effects of DR on both spontaneous and induced tumors. In both models, intakes at or below 9.6 kcal/day were sufficient to strongly delay the time of tumor onset, but more severe DR was required to lower the final tumor incidence.

TABLE 3.11

Induced Tumors in DR Mice: Studies Reported in the 1940's[a]

Tumor	Study[b]	Strain	DR[c]	Carc.[d]	End[e]	%BW[f]	Inc.[g]	Onset[h]
Skin	1	ABC	4	4	22	47	19/44	—/11
	1	ABC	14	14	23	53	0/16	—/—
	1	Swiss	2	2	8	63	18/60	—/7
	2	DBA	2	3	16	66	22/65	—/7
	4	DBA	2	3	20	64	24/69	—/9
	5	DBA	2	3	15	62	71/95	11/5
	6	DBA	2	3	15	55	25/65	15/10
	7	Albino	3[c]	3	12	83	7/87	—/9
	9	C3H	2	3	15	54	6/43	—/10
	10	Rockland	3	3	9	62	48/87	NR
Sarcoma	1	B6	6	6	13	70	27/40	13/11
	2	B6	3	4	16	61	44/79	9/7
	8	Albino	4	6	12	67	62/90	10/9
Leukemia	3	DBA	1	1	LS	54	35/96	7/2

[a]All tumors were induced by benzpyrene except for studies #3 and #9 (methylcholanthrene) and #7 (UV light).

[b]References: (1) Tannenbaum (1940); (2) Tannenbaum (1942); (3) White et al. (1944); (4) Tannenbaum (1944); (5) Tannenbaum (1945a); (6) Tannenbaum (1945b); (7) Rusch et al. (1945a); (8) Rusch et al. (1945b); (9) Tannenbaum and Silverstone (1949); (10) Boutwell et al. (1949).

[c]Age (mo) when DR began. This was not reported in study #7 but was estimated based on 23 g mice entering the study.

[d]Age (mo) when carcinogen applied.

[e]Age (mo) when study ended. "LS" indicates that the mice lived out their LSs.

[f]BW (g) of DR mice as a percentage of the BW of controls.

[g]Incidence of tumor for DR group/incidence for control group. In those studies where various levels of DR were tested, values are for the most severely restricted group.

[h]Onset for DR group/onset for control group. Values give the age at which 25% of the group showed evidence of the disease. "—" indicates that a 25% incidence was not attained. In studies testing many levels of DR, data are from the most severely restricted group. NR, not reported.

Albanes (1987a) analyzed data from 82 cohorts described in 14 reports on induced and spontaneous tumors in DR mice. The average energy restriction was 29 percent below the ad lib level and this was associated with 42 percent fewer tumors in DR mice. Multivariate regression analysis showed that tumor incidence rose with calorie intake independently of fat intake.

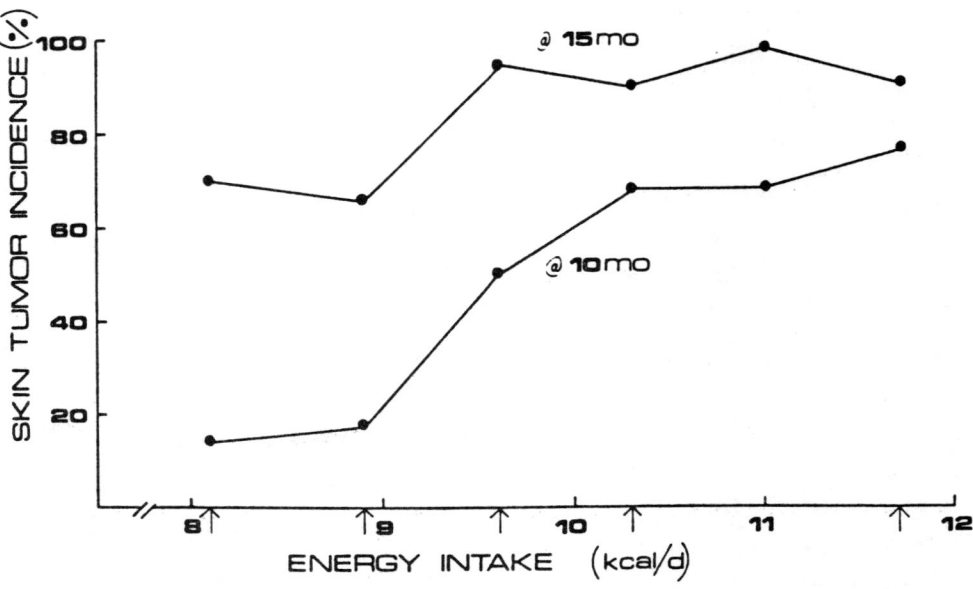

Figure 3.7. Benzpyrene-induced skin tumors at 10 and 15 months of age in DBA mice fed at one of six levels (all less than ad lib) of energy. The DR was started at 2 months of age and benzpyrene applied 1 month therafter. Redrawn from Tannenbaum (1945a).

Does DR Affect Tumor Initiation and/or Promotion?

Study #4 addressed this issue. One hundred 2 month old DBA males were fed normally and another hundred underfed until 5.5 months of age. Benzpyrene was applied twice weekly from 3 to 5.5 months of age, at which time each group was subdivided into normal and DR groups for the promotion period. The study ended at 20 months of age. Table 3.11 compares two of the four final groups: mice which were normally fed during initiation and promotion (N/N, final skin tumor incidence = 69%) and those always restricted (R/R, incidence = 24%). Since the incidence for N/R mice was low (34%) whereas that for R/N was higher (55%), initiation appears less sensitive to DR than does promotion.

Must DR be Started Early in Life to Retard Induced Tumors?

The oldest age at which DR was initiated was 14 months. This prevented skin tumors. Study #1 (Table 3.11) included a group of B6 mice started on ADR at 6 months of age. A mold inhibition of sarcomas was noted. In all other studies DR was started at 4 months or earlier in life.

A recently published abstract (Kritchevsky et al., 1987) describing DMBA-induced mammary tumors in young rats on DR (25% restriction) is relevant here. Calorie intake affected tumor promotion well after DMBA was administered. When DR was started two months post-DMBA, ongoing increases in palpable tumor incidence ceased within the first week and did not increase in the seven weeks thereafter. Conversely, switching a rat from DR to ad lib feeding at that time quickly stimulated tumor growth.

How Does the Quality of the DR Regimen Affect Induction of Tumors?

Four of the studies (#6, 7, 8 and 10) examined this question. In study #6, the inhibition of skin tumors was greater for mice energy-restricted only via carbohydrates than for those restricted in all components. This finding accords with our view that the strongest effects of DR follows the use of isonutrient diets.

A main question concerning diet quality is: How much does restriction of energy compared to restriction of fats contribute to lower incidence and later onset of induced tumors? This question has been the subject of many recent rat studies (see below). Studies #6, 7, 8, and 10 all found that at any given level of restricted energy intake, a high fat diet allowed more tumors than a low fat diet. Such observations have frequently led to the suggestion (often challenged) that dietary fats promote tumors. However, Boutwell et al. (1949) proposed that the higher *net energy value* of a high fat diet could account for its enhancement of carcinogenesis. This suggestion was based on earlier studies (Forbes et al., 1946) showing that as dietary fat increased, the amount of energy expended as heat decreases, so that more energy is retained by the carcass. This is not inconsistent with the notion that the mechanisms underlying DR's effect involve whole animal energy economy and/or metabolic efficiency (see *"Metabolic Efficiency and Energy Intake,"* Chapter 5).

A considerable gap in time separates the above-outlined 1940's work on induced tumors in DR mice from the next series of investigations, which did not occur until the 1980s. All six of these recent studies are summarized in Table 3.12. All involved EDR. In contrast to the heavy emphasis on skin tumors in the 1940s, these newer inquiries examined other models of induced disease. Generally the studies were of brief duration (exception: the radiation-induced leukemia study of Gross & Dreyfuss [#5]) and they reflected a primary interest in DR itself (exception: Beach and co-workers [#1] again used DR mice as inanition controls for mice who ate less when fed a zinc deficient diet).

TABLE 3.12

Induced Diseases in DR Mice: Studies of the 1980's

Study[a]	Disease[b]	Strain	DR[c]	Ind.[d]	End[e]	%BW[f]	Main Findings
1	sarcoma	BALB/c	2	2-4	3-5[e]	87	"Caloric restriction, as evidenced by inanition controls, caused markedly altered tumor incidence and kinetics, making it difficult to quantify those effects from those due to zinc deficiency."
2	cancer	Swiss	1	1	2-10[e]	45	"Calorie restriction at all levels tested (8, 6, 4 and 2 g/day/mouse) with standard pellatized mouse food produced both weight loss in the animals (with and without tumor) and a lowering of the growth rate of all 4 tumors tested growing at a subcutaneous site and/or under the kidney capsule."
3	diabetes	ob/ob	3-4	3-4	4-5	71	"Dietary restriction substantially reduced plasma gastric inhibitory peptide, insulin and glucose concentrations (up to 33%, 25% and 30% of control values respectively), but glucose reached the concentration observed in lean (+/+) mice."
4	melanoma	B6	3[c]	3.5	4.5	73	"Local tumor growth was found to be slower; however, survival after ip injection was no different and the number of pulmonary metastatic colonies after iv injection greater for the underfed mice."
5	leukemia	C3H(f)	3	1	LS	NR	"The fact that reduction of food intake may significantly decrease the incidence of leukemia, and therefore presumably prevent virus activation, is of considerable interest and may have important implications."

TABLE 3.12

(Continued)

Study[a]	Disease[b]	Strain	DR[c]	Ind.[d]	End[e]	%BW[f]	Main Findings
6	hepatocarcinoma	Swiss	1	0	8	60	"The results clearly show that restriction of food intake inhibits promotion and progression of induced liver tumors."

[a]References: (1) Beach et al. (1981a); (2) Giovanella et al. (1982); (3) Flatt et al. (1985); (4) Ershler et al. (1986); (5) Gross and Dreyfuss (1986); (6) Lagopoulos and Stadler (1987).

[b]The diseases were induced as follows. In study #1, the mice were injected with the Moloney sarcoma virus. Study #2 injected mice with cells from malignant human tumor lines. In #3, the mice were fed a savory "cafeteria" diet. Study #4 injected mice with cells from a murine melanoma line. The tumors in studies #5 and 6 were induced by gamma irradiation and a chemical, respectively.

[c]Age in months when DR was started. In study #4, this was not reported and a crude estimate is given based on 24 g mice entering the study.

[d]Age in months when the disease was induced.

[e]Age in months when study ended. For #1, mice were observed for 1 month after innoculation with virus. In study #2, four tumors were studied and the end points of each study varied.

Study #5 (Table 3.12) subjected young mice of both sexes to five consecutive weekly doses of gamma irradiation before instituting DR. Radiation-induced leukemia caused by a transmissible C type virus was monitored (Spontaneous leukemia is rare in this strain.). The study was terminated when the surviving mice were 9 to 14 months old, by which time leukemia incidence was 51 percent for ad lib fed mice (n = 108) vs. 3 percent for DR mice (n = 91). The authors do report an observation which is atypical for modern DR work, excess early mortality in DR mice. This was attributed to infection or cannibalism. The former could stem from malnutrition (from feeding a NPD on a restricted basis). The latter is entirely avoidable by individual housing.

In an extension of the earliest experiments on tumor induction in DR animals, three studies (#1, 2, 4) examined transplanted tumor growth in mice on short-term DR. With such DR, the sarcomas of study #1 regressed whereas the injected human (#2) and mouse (#4) melanomas killed the hosts. Despite slowing tumor growth, DR did not increase survival in any of these studies. Pulmonary metastases *increased* with DR in #4, leading the authors to conclude that the "commonly espoused opinion that moderate calorie restriction benefits physiological homeostasis may need to be reevaluated when one considers tumor-bearing hosts." However, this conclusion must be rejected. The mice were on DR (eating Purina Lab Chow™) for *only 2 weeks* before being injected with B16 melanoma cells under conditions which killed all mice by 30 days thereafter. Thus, the study involved short-term DR using a less than optimal diet regimen fed to mice fighting an aggressive experimental insult. The authors' conclusion would only be tenable if long-term DR via isonutrient diets failed to influence metastasis and survival.

In study #3 short-term DR, carried out by limiting the number of hours the mice fed, retarded the development of morbid obesity (final control BW = 86 g vs. 61 g for DR) and improved several glucoregulatory abnormalities, compared to controls freely fed either a standard diet or a cafeteria diet.

A recent report (Lagopoulos & Stadler, 1987) indicates that EDR (30% restriction) inhibits promotion of diethylnitrosamine-induced liver tumors in Swiss mice. At birth, a single injection of the carcinogen was given (with no more injected thereafter). At 8 months of age, hepatocarcinoma incidence was 100 percent for ad lib-fed mice versus 0 percent for DR mice (a 32% incidence of benign adenomas was reported for DR mice).

Studies with Rats

Dunning et al. (1949) described a delayed onset of diethylstilbestrol-induced mammary cancer in rats fed restricted diets. In 1951, Engel and Copeland reported that DR lowered mammary tumor incidence in rats fed 2-acetylaminofluorene. Both of these studies tested small numbers of restricted rats within ambitious experimental designs (6-8 diet groups/report). Engel and Copeland's result could be explained by the fact that *all* rats (including those eating less food!) ate a diet containing 0.03 percent (by weight) of 2-acetylaminofluorene. Thus, the DR rats ate less carcinogen. These two early studies provided little (if any) new information about DR.

Most of the newer work using rats on DR has involved chemically-induced tumors of the breast or colon. This work has gone in five directions.

Importance of Restriction of Dietary Energy vs. Fat in Inhibiting Chemical Tumorigenesis

This issue was the subject of at least seven recent reports (Kritchevsky et al., 1984 & 1986; Klurfeld et al., 1987a; Thompson et al.,

1985; Boissonneault et al., 1986; Beth et al., 1987; Ip & Sylvester, 1987). Most investigations involved mammary tumors. The studies have clarified the nutritional requisites for DR's inhibition of chemically-induced tumors. Also, the concept of net energy effects of dietary fat has received attention and is clearly important in relation to energy intake and flux in DR animals.

Testing the hypothesis that the enhanced mammary tumor formation in rats fed high-fat diets may be mediated chiefly or in part by an increased caloric intake, Kritchevsky et al. (1984) utilized three different types of dietary regimens (only one of which involved DR) in Sprague-Dawley rats. The carcinogen DMBA was given at 1.6 months of age, and the rats were followed until 4 to 6 months old. Several questions were asked. Does ad lib feeding of a high- vs. a low-fat diet before and/or after administration of DMBA differentially affect tumor incidence? What is the influence of ad lib feeding of a low-fat, high-calorie diet as opposed to a high-fat, low-calorie (high fiber) diet before and/or after giving the carcinogen? Does DR (60% of ad lib) imposed after DMBA still retard cancer even if carried out via a high-fat diet (such that DR rats ate less calories but more than twice the fat consumed by controls)?

The results of this study were striking: only DR completely prevented breast tumors, while the tumor incidence in nine other diet groups ranged from 33 to 67 percent. The high fat intake of the energy restricted rats did not lessen DR's inhibitory action. Clearly the caloric variable needs to be factored into studies of the effect of fat, including different types of fat, on tumor promotion. This variable has been relatively neglected by cancerologists and nutritionists (Cohen, 1987).

Kritchevsky et al. (1986) describe two series of experiments which serve to reinforce the above observations. In the first, rats were fed either a 4 percent corn oil diet ad lib, or a 13.1 percent corn oil diet at 60 percent of the ad lib level, and treated with DMBA. At 4 months post-DMBA, the incidence of mammary tumors was 80 percent for the ad lib, vs. 20 percent for the DR group. Similarly, the incidence of 1, 2-dimethylhydrazine-induced colon cancers was 100 percent for ad lib vs. 53 percent for DR rats at 5 months post-carcinogen. Dietary restriction reduced the number of tumors per tumor-bearing rat from 4 to 1 for breast tumors and from 3.5 to 2 for colon tumors. These same workers reported very similar findings elsewhere (Klurfeld et al., 1987a).

The second series of experiments examined DMBA-induced mammary tumors by feeding cohorts of rats 5, 15 or 20 percent corn oil diets on an ad lib basis, and 20 or 27 percent corn oil diets on a restricted (75% of ad lib energy intake) basis. The total fat intake of the 15 percent fat/ad lib group was the same as that of the 20 percent fat/DR group; and the intake of the 20 percent fat/ad lib group was the same as for the 27 percent fat/DR group. Tumor incidences and tumor yields (= total number of tumors produced) of the two DR groups were similar to the 5 percent fat/ad lib group and lower than those of the other two ad lib groups. Tumor "burden" (= total g of tumor) was about 50 percent lower in the DR rats than in the other groups. Thus, caloric restriction inhibited tumor growth even when the diet was high in fat, and of a type known to promote tumors (Cohen, 1987).

A similar result was reported by Thompson et al. (1985) who gave 1.6 month old Sprague-Dawley rats 1-methyl-1-nitrosourea and then fed PDs containing either 5 or 20 percent fat. For the next 4 months food intake was controlled such that each group ate the same amount of net utilizable energy (50-59 kcal/day). Then, over the next 4 months, the diets were fed ad libitum. During the period of restricted feeding, tumor incidence was not affected by diet. In contrast, the high fat diet produced more tumors than did the low fat diet during ad lib feeding. High fat diets appear capable of enhancing mammary tumorigenesis but only if fed at or near ad lib levels!

An important study, that of Boissonneault et al. (1986), concerned net energy effects of dietary fat on DMBA-induced mammary tumors in Fischer 344 rats, a strain generally not prone to obesity. Rats received ad lib a low fat (5% corn oil) diet until given DMBA at 1.7 months of age, whereupon three diet groups were set up: (1) *LF:* continued on the low fat diet ad lib; (2) *HF:* fed a high fat (30% corn oil) diet ad lib; and (3) HF-R: fed the high fat diet but in a restricted amount calculated to provide net energy equal to the group on LF. In actuality, the rats of the third group did not consume all of their allotment, and hence the "R" designation denotes net energy intake even lower than the LF group.

Table 3.13 shows food, fat and energy intakes as well as BW, carcass energy, and relative net dietary energy for these three groups. Although the HF-R group consumed less food and energy than the LF group, BWs were similar for these two, and carcass energies were higher for HF-R than for LF rats. This result accords with the view that high fat diets result in a greater efficiency of energy utilization. The calculation of net energy was based on an assumption dating to work by Forbes et al. (1946) that under isocaloric conditions a 30 percent fat diet is utilized

11 percent more efficiently than a 5 percent fat diet. Thus, the rats eating 40.8 kcal/day of HF would have the same net energy as others eating 45.3 kcal/day (= 40.8 × 1.1) of LF. Because the LF rats ate 42.2 kcal/day, the HF-R rats were provided with 38 kcal/day (= 42.2 ÷ 1.1) of the HF diet, in order to match net energy intakes. However, the actual intake for the HF-R group, since they did not consume their total allotment, was less, and averaged 34.1 kcal/day. The *relative net energy* values were calculated as the net energy of the diets of the HF or HF-R groups relative to the energy intake of the LF group (viewed as the control). Thus the relative net energy for HF was 45.3 ÷ 42.2, or 1.07; for the HF-R group, it was (34.1 × 1.11) ÷ 42.2, or 0.90.

TABLE 3.13

Relative Effects of Energy and Fat Intakes on Induced Mammary Tumors in Rats[a]

Parameter	High Fat	Low Fat	High Fat-DR
1. Food intake (g/d)	8.0	11.0	6.7
2. Energy intake (kcal/d)	41	42	34
3. Relative net energy	1.07	1.00	0.90
4. Fat net energy (g/d)	2.7	0.6	2.2
5. Carcass energy (kcal)	750	530	630
6. Body weight (g)	220	195	195
7. Body fat (%)	24	16	25
8. Tumor incidence (%)	73	43	7

[a]The high and low fat diets contained 30% and 5% corn oil. Relative net energy is calculated as the net energy of the diets consumed by the High Fat and High Fat-DR groups relative to that of the Low Fat group. Adapted from Boissonneault et al. (1986).

Tumor patterns were markedly influenced by these diets. Final incidences at about 8 months of age were about 70 percent for HF, 40 percent for LF, and 5 percent for HF-R. Other indicators of tumor development (e.g. tumor yield, number of tumors per rat) also showed clear inhibition by the HF-R diet. Tumor incidence was directly related to relative net energy (Figure 3.8). Thus, depending on calorie intake, rats could eat a high fat diet (60% of diet energy as fat via 2.2 g fat/day) and still develop fewer tumors than rats fed a low fat diet (10% of energy as fat, 0.6 g fat/day). Boissonneault et al. (1986) concluded that ". . . tumor appearance does not depend on the percent fat in the diet per se but

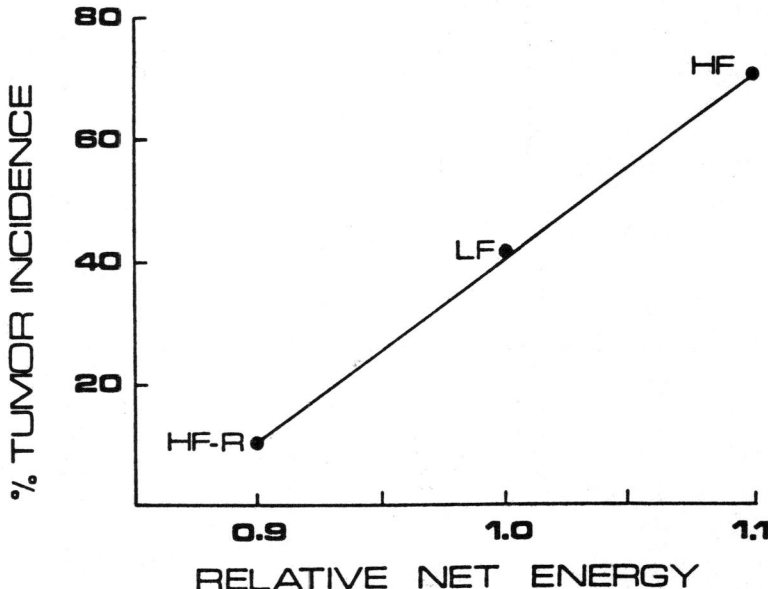

Figure 3.8. Correlation between the calculated relative net energy in the diet and the incidence of palpable DMBA-induced mammary tumors in Fischer 344 rats. Diets and DMBA commenced at 1.7 months of age. HF-R = high fat diet with restricted intake; LF = low fat diet ad lib; HF = high fat diet ad lib. Relative net energy values are the net energy of the HF and HF-R diets relative to the LF diet (see text). Incidence values are for 8 months of age. Redrawn from Boissonneault et al. (1986).

rather on a complex interaction involving energy intake, energy retention, and body size." In this sense, the dietary advice the American public is now receiving from the National Research Council, i.e. to lower fat intake from 42 to 30 percent of total calories, may be simplistic. For additional discussion of net dietary energy and induced tumors, see Pariza (1986).

Very recently, two other groups (Beth et al., 1987; Ip & Sylvester, 1987) also reported that caloric intake is a far more important factor than fat intake in affecting the growth of chemically-induced mammary tumors in rats. This once controversial issue appears settled.

Intestinal Tumorigenesis by Chemicals

Pollard's group at Notre Dame investigated intestinal tumors induced by methylazoxymethanol (MAM), which requires metabolic activation and produces mainly tumors of the small intestine, and by N-methylnitrosourea (MNU), a direct-acting carcinogen leading to colon cancer. Male Sprague-Dawley rats were subjected to EDR via a

NPD (75% of the ad lib level), or (in one study) by ad lib feeding every other day.

The first study (Pollard et al., 1984) showed that DR started ten days after administration of MAM lowered intestinal tumor incidence at day 140 below levels found either in ad lib controls, in rats fed ad lib EOD, or in rats placed on DR on day 63. The tumors ranged from superficial adenomas to adenocarcinomas.

The next study (Pollard & Luckert, 1985) found that DR lowered tumor incidence for MAM-induced but not for MNU-induced tumors in rats evaluated five months after the beginning of carcinogen and dietary treatments. Thus, the carcinogen which requires metabolic activation (MAM) was sensitive to DR while the direct acting carcinogen (MNU) was not. MAM is believed to be activated by alcohol dehydrogenase.

Colon carcinogenesis induced by azoxymethane (an indirect carcinogen) was also inhibited by imposing DR (30% restriction) on Fischer 344 rats (Reddy et al., 1987). The incidence and size of adenomas were sharply reduced and adenocarcinomas were totally prevented by DR. All rats ate a high (23.5%) fat diet.

Radiation-Induced Tumors

Gross and Dreyfuss (1984) studied tumor incidence in X-irradiated Sprague-Dawley rats fed normal or restricted diets in a fashion similar to that of their mouse study (Table 3.12, #5). The EDR was via a NPD (2 pellets/day) and was severe (33% ad lib intake: but recall that Sprague-Dawley rats become obese). All 14 female and 9 male rats fed ad lib developed tumors (including many fibroadenomas) at an average age of 13 months. For DR rats, only 9 of 29 females and 1 of 15 males developed tumors at an average age of 17 months. The suggestion was made that DR may prevent or delay the activation of oncogenic viruses.

In quite a differently oriented radiation study, Prabhu et al. (1978) examined the oral labial mucosa of black hooded male rats during a course of daily UV-irradiation. Dietary restriction was not the primary focus of the study, but rather was employed to produce a thinner lip epithelium in the hope that such would enhance tumor genesis, and yield an improved animal model for squamous cell carcinoma of the lip. Food restriction (a NPD at 50% of ad lib level) was instituted at 3 months of age. UV-irradiation was started after the DR rats had lost 15-20 percent of their BWs. Evidence of epithelial dysplasia was seen in the controls after 1 month of irradiation and increased over the next month whereas dysplasia was rare in DR rats. The mitotic index did not differ with diet until after 2 months of irradiation, at which time the value for DR rats was only 28 percent of controls. Thus DR rats showed less cell turnover following irradiation and this was associated with a decreased likelihood of dysplastic changes. The attempt to increase cancer via DR resulted in changes denoting inhibition.

Hormones and Cancer

Meites' group at Michigan State has studied the possible interplay between endocrine effects of shot-term DR (a NPD at 50% of ad lib level) and chemical carcinogenesis. Injecting 50 day old Sprague-Dawley females with DMBA, they followed the development of mammary tumors over a 6 month period (Sylvester et al., 1981). A 37 day DR regimen instituted 7 days prior to DMBA treatment and continued for 30 days thereafter, and followed by ad lib feeding, resulted in fewer and smaller tumors than occurred in controls fed ad lib thoughout. Food restriction markedly reduced prolactin levels. The benefits of DR were nullified by injecting the animals with estradiol benzoate 1 day prior to and 7 days after DMBA. These results were taken as support for the idea that DR may induce a hormonal deficiency state at the time of tumor initiation, which had lasting tumor inhibitory effects.

Diabetes

In a study by Krishnamacher and Canolty (1985), young male Sprague-Dawley rats made diabetic by streptozotocin injection were fed a PD at one of three energy intake levels (mild, moderate or severe DR) and followed over a 21 day priod. Serum glucose levels of the diabetic rats fell as energy intake decreased.

In conclusion, a number of induced diseases, mainly neoplasia, appear quite sensitive to inhibition by DR. Energy intake per se, and not specific nutrient levels, contributes most significantly to this effect. These models could now be used to clarify the ways by which DR produces these remarkable effects.

SUMMARY

As the food intake of rats and mice is reduced from ad lib levels, the onsets of a broad spectrum of spontaneous and induced diseases are delayed and their overall incidences reduced. As the severity of DR increases, so does the degree of disease inhibition. The evidence to support this assertion mostly concerns carcinogenesis, is long-standing, extensive, and largely descriptive. Both early- and adult-onset DR are effective, and the latter strategy has also been shown capable of retarding the progress of several ongoing diseases. So long as the DR is not accompanied by deficiency of essential nutrients (i.e., especially if isonutrient diets are employed) these beneficial effects can be achieved, as shown elsewhere in this book (Chapters 2 and 4) without sacrifice of any essential physiologic functions, and in fact with improvement in the large majority of functions so far measured.

CHAPTER 4

DIETARY RESTRICTION: EFFECTS ON BIOLOGICAL PARAMETERS

INTRODUCTION

IN ADDITION to LS extension and disease prevention and/or retardation, DR affects a great spectrum of biologic parameters. Certain of these may turn out to qualify as basic changes underlying DR's impact on LS and diseases. Again, the DR work is rodent-dominated with scant data on biological effects in lower animals (but see "STUDIES IN INVERTEBRATES," Chapter 2) and no more than indirect or inferential evidence for primates (see Chapter 6).

Here we review the rodent data, beginning at the molecular level, proceeding to the effects of DR on the immune system, then on a diverse set of other "physiologic" phenomena and finally to a consideration of how DR influences learning and behavior. Our focus is on *long-term* DR (defined here as at least 1 month of DR) via regimens proven or likely to extend maximum LS. The vast literature on starvation, short-term DR, ad lib low protein diets, and various forms of frank malnutrition may be referred to on occasion, but the focus is on proven (or probably) effective long-term DR regimens.

The biological parameters to be considered can be divided into those changing normally with age (which would include the "biomarkers" of aging) and those which do not change. Hopefully, future longitudinal aging studies will distinguish between those age-sensitive parameters which can predict subsequent LS (on the basis of multi-cause mortality, and not simply from increased risk to a specific disease), and those which cannot. For those parameters which change with age, "negative" (i.e., unchanged) findings in DR rodents may be as important as positive. Perhaps the animals would live still longer if DR-resistant parameters could be affected by other means. On the other hand, the lack of a DR effect on an age-sensitive index might signal that these "biomarkers" are noncausal in aging.

MOLECULAR PARAMETERS

Collagen

Collagen was the first molecular marker to be examined in DR rodents, coinciding with an early appreciation that with increasing age of the organism, collagen fibers become more stable to external influences (for review, see Balazs [1977]). Typically, a decline with age occurs in the amount of collagen extractable by salt solutions or acetic acid from most connective tissues. Also, old tissue is less flexible when mechanically stressed. The molecular basis for these changes apparently resides in the formation of cross-links between fibrils. The DR-collagen studies are "molecular" only in that inferences about a molecule were obtained; however, the data have been derived from non-molecular, "low-tech" methods.

Studies in young, growing guinea pigs by Gross (1958) evidenced a profound sensitivity of collagen formation to quantity of diet. Short term-DR or fasting reduced the amount of neutral-salt extractable collagen to very low levels. Two days of fasting halved the amount of extractable collagen. Short-term ad lib feeding brought a rapid return to pre-DR values.

The main findings on collagen in rodents on long-term DR are summarized in Table 4.1. Chvapil and Hruza (1959) found that low food intake retards collagen aging as judged by fibril contractility and relaxation properties. Later work showed that the breaking time of collagen fibrils increased with age and fell with DR. Everitt's data (1971, Figure 4.1) indicates that rats fed more than 15 g of food per day showed increasingly longer tail tendon breaking times than rats fed less. Some evidence (study #4) indicates that a lower tail temperature in DR rats may contribute to these findings. Harrison's group (#8, 9) has confirmed that DR retards collagen aging in mice. Study #9 is especially noteworthy in that a variety of potential biomarkers of aging were measured in DR and control mice (see "Other Physiologic Parameters," this Chapter). Molecular explanations of DR's affect on collagen aging have not been advanced.

TABLE 4.1
Effects of Dietary Restriction on Collagen Aging

Study[a]	Animal	Diet[b]	Effect of DR
1	Wistar rat	NPD[b]	"Younger tail coll. based on contractility/relaxation.
2	Wistar rat	NPD, IF	Same as above.
3	Wistar rat	NPD, 66% ad lib	↓ breaking time of tail coll. in 7M urea.
4	S-D rat	NPD, 9 g/day	Same as #1, but may be due to ↓ tail temperature.
5	Wistar rat	NPD, 3-21 g/day	Same as #3.
6	Wistar rat	NPD, 50% ad lib	Delayed accum. of coll. in lungs, liver, heart and kidneys.
7	Wistar rat	NPD, 50% ad lib	↑ % of skin coll. extractable by 6M urea after EDR (but not ADR).
8	B6 mouse	NPD, 66% ad lib	↓ tail coll. denat. time in +/+ and ob/ob.
9	B6, B6CBA mice	Same as #8	↓ tail coll. denat. time

[a]References: (1) Chvapil and Hruza (1959); (2) Chvapil and Holeckova (1962); (3) Giles and Everitt (1967); (4) Hruza and Hlavackova (1969); (5) Everitt (1971); (6) Deyl et al. (1971); (7) Svojtkova et al. (1972); (8) Harrison et al. (1984); (9) Harrison and Archer (1987a).

[b]Abbreviations: coll., collagen; denat., denaturation; IF, intermittent feeding; ↑, increase; ↓, decrease. In #1, food intake was not reported.

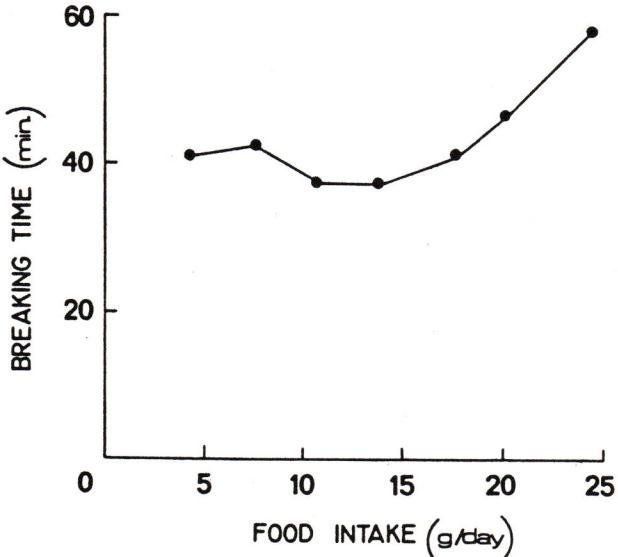

Figure 4.1. Effect of food intake on the breaking time of tail tendon fibers from 10 month old Wistar rats. Data give breaking time in 7M urea for fibers from rats maintained at different food intake levels for 9 months. Adapted from Everitt (1971).

Enzymes and Metabolites

Does LS-prolonging DR affect the activities of certain enzymes and the levels of key metabolites? While a substantial literature describes effects of various types of restricted feeding on these parameters, most of it deals with very short-term studies, e.g. starving a rat or mouse for a day or two and assaying liver enzyme activities. Much less is known about long-term DR regimens which slow aging. We will discuss the long-term data in an organ-by-organ fashion. A brief discussion of fasting and short-term DR results follows.

Our organization of the enzyme data is patterned after that of Wilson's careful review of the largely conflicting information on age changes in mammalian enzyme activities (Wilson, 1981). She enumerates pitfalls which threaten any combined analysis of biochemical data from many different laboratories. In terms of the present discussion, one must consider possible differences due to: animal age, sex, species or strain; tissue preparation and media; nature of the DR regimen and the possibility of malnutrition. Regarding tissue preparation, most of the DR investigations, but excepting those on xenobiotic-metabolizing enzymes (which generally use microsomal fractions), deal with whole homogenates of organs. The latter sometimes contain interfering molecules (inhibitors, activators, cofactors).

Another concern is whether it is best to express data on enzyme activity or metabolite content on the basis of protein content, wet weight, tissue nitrogen, or DNA in animals differing in body size and composition. This problem of appropriateness of reference base appears repeatedly in DR studies (e.g. with metabolic rate measurements).

A final and perhaps most serious concern is that none of the studies have taken into account the important work of Adelman and colleagues (Adelman, 1975), to the effect that aging, and very likely DR, may affect induction time, level reached, and overall kinetics of enzyme activities. One-shot determination of basal activity level (which most of the DR enzyme work has been) may present a very incomplete, even misleading picture.

Long-Term DR

Table 4.2 summarizes enzyme activities and metabolite levels as reported in 23 long-term DR investigations. The data are alphabetized by tissue of origin. Except for one rabbit study (reference #20), all work involved either rats or mice. Only 6 reports (references #6, 7, 10, 13, 14,

17) used DR regimens proven in that particular animal colony to extend maximum LS. Seven studies (references #5, 7, 10, 13, 14, 21, 23) employed vitamin- and mineral-enriched diets. About half the data concern liver, with less information available on brain, kidney and skeletal muscle. Little is known in terms of DR about complex metabolic pathways. Enzymes in adipose tissue, heart, intestine and spleen have been little studied in DR animals. We could find no data pertaining to any tissue not in Table 4.2.

(1) Data on *adipose tissue* are scant. Activities of NADPH generating enzymes in adipose tissue were *markedly* increased by a 1.6 month period of EDR (50% restriction) imposed on Sprague-Dawley rats (see Table 4.2 for references). The investigators stated that activities of these enzymes typically rise with anabolic processes which consume NADPH (e.g. lipogenesis), and fall with starvation. A relationship between the rise in activity levels for these enzymes and for xenobiotic-metabolizing enzymes was emphasized. Another study indicated that adipocyte lipoprotein lipase activity falls sharply with DR.

(2) Data on enzymes in the "DR *brain*" are also sparse, a notable knowledge gap. Brain homogenates from DR mice showed lower than control activities of lysosomal enzymes and of SOD (references #3, 4). London et al. (1985) studied three enzymes reported to show age-related changes in rat brain which are known to reflect the integrity of cholinergic, gamma-aminobutyric acid-ergic, and catecholaminergic neurons. The analysis was conducted region-by-region (cerebral cortex, cerebellum, hippocampus, and striatum) on brains from 6 and 24 month old animals on control and DR diets, and from 30 month old animals on DR. Choline acetyltransferase activity fell with aging but less so in 24 month old DR rats than in controls. Rats on DR showed higher activities in all regions except the cerebral cortex. Cholinergic function did not increase after a 2 week DR regimen.

(3) The effect of DR on enzymes and metabolites in *heart* muscle is nearly unstudied (see Table 4.2).

(4) Analysis of *intestinal* homogenates from DR mice revealed lower activities for two lysosomal enzymes when feeding was at 50 percent of ad lib; moreover, the same research group found that ad lib feeding of a 6 percent protein diet (which also slowed growth) did not influence activities of the enzymes (reference #3). Shao et al. (1987) reported in a recent abstract that intestinal alkaline phosphatase activity falls with age in ad lib fed NZB and B/WF$_1$ females, and that DR retards this change.

TABLE 4.2
Influences of Long-Term Dietary Restriction on Enzyme Activities and on Levels of Metabolites[a]

Tissue	Function	Enz. or Metabolite[b]	Species	Activity[c]	Tissue Prep.[d]	Nature of DR[e] Diet	%AL	DUR	Effect[f]	Ref.[g]
ADIPOSE	NADPH generation	G-6-PDH	rat	protein	1,000g inf.	PD	50	1.6	1440%	2
		6-PGDH	rat	protein	1,000g inf.	PD	50	1.6	1295%	2
		malic enzyme	rat	protein	1,000g inf.	PD	50	1.6	1339%	2
	Lipolysis	lipoprotein lipase	rat	wet wt.	tis. powder[d]	PD	60	4	164%	21
BRAIN										
Whole Brain	Citrate cycle	malic DH	mouse	DNA	homogenate	PD	70[e]	24	NSD	19
	Respiratory	cytochrome c oxidase	mouse	protein	mitochondria	PD	40	4	NSD	13
	Hydrolytic	acid phosphatase	mouse	protein	mitochondria	PD	?[e]	9	126%	3
		acid phosphatase	mouse	protein	mitochondria	PD	50	9	128%	4
	degradative	cathepsin	mouse	protein	mitochondria	PD	?[e]	9	138%	3
		cathepsin	mouse	protein	mitochondria	PD	50	9	139%	4
	Radical Scavenging	SOD	mouse	wet wt.	post-mito sup.	PD	50	12	122%	4
Cerebral Cortex	Neurotransmission	choline acetyltransferase	rat	protein	sonicate	NPD	62	23	NSD	17
	Neurotransmission	L-glutamic acid DC	rat	protein	sonicate	NPD	62	23	NSD	17
	Neurotransmission	tyrosine hydroxylase	rat	protein	14,000g sup.	NPD	62	23	155%	17
Cerebellum	Neurotransmission	choline acetyltransferase	rat	protein	sonicate	NPD	62	23	NSD	17
	Neurotransmission	L-glutamic acid DC	rat	protein	sonicate	NPD	62	23	NSD	17
	Neurotransmission	tyrosine hydroxylase	rat	protein	14,000g sup.	NPD	62	23	NSD	17
Hippocampus	Neurotransmission	choline acetyltransferase	rat	protein	sonicate	NPD	62	23	145%	17
	Neurotransmission	L-glutamic acid DC	rat	protein	sonicate	NPD	62	23	NSD	17
	Neurotransmission	tyrosine hydroxylase	rat	protein	14,000g sup.	NPD	62	23	NSD	17
Striatum	Neurotransmission	choline acetyltransferase	rat	protein	sonicate	NPD	62	23	133%	17
	Neurotransmission	L-glutamic acid DC	rat	protein	sonicate	NPD	62	23	NSD	17
	Neurotransmission	tyrosine hydroxylase	rat	protein	14,000g sup.	NPD	62	23	NSD	17
HEART	Citrate cycle	malic DH	mouse	DNA	homogenate	PD	70[e]	32	NSD	19
INTESTINE	Hydrolytic degrad.	acid phosphatase	mouse	protein	homogenate	PD	?[e]	9	NSD	3
		acid phosphatase	mouse	protein	homogenate	PD	50	9	127%	4
		cathepsin	mouse	protein	homogenate	PD	?[e]	9	NSD	3
		cathepsin	mouse	protein	homogenate	PD	50	9	133%	4

TABLE 4.2
(Continued)

Tissue	Function	Enz. or Metabolite[b]	Species	Activity[c]	Tissue Prep.[d]	Nature of DR[e] Diet	%AL	DUR	Effect[f]	Ref.[g]
KIDNEY	Respiratory citrate cycle	ATPase	rat	protein	NR	PD	50	2	NSD	12
		succinate DH	rat	wet wt.	homogenate	NPD	50	2.5	NSD	15
		succinate DH	rat	wet wt.	homogenate	NPD	50	3.2	NSD	16
		succinate DH	mouse	wet wt.	homogenate	PD	65[e]	6	↑110%[f]	18
		succinate DH	mouse	wet wt.	homogenate	PD	85[e]	5	NSD	18
		succinate DH	mouse	DNA	homogenate	PD	70[e]	32	↑24%	19
		malic DH	mouse	wet wt.	homogenate	PD	85[e]	6	NSD	18
		malic DH	mouse	wet wt.	homogenate	PD	85[e]	5	NSD	18
		malic DH	mouse	DNA	homogenate	NPD	70[e]	32	NSD	19
	Hydrolytic degr.	alkaline phosphatase	rat	wet wt.	homogenate	NPD	50	2.5	↑28%	15
		alkaline phosphatase	rat	wet wt.	homogenate	NPD	50	3.2	↑22%	16
	Protein metab.	amino acid oxidase	rat	wet wt.	homogenate	PD	50	2.5	NSD	15
		cathepsin	mouse	DNA	homogenate	PD	70[e]	32	↑34%	19
LIVER	Carbohydrate metab.	glucokinase	rat	wet wt.	homogenate	NPD	60[e]	20	NSD	11
		glucokinase	rat	protein	cytosol	PD	60	6	↓?[f]	23
	Glycolysis	phosphofructokinase	rat	wet wt.	homogenate	NPD	60[e]	20	NSD	11
		aldolase	mouse	DNA	homogenate	PD	70[e]	29	↑28%	19
	Hexose shunt	G-6-PDH + 6-PGDH	rat	protein	cytosol	PD	55	1	↑110%	1
		G-6-PDH	rat	protein	15,000g sup.	PD	50	1.6	↑97%	2
		G-6-PDH	rat	protein	100,000g sup.	PD	70	14.5	NSD	22[a]
		G-6-PDH	rat	protein	100,000g sup.	PD	60	6	↑44%	23
		6-phosphogluconate DH	rat	protein	100,000g sup.	PD	70	14.5	NSD	22[a]
		6-PGDH	rat	protein	15,000g sup.	PD	50	1.6	↑99%	2
	NADPH generation	malic enzyme	rat	protein	cytosol	PD	55	1	↑60%	1
		malic enzyme	rat	protein	15,000g sup.	PD	50	1.6	↑79%	2
		malic enzyme	rat	protein	100,000g sup.	PD	70	14.5	NSD	22[a]
		malic enzyme	rat	protein	cytosol	PD	60	6	↑41%	23
	Citrate cycle	malic DH	rat	protein	15,000g sup.	PD	50	1.6	NSD	2
		malic DH	mouse	protein	homogenate	PD	65[e]	6	NSD	18
		malic DH	mouse	protein	homogenate	PD	85[e]	5	NSD	18
		malic DH	mouse	DNA	homogenate	PD	70	33	↑24%	19

TABLE 4.2
(Continued)

Tissue	Function	Enz. or Metabolite[b]	Species	Activity[c]	Tissue Prep.[d]	Nature of DR[e] Diet	%AL	DUR	Effect[f]	Ref.[g]
		isocitrate DH	rat	wet wt.	15,000g sup.	PD	50	1.6	NSD	2
		isocitrate DH	rat	wet wt.	homogenate	NPD	60[e]	20	NSD	11
		citrate synthase	rat	wet wt.	homogenate	NPD	60[e]	20	120%	11
		a-ketoglutarate DH	rat	wet wt.	homogenate	NPD	60[e]	20	120%	11
		succinate DH	rat	wet wt.	homogenate	NPD	50	2.5	132%	15
		succinate DH	rat	wet wt.	homogenate	NPD	50	3.2	136%	16
		succinate DH	mouse	wet wt.	homogenate	PD	65[e]	6	126%[f]	18
		succinate DH	mouse	wet wt.	homogenate	PD	85[e]	5	NSD	18
		succinate DH	mouse	DNA	homogenate	PD	70[e]	33	157%	19
	Respiratory	Cyt. c oxidase activity	rat	wet wt.	homogenate	PD	60[e]	20	130%	11
		Cyt. c oxidase activity	mouse	wet wt.	mitochondria	PD	40	4	125%[f]	13
		Cyt. c content	rat	wet wt.	homogenate	NPD	60[e]	20	120%	11
		Cyt. $a+a_3$ content	rat	wet wt.	homogenate	NPD	60[e]	20	120%	11
		ATPase	rat	protein	NR	PD	50	2	135%	12
		ATPase	rat	nitrogen	homogenate	PD	39	33	18%	10
	Metabolic regulation	adenylate cyclase	rat	protein	homogenate	PD	60	23	130%	7
	Beta-oxidation	3-hydroxyacyl-CoA DH	rat	wet wt.	homogenate	NPD	60[e]	20	NSD[f]	11
		palmitoyl CoA oxidation	mouse	protein	600g sup.	PD	50	11	NSD[f]	14
	Protein metab.	glutamic-pyruvate TA	rat	protein	15,000g sup.	PD	50	1.6	NSD	2
		glutamic-oxaloacetic TA	rat	protein	15,000g sup.	PD	50	1.6	NSD	2
		histidase	rat	nitrogen	homogenate	PD	39	33	135%	10
		amino acid oxidase	rat	wet wt.	homogenate	PD	50	2.5	135%	15
		tryptophane oxygenase	rat	nitrogen	homogenate	PD	50	1.5	NSD	9
		quinolate PRT	rat	protein	homogenate	PD	50	1.5	141%	9
		nicotinate PRT	rat	protein	homogenate	PD	50	1.5	157%	9
		nicotinamide nucs.	rat	wet wt.	homogenate	PD	50	1.5	153%	9
		picolinate carboxylase	rat	wet wt.	homogenate	PD	50	1.5	115%	9
	Purine catabolism	xanthine oxidase	mouse	protein	cytosol	PD	50	23	NSD[f]	14
		xanthine DH	mouse	protein	cytosol	PD	50	23	144%[f]	14
	Lipid synth.	3HMG-CoA reductase	rat	protein	microsomes	PD	60	23	157%	7
		acetyl-CoA carboxylase	rat	protein	100,000g sup.	PD	70	14.5	NSD	22[a]

TABLE 4.2
(Continued)

Tissue	Function	Enz. or Metabolite[b]	Species	Activity[c]	Tissue Prep.[d]	Nature of DR[e]			Effect[f]	Ref.[g]
						Diet	%AL	DUR		
	Xenobiotic metab.	fatty acid synthase	rat	protein	100,000g sup.	PD	70	14.5	NSD	22[a]
		aniline hydroxylase	rat	wet wt.	microsomes	PD	55	1	142%	1
		PCMA-N-demethylase	rat	wet wt.	microsomes	PD	55	1	173%	1
		p-nitrobenzoate reductase	rat	wet wt.	microsomes	PD	55	1	131%	1
		cytochrome P-450 content	rat	wet wt.	microsomes	PD	55	1	138%	1
		cytochrome P-450 content	rat	protein	microsomes	NPD	50	1.5	117%[f]	8
		cytochrome P-450 content	mouse	protein	microsomes	PD	50	23	NSD[f]	14
		cytochrome P-450 content	rabbit	protein	microsomes	NPD	50	5	144%	20
		cytochrome C reductase	mouse	protein	microsomes	PD	50	23	NSD[f]	14
		cytochrome C reductase	mouse	protein	microsomes	PD	70[e]	28	194%	19
		aryl hydrocarbon hydroxylase	mouse	protein	microsomes	PD	50	23	NSD[f]	14
		7-ethoxycoumarin 0-deethylase	mouse	protein	microsomes	PD	50	23	136%[f]	14
		p-nitroanisole	mouse	protein	microsomes	PD	50	23	NSD[f]	14
		aminopyrene N-demethylase	rat	protein	microsomes	NPD	50	1.5	113%[f]	8
		acetanilide hydroxylase	rat	protein	microsomes	NPD	50	1.5	148%[f]	8
		glutathione-S-transferase	rat	protein	cytosol	NPD	50	1.5	116%	8
		glutathione-S-transferase	mouse	protein	cytosol	PD	50	23	NSD[f]	14
		epoxide hydrolase	mouse	protein	cytosol	PD	50	23	NSD[f]	14
		malathion carboxylesterase	mouse	protein	microsomes	PD	50	23	NSD[f]	14
		biphenyl-4 hydroxylase	rat	wet wt.	10,000g sup.	PD	50	1.6	155%	2
		4-MUG-transferase	rat	wet wt.	10,000g sup.	PD	50	1.6	120%	2
		p-nitrobenzoate reductase	rat	wet wt.	10,000g sup.	PD	50	1.6	121%	2
		ethylmorphine N-demethylase	mouse	DNA	homogenate	PD	70[e]	28	1210%	19
		glucuronyl transferase	rabbit	protein	microsomes	NPD	50	5	133%	20
		sulfuryl transferase	rabbit	protein	microsomes	NPD	50	5	NSD	20

TABLE 4.2
(Continued)

Tissue	Function	Enz. or Metabolite[b]	Species	Activity[c]	Tissue Prep.[d]	Diet	Nature of DR[e] %AL	DUR	Effect[f]	Ref.[g]
	Hydrolytic degradative	acid phosphatase	mouse	protein	homogenate	PD	?[e]	9	131%	3
		acid phosphatase	mouse	protein	homogenate	PD	50	9	141%	4
		acid phosphatase	rat	protein	homogenate	PD	50	7	NSD	5
		alkaline phosphatase	rat	nitrogen	homogenate	PD	39	33	1111%	10
		alkaline phosphatase	rat	wet wt.	homogenate	NPD	50	2.5	NSD	15
		alkaline phosphatase	rat	wet wt.	homogenate	NPD	50	3.2	NSD	16
		cathepsin	mouse	protein	homogenate	PD	?[e]	9	NSD	3
		cathepsin	mouse	protein	homogenate	PD	50	9	133%	4
		cathepsin	rat	protein	homogenate	PD	50	7	NSD	5
		B-galactosidase	rat	protein	homogenate	PD	50	7	NSD	5
		arylsulphatase	rat	protein	homogenate	PD	50	7	152%	5
	Neurotransmission	cholinesterase	mouse	wet wt.	homogenate	PD	65[e]	6	NSD	18
		cholinesterase	mouse	DNA	homogenate	PD	70[e]	33	121%	19
	Radical scavenging	SOD	mouse	wet wt.	post-mito. sup.	PD	?[e]	9	189%	3
		SOD	mouse	wet wt.	post-mito. sup.	PD	50	12	119%	4
		SOD	rat	NR	specific mRNA in nuclei	NR	60	35	175%[f]	6
		SOD	mouse	protein	600g sup.	PD	50	23	NSD[f]	14
		catalase	rat	NR	specific mRNA in nuclei	NR	60	35	150%[f]	6
		catalase	rat	nitrogen	homogenate	PD	39	33	118%	10
		catalase	mouse	protein	600g sup.	PD	50	23	164%[f]	14
		glutathione peroxidase	mouse	protein	600g sup.	PD	50	11	NSD[f]	14
MUSCLE										
Gastrocnemius	Carbohydrate metab.	glucokinase	rat	wet wt.	3500rpm sup.	NPD	60[e]	20	NSD	11
	Glycolysis	phosphofructokinase	rat	wet wt.	3500rpm sup.	NPD	60[e]	20	NSD	11
	Citrate cycle	isocitrate DH	rat	wet wt.	3500rpm sup.	NPD	60[e]	20	NSD	11
		citrate synthase	rat	wet wt.	3500rpm sup.	NPD	60[e]	20	NSD	11
		a-ketoglutarate DH	rat	wet wt.	3500rpm sup.	NPD	60[e]	20	NSD	11

TABLE 4.2
(Continued)

Tissue	Function	Enz. or Metabolite[b]	Species	Activity[c]	Tissue Prep.[d]	Nature of DR[e] Diet	% AL	DUR	Effect[f]	Ref.[g]
	Respiratory	Cyt. c oxidase activity	rat	wet wt.	3500rpm sup.	NPD	60[e]	20	NSD	11
		Cyt. c content	rat	wet wt.	3500rpm sup.	NPD	60[e]	20	NSD	11
		Cyt. $a+a_3$ content	rat	wet wt.	3500rpm sup.	NPD	60[e]	20	NSD	11
	Beta-oxidation	3-hydroxyacyl-CoA DH	rat	wet wt.	3500rpm sup.	NPD	60[e]	20	NSD	11
"Thigh"	Respiratory	ATPase	rat	protein	NR	NPD	50	2	NSD	12
SPLEEN	Citrate cycle	malic DH	mouse	DNA	homogenate	PD	79[e]	24	134%	19

[a]Feeding started before 3 months of age except for #11 (10 mo), #16 (12 mo), #18 (17 mo), #21 (16 mo) (others started on DR when weaned). In #22, both obese and lean Zucker rats were studied. The values above are for the lean rats.
[b]Abbreviations: G-6-PDH = glucose-6-phosphate dehydrogenase; 6-PGDH = 6-phosphogluconate dehydrogenase; SOD = superoxide dismutase; PCMA = p-chloromethylaniline; MUG = methylumbelliferone glucuronyl; 3-HMG-CoA reductase = 3-hydroxy-3-methylglutaryl coenzyme A reductase; TA- = transaminase; DC = decarboxylase.
[c]Indicates the basis of expression of specific activity.
[d]Indicates how the tissue was prepared for study. inf. = Infranatant; sup. = supernatant; tis. = tissue (in #21 the epidymal fat pad was delipidated and enzyme activity measured in acetone-ether powders).
[e]"% AL" is the percent of the ad lib intake level fed to rodents on DR. "DUR" is the duration of DR in months. In study #3, a 6% protein diet was fed ad lib to female Swiss mice. Body weights were 30% less than for controls fed a 24% protein diet after 3 months of weaning-onset feeding but were not different at 9 months of age. Study #11 reports that the DR rats were "...permitted free access to food but on alternate days or about 60% of the amount consumed by *ad libitum* fed rats." A 40% drop in food intake does not typically follow EOD feeding and appears more unlikely in that BWs of DR mice were 77-86% those of controls at 18, 24 or 30 months of age. Influences of this regimen on LS were not reported. Mice were also restricted via an EOD protocol in study #18. DR started at either weaning and lasted 6 months or started at 17 months and lasted 5 months. Food intakes and LSs were not reported but BWs suggest significant DR occurred. In study #19, EOD feeding from weaning of B6D2F$_1$ male mice led to a 30% drop in food intake and improved survivorship at 32 months (30% of controls living vs. 63% of the EOD group). The lack of maximum LS data here make it difficult to evaluate the efficacy of this EOD regimen.
[f]Indicates the effect of DR relative to the control group. Study #6 was reported as a meeting abstract and the authors state that the DR data are preliminary. Note that this study differs from the others in that enzyme activities per se were not measured but rather specific mRNA levels coding for the enzymes. For study #8 the data listed are for males. Females responded oppositely (*dex.* in P-450 content and all enzyme activities except glutathione-S-transferase [which fell with DR in both sexes]). Our work (#13, 14) did not use ad lib fed controls but rather mice fed 75% of the ad lib level. In study #18 the higher succinate DH activity for restricted mice was only observed when the DR mice were killed after fasting 24 hours. In study #23, glucokinase was not detectable in samples from DR rats but was readily measured in control cytosol fractions.
[g]References: (1) Sachan (1982); (2) Sachan and Das (1982); (3) De et al. (1983); (4) Chipalkatti et al. (1983); (5) Solomon et al. (1984); (6) Richardson et al. (1987a); (7) Yu et al. (1984a); (8) Hasmi et al. (1986); (9) Satyanarayana and Rao (1977); (10) Ross (1969); (11) Rumsey et al. (1987); (12) Mohan and Rao (1985a); (13) Weindruch et al. (1980); (14) Koizumi et al. (1987a); (15) Barrows et al. (1965); (16) Barrows and Roeder (1965); (17) London et al. (1985); (18) Barrows and Kokkonen (1978); (19) Barrows and Kokkonen (1985); (20) Prasad et al. (1981); (21) Panemangalore et al. (1986); (22) Cleary et al. (1987); (23) Ruggeri et al. (1987).

(5) Very limited information is available about the effect of DR on *kidney* enzyme activities. Succinate dehydrogenase activity increased with DR in 2 (references #18, 19) of 5 studies. Malic dehydrogenase was not DR-sensitive (references #18, 19). Alkaline phosphatase activity was higher in homogenates from rats fed at half the ad lib level for about 3 months (references #15, 16).

(6) Data on biochemistry of the *liver* are relatively plentiful and suggest that DR can alter enzyme activities. However, the data generally are not focussed on specific aspects of metabolism, so that only meager information exists about most metabolic pathways.

Although one group (references #1, 2) reported that 1.0-1.6 months of DR nearly doubled the activities of hexose shunt enzymes and of malic enzyme (all involved in NADPH generation), two other studies of longer duration, albeit at less severe DR levels, revealed either no influence of DR (reference #22) or lower activities (#23) of these enzymes in preparations from DR livers. Activities of certain citrate cycle enzymes may increase with DR. Four (#15, 16, 18, 19) of five reports described 26-157 percent increases in succinate dehydrogenase activity in liver homogenates from DR rodents. Alpha-ketoglutarate dehydrogenase and citrate synthase activities increased with DR by 20 percent in one study (#11). Malic dehydrogenase was uninfluenced by DR in two studies (#2, 18) but rose 24 percent in another (#19). Isocitrate dehydrogenase activity proved insensitive to DR (#2, 11).

As for respiratory molecules, the activity of cytochrome c oxidase in whole liver homogenates was increased 30 percent in rats restricted from 10 to 30 months of age (#11) but was decreased by 25 percent in our study of isolated mitochondria from mice on severe EDR until 5 months of age (#13). In the former study, the content of cytochrome c and cytochrome $a + a_3$ in the homogenates was 20 percent higher in the DR rats.

Activities of liver enzymes involved in protein metabolism are, for the most part, either unchanged or lowered by DR. These scant data seem at odds with the prevailing view that DR increases protein turnover (see "PROTEIN SYNTHESIS, DNA, CHROMATIN, GENE EXPRESSION, DNA REPAIR," Chapter 5). Note that the five enzymes in reference #9 (3 decreased, 1 increased, 1 unchanged by DR) are involved in converting tryptophan to nicotinamide nucleotides.

As summarized in Table 4.2, much data exist on the effect of DR on xenobiotic metabolizing enzyme content and activities in liver microsomal preparations. Values typically either increase or remain unchanged with DR. Most of the increases follow brief DR (i.e. 1 to 2 months) whereas longer DR was often without influence.

As shown in the table, no clear pattern emerges regarding DR's impact on hydrolytic degradative enzyme activities in liver homogenates.

Information is rapidly accumulating on radical scavenging enzymes in livers of rodents on DR. Data on SOD do not offer a clear picture: SOD activity was 89 percent higher in post-mitochondrial supernatants from 10 month old, but not 7 month old mice fed a 6 percent protein diet ad lib (reference #3). The same investigators observed that 12 months of 50 percent DR lowered SOD activity by 19 percent (#4). We observed no effect of EDR on SOD activity in a long-lived mouse strain (#14), which agrees with observations in 6 month old B/WF$_1$ mice on EDR (Kubo et al., 1987b). In contrast, Richardson's laboratory recently reported (#6) a 75 percent increase in levels of mRNA specific for SOD, and a 50 percent increase in catalase-specific mRNA in 36 month old rats on EDR. The latter observation does accord with our finding of a 64 percent increase in catalase activity in livers of DR mice. Another report on catalase was that of Ross (#10): 33 month old DR rats displayed 18 percent higher activities when the basis of expression was unit nitrogen. In the B/WF$_1$ mice studied by Kubo et al. (1987b), catalase activity did not vary in a predictable way with caloric intake.

(7) Enzyme activities in skeletal *muscle* have not been observed to change with DR. Nearly all available data are from a single report (#11).

(8) The *spleen* and other immune system tissues have been virtually ignored enzymologically in DR rodents.

Ross' 1969 report (#10) contains much valuable information on the complexities of data expression in the DR model. He studied DR's impact on liver composition, activity levels of four enzymes (catalase, ATPase, histidase, and alkaline phosphatase), and how activities at different ages correlated with LS in male Sprague-Dawley rats. Activities were measured in homogenates and expressed per unit weight (wet, dry, or fat-free), per unit nitrogen, per cell and per organ. Five diets (4 PDs and 1 NPD) were tested at energy intakes ranging from 20 to 60 kcal per day. A great deal of data (13 tables, 21 figures) were collected and a careful analysis of the many age- and diet-related effects led Ross to the following conclusions:

"For each of the enzymes studied, the activity levels were found to vary with the age of the rat and the diet fed. Similarly, the volume of the individual hepatocyte and the total number of hepatocytes also varied throughout the life of the rat and were significantly influenced by the dietary regimen imposed. When parameters other than age were used as a basis of comparison, these discrete multiple patterns disappeared. The levels of activity of each of the enzymes, irrespective of age or diet, formed a single, continuous slope when related to nitrogen content, number of hepatocytes, hepatocytic volume, body weight and caloric intake. The progressive changes with age in the activity level of the organ or of the cell, represent an adaptation to the change in requirements of a larger animal or a larger cell. Rapid growth rates, structural or biochemical, are not commensurate with prolonged life span. The dietary regimen which evoked the greatest rate of change with age was most detrimental and such rats had the shortest life expectancy. With long-term caloric restriction, the levels of any of the biochemical constituents as well as of cell and animal size, were more like that of the young rat, and the longest life spans were obtained."

In Table 4.2, data from Ross' study (#10) are given by comparing values for a DR and a control group fed PDs for 33 months. The restricted group ate a 22 percent casein, 54 percent sucrose, 14 percent corn oil diet at 20 kcal per day. Controls ate 55 kcal per day (ad lib is around 75 kcal/day) of a 30 percent casein, 61 percent sucrose, 5 percent corn oil diet. Adult BWs for DR rats averaged 150 g vs. 400 g for controls. LSs were not directly reported but life expectancy values suggested that this population responded to DR in a fashion typical of Ross' colony (see Table 2.4, references #7, 8 and 9). Note that the statistical significances of differences between average values were not reported. Our statements (given below) of the statistical significance of differences between averages which Ross reported are based on calculating Z values and determining the probability of significant differences (two-tailed test).

Table 4.3 shows the robust effects of DR on composition of the liver of 33 month old DR and control rats. Liver weight and BW were decreased 60 percent by DR. The number of hepatocytes was halved by DR and the average volume of hepatocytes was 20 percent lower. The DR rats had 25 percent more hepatocytes per g liver than controls and there was 60-70 percent less total fat and nitrogen in DR than in control livers.

Figure 4.2 gives ATPase and catalase activities expressed as units per liver versus age for DR and control rats. Lower enzyme activities per liver of DR rats paralleled the degree of liver weight reduction. Late-life decreases in activities only occurred for the control group. Activities of histidase and alkaline phosphatase did not show late-life decreases in either group, regardless of the mode of reference.

TABLE 4.3
Influences of Dietary Restriction on Liver Composition in Rats[a]

Parameter	Units	Control	DR	Effect of DR
Body wt.	g	383 ± 16	150 ± 4	↓61%
Liver wt.	g	10.2 ± 0.3	4.2 ± 0.1	↓59%
Hepat./liver	no. $\times 10^{-6}$	2134 ± 132	1111 ± 39	↓47%
Hepat./g liver	no. $\times 10^{-6}$	209 ± 11	263 ± 10	↑26%
Ave. hepat. vol.	μ^3	3925 ± 214	3161 ± 146	↓20%
Liver fat	%	6.7 ± 1.1	4.6 ± 0.2	↓31%
Liver fat (total)	$g \times 10^2$	70 ± 14	20 ± 1	↓72%
Liver fat (/hepat.)	$g \times 10^{11}$	32 ± 5	18 ± 1	↓44%
Liver N (/wet wt.)	mg/g	37 ± 1	38 ± 1	NSD
Liver N (total)	mg	374 ± 10	159 ± 4	↓58%

[a] Data ($\overline{X}$ ± SEM for n of 10 of more) are from Ross (1969) for 33 month old rats. Abbreviations: Hepat. = hepatocyte; vol. = volume; N = nitrogen; NSD = no significant difference.

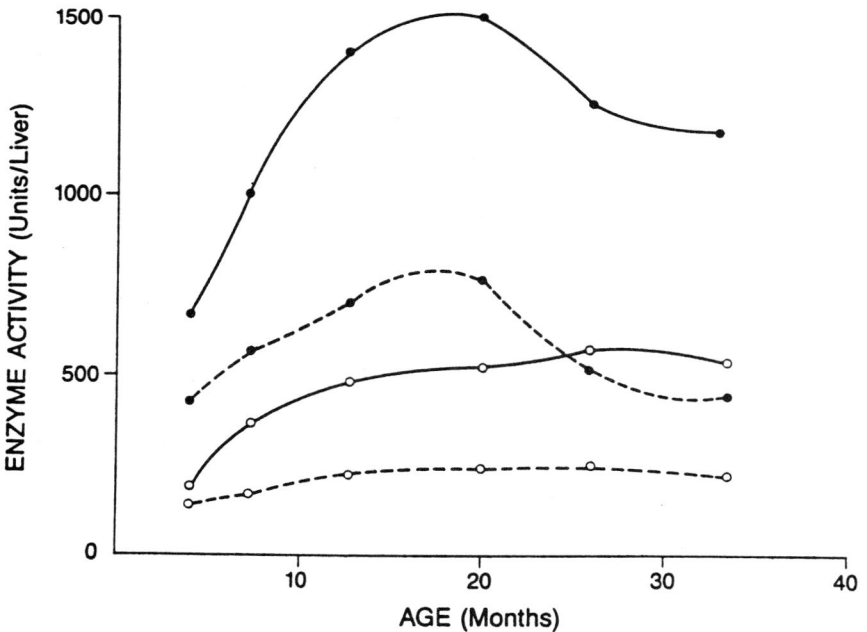

Figure 4.2. Activities (units/liver) of ATPase (———) and catalase (-----) in liver homogenates from DR (o) and control (•) Sprague-Dawley rats. Activities of ATPase are units $\times 10^{-2}$. Redrawn from Ross (1969).

Were influences of DR on ATPase activity apparent when the data were expressed in other ways? Figure 4.3 shows ATPase activity expressed per hepatocyte, per nitrogen (N), and per wet weight. Late-life declines were mild but real. Activities per hepatocyte must be interpreted knowing that the average volume of DR hepatocytes was 20 percent less than that of controls (Table 4.3). Activities per N or per wet weight for 33 month old DR rats were significantly greater ($p < .01$) than for age-matched controls. ATPase is of interest because of its central role in oxidative phosphorylation as a component of ATP synthase (which comprises about 15 percent of total inner membrane protein) (see "ENERGY METABOLISM," Chapter 5).

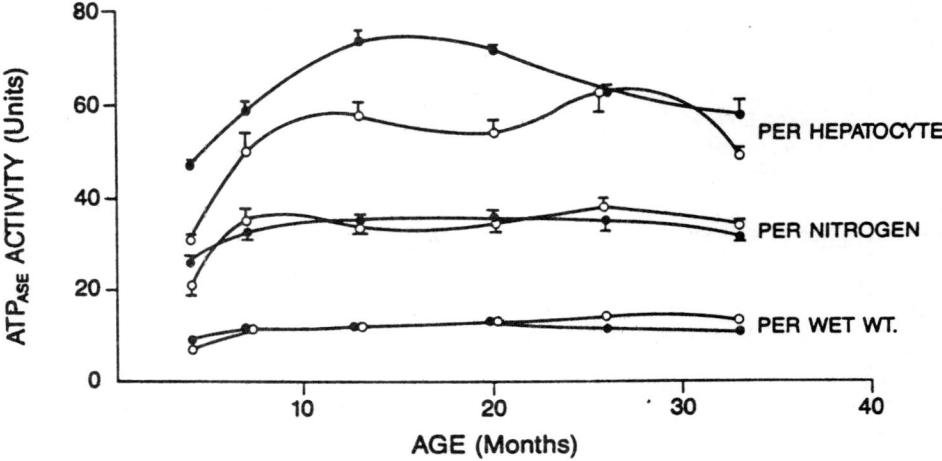

Figure 4.3. ATPase activity in liver homogenates from DR (o) and control (•) Sprague-Dawley rats. As indicated in the figure, activity is expressed in three ways: units $\times 10^6$/hepatocyte, units $\times 10^1$/mg nitrogen, or units/mg wet weight. Values are mean ± SEM for at least 10 rats. The SEMs for activity/wet weight are not shown (11 of the 12 values were < 0.5). Drawn from data tabulated in Ross (1969).

Catalase is emerging as an enzyme of special interest in DR studies, in part due to recent studies suggesting that DR may *selectively* upregulate the activity of this enzyme (Koizumi et al., 1987a). Figure 4.4 shows Ross' earlier catalase data, expressed in three ways (per hepatocyte, per N and per wet weight) other than per liver for control and DR rats. During the first 20 months of life, activity values for controls were greater than for DR mice. At 20-26 months, all three curves reversed. (This "reversal effect" occurs for other age-sensitive parameters in rodents subjected to EDR [Gerbase-DeLima et al., 1975].) Catalase

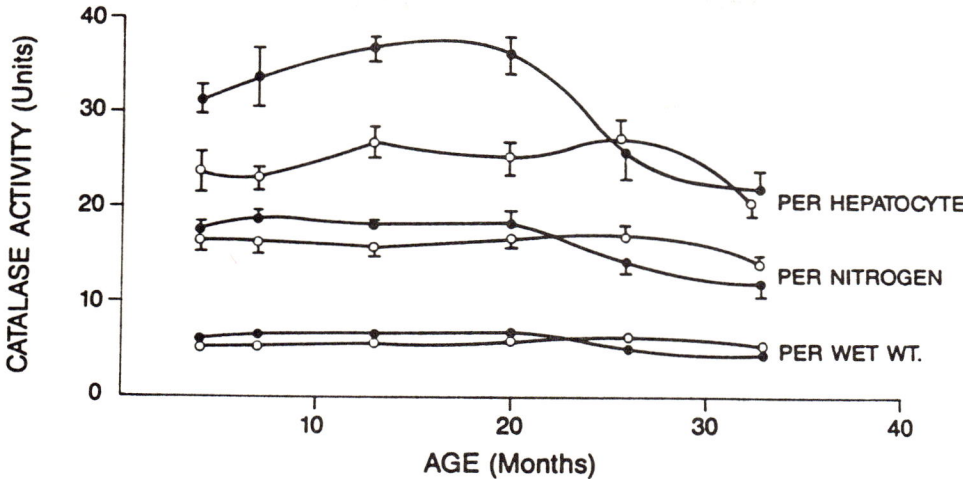

Figure 4.4. Catalase activity in liver homogenates of DR (o) and control (•) Sprague-Dawley rats. As indicated in the figure, activity is expressed in three ways: units $\times$ 10^8/hepatocyte, units $\times$ 10^1/mg nitrogen, units $\times$ 10^2/mg wet weight. Values are mean $\pm$ SEM for at least 10 rats. The SEMs for activity/wet wt. are not shown (all 12 values were < 0.4). Drawn from data tabulated in Ross (1969).

activities fell with aging in both diet groups. Comparing values at 20 months to those at 33 months, one finds that the control group displayed activity decreases of 30-40 percent per hepatocyte or per N or per wet weight, while in DR rats the same indexes fell by only 13-20 percent. At 33 months, activity values for DR rats exceeded those of controls when expressed per wet weight (5.2 $\pm$ 0.3 (SEM) vs. 4.4 $\pm$ 0.4) and per N (13.8 $\pm$ 0.7 vs. 11.7 $\pm$ 0.9). Both of these differences approached but did not reach statistical significance (0.10 > p > 0.05). Values per hepatocyte did not differ in late life, but one recalls that hepatocyte volume averaged 20 percent less for DR rats. Ross' overall data suggest that liver catalase activity falls with age and that DR attenuates this decline.

In a collaborative study with Koizumi (Koizumi et al., 1987a) (Table 4.2 [#14]; Table 4.4), we compared livers of 12 and 24 month old mice fed control (C, 95 kcal/week) and restricted (R, 55 kcal/week) diets since 3 weeks old. The enzyme activities measured included several xenobiotic metabolizers, radical scavengers (catalase, SOD, glutathione peroxidase), superoxide sources (xanthine oxidase, peroxisomal β-oxidation of palmitoyl-CoA), and glucose 6-phosphatase. Lipid peroxidation was also measured. The strongest dietary effect was an increased catalase activity for DR mice (group R: 42% higher at 12 months, 64% at 24 months). Lipid peroxidation was clearly lower in group R at 12 months (a 30% decrease) and somewhat lower (13%) at 24 months than in controls. Similarly, in 12 month old control and DR mice injected with either the P-450 inducer β-naphthoflavone (β-NF in corn oil) or with corn oil alone, DR mice showed higher catalase activity (40-44%) and lower lipid peroxidation (43-46%) in both β-NF-injected and vehicle-injected groups. These data suggest that if free radical damage is involved in aging, it may be a particular kind of damage that is in part prevented by a selective increase in catalase activity.

TABLE 4.4

Effects of Dietary Restriction and Age on Activities of Superoxide Dismutase, Catalase and β-Oxidation, and on Lipid Peroxidation in Mice[a]

Diet	Age	SOD	Catalase	β-Oxidation	Lipid Peroxidation
C	12	43 ± 14^A	210 ± 29^C	2.2 ± 0.8^A	27 ± 4^{AB}
R	12	43 ± 8^A	298 ± 31^B	1.7 ± 0.5^A	19 ± 2^C
C→R	12	41 ± 3^A	198 ± 31^C	ND	24 ± 3^B
C	24	39 ± 4^A	212 ± 15^C	ND	31 ± 6^A
R	24	39 ± 7^A	347 ± 67^A	ND	27 ± 5^{AB}

[a] Ages are in months, other values are means ± SD. Abbreviations: SOD, superoxide dismutase; ND, not determined; pro, protein; C, control; R, restricted; C→R, C diet until 1 week before assay when switched to R. The number of mice studied in each diet-age group was: C-12 mo=10, R-12 mo=10, C→R-12 mo=6, C-24 mo=8, and R-24 mo=5. The values for SOD (units/mg pro), catalase (umol/[mg pro·min]), and β-oxidation (palmitoyl CoA oxidation in nmol/[mg/pro·min]) are enzyme activities whereas those for lipid peroxidation (pmol/[mg pro·h]) give the amount of MDA formed in the TBA test. Means in each column not sharing a common superscript letter were significantly different (P=0.05). Adapted from Koizumi et al. (1987a).

It may be important that H_2O_2, the substrate for catalase, is a potent inducer of single strand breaks in DNA (Cantoni et al., 1987). Also, the partial post-translational inactivation of certain enzymes with age (Rothstein, 1987) may be mediated through mixed function oxidases and involve mainly the production of H_2O_2 (Oliver et al., 1987).

How DR increases catalase activity in mice needs further investigation. It may not be simply a response to increased H_2O_2 production, since most agents which increase H_2O_2 cause peroxisomal proliferation, and, based on the lack of effect on β-oxidation (no change in palmitoyl CoA oxidation), this seems not to occur in DR mice. One explanation could stem from DR's raising NADPH levels in cells (Table 4.2, #1, 2). NADPH is bound to catalase and is needed to prevent and reverse the accumulation of an inactive form of catalase generated by exposure to H_2O_2 (Kirkman et al., 1987). These and other possibilities are further discussed in Chapter 5 (see *"Increased Free Radical Neutralization by DR"*).

Rumsey et al. (1987: #11, Table 4.2) investigated the bioenergetic status of liver and gastrocnemius muscle from Fischer 344 rats following adult-onset (10 month) regimens of either DR (EOD feeding) or treadmill running. At 18, 24 and 30 months of age, three types of parameters were measured in homogenates: activities of several regulatory enzymes of the respiratory chain, citrate cycle, β-oxidation and glycolysis; cytochrome c and $a + a_3$ content; and mitochondrial respiratory rates (O_2 consumption: see "Metabolic Rate," this Chapter.). In control rats aging decreased activities of citrate synthase and 3-hydroxyacyl-CoA-dehydrogenase in both tissues, and the content of cytochrome c in the liver. More youthful indices were observed at all ages for muscle from exercised rats and for liver from DR rats. The authors suggested that the EOD-fed rats adapted to chronic episodes of gluconeogenic activity by increasing the number of liver respiratory assemblies.

But the main conclusion of the above report relates to the O_2 consumption studies. Substrate oxidation rates did not fall overtly with age in the liver (They did fall in muscle.), leading to the conclusion that the liver's capacity for ATP synthesis was unimpaired and that ". . . energy metabolism in the senescent animal was fully competent to meet its needs and age-related declines in energy metabolism are secondary to the aging process." This conclusion ignores the metabolic lesion in muscle while assuming that O_2 consumption rates of homogenates mirror *in vivo* production/use of ATP. (See "EVOLUTIONARY PERSPECTIVE" in Chapter 5 for discussion of possible significance of differential metabolic effects of DR in skeletal muscle vs. other tissues.).

Short-Term DR

Short-term DR studies are less pertinent to our inquiry than long-term ones. Short-term DR (defined here as starvation or as underfeeding for less than 1 month) probably does not affect aging, and many biological effects of long-term DR may well be unique to a long-term regimen. For example, Table 4.4 shows that long-term DR raised catalase activity and lowered lipid peroxidation, while DR for 8 days had no effect. Similarly, London et al. (1985) observed that 2 years but not 2 weeks of DR could favorably influence certain age-sensitive neurochemical indexes. Short-term DR studies tend to focus on the initial adaptation of a young, previously rapidly growing animal, and may not reflect the steady-state outcome of long-term DR.

Despite the above, short-term DR data cannot be entirely ignored. Some changes evoked thereby do persist into the long-term (e.g. low serum T_3 levels) and may signal long-term results. Also, because some long-term DR findings point towards influences on active oxygen production/scavenging, it is worth inquiring whether similar results obtain in short-term studies. We will therefore review selected metabolic outcomes of short-term DR.

Catalase activity increased markedly while SOD activity did not change in skeletal and cardiac muscles after an 18 day starvation period (40% loss of BW) was imposed on 12 month old rats (Lammi-Keefe et al., 1981). The investigators also found the same result after a severe (2-3 g of food/rat · day) 16 day EDR regimen (Lammi-Keefe et al., 1984). In an additional population from the latter study, the reduced growth rate caused by feeding a low protein diet was not associated with raised catalase activity.

Active oxygen defenses were studied in several tissues (heart, liver, kidney, pancreas) of mature female rats starved for 72 hours (Wohaieb & Godin, 1987). Catalase activities increased in the heart and pancreas but fell in the liver. Activities of SOD increased in the kidney and pancreas and decreased in the heart. Other workers have also found that liver catalase activities of rats fasted for 24 hours are lower (29%) than for fed rats (Isaacs & Binkley, 1977). The effect of long-term DR on liver catalase is thus opposite to that of short-term fasting. Liver cAMP levels were increased seven-fold by the day long fast.

Rats subjected to either severe DR (25% of ad lib) or a low protein (3% casein) diet for a 6 day period were tested for tolerance to hyperoxic stress (Deneke et al., 1985). The DR and ad lib fed rats lived longer (death was from lung edema) after oxygen exposure than did the protein restricted ones. Lung catalase activity per dry weight was not influenced by this DR regimen whereas lung content of glutathione was lower in the underfed group, leading the authors to conclude that ". . . other factors are necessary for explanation of the relative oxygen tolerance of feed-restricted animals with reduced levels of glutathione in the lung."

Gold and Costello (1975) studied the effects of a 7-day period of severe DR (25% of ad lib) on liver, kidney and heart mitochondrial function in young adult rats. Activities of several citrate cycle enzymes were reduced on a tissue-specific basis, but most severely in the heart. Other parameters found to be lower in the semi-starved group were pyruvate (in plasma) and citrate (in liver and kidney).

In weanling male rats restricted to 6 g per day for 3 weeks and compared to ad lib fed controls for 11 enzyme activities and levels of 7 metabolites in the gastrocnemius muscle, Howarth and Baldwin (1971) found that some parameters fell (activities of glucose-6-phosphatase and lactate, malate, and isocitrate dehydrogenases), others rose (levels of ADP, glucose-6-phosphate and pyruvate) and still others remained unaltered (levels of glucose, ATP and lactate; activities of certain enzymes including pryuvate kinase and glucose-6-P isomerase). The study primarily addressed biochemical changes associated with the inhibition of muscle growth.

Wulf and Cutler (1975) investigated the thermal stability of glucose-6-phosphate dehydrogenase in young and old mice. The percentage of thermolabile enzyme in brain, liver and spleen rose from 0-5 percent in young to 10-15 percent in old mice. But when old mice were starved for 40 hours, the percent of thermolabile glucose-6-phosphate dehydrogenase fell to youthful values, leading to the suggestion that protein degradation may be an effective way to remove altered proteins. One recalls that glucose-6-phosphate dehydrogenase (the first enzyme in the hexose shunt and therefore a main NADPH generator) increased with longer-term DR (Table 4.2).

Neuroendocrine

Many neuroendocrine changes appear to be associated with long-term DR. One or more of these could be fundamental in explaining the mechanism of DR's actions in retarding aging (see "NEUROENDOCRINE INTERPRETATION," Chapter 5). The term "pseudohypophysectomy" was coined by Pomerantz and Mulinos (1939) to describe their observations in starved or 50 percent underfed rats. The small size and altered histological appearance of ovaries, uteri and mammae from 17 month old C3H mice on EDR (66% of ad lib) was viewed as consistent with psuedohypophysectomy by Huseby et al. (1945). However, the notion that DR may retard aging via nutritional Hx (Everitt, 1973; Segall, 1979) has been challenged as too simplistic (Merry & Holehan, 1985a).

We shall consider "Reproductive," then "Nonreproductive" aspects of DR's neuroendocrine influences. Again, we focus on rodent work involving long-term (> 1 month) DR regimens proven to extend LS.

Reproductive Aspects

The onset of puberty in both sexes, and the length of the reproductive LS, at least in females, are sensitive to DR. (These are discussed in Chapter 2 ["*Growth, Puberty Onset and Health.*"] and later in this Chapter [Reproductive Senescence"].) Surprising species differences do occur in relation to cycling and DR: female rats on a LS-prolonging DR regimen in the colony of Merry show normal 5 day estrus cycles (Holehan & Merry, 1985a) whereas DR mice in our UCLA colony (unpublished data) and in other mouse colonies (e.g. Boutwell et al., 1948; Nelson et al., 1985) do not cycle. Available molecular data pertinent to DR's impact on reproduction (still quite limited but expanding) do not explain these "whole animal" phenomena. (A potential negative outcome of today's heavy emphasis on molecular biology is that few and fewer scientists study whole animals. Thus, detailed molecular information is becoming available on undiscovered organismic responses!)

Merry, Holehan and their colleagues have published several reports which begin to clarify EDR's impact on hormone levels. Their DR rats were fed a NPD at half the ad lib level, achieving a maximum 10th decile of survivorship of about 45 months. Their findings on reproductive hormone levels early in life include the following.

(1) In male EDR rats, the pubertal peak of serum testosterone was delayed by 20 days and the peak height reduced to 30 percent of that of ad lib fed controls (Merry & Holehan, 1981; Figure 4.5). Only in the ad lib group did testosterone levels fall in late-life. Levels of LH were higher in DR rats. Serum FSH content was lower in DR rats between 30 and 70 days of age. As judged by fertility, puberty was delayed by 10-20 days in the DR group.

(2) Ninety percent of ad lib fed female rats displayed open vaginas and first estrus by 37 days of age, whereas these criteria of puberty were not satisfied for 90 percent of the DR group until 147 days (Holehan & Merry, 1985a). Pre-pubertal serum levels of FSH and progesterone tended to be reduced by DR, while the concentration of estradiol-17β was increased.

(3) The hormonal profile of the estrus cycle was found to be modified in underfed rats (Holehan & Merry, 1985b). As shown in Figure 4.6, the

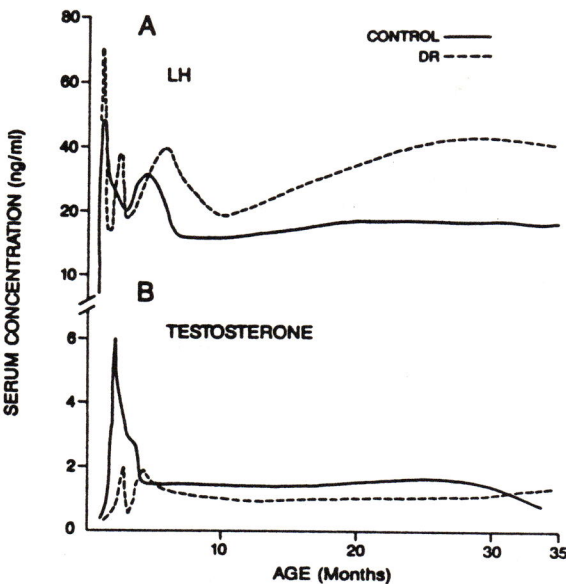

Figure 4.5. Influences of aging and DR on serum levels of LH and testosterone in male Sprague-Dawley rats. Control, ———. DR, -----. Adapted from Merry and Holehan (1981).

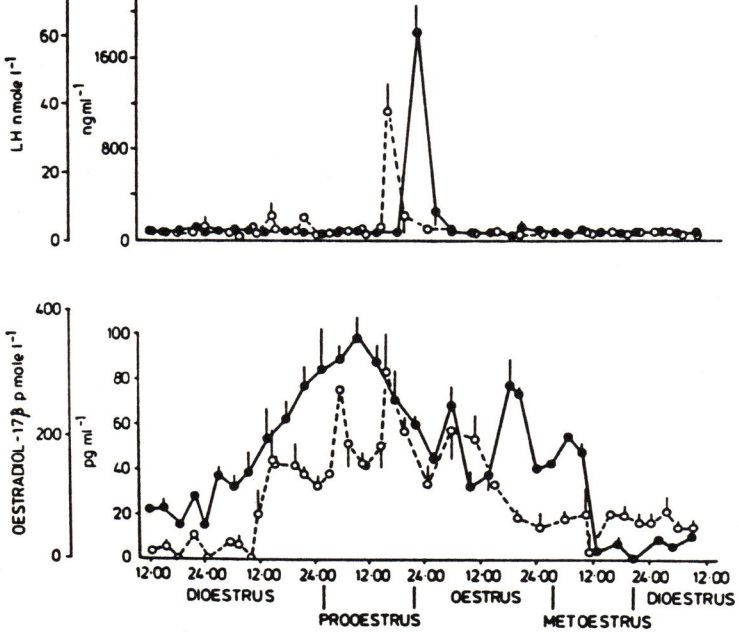

Figure 4.6. Serum levels of LH and estradiol-17β over the 5 day estrous cycle in 6 month old DR (o-----o) and ad lib (●———●) Sprague-Dawley rats. From Merry and Holehan (1985a), with permission.

peak in serum LH occurred 6.5 hours earlier in the cycle in DR than in ad lib-fed rats. The figure also shows that the peak in estradiol-17β was delayed and blunted by DR. Serum progesterone and FSH levels were oppositely affected by DR with the former lower and the latter higher than in controls.

How does DR influence the hormonal profile of female rats later in life, i.e., during reproductive decline? Gauging reproductive decline on a three stage scale based on vaginal cytology, Merry et al. (1985) measured serum levels of FSH, LH, prolactin, progesterone and estradiol-17β in aging DR and control rats. With only two exceptions (lower prolactin and FSH during Stage 2 in the DR group), the hormonal changes associated with the eventual decline of the extended reproductive LS of DR rats resembled those of controls. A decline in serum prolactin was also observed in 4 and 16 month old female Sprague-Dawley rats subjected to 10 weeks of ADR, which was associated with regression of mammary tumors in the older rats during the period of ADR (Quigley et al., 1987).

To better understand the hormonal differences, ovarian follicles from DR and control rats were isolated and steroid release was measured (Holehan & Merry, 1985c, 1986). Release of estradiol-17β after stimulation with LH (but not with testosterone) was higher in proestrus follicles from DR rats. Follicles from ad lib-fed rats showed the following age-related changes: by 1 year of age the LH- or testosterone-induced stimulation of estradiol-17β was increased throughout the cycle, while progesterone metabolism, as estimated by 20α-dihydroprogesterone levels, fell. These age changes commenced much later in life (20 months) in the DR group, and were less severe.

Only a few other studies are on record concerning the effects of long-term DR on reproduction. Five months of DR in rabbits led to an increased level of cytosol progesterone receptors, but no changes in their affinity, and no changes in plasma sex hormone binding globulin (Prasad et al., 1981). Grewal et al. (1971) limited young adult male Sprague-Dawley rats to half the ad lib intake level for 5 months. Serum testosterone levels were reduced by DR after 2 months, but had returned to control levels by 5 months. An actual return to ad lib feeding led to quite high testosterone levels. The standard errors given indicate that the testosterone data were highly variable from rat to rat. The concentration of sperm in the testes and epididymides was unaltered by DR. In rats fed 70 percent as much as ad lib controls, testes weight was unchanged and serum testosterone levels were increased about 2-fold (Snyder & Wostmann, 1987).

Work from three other laboratories describes neuroendocrine effects in relation to reproduction following brief EDR periods of 1 to 2 months.

Segall et al. (1978) studied brain monoamines and pituitaries in tryptophane-deficient (T−) rats and in pair-fed ones eating the same low calorie intake as the T− group chose spontaneously, but via a T+ diet. This was *severe* DR (4.5 g/day, killing about half of the animals in 30 days)! A third cohort was fed a T+ diet ad lib. Feeding lasted 1-2 months. Dopamine, norepinephrine and serotonin levels were measured in cerebral hemispheres, mesencephalon plus diencephalon, and in pons plus medulla oblongata. The rats fed the T+ diet on a restricted basis showed higher levels of serotonin in the cerebral cortex (but nowhere else) than did controls. Dopamine and norepinephrine levels were not influenced by severe DR. The histologic picture of pituitaries from rats fed either the T− diet or pair-fed the T+ diet in restricted amounts was one of decreased cell size and fewer basophilic cells (which secrete gonadotropic and thyrotropic hormones).

A second brief (6 week) EDR study was that of Pierpaoli (1977) who fed outbred mice an NPD at half the ad lib level. Serum estradiol-17β, progesterone and thyroxine levels were reduced 19 to 34 percent by DR. Upon return to free feeding, certain group differences were still observed (although not always in the original direction). Pierpaoli considered his findings as preliminary but supporting Dilman's hypothesis (Dilman, 1971) that an age-related increase in the hypothalamic threshold to feedback regulation causes aging.

In a third brief EDR study, Sisk and Bronson (1986) severely restricted (4 g/day) male Sprague-Dawley rats until 60 days of age. At this time the BWs of the DR group averaged one-fourth that of controls. DR reduced the frequency of LH and GH pulses and the amplitude of GH pulses. Serum FSH levels were slightly reduced by DR. When switched to ad lib feeding, the normal hormone profile was attained or approached rapidly.

We will not attempt an in-depth survey of how DR lasting less than 1 month impacts on reproductive endocrinology (but see discussion in Holehan & Merry [1986]). However, findings of possible relevance to longer-term DR include the following.

(1) An important brief underfeeding study spanning both reproductive and non-reproductive endocrinology was carried out by Meites'

group (Campbell et al., 1977). Young adult male Sprague-Dawley rats were either starved for 7 days, starved for 7 days and then fed 25 percent of ad lib for 14 days, refed for 7 days after being subjected to the regimen just described, or fed ad lib. Starvation and underfeeding periods markedly lowered serum levels of all hormones measured except FSH (Figure 4.7). Refeeding led to very high levels of FSH and LH whereas TSH, prolactin and GH resisted restoration. After LHRH + TRH injection, serum LH and TSH increased in all groups. Prolactin and FSH rose in starved but not in rats eating one-fourth of ad lib. Growth hormone did not rise in any group after LHRH + TSH injection. The conclusion: anterior pituitary hormone release falls with severe very short-term DR and this appears due to decreased hypothalamic stimulation of the pituitary. The pituitary itself remains capable of a normal response.

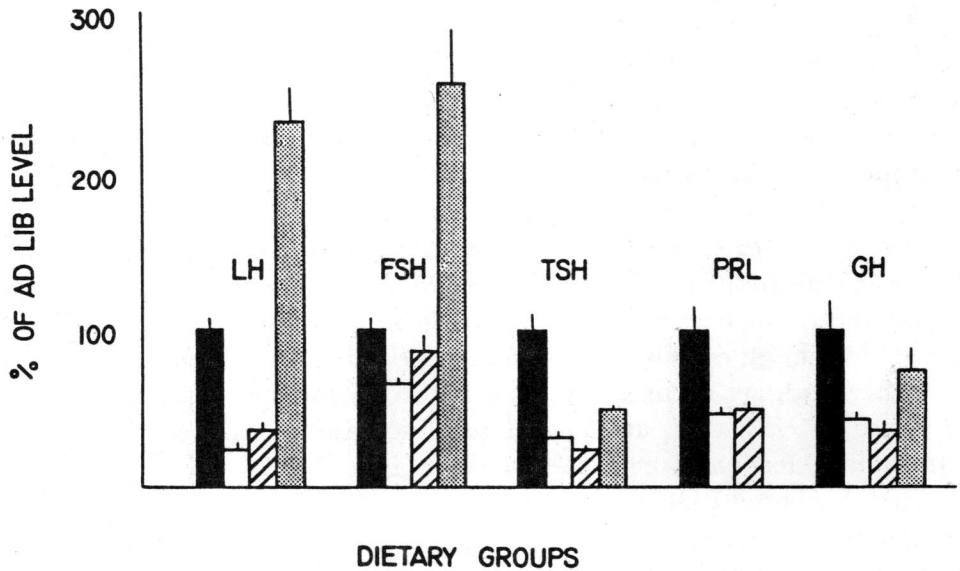

Figure 4.7. Effects of short-term DR on serum hormone levels of Sprague-Dawley rats. Data are graphed as the percent change from the hormone levels of controls fed ad lib. The dietary regimens were: AL (■), ad lib fed controls; AS (□), acutely starved for 7 days; CS (▨), starved for 7 days and then given 25 percent of the ad lib intake for 14 days; RF (▩), refed at ad lib level after the CS regimen. Vertical bar is 1 SEM. Adapted from Campbell et al. (1977), with permission.

(2) Young adult male rats starved for 7 days showed lower serum levels of FSH and LH but did not differ from controls in pituitary content of these molecules (Root & Russ, 1972). Starvation apparently

inhibited gonadotropin release but not synthesis. A hypothalamic cause was suggested.

(3) Compared to unrestricted controls, young adult male rats underfed (50% of ad lib) for 20 days showed 42 percent lower serum levels of testosterone and 29 percent lower levels of LH (Howland, 1975). Levels of FSH were not DR-sensitive in either serum or pituitary. The pituitary concentration of LH was higher (25%) in the DR group.

(4) Adult female rats were fed one-fourth of the ad lib level for 21-30 days to provide an animal model for "human emaciation" (Matsubara et al., 1986). This severe DR reduced the serum and pituitary LH concentrations but did not change serum LHRH levels. The hypothalamic content of LHRH was higher in the underfed group. Why hypothalamic LHRH (and probably other RHs) is not being released in semi-starved rats is unknown.

(5) Serum levels of FSH rose while LH fell in adult female rats fed at half of ad lib for 16 days (Knuth & Friesen, 1983). This protocol led to irregularities in estrus cycles. Compared to controls, the pituitaries from the restricted rats contained more FSH, but similar amounts of LH. Nevertheless, the LH response to injected LHRH for the DR rats was only 15 percent that obtained in proestrus controls, which finding goes against the hypothalamic notion cited in (1) above that the pituitary of an underfed animal would in fact produce if it were properly stimulated.

Non-Reproductive Aspects

Thyroid Axis. The thyroid axis deserves special attention in trying to find the mechanism of DR's action. Although the precise actions of thyroid hormone remain somewhat cloudy, the prevailing view (Smith et al., 1983; Sherwin, 1985) is that T_3 binds to high-affinity, low capacity nuclear receptors. The biologic activity of T_3 is far greater than that of T_4. Circulating T3 is formed chiefly by liver and kidney microsomal T_4-5'-deiodinase acting on T_4 released by the thyroid, but some T_3 is also directly released from the thyroid. The union of T_3 with receptors promotes the synthesis of specific mRNAs (Table 4.5 [over 100 enzyme activities rise with T_3 treatment!]).

T_3 stimulates oxygen consumption and heat production in a number of tissues (Exceptions are adult brain, lymph nodes, and gonads.). This increased consumption was once solely ascribed to uncoupling of oxidative phosphorylation, but may also involve other events (e.g. energy needed for new protein synthesis or Na/K ATPase activity). In any

TABLE 4.5

Some of the Many Proteins Whose Synthesis Is Induced
or Activity Increased by Thyroxine[a]

Arginase	Glycerol phosphate DHase
β-adrenergic receptors	Growth hormone
Cytochrome oxidase	Na/K ATPase
Glucagon receptors	NADPH-cytochrome C reductase
Glucokinase	Malic enzyme
Glucose-6-phosphate DHase	PEP carboxykinase
Glucose-6-phosphate	Pyruvate carboxylase

[a] Adapted from Smith et al. (1983). Abbreviations: DHase, dehydrogenase; PEP, phosphoenolpyruvate.

event, all of these pathways involve major investments in *energy*, the essential item which is being restricted in LS-prolonging DR. An increased efficiency of mitochondrial energy generation (with less generation of active oxygen products) or a decreased rate of energy usage per animal or per "critical organ mass" may be fundamental in the effects achieved by DR.

Dietary restriction strongly and consistently depresses thyroid axis activity in diverse animals. Fasting or underfed humans usually show normal T_4 and TSH levels but decreases in serum T_3 (Sherwin, 1985). One year old steers underfed such that BWs were maintained for a 5 month period (while controls gained a mere 115 kg) had lower serum levels of T_4 and T_3 (with the T_3 drop being far more robust) (Blum et al., 1985). Nikitin (1979) reported a decrease in synthesis and secretion of iodine-containing hormones of the thyroid gland. Merry and Holehan's rats (Figure 4.8, Merry & Holehan, 1985a) and our mice (unpublished observations) both show about 50 percent lower serum T_3 levels than controls. Plasma T_4 levels were marginally and inconsistently depressed in the former study leading to the conclusion that DR reduces the peripheral conversion of T_4 into T_3 more strongly than it impacts on neuroendocrine regulation involving TRH and TSH. Holehan and Merry (1986) cite their own unpublished data plus a report by van Doorn et al. (1984) as supporting their view. In the latter study, athyreotic thyroxine-maintained rats underfed by one-third for 20 day showed lower local production of T_3 in several tissues than did full fed controls.

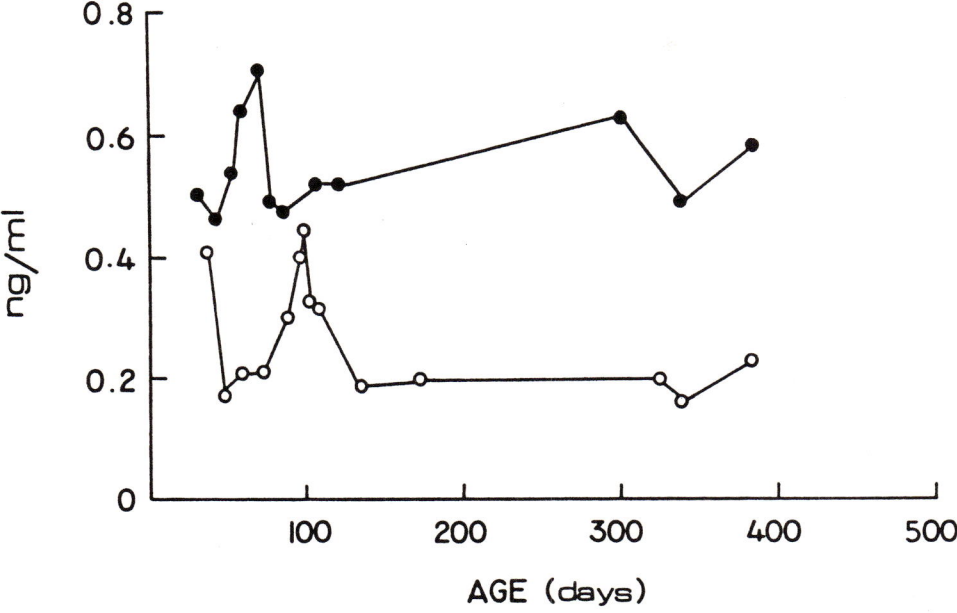

Figure 4.8. Plasma T_3 levels over the first year of life in DR (o) and ad lib (•) male Sprague-Dawley rats. Adapted from Merry and Holehan (1985a), with permission.

Ooka (1979) did not observe any reduction in the local conversion of T_4 to T_3 in DR animals. Rats were fed at one-third of the ad lib level and liver and kidney homogenates studied *in vitro* as a function of age. In controls, a clear pubertal peak in the rate of T_3 production was found, plus some tendency for a late-life decline. Food restriction beginning at 1 month of age and carried out for 1 month did not affect T_3 production; however, when DR rats were refed, higher than control values resulted. If DR ran from 3 to 4 months of age, a return to ad lib feeding was not followed by a rise in conversion activity.

Milder EDR (70% of ad lib) only marginally reduced serum T_3 and T_4 levels in young adult rats and did not affect these measures in late life (Snyder & Wostmann, 1987).

Evidence that the binding of T_3 to its nuclear receptor is reduced in livers from rats starved for 2 to 3 days (Burman et al., 1977; DeGroot et al., 1977) suggests the possibility that the low T_3 levels of chronic DR in fact understate a more severe hypothyroid state. And yet DR rodents are extremely active (see "LEARNING AND BEHAVIORAL PARAMETERS," this Chapter) and do not show any basal metabolic decrement per lean body mass when compared to controls (see "Metabolic Rate," this Chapter).

Does underfeeding affect brain regulation of the thyroid? Little is known about long-term DR in this regard. Armario et al. (1987) found that rats fed at two-thirds of the ad lib level for 1 month have circulating TSH levels half that of controls. Ooka et al. (1978) imposed quite severe EDR (20% mortality/month in this 2 month study) and observed lower serum levels of TSH, T_4 and T_3. As discussed above, starvation and short-term underfeeding of rats reduce serum TSH levels, but these rise after TRH injection, supporting the idea that underfeeding interferes with hypothalamic stimulation of an otherwise capable pituitary gland (Campbell et al., 1977).

Other nutrients besides calories affect T_3 levels. Glass et al. (1978) reported that calorie-restricted rats fed a high protein (36% casein) diet for 5 weeks showed low serum T_3 levels (45 ng/dl), whereas rats fed a diet containing 18 percent casein but equally restricted in calories had T_3 levels (70 ng/dl) not differing from full-fed rats on the latter diet. Although these studies involved only short-term DR, the finding that T_3 levels were affected mainly by the diet's protein:carbohydrate ratio, rather than calorie content, may signal some caution in interpreting the long-term DR data, since most DR diets contain less carbohydrate. Indeed, in isonutrient diets, it is mainly the carbohydrate that is reduced. Studies in humans on very low calorie diets (600-800 kcal/day) have also suggested that T_3 is much more sensitive to the carbohydrate content than the calorie content (Jung et al., 1980), although in these studies T_3 may be more sensitive to the *change* in carbohydrate than to its absolute amount. But other studies in humans on very low calorie diets have shown T_3 to vary with the calorie content itself and to be independent of the proportions of carbohydrate or protein (O'Brian et al., 1980).

Cox et al. (1984) fed an 18 percent casein diet either ad lib or in restricted (8 g/day) amounts to growing rats for 14 days. Diets with 9 and 4.5 percent protein were also tested, but only fed ad lib. Free T_3 (= T_3 not bound to proteins) was measured because the authors hypothesized that protein-energy malnutrition will increase the binding capacity of T_3. The hypothesis proved correct. The concentration of free T_3 was low in the energy-restricted and 4.5 percent protein diet-fed rats. Total T_3 was higher than controls in the 4.5 percent protein group and was unchanged in the energy-restricted group. Only the free T_3 level correlated with metabolic rate (O_2 consumption), leading the authors to suggest that free rather than total T_3 is the best index of thyroid status in protein-energy malnourished rats.

In summary, the thyroid axis does influence diverse aspects of metabolism and is quite sensitive to DR. Energy-related processes (e.g. metabolic rates of whole animals, tissues or mitochondria; heat production; protein synthesis rates) are clearly under thyroidal influence. Our attempt to provide an energy-related explanation for the "DR effect" (see "ENERGY METABOLISM," Chapter 5) is in part stimulated by these strong thyroidal effects of DR.

Growth Hormone (GH) and Somatomedins. Released in a pulsatile fashion by the anterior pituitary, GH is chiefly regulated by two hypothalamic peptides: GH-releasing factor (GH-RF) and GH release-inhibiting hormone (also called somatostatin). Pituitary synthesis of mRNA coding for GH is stimulated by T_3 (Spindler et al., 1982). Growth hormone binds to plasma membrane receptors, exerting both direct (e.g. lipolysis, anti-insulin) and indirect effects. The latter are caused by release of somatomedins (a family of peptides some of which are insulin-like growth factors) which in part mediate GH's growth-promoting effects, and are lowered by short-term DR (Phillips & Vassilopoulou-Sellin, 1979). Insulin-like growth factors may also signal the CNS to reduce both GH secretion (possibly via somatostatin) and food intake (Tannenbaum et al., 1983).

Serum GH levels during long-term DR have not been well studied. The underfed steers of Blum et al. (1985) showed 2- to 4-fold higher GH levels than were observed in controls. However, the data were from a single morning bleeding so the values remain problematic due to GH's pulsatile secretion. Merry and Holehan (1985a) reported initial data on serum GH levels from cannulated rats sampled every 20 minutes. No clear DR effect was seen in 4 to 5 month old rats, and considerable rat-to-rat variation occurred independently of diet. Growth hormone treatment of young rats accelerated BW gain in ad lib-fed but not in DR rats. Thus, slower growth in DR rats was not due to GH deficiency.

Levels of GH in male Sprague-Dawley rats subjected to short-term DR formed the topic of four reports. Feeding rats at half the ad lib level during the second month of life, Sorrentino et al. (1971) found in the DR group a 4-fold fall in pituitary GH content, a 2-fold fall in pituitary GH concentration, and a 10-fold fall in serum GH levels compared to controls. Similarly, rats fed 65 percent of ad lib for 1 month showed very low serum levels of GH (Armario et al., 1987). Campbell et al. (1977) starved one group of adult rats for 7 days and in a second group followed a 7 day starvation period with feeding at one-fourth of ad lib for 2 weeks.

Both groups displayed serum GH levels less than half that of controls. Rats starved for 3 days showed sharply lower amplitudes and durations of GH secretion episodes (normally every 3.3 hours) (Tannenbaum et al., 1978). That this depression with starvation was partially due to somatostatin was suggested by the observation that fasted rats injected with antibodies to somatostatin had GH levels 3-fold higher than non-antibody treated, fasted controls.

It seems quite clear that with DR the organism has less need to invest its limited energy resources in synthesizing anabolic hormones.

ACTH and Corticosterone. The secretion of adrenocorticotropic hormone (ACTH) by the pituitary is mainly regulated by hypothalamic corticotropin releasing factor (CRF). Binding to adrenal plasma membrane receptors, ACTH activates adenylate cyclase, stimulating adrenal cortical growth and steroid synthesis by increasing the conversion of cholesterol to pregnenolone. Several biochemical changes are then induced to favor steriodogenesis.

We are unaware of any reports in English on the effect of long-term DR on pituitary ACTH content and release, and only scant data are extent describing plasma levels of corticosterone in DR animals. An English summary of a Russian report (Nesterenko et al., 1977) states that a diet with adequate protein but with "insufficient caloric content" inhibited age-related declines in hypothalamic CRF activity, ACTH secretion, and pituitary response to CRF in rats.

Gallo and Weinberg (1981) fed male adult Sprague-Dawley rats 80 percent of the ad lib level per BW for 11 weeks. The food was presented either in the early morning, late evening or continuously (via an automated feeder). Corticoid levels of ad lib fed controls varied in a circadian rhythm, with lowest values at 0800 hours and a peak at 2000 hours. Restricted rats fed in the morning showed a 12 hour shift in timing of the peak. The machine-fed rats displayed no rhythmicity at all. Peak corticoid levels were not influenced by DR. Pre- and post-feeding corticoid levels did not differ in ad lib fed rats whereas all DR groups showed definite post-feeding lowering of serum corticosterone.

Armario et al. (1987) observed a similar rhythmicity in ad lib fed rats. Diet restriction (65% of ad lib for 1 month) raised peak circulating corticosterone levels and modified the circadian rhythms of corticosterone and ACTH.

Merry and Holehan (1985a) published preliminary findings on the adrenal axis in their male rats. Absolute adrenal weight was lowered by

DR but the adrenal/BW ratio was higher in the DR group at most ages. A stress (move from animal quarters to laboratory) raised plasma corticosterone of ad lib fed rats to a greater extent than in DR rats during the first year of life, but differences were not observed thereafter (Figure 4.9). Refeeding the DR rats for 7 days prior to assay partially restored the response deficit of the first year. When DR rats were infused with ACTH, a rapid rise in corticosterone took place. Thus, a failure to increase ACTH levels in response to the stress probably caused the observed differences.

Starvation was reported initially to stimulate and later (after 4-14 days) to mildly dampen adrenal axis activity in adult rabbits (Bouille & Assenmacher, 1970). In rats, 7 days of starvation resulted in an increase in bioassayable CRF in the hypothalamus, a marginal fall in bioassayable ACTH in the pituitary, and higher plasma corticosterone than in controls (Chowers et al., 1969).

Insulin and Glucagon. As might be expected on the basis of the well-known association of obesity with hyperglycemia, hyperinsulinemia and insulin resistance, long-term DR profoundly impacts on age-related changes in glucose regulation. Data on regimens actually proven to extend maximum LS are largely confined to those from Masoro's laboratory.

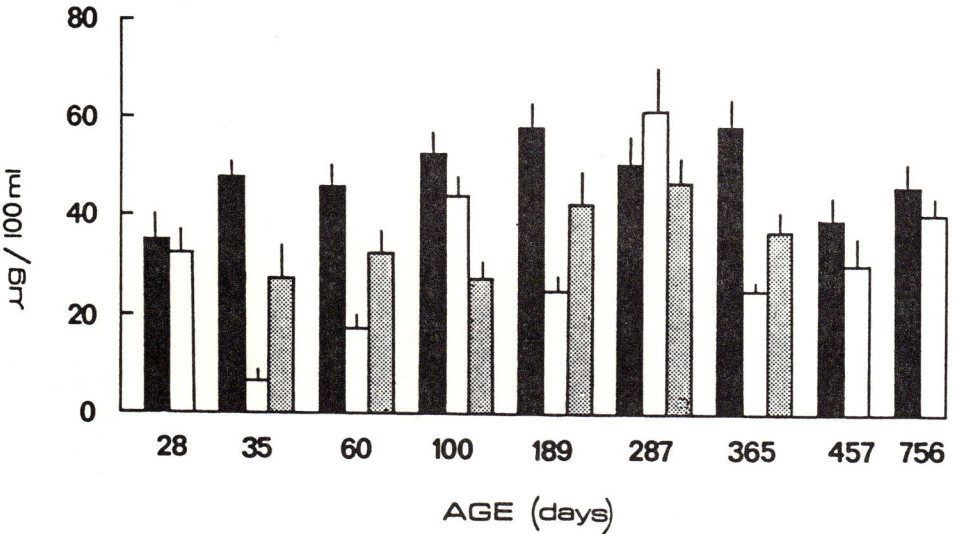

Figure 4.9. Plasma corticosterone levels in male Sprague-Dawley rats as a function of age and diet. These are stress-induced levels (rats moved from colony to laboratory and then bled). Diets: ■ = ad lib; □ = DR; ▨ = DR rats returned to ad lib feeding for 7 days. Adapted from Merry and Holehan (1985a), with permission.

Masoro et al. (1983) described plasma levels of glucose, insulin and glucagon in rats fed the same diets as those studied for LS (see Table 2.4, #21, wherein four of the five groups tested are summarized). Data were for single bleedings (intraday variation not studied). As shown in Figure 4.10, glucose levels peaked in all diet groups at 18 months of age and were lowest in the two groups on DR (onset of 6 weeks or 6 months). Insulin levels increased in all groups but remained lowest in the two DR groups. Glucagon rose with age through 24 months but, contrasting to the situation for glucose and insulin, was uninfluenced by DR. The "glucostatus" of these rats was also studied by Yu et al. (1984a) who found that post-absorptive concentrations of liver glycogen were 2- to 3-fold higher in the two DR groups than in the ad lib groups at all ages tested.

There are many reports on the responsiveness of rat adipose cells to glucagon or insulin as a function of aging and DR. According to Bertrand et al. (1980b) glucagon-stimulated lipolysis of adipocytes did not occur after 6 months of age in ad lib fed rats (agreeing with prior reports) whereas fat cells from DR rats as old as 36 months still responded (Figure 4.11). The effect was not due to differences in cell volume. Voss et al. (1982) studied the events occurring early in life (from 6 to 15 weeks of age) in fully fed rats that might be causal to this age deficit, as well as DR's influence thereon. Adenylate cyclase activity paralleled lipolysis. No evidence was found for low amounts of the enzyme in "ad lib adipocytes." Phosphodiesterase activity rose with age to a greater extent in adipocytes from the fully fed group. The authors concluded that DR probably impinges on receptor-plasma membrane phenomena. Most recently, Bertrand et al. (1987) reported that ADR (6 month onset) caused the recovery of both glucagon- and epinepherine-stimulated lipolysis.

Cooper et al. (1977) observed that EDR but not brief ADR (from 12 to 15 months of age) opposed age-related declines in glucagon-stimulated adenylate cyclase activity in rat adipocytes. Other hormones (e.g. ACTH, epinepherine) which increase the activity of this enzyme did so to a greater extent in adipocytes from EDR rats than from age-matched controls.

Insulin-sensitive phosphodiesterase activity in fat cells of 8 week old rats fed at 35 percent of the ad lib level for 4 weeks was studied by Suzuki et al. (1987). Enzyme activation was higher in cells from underfed than fully fed rats. The increase in insulin sensitivity appeared due to greater insulin binding per unit of cell surface area. Thus, in adipocytes

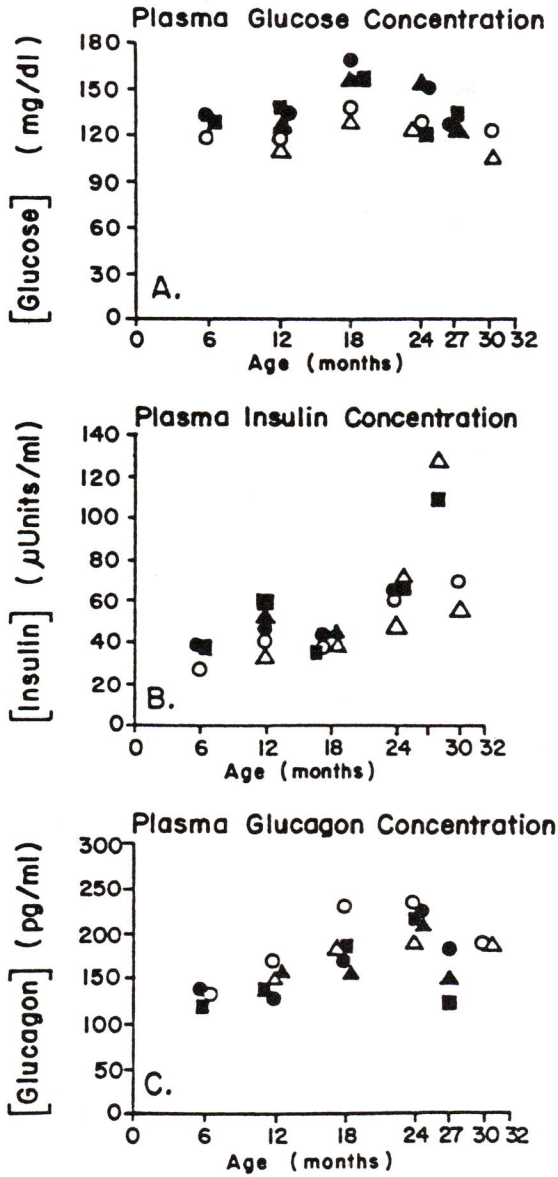

Figure 4.10. Influence of diet and age on plasma concentration of glucose (panel A), insulin (panel B), and glucagon (panel C) in male Fischer 344 rats. The diet groups were: Group #1 (●) = ad lib throughout life; #2 (o) = 60 percent of ad lib from 6 weeks of age; #3 (▲) = 60 percent of ad lib until 6 months of age and then fed ad lib; #4 (△) = ad lib until 6 months and then fed 60 percent of the ad lib level; #5 (■) = low protein (12.6% casein) diet ad lib. Adapted from Masoro et al. (1983), with permission.

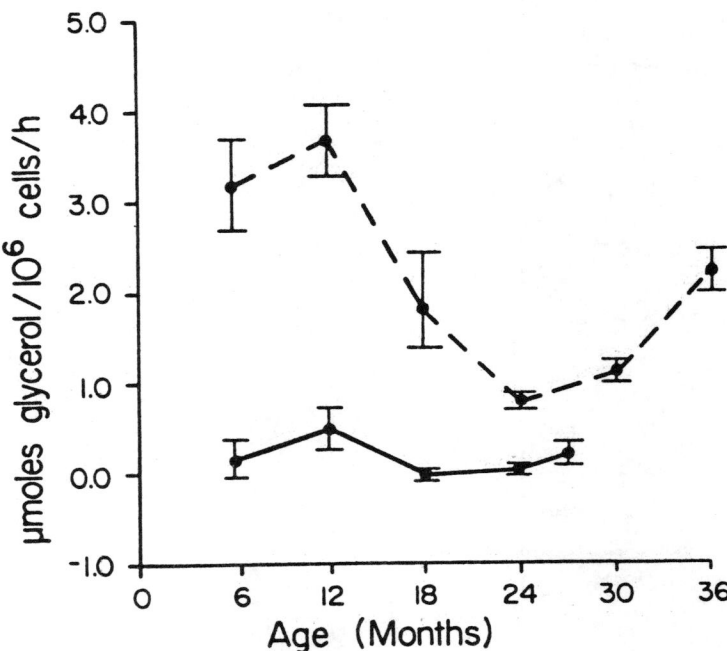

Figure 4.11. Effects of age and DR on the lipolytic response of epidiymal adipocytes to glucagon. Male Fischer 344 rats were studied. DR, -----; ad lib control ———. From Bertrand et al. (1980b), with permission.

of rats the activity of insulin-stimulated phosphodiesterase (which leads to lipogenesis) is increased by DR, whereas that of glucagon-stimulated phosphodiesterase (leading to lipolysis) is lowered.

Rat adipocytes were also studied by DiGirolamo et al. (1984). Their abstract describes influences of DR and aging (from 3 to 24 months) on diverse aspects of fat cell metabolism. Commenced at 3 months of age, DR was maintained at either 50 or 75 percent of ad lib. The basal conversion of glucose to fatty acids fell early in life in all diet groups. Basal glyceride synthesis increased until 12 months of age in adipocytes from ad lib rats, and was reduced by DR. The rate of age-related decline in insulin-induced glyceride synthesis was retarded by DR. The antilipolytic effect of insulin declined with aging in DR and ad lib groups whereas the age-related decline in epinephrine-induced lipolysis occurred only in ad lib fed rats. Thus, DR corrected only some of the age-related deficits.

Holloszy's group at Washington University studied insulin resistance of adipocytes from 12 and 28 month old ad lib fed, sedentary rats and from age-matched rats started on exercise (running) or on ADR (underfed to weigh as much as the running rats) at 6 months of age (Craig et al., 1987). The sedentary controls became obese. They developed large, insulin-resistant fat cells. The runners had small, insulin-responsive fat cells. Cells from the ADR rats displayed intermediate values. Aging (12→28 months) did not influence these parameters in any group. Thus, adipocyte hypertrophy associated with obesity (and not aging *per se*) leads to insulin resistance, and this can be prevented by exercise and, to a lesser extent, by ADR.

Cleary et al. (1987) imposed moderate EDR (70% of ad lib) on lean and obese Zucker rats for 11-15 months, and, besides liver enzymes (see Table 4.2, #22), measured serum insulin and glucose levels and adipocyte glucose metabolism. The serum parameters were not influenced by DR. Insulin-stimulated glucose metabolism (CO_2 production was measured) in adipocytes from lean DR rats was about 2-fold that of lean controls, but was insensitive to DR in the obese genotype. The effect of age on this parameter was not determined (all rats were 12 months old). The conversion of glucose to glyceride-glycerol was not affected by DR.

Other studies on insulin and glucagon in DR rodents did not focus on adipocytes. A report by Cohn and Joseph (1970) compared growing rats fed at 80 percent of ad lib for 4 weeks to ad lib controls. The DR rats were more reactive to the hypoglycemic effects of insulin and could dispose of a glucose load at a rapider rate.

Eve and Gerald Reaven and colleagues at Stanford have explored pancreatic structure, function and insulin action in male Sprague-Dawley rats underfed since weaning but in an unusual way: a standard NPD was mixed with cellulose in a 1:2 ratio and fed ad lib. Controls were freely fed the NPD. It is not known whether this type of DR ("caloric dilution") influences LS.

At 12 months of age, rats on this "caloric dilution" type of EDR and other rats fed the NPD ad lib but given access to a running wheel showed a 3-fold decrease in serum insulin and triglycerides compared to sedentary, ad lib fed controls (Reaven & Reaven, 1981a). Body weights at 10-12 months of age for both the EDR and ad lib running groups averaged 500 g, vs. 750 g for controls. Daily caloric intakes approximated 125 for the exercised rats, 110 for the sedentary controls and 80 for those eating the calorie-diluted diet. Pancreatic islets from 12 month old sedentary controls were multi-lobulated and fibrotically enlarged whereas neither of the other two groups displayed these changes (Reaven & Reaven, 1981b).

In another study, "caloric dilution" DR lowered plasma insulin levels after an oral glucose load, and also lowered insulin resistance (Reaven et al., 1983a). The average volume of collagenase-isolated islets increased 2.5-fold between 2 and 12 months of age in controls fully fed a standard diet or a high (60%) sucrose diet, but not in DR rats (Figure 4.12). An age-sensitive but not DR-sensitive parameter was glucose-stimulated insulin secretion per volume of pancreas.

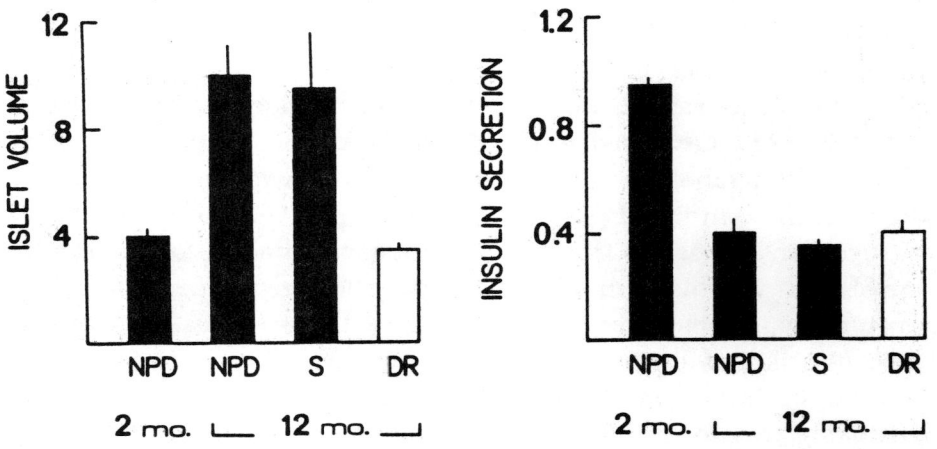

Figure 4.12. Islet volume ($\times 10^6 \mu^3$) and glucose-stimulated insulin secretion (mU/min/volume of islet) in 2 month old Sprague-Dawley rats fed a NPD, and in 12 month old rats fed for a 10.5 month period either a standard NPD, a sucrose-enriched diet (S), or a calorically restricted (DR) diet. ■, ad lib feeding; □, DR. Adapted from Reaven et al. (1983a), with permission.

Reaven et al. (1983b) studied glucose-stimulated insulin release from the perfused pancreas of rats fed the control or DR regimen, and from others fed a high sucrose (66%) diet ad lib. Twelve month old rats were compared with 2 month old controls. Pancreas dry weights were lowest in the 2 month old rats (ave. = 0.27 g), higher (0.34 g) in the DR group, and highest (0.45 g) in the ad lib groups. The differences appeared due to variations in islet cell content. Compared to the other groups, the maximum insulin release per pancreas was reduced 40 percent in DR rats. The maximum insulin release per g of pancreas or per µg of islet cell mass in 12 month old rats fed any of the three diets was only 30 percent that of the 2 month old rats. The fully fed rats appeared to battle a declining β cell response by increasing the number of β cells.

In another study from the same laboratory (Mondon et al., 1986), 12 month old ad lib fed rats weighing 650–700 g were subjected to either a calorically-diluted diet or to exercise for a 4 month period. Over this term the controls gained another 150 g while the treated rats lost 0-100 g. Insulin-stimulated glucose uptake continued its age-related fall in fully fed rats; however, glucose-uptake was much higher in 16 month old rats in both dieted and exercised groups.

The above studies indicate that caloric dilution strongly influences glucose homeostasis. It is not excluded, however, that the benefits in the DR group might be caused in part by a high fiber intake. Nonetheless, the pancreas of an underfed Sprague-Dawley rat is not subjected to the extreme metabolic demands chronically imposed on that of a fully-fed, obese control. The need for cells to proliferate (and invest energy to do so) in the pancreas and elsewhere appears reduced by DR. The "energy-efficiency" of the whole animal may increase with DR (i.e. less energy directed toward new synthesis; less cells to maintain) and perhaps also efficiency of its energy-generating system (see *"Metabolic Efficiency and Energy Intake,"* Chapter 5).

Catecholamines. Landsberg and Young (1985) present a good case for the sympathoadrenal system's playing a key role in a mammal's response to underfeeding. Norepinephrine turnover is a reliable index of sympathetic activity (whereas serum levels of norepinephrine and epinephrine are not). Fasting or brief underfeeding in rodents and humans lowers norepinephrine turnover. Overfeeding increases turnover. Some evidence suggests that insulin-mediated glucose metabolism within critical ventromedial hypothalamic centers may produce an enhanced sympathetic outflow. That catecholamines are of major importance in the body's energy strategies is also supported by evidence that brown adipose tissue thermogenesis is mediated by the sympathetic nervous system.

Knowledge about long-term DR's impact on catecholamines is scarce. Existing reports do not explore the central metabolic aspects just discussed, but instead describe age-sensitive physiologic responses in various target tissues as a function of age and DR. Yu et al. (1980) reported that the age-related fall in epinephrine-promoted lipolysis in rat adipocytes is attenuated by DR. Scarpace and Yu (1987) observed that DR retards losses with age of β-adrenergic receptor levels and isoproterenol-stimulated adenylate cyclase activity in rat lung. These findings agree with an earlier observation in cultured vascular smooth muscle cells from either DR or ad lib rats, where epinephrine-induced increases in cAMP fell more sharply with age in cells from the ad lib animals (Volicer et al., 1983). Finally, Katz et al. (1987) reported that β-adrenergic responsive glycogenolysis in hepatocytes increases with age (6 to 24 months), but more markedly in ad lib fed than in DR rats.

Parathyroid Hormone (PTH) and Calcitonin. Kalu and colleagues at San Antonio explored calcium homeostasis in male Fischer 344 rats subjected to DR. The restricted diet was enriched to provide daily intakes of calcium, phosphorus and vitamin D equivalent to those of controls. Aside from the work of these investigators, little appears known on DR's influence on calcium regulation.

The effect of DR on PTH, which increases serum Ca^{++} by actions in bone, kidney and GI tract, was the subject of two reports (Kalu et al., 1984a & 1984b). DR started at 6 weeks or 6 months of age prevented two late-life occurrences of an ad lib lifestyle: (1) a rapid 7-fold increase in PTH starting at 20 months of age (Figure 4.13) and, (2) senile bone loss. Low protein diets or DR maintained only from 6 weeks to 6 months of age were largely ineffective in preventing these two changes. The suggestion was made that late-life disruptions in calcium homeostasis in fully fed rats may relate causally to the chronic nephropathy afflicting some strains of ad lib fed rats.

Calcitonin inhibits osteoclastic bone resorption and lowers plasma calcium. Levels of calcitonin in serum and thyroid were also studied in rats from the same five diet groups (see Figure 4.13 for explanation of groups) (Kalu et al., 1983b). Calcitonin levels rose progressively with age in all groups, with late-life increases being rapid in the ad lib group and very mild in the DR groups (Figure 4.14). Surprisingly, the inhibitory effect of ADR on the rise of calcitonin was more profound than that of EDR. As with PTH, rats fed a low protein diet ad lib or underfed only early in life showed control-like values. Neither aging nor DR influenced serum calcium levels. In a separate study on Wistar rats, Kalu (1984) found that DR but not dehydroepiandrosterone (DHEA) injection could reduce serum levels of calcitonin. How DR alters calcitonin levels is quite unclear but it is noteworthy that DR's depression of the thyroid extends beyond the follicular cells.

Brain Receptors. It is easy to envision receptor losses in old brains as having severe biologic consequences. Contained in three reports from the Gerontology Research Center of the NIA, the published data on brain receptors in long-term DR rodents concerns male Wistar rats on an EOD restriction plan. Levin et al. (1981) found that the age-related loss in striatal dopamine receptors was retarded by DR. The concentration of dopamine receptors in 24 month old DR rats was 50 percent greater than that of age-matched controls, and resembled that of 3 to 6

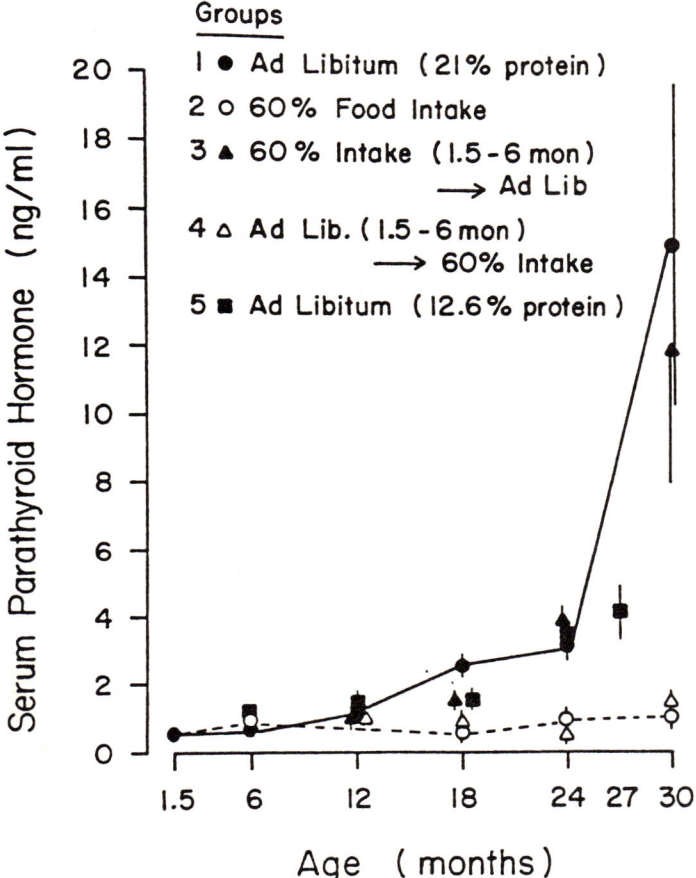

Figure 4.13. Effects of aging and diet on serum PTH levels in Fischer 344 rats. Adapted from Kalu et al. (1984a), with permission.

month old controls. In an extension of these investigations, Roth et al. (1984) studied young, middle aged and old mice. Figure 4.15 shows that DR rats maintained receptor levels during the first year of life, while controls did not. At 30 months of age, the DR rats reached the levels of the 24 month old controls. Short-term DR (2 weeks of EOD feeding) starting at 24 months did not alter dopamine receptor levels. In still a third study, London et al. (1985) (see Table 4.2, reference #17 for enzyme data) showed that 24 month old EOD rats have a higher density of striatal muscarinic binding sites which, together with higher activities of choline acetyltransferase, was interpreted to signify enhanced cholinergic transmission in the old DR rat brain compared to age-matched controls.

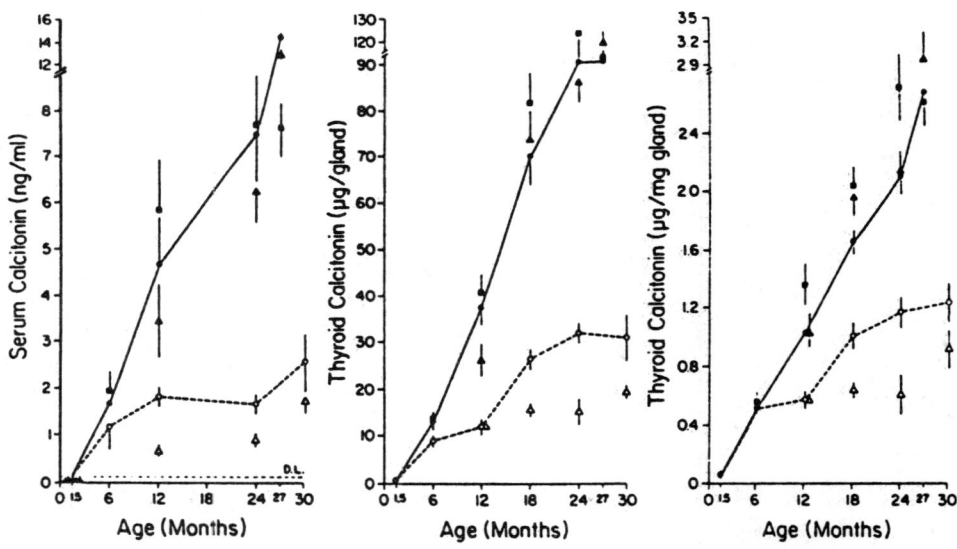

Figure 4.14. Effects of aging and diet on serum and thyroid calcitonin content in male Fischer 344 rats. See Figure 4.13 for designation of diet groups. Adapted from Kalu et al. (1983b), with permission.

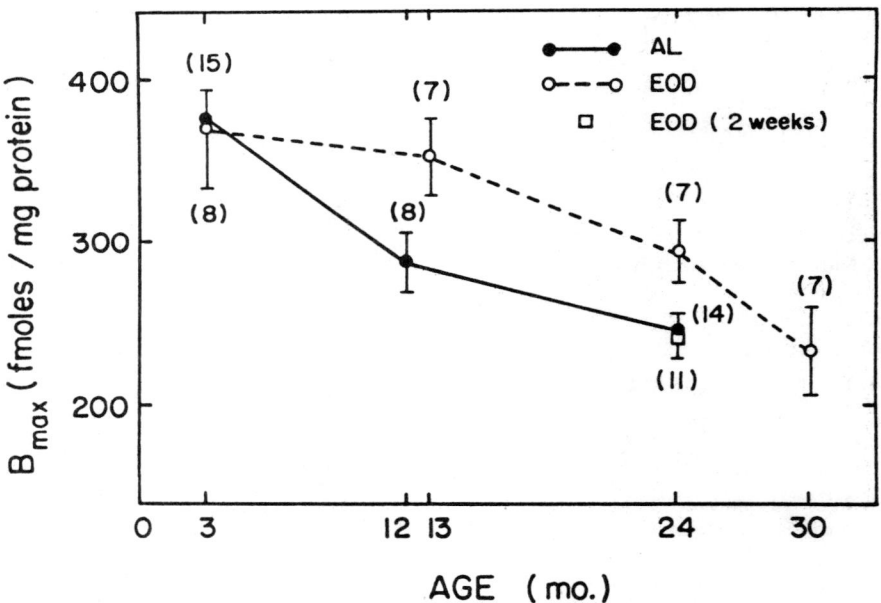

Figure 4.15. Effects of aging and DR on dopamine receptor concentrations in the striata of male Wistar rats. AL (●———●), ad lib fed; EOD (o-----o), fed every other day; EOD (2 weeks) (□), 24 month old rats fed every other day starting 2 weeks before sacrifice. From Roth et al. (1984), with permission.

With Drs. Patrick May and Caleb Finch, we have attempted to confirm in mice this DR-mediated saving of striatal dopaminereceptors. However, our preliminary results do not show any influence of DR on this age-sensitive parameter.

Synopsis

Table 4.6 summarizes extent data on the endocrine effects of long-term, LS-prolonging DR. It also indicates the effects of normal aging on these parameters, based on the review of Cole et al. (1982). The list is short because few solidly established indexes of neuroendocrine aging exist for rodents and DR data are even fewer.

TABLE 4.6

Influences of Dietary Restriction on Neuroendocrine Aging[a]

Age-Sensitive Parameter	Effect of DR
♀ hormonal changes and reproductive decline	↑ age of onset
↓T_4 levels in serum	<−>, ↓
↓T_3 levels in serum	↓
↑glucose and insulin levels in serum	↓
↓glucose tolerance	↑
↑insulin resistance	↓
↓glucose-stimulated insulin secretion/unit pancreas	<−>
↑glucagon levels in serum	<−>
↓glucagon-stimulated lipolysis in adipocytes	↑
↓epinepherine-stimulated lipolysis in adipocytes	↑
↑PTH levels in serum	↓
↑calcitonin levels in serum	↓
↓concentration of striatal dopamine receptors	↑, <−>

[a]Data for DR are from long-term studies using regimens shown or highly likely to extend maximum LS (see text for references). The effect of DR is that relative to ad lib fed controls. The effect of aging is the one arrived at for rats in the review of Cole et al. (1982) or, for later DR studies, the effect of age on responses of normally fed controls. Symbols: ↑, increase; ↓, decrease; <−>, no effect.

Nucleic Acid Content, Expression and Repair

The nucleic acid content in cells from rodents underfed for many months, but not noticeably malnourished in the sense of essential nutrient deficits, is the subject of several reports. (We do not cover the large literature on frank malnutrition.) Certain of the DR reports also describe protein parameters. In these instances, both will be discussed. Not a great deal is known about gene expression in the DR model; however, based on abstracts of meeting reports, this will soon change. Likewise, there are few publications relating to DNA repair of cells from rodents subjected to long-term DR but several laboratories are now studying this aspect of caloric restriction.

Content

Srivastava and colleagues at the University of Montreal have published four studies in this area.

(1) Female rats fed at half ad lib level for 5 months showed changes in nucleic acid metabolism in liver, brain and kidney (Srivastava et al., 1972). Because the focus here was on the response of an underfed rat to the additional metabolic demands of gestation and lactation, DR and controls were mated at 3 months of age with young, fertile males. Liver and kidney weights fell with DR. Brain weight was stable. Total DNA and RNA content fell in each of these three organs. In contrast, the amount of RNA per cell was *increased* by DR in liver and brain. Cell weight increased with DR in all organs. Protein content per organ fell but protein per cell rose. When rats were injected with ^{14}C-leucine and 6-^{14}C-orotate, the incorporation of ^{14}C-leucine per mg RNA increased in liver and kidney and decreased in brain with DR, whereas the incorporation of labelled orotate per mg RNA increased dramatically with DR in all three organs. Thus, protein and RNA synthesis rates were increased in the DR group.

(2) Liver RNA metabolism was studied in female Sprague-Dawley rats underfed (50% DR) a NPD for 13 months (Srivastava et al., 1978). Liver weights and BWs reflected the degree of underfeeding. The RNA/DNA ratio fell and rates of synthesis and degradation of liver RNA rose with DR. The largest effects of DR were on tRNA and 4-18S RNA fractions.

(3) A more recent study of liver nucleic acid and protein metabolism in EDR rats on a vitamin- and mineral-enriched PD tested animals restricted by 10, 30 or 50 percent for 24 weeks (Shatenstein et al., 1985). Table 4.7 gives data for control (ad lib fed) and DR (50% of ad lib) rats. Liver growth and the rate of accumulation of RNA, DNA and protein were slowed by DR. Free amino acid and nucleotide pool sizes fell. Rates

TABLE 4.7

Influences of Dietary Restriction on Nucleic Acid and
Protein Metabolism in Rat Liver[a]

Parameter, units	Ad Lib	DR	Effect of DR[b]
1. Body wt., g	290	164	↓43%
2. Liver wt., g	7.0	3.5	↓50%
3. Total RNA, mg	45	22	↓51%
4. Total DNA, mg	26	14	↓46%
5. Total protein, mg	1700	910	↓46%
6. Protein: DNA	66	68	NSD
7. Free amino acid pool size[c]	324	152	↓53%
8. Free nucleotide content (mg)	183	83	↓55%
9. Protein synth. (^{14}C-leu./mg pro.)	434	364	NSD
10. RNA synth. (^{3}H-orotate/mg RNA)	10,500	10,900	NSD

[a] Data adapted from Shatenstein et al. (1985) are for female Sprague-Dawley rats fed 50% of ad lib intake for 24 weeks post-weaning.
[b] Gives the effect of DR as a percentage change from the value for ad lib controls. NSD, no significant difference.
[c] Based on absorption at 280 nm.

of RNA and protein synthesis were not much influenced by DR in this study.

(4) Srivastava and Thakur (1987) reported in an abstract that 30 or 50 percent EDR imposed on female rats returned the levels of RNA and protein synthesis in livers from 11 and 22 month old rats to the levels of 1 to 3 month old controls. It appears from their brief report that protein synthesis rose with age in the control group, whereas it is difficult to judge how age influenced RNA synthesis.

Barrows and Kokkonen studied mice underfed by their EOD regimen. At 7 months of age, the protein content per mg of DNA in liver and kidney was not influenced by EOD feeding (Barrows & Kokkonen, 1978). Likewise, EOD-fed and control groups showed similar amounts of DNA per mg tissue. In sharp contrast to most data for DR rats, liver weight did not fall with DR, despite the fact that the EOD regime lowered BW by 30 percent. A more recent study (Barrows & Kokkonen, 1985) of B6D2F$_1$ hybrid mice also measured DNA and protein content of liver and kidney after EOD feeding, but included other organs (spleen, heart, brain). Also the DR was to 33 months. The authors concluded that aging and EOD-feeding reduced cell size in the liver but not elsewhere.

Rats subjected to EDR in Merry's colony have been described in several recent reports on the content and synthesis of nucleic acids and proteins.

(1) Total DNA, RNA, and protein in livers, kidneys, hearts and thymuses at 9 ages (21 days to 25 months) were quantitated in rats by Merry and Holehan (1985b) (Figure 4.16). Early-onset DR decreased the content of these molecules in these organs at all ages, except for the thymus where the DR curves reached or exceeded control levels at 1

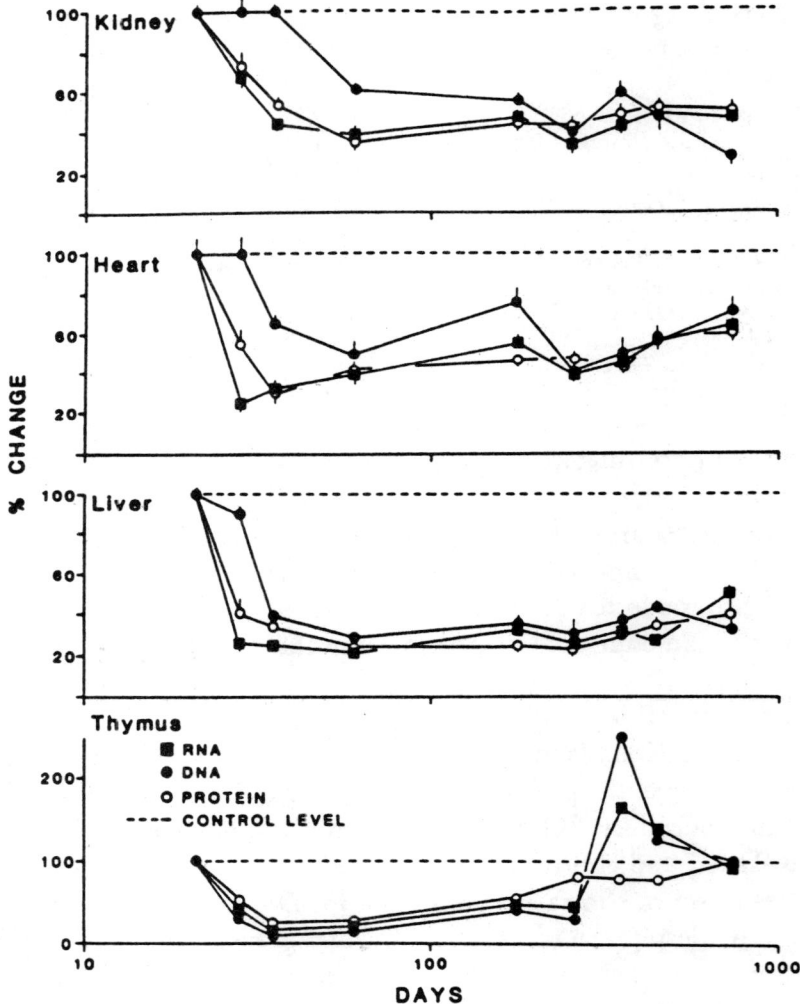

Figure 4.16. Relative changes in RNA, DNA and protein content in tissues from male Sprague-Dawley rats on DR (50% of ad lib) as a function of age (log scale). From Merry and Holehan (1985b).

year of age. Ratios among the DNA, RNA and protein values were calculated. The authors stated: "The capacity for protein synthesis (RNA/DNA ratio) was decreased by restricted feeding and was associated with a reduced protein/DNA ratio indicative of reduced cell size during the first six months of life. The translational activity per ribosome (protein/RNA ratio) was not disturbed by undernutrition in any of the tissues studied." The lower RNA/DNA and protein/DNA ratios in DR rats were largely early life (first year) effects.

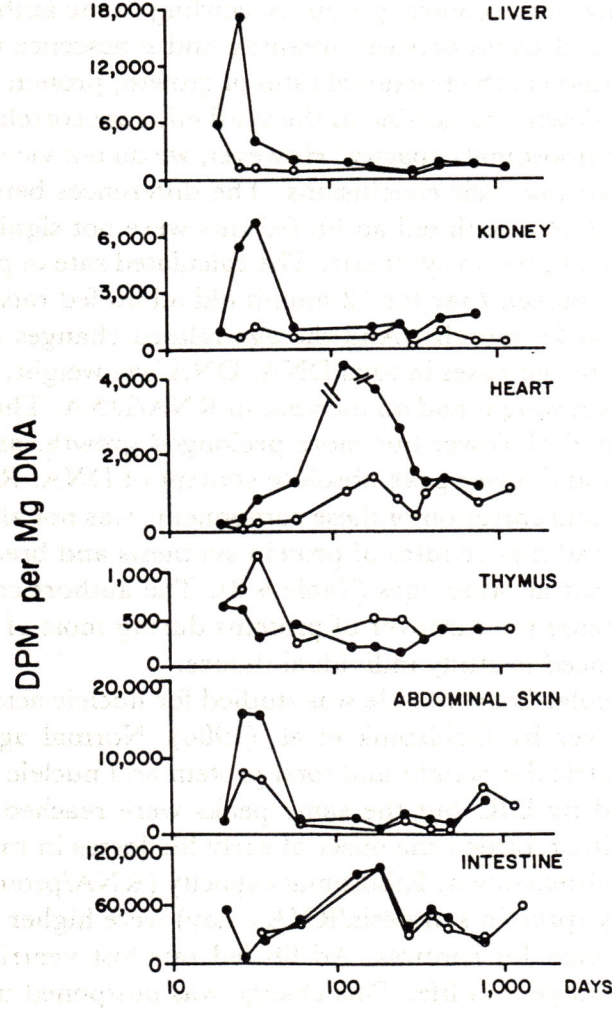

Figure 4.17. DNA synthesis (^{3}H-thymidine incorporation) as a function of age (log scale) in tissues from male Sprague-Dawley rats fed either restricted (o) or ad lib (•) diets. Adapted from Merry and Holehan (1985b), with permission.

In vivo DNA synthesis (^{3}H-thymidine uptake) was measured in the same tissues as well as in skin and intestine over the LS. As shown in Figure 4.17, DR suppressed first year peaks in all tissues except thymus and intestine. Thymus again differed by having *higher* DNA synthesis with DR. Late-life declines in DNA synthesis were not apparent.

(2) Lewis et al. (1985) determined whole body content of nucleic acids and proteins as well as protein turnover rates in rats of diverse ages injected with ^{3}H-phenylalanine before sacrifice. The findings of this important study are summarized in Table 4.8. We must first consider the effects of aging in the control group. According to the authors, "Normal developmental changes between weaning and senescence included progressive decreases in the fractional rates of growth, protein synthesis and protein breakdown; the decline in the synthetic rate correlating with decreases in the ribosomal capacity." However, we do not view their data as entirely supporting their conclusions. The differences between the values for 12 and 24 month old ad lib fed rats were not significant for the fractional rate of protein synthesis. The calculated rate of protein breakdown was 8.1 percent/day for 12 month old ad lib fed rats compared to 10.9 percent at 24 months. And the age-related changes in the second year of life were decreases in total DNA, DNA/wet weight, total protein, and protein/wet weight and an increase in RNA/DNA. The main effects of DR consisted of slower but more prolonged growth, and a retarded accumulation and lower peak absolute content of DNA, RNA and protein. But the concentration of these components was not altered by DR. Rats on DR had higher rates of protein synthesis and breakdown at 12 months, but not at other ages (Table 4.8). The authors concluded that DR may increase the turnover of proteins during most of life, and emphasized the need to study individual tissues.

(3) Ventricular heart muscle was studied for nucleic acid content and protein turnover by Goldspink et al. (1986). Normal age-specific increases in ventricular weight and total protein and nucleic acid contents were retarded by DR, but the same peaks were reached 1 year later. Early-onset DR retarded the onset of early life losses in rates of protein synthesis and breakdown. Ribosomal capacity (RNA/protein) and ribosomal activity (protein synthesis/RNA · day) were higher for adult and old DR rats than for controls. Ad lib fed rats lost ventricular protein over the second year of life. This change was postponed until the third year by DR.

(4) These same parameters were considered in fast (anterior tibialis) and slow (soleus) types of skeletal muscles by El Haj et al. (1986).

TABLE 4.8

Effects of Aging and Dietary Restriction on Whole Body Nucleic Acid and Protein Contents and on Protein Turnover in Rats[a]

Parameter	Effect of Age		Effect of EDR by Age		
	1.7→12	12→24	1.7	12	24
BW(g)	↑52%	↑9%	↓67%	↓56%	↓43%
Total RNA (mg)	-	-	↓72%	↓39%	↓21%
RNA/wet wt. (µg/g)	↓50%	-	-	-	-
Total DNA (mg)	↑17%	↓23%	↓68%	↓49%	↓35%
DNA/wet wt. (µg/g)	↓40%	↓32%	-	-	-
RNA/DNA	↓12%	↑32%	-	-	-
Total protein (g)	↑126%	↓24%	↓70%	↓51%	↓26%
Protein/wet wt. (%)	-	↓30%	-	-	-
Fractional rate of protein synth. (%/day)	↓65%	-	-	↑45%	-
Total protein synthesized (g/day)	-	-	↓70%	-	-
Total protein synthesized (g/day·kg BW)	↓61%	-	-	↑61%	-
Total protein synthesized (g/day·g RNA)	↓24%	-	-	-	-
RNA/protein ("ribosomal capacity," mg/g)	↓56%	-	-	↑23%	-
Calculated rate of breakdown (%/day)	↓62%	-	-	↑60%	-

[a] The "Effect of Age" is for ad lib fed rats. "1.7→12" gives the percent change from 1.7 to 12 months of age in ad lib fed controls, thereby showing the relative change during the growth period. "12→24" indicates the percent change from 12 to 24 months of age in ad lib fed controls, thereby giving changes from middle to later adulthood. The "Effect of EDR by Age" shows the percent change in the DR group at that age relative to age-matched controls. As DR began at 22 days, the 1.7 month value is the result of only 1 month of DR. "-" indicates no significant difference. Protein synthesis was measured after injection of ^{3}H-phenylalanine. The fractional rate of protein synthesis was calculated from the CPM of both the free and protein bound phenylalanine in the whole bodies. Total rate of protein synthesis = (fractional rate) × (protein content). Adapted from Lewis et al. (1985).

Again, DR slowed muscle growth as mirrored by 50 percent decreases in DNA, RNA and protein contents. Late-life declines in mass of these skeletal muscles were mild compared to those in the heart. Total protein synthesis (mg/day or mg/RNA · day) was reduced by DR, but fractional protein synthesis (%/day) was largely insensitive to DR. Ribosomal activity (mg protein synthesized/mg RNA · day) did not fall with age; however, it was reduced by DR at several ages. The ribosomal capacity (RNA/protein) fell with aging in controls but not in DR rats. Protein turnover tended to be lowered by DR. Acute starvation (malnutrition) caused muscle atrophy. By contrast, long-term DR slowed muscle growth, but did not cause atrophy.

(5) A recent report from this group (Goldspink et al., 1987) describes these same parameters for the diaphragm and extensor digitorum longus muscles. Both muscles showed post-weaning decreases in fractional rates of growth, protein synthesis and protein breakdown, which progressed with age. Muscle growth was retarded by EDR. In later life, muscle sizes and total (not fractional) protein synthesis rates were lower in rats on EDR. As was the case in the study of El Haj et al. (1986) on other skeletal muscles, protein turnover was generally lowered by DR, an opposite effect to this group's findings for heart, whole body, lymphocytes, renal cells, and small intestine.

In summary, DR in rats generally: (1) reduces nucleic acid and protein content of the whole body and its organs, (2) increases the fractional rates of protein synthesis and breakdown in whole bodies and heart muscle but tends to reduce these in skeletal muscle, and (3) increases ribosomal activity in heart muscle and lowers it in skeletal muscles. Clearly the effects of DR can differ from tissue-to-tissue. Further studies on protein metabolism in DR animals are discussed in a later section (see "Protein Content, Synthesis, and Turnover," this Chapter).

Expression

Recent work reported in abstracts from the 1987 FASEB meeting as part of a symposium "Aging and Food Restriction: Mechanisms and Correlations" indicates that DR can retard severe age-related losses in gene expression. Richardson et al. (1987a) reported that liver preparations from ad lib fed Fischer 344 rats showed decreases from 6 to 30 months of age in the expression (as indicated by synthesis, mRNA levels, and transcription) of α2u-globulin (90% decrease) and of SOD and catalase genes (60% falls). Rats on EDR studied at 18 months of age showed much higher levels of gene expression than age matched controls. The higher levels were 180-300 percent for α2u-globulin, 50 percent for catalase, and 80 percent for SOD (see Table 4.2, #6). Quite recently, Richardson et al. (1987b) fully reported their findings on α2u-globulin expression.

Good's group (Risley et al., 1987) studied the intestinal epithelial cells of mice from short-lived strains. The microsomal fractions from DR mice did not show (or showed less of) 2-4 strong protein bands present in ad lib fed mice, a finding which could signal an impact of DR on gene expression.

Repair

Experiments done in our laboratory (Licastro et al., 1986 & 1988) measured DNA repair in splenocytes from $C3B10RF_1$ mice fed normal or restricted diets. Spleen cells were UV-irradiated and DNA repair estimated by measuring ^{3}H-TdR incorporation in the presence of hydroxyurea (unscheduled DNA synthesis). The results (Table 4.9) indicate that repair fell with age in all groups; however, higher values were observed for late middle-age to old DR animals than in age matched controls. Ad lib feeding of a NPD yielded the least repair.

Similarly, very recent findings from Richardson's laboratory describe a 30 percent increase in UV-induced unscheduled DNA synthesis in liver and kidney cells from Fischer 344 rats on DR (Weraarchakul & Richardson, 1988). Additional recent studies on DNA repair are commented on in Chapter 5 (see "DNA Repair").

TABLE 4.9

Effect of DR on DNA Repair After UV Irradiation in Spleen Cells From Young and Old Mice[a]

Diet Group	Age (mo)	n	DNA Repair
1. NPD, ad lib	3-7	12	3.4 ± 0.4
	18-27	13	1.8 ± 0.2
2. PD, 95 kcal/week	5-7	6	4.7 ± 0.6
	21-28	14	2.3 ± 0.1
3. PD, 55 kcal/week	4-7	9	4.3 ± 0.4
	19-30	17	3.0 ± 0.3
	45	3	1.9 ± 0.2

[a] DNA repair has been expressed as a stimulation index: (cpm of cultures treated with UV plus hydroxyurea) ÷ (cpm of cultures treated with hydroxyurea only). Values are mean ± SEM as adapted from Licastro et al. (1986 & 1988).

Protein Content, Synthesis and Turnover

Evidence discussed above from studies including both nucleic acids and proteins, indicates that DR reduces the total protein content of organs. Effects on protein synthesis seem to be tissue-specific. Other work that is limited to protein metabolism also provides much information about long-term DR.

Content

Whole body protein metabolism was studied in male EDR (50% of ad lib) and control (80% of ad lib) Wistar rats from 21 months of age to death by Fujita and Ichikawa (1986). Controls were mildly underfed to avoid complicating the experiment with late-life decreases in ad lib intakes. In this study, LSs were only mildly increased by EDR (average LS = 31 months for controls and 33 months for DR animals). Figure 4.18 shows data on BW, food intake and nitrogen related variables. Late-

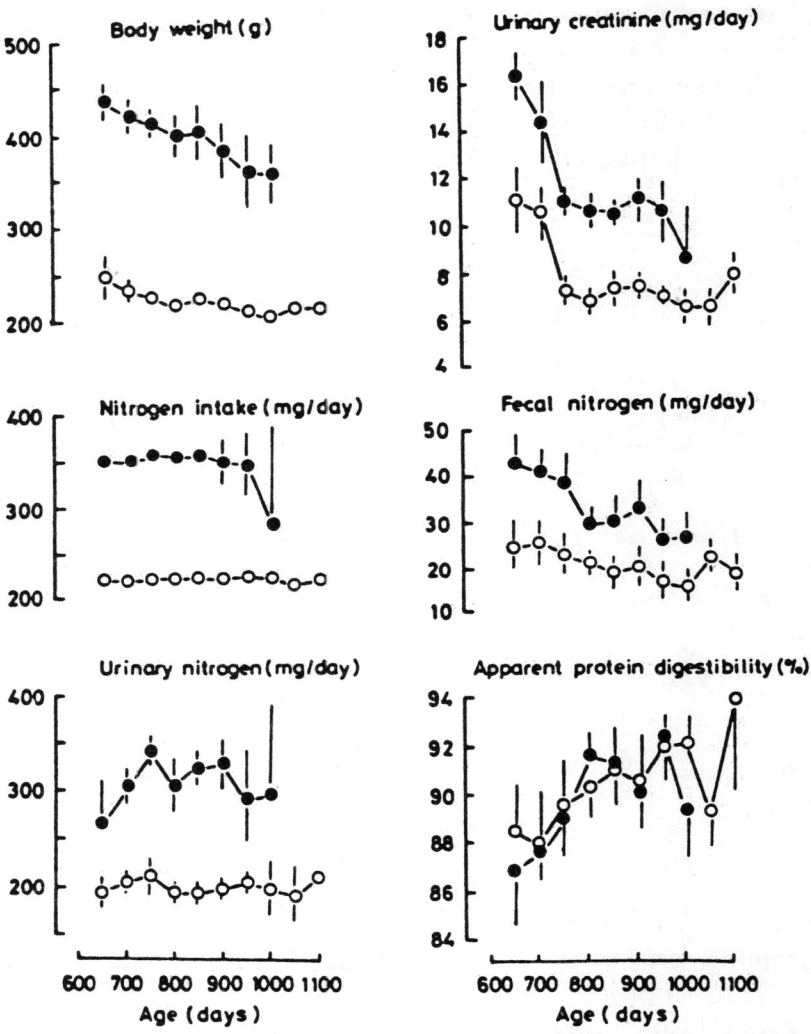

Figure 4.18. Changes with age in BW, nitrogen intake and excretion, and protein digestibility in male Wistar rats fed either restricted (o) or control (•) diets. Values are mean ± SD. From Fujita and Ichikawa (1986), with permission.

life losses in BW for controls *preceded* decreases in food intake suggesting the importance of age-related metabolic changes and diseases (not just lowered food intake) in BW loss in old age. Urinary creatinine, a crude index of skeletal muscle mass, declined in both DR and control groups, though more so in controls. Fecal nitrogen fell due to a decrease in fecal weight (not in fecal nitrogen concentration). Protein digestibility was not influenced by DR. Nitrogen balance (Figure 4.19) was highly variable, especially in controls. Average nitrogen balance after 650 days was −11.5 mg nitrogen/day for controls and −1.3 mg nitrogen/day for the DR group; however, this apparent difference was largely due to a sudden drop in food intake for the three longest-lived control animals and

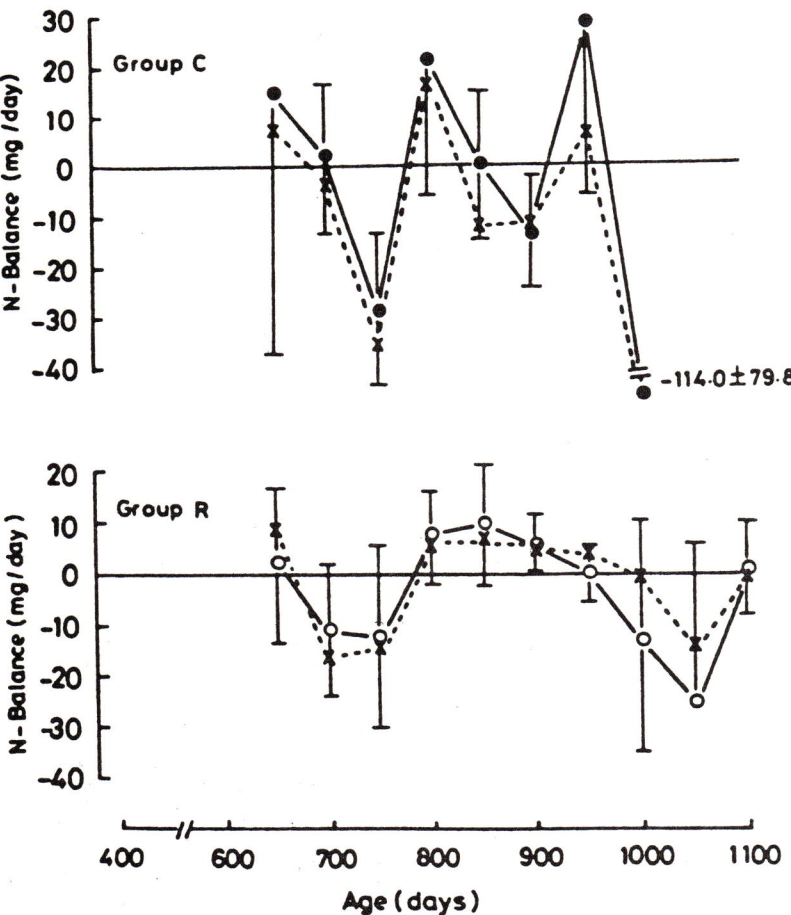

Figure 4.19. Changes with age in nitrogen balance in later life in male Wistar rats fed either restricted (o) or control (•) diets. Values are mean ± SD. From Fujita and Ichikawa (1986), with permission.

170   *The Retardation of Aging and Disease by Dietary Restriction*

was not due to an increased loss of urinary nitrogen. Thus, nitrogen metabolism at the whole body level did not change consistently even quite late in life. Most recently, this group reported that the main cause of late-life losses in BW is an increase in energy expenditure due to an increase in basal metabolic rate (not activity) (Ichikawa & Fujita, 1987).

Imposing 50 percent EDR of Purina Lab Chow™ on female rats for 3 months, Dutta et al. (1981) found that EDR did not decrease total serum protein or albumin levels but did decrease levels of alpha and gamma globulins.

Protein content in female $C3B10RF_1$ mice on EDR in our colony was investigated in two collaborative studies. the first study showed that, as studied in 2, 11 or 30 month old mice, EDR retarded age-related losses of gamma crystallins in the eye lens (Leveille et al., 1984) (Figure 4.20). Mechanisms underlying this loss or its inhibition by DR are unclear; however, levels of this structural protein decrease with aging in humans and may conribute to the genesis of cataracts. The second study (unpublished) was undertaken to determine the levels of oxidatively modified liver proteins in normal and DR mice. Female $C3B10RF_1$ mice 14

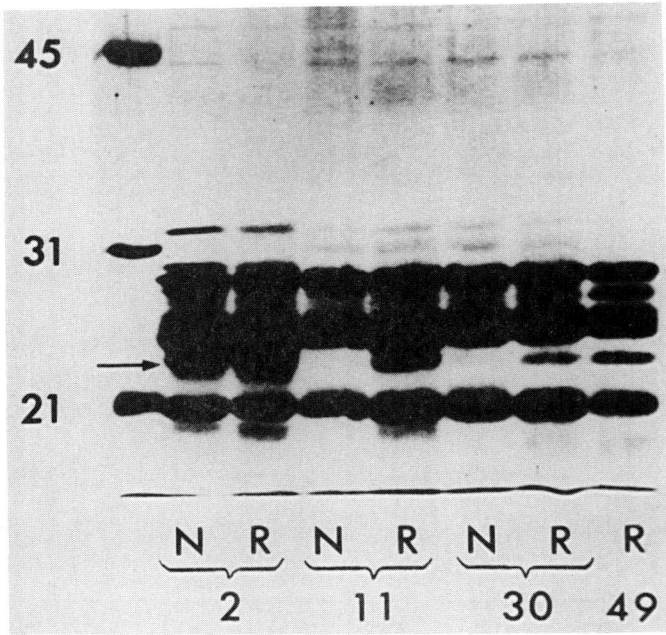

Figure 4.20. Soluble proteins from the eye lens of normally-fed (N) and restricted (R) $C3B10RF_1$ female mice as resolved by polyacrylamide gel electrophoresis. Numbers on the X-axis indicate mouse age in months. Numbers on the Y-axis give molecular weights (kD). From Leveille et al. (1984).

months of age were sent to Earl Stadtman's laboratory at the NIH. DR showed no effect on levels of such proteins. Stadtman's group has suggested that oxidative changes in enzymes (brought about chiefly by mixed function oxidases) may lead to the accumulation of inactive or defective enzyme molecules in old age (Oliver et al., 1987). Older mice need to be studied in relation to this hypothesis.

Synthesis and Turnover

Richardson's laboratory first provided data suggesting that DR opposes the age-related decline in *vitro* protein synthesis. They fed rats a DR regimen identical to that used by Masoro's group. Richardson and Cheung (1982) reported that spleen cells from two 19 month old EDR rats synthesized more total protein and interleukin 2 (IL-2) than did cells from age-matched controls. They proposed that an age-related decline in protein synthesis leads to a fall in protein turnover, and suggested that this latter decrement is the molecular basis for many age-related physiologic changes.

Other findings from Richardson's group supporting this view are as follows:

(1) Hepatocyte protein synthesis fell sharply during adulthood in control rats, such that activities at 19 months of age were only half that at 4 months of age (Birchenall-Sparks et al., 1985). Rats on DR showed no decrease in this measure through 19 months of age. Dietary restriction lowered the protein content per hepatocyte but did not affect RNA levels. The content of DNA per hepatocyte increased with age, and at 19 months (the oldest age tested) was lower in cells from DR than from control animals.

(2) Isolated kidney cells from four 19 month old DR rats synthesized protein at a 45 percent higher rate than cells from age-matched, ad lib fed rats (Ricketts et al., 1985). For controls the rate fell 63 percent between 4 and 23 months of age, and did not decline thereafter. The degree of proteinuria was lower in DR rats.

(3) Richardson (1985) reported in a review article that cell-free protein synthetic activity of testicular tissue fell in control animals in mid-adulthood but not in DR animals (Fig. 4.21).

(4) Sparks et al. (1983) reported in an abstract that cell-free protein synthetic activity in the brain falls with age and is not influenced by DR.

Findings on protein synthesis and turnover from other laboratories include:

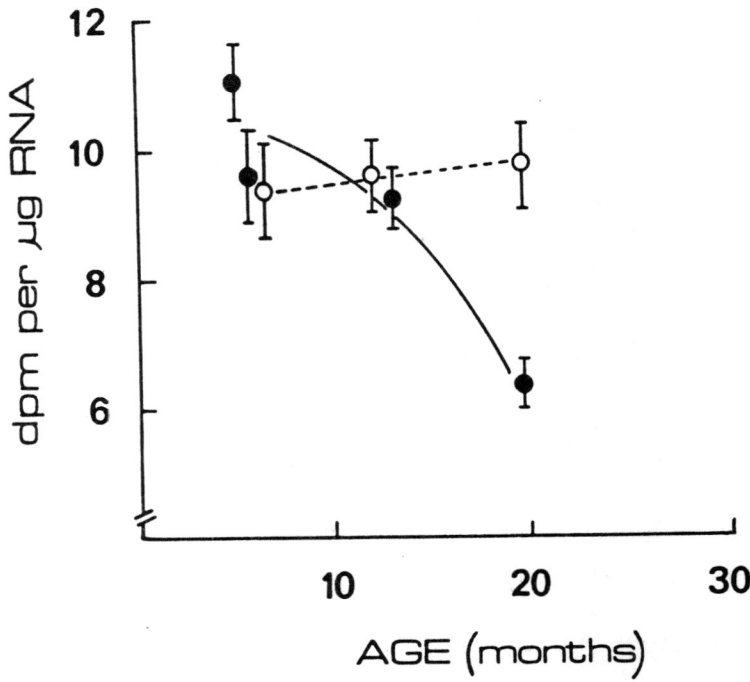

Figure 4.21. Effects of aging and DR on protein synthesis in testicular tissue from Fischer 344 rats fed either restricted (o-----o) or ad libitum (•———•) diets. From Richardson (1985), with permission.

(1) Liver slices from rats fed a PD at half of the ad lib level for 11 weeks incorporated only 40 percent as much ^{14}C glycine as did control slices (Barrows et al., 1965). Based on determination of the half-life of protein *in vivo*, Barrows and Kokkonen (1987) reported a *decrease* in liver protein synthesis in DR mice.

(2) Ward (1987) studied protein synthesis and turnover in perfused livers of EDR and control rats. Both parameters declined with age, starting at about 6 months. The losses were not prevented by DR; however, protein synthesis and degradation rates were maintained in the DR liver at levels at least 40 percent greater than in the ad lib liver. Thus, DR raised protein turnover rates in these experiments.

(3) Thyroid hormones affect the synthesis and breakdown of protein. In skeletal muscle of thyroidectomized rats the rate of protein synthesis falls because of a loss of total RNA and not because of any drop in RNA activity (Brown et al., 1981). Protein degradation rates likewise are lowered by thyroidectomy. These findings seem incongruous with reports of

increased protein turnover with DR, because DR is clearly a hypothyroid state.

(4) In a recent study in which EDR and control rats were injected with a labeled amino acid and the amount of label in liver proteins estimated 10 minutes later, Merry et al. (1987) reported that in DR rats the fractional rate of protein synthesis was depressed at ages 7 and 103 weeks but was not significantly altered at other times. Protein turnover in heart was increased in DR animals (Goldspink et al., 1986), and decreased in skeletal muscle tissue (El Haj et al., 1986; Goldspink et al., 1987). It was also decreased in the lung (Goldspink & Merry, 1988). The progressive loss of translational efficiency with age was slowed by DR.

(5) An age-related increase in heat-labile (i.e., altered) aminoacyl tRNA synthetases in mouse liver and brain was observed which was reversed and retarded in these respective organs by 70 days of ADR started at 23.5 months of age (Takahashi & Goto, 1987).

Thus, data on protein parameters in the DR rodent are limited and largely of recent origin. Although there may be some disagreement between *in vivo* and *in vitro* studies, support for increased protein turnover in some tissues with DR is mounting and the suggestion has been advanced that this may be central to DR's mode of action. But whether or not this provides a fundamental, primary explanation for DR remains an open question (see "PROTEIN SYNTHESIS, DNA, CHROMATIN, etc. . . .," Chapter 5).

Lipid Content and Peroxidation

On *a priori* grounds, lipid content ought to be influenced by DR. If the DR regimen is not fat-enriched, fat intakes are less for DR animals than for controls, which situation should reduce the amount of peroxidizable lipid in the former. The restriction of energy intake, an essential part of *all* good DR regimens, should also influence lipid content by limiting the energy available for storage as lipid. Alterations in intakes of micronutrients might also alter lipid metabolism.

Lipid peroxidation and lipofuscin content are indicators of the "peroxidative tone" of the animal (Ball et al., 1986). Determinations of lipid peroxides in tissue samples have been most frequently made by the thiobarbituric acid (TBA) assay which spectrophotometrically measures TBA-reactive substances, among them malondialdehyde (MDA), a decomposition product of lipid hydroperoxides (Marshall et al., 1985). But

MDA is only one of several TBA reactive substances (e.g. sugars, hemoglobin) in tissues. Further, the amount of MDA produced in the TBA reaction is not simply equal to the concentration of lipid hydroperoxides, but varies in the efficiency of conversion of hydroperoxide to MDA from 2.7 to 4.6 percent. As a sensitive and specific assay of lipid hydroperoxides, the TBA has its shortcomings.

Lipid Content

Several reports provide information on lipid content after long-term DR. Most data are for adipose tissues, sera, livers and whole animal bodies, and suggest that several changes in lipid content taking place during adulthood are retarded or prevented by DR.

Ross (1969) reported reduced levels of hepatic lipids in EDR rats fed as previously described (Table 2.4, #7; Table 4.2 #10). Food restriction did not strongly alter the percent of liver fat, but did reduce the total fat content (30% of control value) and the amount of fat per hepatocyte (70% of control value).

Nolen (1972) determined serum cholesterol and phospholipid levels, liver lipids and adipose tissue fatty acid composition for rats fed as described earlier (Table 2.6, #6). All diets contained high levels (17%) of soybean oil. Serum lipid levels were not affected by DR. At 24 months of age, livers from males (but not females) restricted only during the first 3 months, and then fed ad lib, showed higher total lipid and cholesterol levels than either ad lib or always restricted rats. Dietary influences on lipids in the livers of females were not striking. Adipose tissue fatty acids (16:0 = palmitic, 16:1 = palmitoleic, 18:0 = stearic, 18:1 = oleic, 18:2 = linoleic, 18:3 = linolenic) were quantitated. The overall effect of aging was to reduce proportionately the saturated fatty acids and to increase the level of monounsaturated fatty acids. Underfeeding initiated at 1 or 3 months of age tended to reduce these differences. Polyunsaturated fatty acids were clearly lower with advancing age, but higher for DR rats.

Influences of aging and DR on serum levels of cholesterol, phospholipids and triglycerides in the male Fischer rats were studied by Liepa et al. (1980). Age-related increases in all three parameters were held in check by DR (Figure 4.22). Postabsorptive free fatty acid concentrations fell with aging in ad lib fed controls, a loss partially prevented and long delayed by DR.

Yu et al. (1984a) observed that cholesterol and triglyceride concentrations increased with aging in the livers of ad lib fed rats. These increases

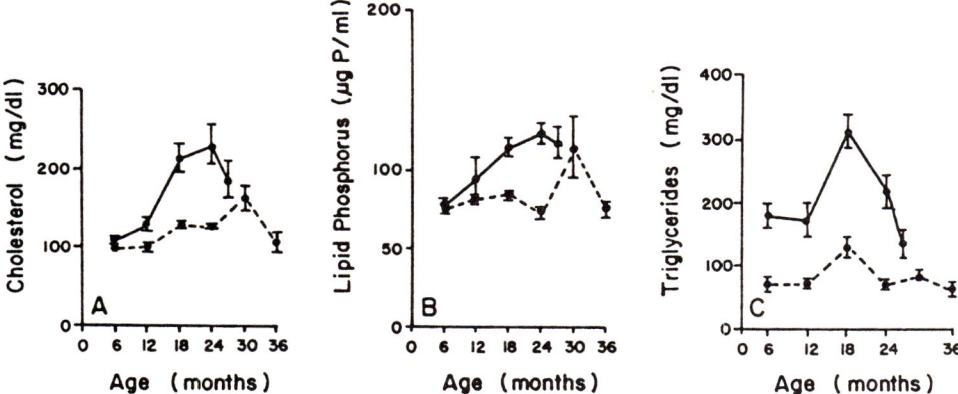

Figure 4.22. Serum levels of cholesterol (Panel A), phospholipids (Panel B) and triglycerides (Panel C) in male Fischer 344 rats fed either ad libitum (———) or restricted (-----) diets. From Liepa et al. (1980), with permission.

were partially inhibited by DR started at 6 weeks or 6 months of age. The phospholipid content of liver was uninfluenced by either aging or DR.

Sachan and Das (1982) mainly studied enzymes (Table 4.2, #2) but also described serum lipids in rats after 1.6 months of EDR. Concentrations of total lipids, polar lipids and neutral lipids were roughly halved by DR. A 2-fold increase in the level of linoleic acid (18:2) was found in sera from DR rats. Thus, the underfed rats were very likely not deficient in essential fatty acids.

Taylor et al. (1974) imposed EDR (an NPD at 55% of ad lib) on Wistar rats for 3 months. In their study, restriction did not alter serum or adipose tissue levels of free fatty acids.

Only the report of Mark et al. (1984b) addressed the effects of long-term DR on prostaglandin metabolism. Five month old MRL/n mice (physiologically normal congenic partners of the autoimmune-prone MRL/lpr mouse) were fed 10 kcal/day of a 5 percent corn oil diet and were compared to mice of the same strain fed 20 kcal/day (nealry ad lib) of either a 5 or 20 percent corn oil diet. The 10 kcal/day intake lowered serum cholesterol. Thromboxane B_2 production by platelets was not altered by this degree of DR. But arachidonic acid-stimulated PGI_2 production by heart tissue was 3-fold higher in the DR group than in the group fed the low fat diet ad libitum. In general, diets producing high levels of serum cholesterol lowered PGI_2 production by the heart, and raised thromboxane B_2 production by platelets.

Two short-term studies on male Sprague-Dawley rats contain information on serum cholesterol composition. Schneeman et al. (1986) carried out EDR for 21 days such that the final BW was 70 percent that of controls. Dietary restriction reduced VLDL triglyceride and HDL cholesterol levels. Imposing a 50 percent restriction of an undescribed "standard cholesterol-free diet" on adult rats, Corraze et al. (1985) observed that DR Initially *increased* serum cholesterol levels over those of an ad lib fed group, but that this difference vanished by 2 months, at which time the experiment was terminated.

Lipid Peroxidation and Lipofuscin

Evidence is rapidly mounting to suggest that long-term DR lowers levels of lipid peroxides and lipofuscin. These data lend indirect support for a role of peroxidative damage in the aging process. Again, the quantitation of lipid peroxidation has been done by the TBA assay and, as just discussed, this assay has drawbacks. Whether DR reduces the production of active oxygen, enhances its detoxification, or both, or neither, is not yet established.

Enesco and Kruk (1981) fed weanling male Swiss albino mice either a 4 or 26 percent casein PD ad lib until 1 year of age. Lipid peroxidation products were extracted from brains and hearts at various ages. Fluorescence of these extracts was measured as an index of lipofuscin levels. One notes that their 1 year old "controls" were huge, *averaging* about 60 g in BW (We have never encountered any mouse this heavy in the strains we have studied.) vs. 25 g for the low protein group. Significantly less fluorescence was detected in brains from the group fed the low protein diet at 3, 5, 7 or 12 months of age (18-52% decreases). In hearts, the only effect of underfeeding was a reduction (25%) in lipofuscin at 12 months of age.

Two studies of Chipalkatti, De and Aiyar, discussed earlier regarding enzyme activities (Table 4.2, #3 & 4), also contained data on lipid peroxidation and lipofuscin in DR mice. In #3 (Table 4.2), female Swiss mice were given either a 6, 12 or 24 percent protein diet from time of weaning. The low protein diets retarded growth, but in sharp contrast to the study just discussed, final BWs after 9 months averaged 25-28 g in all groups. Liver homogenates from 1 year old mice fed the 6 or 12 percent protein diets contained 25 percent less lipid peroxides than those on the 24 percent diet. Lipofuscin content of heart, brain and intestine increased with the level of protein intake. In study #4, weanling Swiss female mice were fed either ad libitum or half of ad lib intake until 12 months of age. Figure 4.23 shows that the content of cardiac lipofuscin rose during the first year of life to a greater extent in the control than in the EDR group. An increase of lipofuscin occurred also in the brain, and this was less sensitive to EDR's inhibitory action. Lipid peroxidation in liver homogenates was decreased 40-45 percent by EDR at 6 and 12 months of age. Because SOD activity was increased by a low protein diet (study #3) but not by 50 percent DR (study #4), no strict association between SOD activity and lipid peroxidation can be inferred from these data.

Our own study (Koizumi et al., 1987a) (Table 4.2, #14; Table 4.4) showing 40 to 65 percent increases in liver catalase activity and 13 to 40 percent decreases in liver lipid peroxidation (MDA formation) in DR animals, differed from the earlier investigations by using a DR regimen proven to extend LS, and by including old mice among the animals tested.

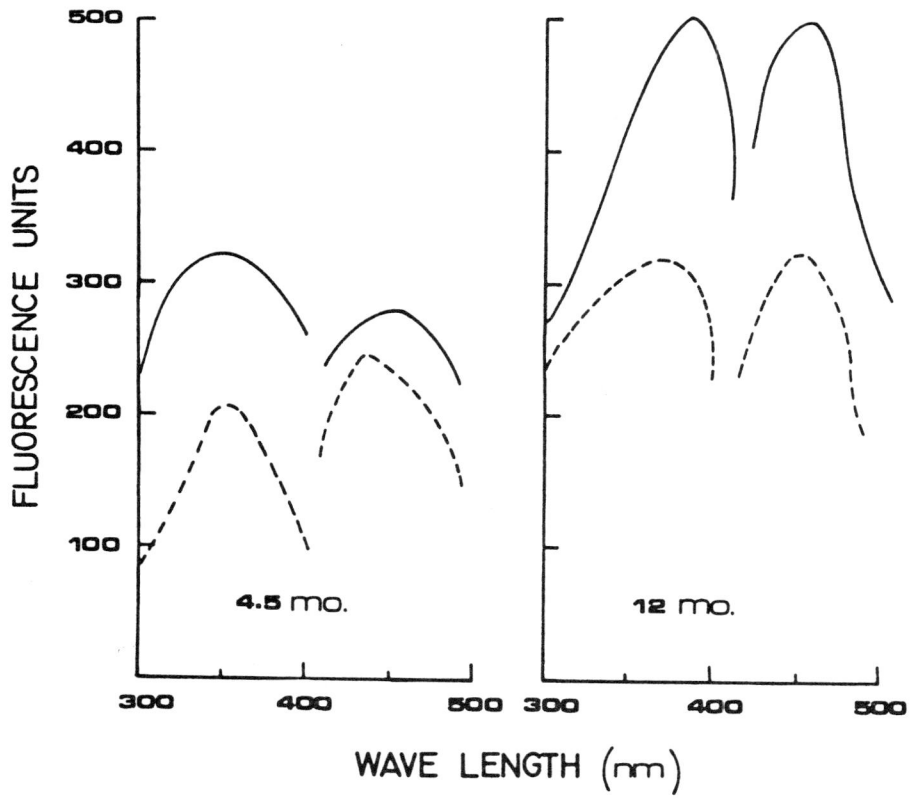

Figure 4.23. Heart lipofuscin content in 4.5 and 12 month old Swiss female mice fed either an ad lib (———) or a restricted (50% of ad lib, -----) diet. From Chipalkatti et al. (1983), with permission.

Abstracts presented by the San Antonio group at recent meetings confirm and extend these findings (Laganiere & Yu, 1986; Laganiere et al. 1987). The investigators studied subcellular fractions of livers from DR and control rats. They observed that: (1) membrane lipid hydroperoxide content increased with age in both groups but was 2-fold less in DR rats at 6 and 24 months of age; (2) the ratio of unsaturated:saturated fatty acids in membranes decreased with age, and this decrease was prevented by DR; (3) cytosolic levels of antioxidants (glutathione, ascorbic acid) and activities of protective enzymes (catalase, glutathione reductase and transferase) fell with aging in the control group. Food restriction completely stopped the loss in glutathione and raised the activities of all three enzymes during the second year of life.

Laganiere and Yu (1987) recently published a full report on this work. Mitochondrial and microsomal membranes from livers of DR rats showed much lower levels of endogenous and enzyme-dependent lipid hydroperoxides. Both parameters rose with aging. Food restriction increased the content of linoleic acid and decreased that of docosapentaenoic acid in both membranes.

Preliminary data on aging in both germfree and conventionally housed Wistar rats fed either ad lib or restricted diets were reported by Wostmann et al. (1986). Serum MDA levels were lower in DR rats.

Therefore, DR appears to reduce the rate of age-related accumulation of lipid peroxidation and lipofuscin. The results support but certainly do not prove an important role of free radicals/active oxygen in aging processes. A clearer picture awaits the implementation of assays providing precise detection of the active oxygen species produced and the damage they may inflict.

Other Serum Components

Pickering and Pickering (1984) fed weanling Wistar rats of each sex a NPD either ad libitum or at several levels of DR for a 5 week period and measured a wide variety of parameters (clinical chemistry, hematology, organ weights). Underfeeding was associated with increased hemoglobin concentration, erythrocyte count, hematocrit and plasma chloride. Study of urine showed that restricted rats excreted an increased volume of more alkaline urine of lower specific gravity and containing more triphosphates than rats fed ad lib.

Sachan and Das (1982) reported that 1.6 months of EDR (50% ad lib) lowered serum levels of glucose, uric acid and fats in male Sprague-

Dawley rats. Unaltered parameters included calcium, phosphorus, total protein, albumin, total bilirubin and several serum enzymes.

IMMUNOLOGIC PARAMETERS

Dietary restriction strongly influences the immune system. It retards age-related changes in most immune parameters thus far measured. This action may at least in part explain the good health observed in old DR animals. We shall here focus on results obtained in rodents fed diets calorically restricted but still adequate in essential nutrients, and disregard the large literature on how *mal*nutrition devastates the immune system. Certain studies on ad lib low protein diets which did not produce overt malnutrition also merit consideration.

The immunogerontologic DR work has largely concerned mice. Publications began to appear in the early 1970s with most work from two laboratories. Good, Fernandes and colleagues reported most of what is known about short-lived strains, while our laboratory studied long-lived ones. Good's group first focussed on feeding low protein diets ad lib but later switched to restricted feeding of a complete diet. We have always taken the latter approach.

We will discuss five aspects of immunologic aging in relation to DR: (1) thymus, (2) cell numbers, proportions and subpopulations, (3) immune response capacities, (4) autoimmunity, and (5) lymphoid biochemistry.

Thymus

Thymic weight, structure and age involution are markedly altered by DR in mice. We measured thymus weights at 6, 16 and 24 weeks of age for female B10C3F$_1$ mice fed EDR or "control" (80% ad lib) regimens (Weindruch et al., 1979). (Our "controls" are in fact somewhat restricted, just enough so that all "control" animals eat all of what is offered them.) At 6 weeks of age the average thymus weight for DR mice was one-seventh that of controls (Figure 4.24). Over the next 10 weeks the control thymuses lost 60 percent of their mass while the average weight of a DR thymus increased. Thus, there was no real effect of DR on weights at 16 or 24 weeks of age. At this latter age, the thymus:BW ratio for the DR group exceeded that of controls.

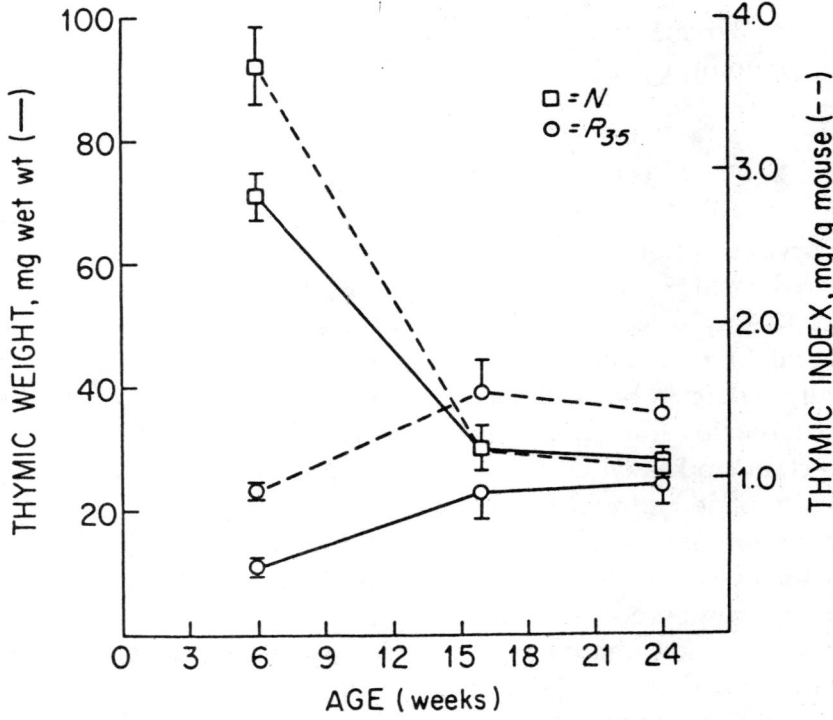

Figure 4.24. Thymus weight (mg, ———) and index (mg thymus/g mouse, - - - - -) in normally-fed (□) and diet restricted (o) B10C3F$_1$ female mice. From Weindruch et al. (1979).

In a subsequent study we determined by point counting volumetry the quantitative histologic make-up of thymuses from the 24 week old mice (Weindruch & Suffin, 1980). The fraction of thymus volume occupied by cortex is known to fall as the thymus involutes. Volume fraction ratios of cortex:medulla were about 2:1 for the DR group and 1:1 for controls, suggesting retardation of involution. The cortex of DR thymuses contained a greater volume fraction of lymphoid cells (60% of cells were lymphoid) than control cortexes (45% of cells were lymphoid). Food restriction did not influence the fraction of medullary volume populated by lymphoid cells. Stromal components occupied a very small part of the thymus. They were unaltered by DR. Thus, thymuses from 6 month old DR mice appeared histologically "younger" than those from age-matched controls.

Effects of 10 weeks of DR (50% of the ad lib intake of a NPD) started at 1 or 8 months of age on thymus mass and cell division in outbred rats were described by Franklin et al. (1983). Early-onset DR did allow for

BW gain, and lowered the following thymic parameters: (1) weight (by 30%), (2) mitotic index (by 20%) and, (3) cell density (as judged by number of cells in the microscopic field). If started at 8 months of age, ADR resulted in a 20 percent loss of BW, a 70 percent loss in thymus weight, and decreased cell density; but no alteration in mitotic rate, which was already depressed by age in the control group. Thymuses of older rats were more sensitive to DR, perhaps because these rats had been fed ad libitum until 8 months of age.

Other work has examined thymic factor and hormone levels in underfed rodents.

Chandra's group (Chandra et al., 1980; Heresi & Chandra, 1980) found that weanling rats exposed to 4 weeks of malnutrition (a 70% restriction of a NPD) exhibited very low serum thymic factor activities. They employed as bioassay the serum's capacity to produce mature T cells from splenocytes of thymectomized mice, as judged by levels of cells which rosetted with sheep red blood cells (SRBC).

We provided Allan Goldstein's laboratory with serum samples from C3B10RF$_1$ females of diverse ages (2, 7, 19, or 26 months) fed either control (80% of ad lib) or EDR (50% of ad lib) regimens and from 3 week old weanlings. Levels of thymosin$_{\alpha 1}$ were determined by radioimmunoassay (Weindruch et al., 1988). The average thymosin$_{\alpha 1}$ level was highest (60 ng/ml) at 3 weeks of age. It fell sharply thereafter, such that 2 month old mice fed either diet averaged 20 ng/ml. Any age-related declines after 2 months of age were mild and statistically significant only for DR mice bled 2 to 4 hours (but not 24-48 hours) postfeeding (Figure 4.25). Thymosin$_{\alpha 1}$ levels were slightly lower in DR sera in one experiment in which 19 month old mice were tested but not in another using 26 month old ones. Thus, age declines in this thymic hormone occurred early in life and appeared uninfluenced by DR.

In view of the often suggested similarities between DR and hypophysectomy (Hx), it is important to consider the report by Harrison et al. (1982) on thymic aging in hypophysectomized B6 mice. Surgery was performed on animals 8-9 months of age (Endocrine supplementation was started immediately.) and assays conducted at 15 months of age. The outcome of this experiment was very different from that reported for Hxed rats by Everitt's group (see *"Early-Onset Dietary Restriction (EDR),"* Chapter 2), who observed that Hxed rats eat less but live longer than controls. Harrison's group found that food intake was not reduced by Hx in mice but in fact increased by 18 percent. Nevertheless, the

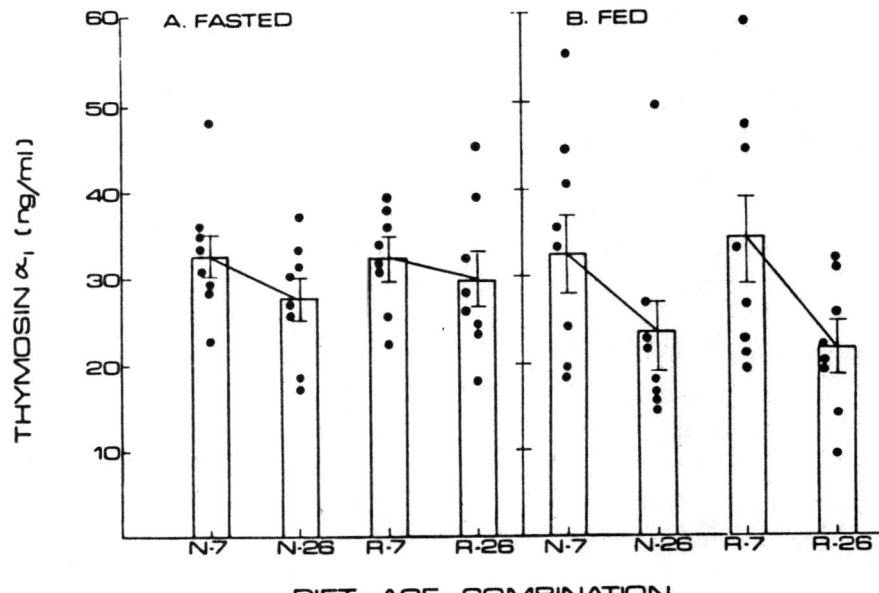

Figure 4.25. Serum thymosin$_{\alpha 1}$ levels in normally-fed (N) and restricted (R) female C3B10RF$_1$ mice. Adult (7 month, N or R) and old (26 month, N or R) mice were tested. Each symbol gives data for an individual mouse. The same 8 mice were tested for each diet-age combination after 24-48 hours of fasting and 2-4 hours post-feeding. Adapted from Weindruch et al. (1988).

Hxed mice weighed 24 percent less than controls, and looked younger as well (sleeker coats, more active). Hypophysectomy resulted in larger thymus weights (34 vs 25 mg) and a larger cortex:medulla ratio (4.5 vs. 2.4). Several (but not all) of the age-sensitive immune responses tested were "younger" in the Hxed group. However, the LS of the Hxed mice was somewhat curtailed. This failure of Hx to extend LS could have resulted from the increased food intake following the procedure, complications from the surgery, shortcomings in the hormone replacement regimen, or unknown factors. Unfortunately, causes of death in Hxed and control mice were not reported.

The effects of low protein diets on the thymus have also been studied. Bell and co-workers (1976, 1977) fed a 4 percent protein diet ad lib to weanling mice for 1 month and found that lymphoid tissue loss was more severe in the thymus than in the spleen or mesenteric lymph nodes. Cortical cells were chiefly lost (unlike our own observations just described for mice restricted in energy but not protein intake). Refeeding of an 18 percent protein diet led to vigorous thymic growth.

Genotype profoundly affected the BW response of weanlings to the low protein diet. After 2 weeks of eating the low protein diet, BALB/c mice had increased their BWs by 15 percent whereas B6 mice lost 15 percent of their starting BW.

All of the above argues that thymocyte replication and numbers decrease with DR. Whether the same obtains for thymic epithelial cells is unknown, but of interest in view of Hirokawa's study (1978) of mouse thymuses. He demonstrated three types of thymic epithelial cells, differing in radiosensitivity and age-dependent decreases in numbers. The most radiosensitive cell type was the first to be lost (at 1 month of age), and is believed to be essential for the differentiation and peripheralization of T cells in early life. Perhaps DR retards losses of some type(s) of thymic epithelial cells (probably not those which produce thymosin$_{\alpha 1}$) and thereby maintains certain aspects of T cell differentiative capacities in a "younger" state.

Based on what DR data are available, the thymus appears quite sensitive to a LS-prolonging DR regimen. The cortex-depleting action of classical protein/energy malnutrition is demonstrably opposite to what follows "undernutrition without malnutrition." That the thymus shows dramatic structural and functional losses with age should not be overlooked when considering the nature of DR's impact on aging. Add to this the unique dual immune-neuroendocrine role of the thymus and one can understand why it has aroused the fancy of many a theorizing gerontologist. Future aging studies of the "DR thymus" emphasizing topics like quantitation of lymphoid and reticuloepithelial cells and their subpopulations, immune and neuroendocrine interactions, T cell differentiation capacities, and gene expression should yield valuable data.

Cell Numbers, Proportions and Subpopulations

Dietary restriction greatly reduces cell numbers in spleen, lymph nodes and blood. Declines in thymus weight (and cell number) are dramatic soon after DR is started but, as just discussed, are not universal long-term outcomes. Data from our laboratory (Table 4.10) illustrate certain of these changes. Nucleated cell yields from the spleen and pooled lymph nodes were 40 percent that of controls. Nucleated white cell counts in blood were only 20 percent as high as for controls. Mice on DR are strikingly lymphopenic as their already reduced white cell numbers are comprised of only 40 percent lymphocytes, vs. 65 percent lymphocytes for blood from controls.

TABLE 4.10

Influence of Dietary Restriction on Lymphoid Cell Numbers[a]

Lymphoid Organ	Age (mo)	Cell Yield ($\times 10^{-6}$)	
		Control	Restricted
Spleen	12	86 ± 7	32 ± 4
Lymph nodes	12	11 ± 2	5 ± 1
Blood	6	5975 ± 1075	1025 ± 275

[a] Data are means ± SEM for female C3B10RF$_1$ mice (n=6-7). Data for spleen and pooled peripheral lymph nodes (brachial, inguinal and axillary are from Weindruch et al. (1982c) for mice fed either a control PD (80% of ad lib) or a restricted (50% of ad lib). Data for blood leukocytes are our unpublished observations and give the number of nucleated cells per mm^3 of blood for controls fed a NPD ad lib and for DR mice (50% restriction of a PD).

A drop in circulating leukocytes and lymphocytes with DR was described long ago but has been little appreciated. Boutwell et al. (1948) found that DR (half of ad lib) in mice reduced total leukocyte and lymphocyte counts by 45 and 76 percent, respectively. McCay (1952) stated that blood from his rats contained only two-thirds as many leukocytes as in controls.

It is surprising that such low numbers of circulating leukocytes (and especially lymphocytes) in DR animals are associated with good health and extremely long LSs. The immune system of the DR rodent appears to require the use of very little of its potential "immunocellular fleet"; however, studies on induced immune responses show that DR animals can respond robustly upon stimulation. Improved late-life immunity may be due in part to DR rodents having produced (and destroyed) far fewer lymphoid cells over their lives, leaving a greater ability to generate good lymphoid cells in old age (see "THE BASAL/INDUCED ACTIVITY HYPOTHESIS," Chapter 5).

We reported that the percentage of splenocytes bearing the Thy-1$^+$ marker of T cells is 2-fold higher than for controls following several months of either EDR (Weindruch et al., 1982c) or ADR (Weindruch et al., 1982a). Absolute levels of T cells were 2-fold higher in control spleens than in the tiny DR spleens.

Later work with John Wells at UCLA (unpublished observations) sought to quantify T cell Lyt-1$^+$ and Lyt-2$^+$ subpopulations in splenocytes from C3B10RF$_1$ females fed control and EDR regimens. We have discussed Lyt subpopulations elsewhere (Weindruch et al., 1982c). PHA-responsive T cells are predominately Lyt-$1^+2^+3^+$ (= 25-35% of spleen and lymph node T cells in mice) whereas ConA-responsive T cells are Lyt-$1^+2^-3^-$ (65-75% of splenic and lymph node T cells in mice). The latter population includes IL-2-secreting T helper cells. Our findings (Table 4.11) showed that adult mice on EDR possess a 30 percent greater frequency of Lyt-1^+ cells than do controls. A marginal rise with DR in Lyt-2^+ expression was also seen. Very little mouse-to-mouse variation was observed. These data would suggest that DR preferentially increases proportions of Lyt-$1^+2^-3^-$ helper T cells. Interestingly, mice on EDR also showed a population of Lyt-1^+ cells which were small in size, very brightly fluorescent, and not seen in control spleens. The nature of these cells has not been established.

TABLE 4.11
Influences of Dietary Restriction on Spleen Lymphocyte Lyt Subpopulations[a]

Diet	Cells/Spleen (X10^{-6})	% Lyt-1^+	% Lyt-2^+
Control	90 ± 6	60 ± 3	29 ± 2
Restricted	45 ± 5	78 ± 1	35 ± 2

[a] Values are mean ± SEM for 5-10 month old C3B10RF$_1$ mice (n=10) and are our unpublished observations. Controls were fed a PD at 80% of the ad lib level. Restricted mice were fed at 50% of the ad lib level. Nucleated splenocytes were passed through a nylon wool column. The T cell-enriched eluate was stained with fluoresceinated monoclonal antibodies to either Lyt-1 or Lyt-2 and quantitated on the cell sorter.

A prospective study on associations between levels of T cell subsets in the blood and the LSs of individual mice was reported by Boersma et al. (1985). Proportions of Thy-1^+ and Lyt-2^+ peripheral blood lymphocytes in aging individual CBA and B6 mice were determined. Levels of Thy-1^+, Lyt-2^- cells fell with age, suggesting diminution with age in numbers of T helper lymphocytes. For individual CBA mice a direct relation between the relative number of Thy-1^+, Lyt-2^- cells at a certain age and the time remaining to live was obtained. This observation is intriguing in view of the possibility that DR selectively raises this cell type! Proportions of Lyt-2^+ T cells in CBA mice increased slowly with aging, and underwent a rapid increase during the months before death. In B6 mice, age-related changes in T cell proportions were more variable but rapid late-life changes did signal that death was near. Longitudinal immunologic/LS studies of this nature are required to identify immune indexes correlating with, and possibly contributing to, differences in LSs.

Fernandes (1987) described splenic lymphocyte subsets in female B/WF$_1$ mice fed since weaning either a 5 or 20 percent corn oil diet ad lib, or the 5 percent corn oil diet at half of the ad lib level. Diet-induced changes at 4 months of age were minimal. All mice showed the following values: Thy-1$^+$, 45 percent; Lyt-1$^+$, 50 percent; Lyt-2$^+$, 15 percent; Ig$^+$, 25 percent. By 8 to 12 months of age some differences were noted between DR and control animals: 47 percent of splenocytes of DR mice were Thy-1$^+$ vs. 33 percent for controls freely fed the low fat diet. Corresponding values were 61 vs. 43 percent Lyt-1$^+$, 14 vs. 9 percent Lyt-2$^+$, and 29 vs. 38 percent Ig$^+$. Values for mice fed the high fat diet ad lib were similar to those for animals freely fed the low fat diet. Thus, with the development of autoimmunity in normally fed mice, splenic T cell levels declined in relation to B cells. DR retarded the alterations in this ratio. Also, Ly-1 B cells (which occur in lower proportions in normal mouse strains than in autoimmune strains) were reduced by DR. These effects of DR (including disease retardation) were duplicated by feeding diets with 20 percent fish oil instead of corn oil.

Thus, evidence suggests that DR retards age-related changes in T cell subset proportions in both long- and short-lived strains of mice. The helper cell sector appears especially vulnerable to decrease with age, but is increased by DR. These effects of DR on T cell subsets very likely contribute to several alterations in the immune responses discussed in the next section.

Immune Response Capacities

As previously noted, most of what is known about the immunogerontologic effects of DR concerns declining immune responses of mice, and is fairly evenly divided between short- and long-lived strains. *In vitro* testing has predominated. Little is known about DR's impact on whole animal resistance to insult. The main findings for long-term DR regimens proven to extend LS are grouped in Table 4.12.

It is appropriate to turn first to low protein diets, as these were used by Good's group (then at the University of Minnesota) in their initial studies, which revealed that low protein/low energy intakes could

TABLE 4.12
Effects of DR on Age-Sensitive Immune Response Capacities in Mice[a]

Immune Parameter[b]	Strain	Cell	Nature of DR[c] %AL	DUR	Eff. of DR[d]	Ref.[e]
1. Lymphocyte prolif.						
PHA-induced	C3B10RF$_1$	Spl.	50	12	↑140%	1
	C3B10RF$_1$	LN	50	12	NSD	1
	C3B10RF$_1$	Spl.	40	30	↑1600%	2
	C3B10RF$_1$	Spl.	60	8*	↑150%	3
	B6	Spl.	65[d]	6	↑20%	4
	CBA	Spl.	85[e]	5*	↑40%	4
	B/WF$_1$	Spl.	50	11	↑870%	5
	B10C3F$_1$	Spl.	60	35	↑550%	6
	B10C3F$_1$	Spl.	60	7	↑65%	7
ConA-induced	C3B10RF$_1$	Spl.	50	6	NSD	1
	C3B10RF$_1$	Spl.	40	30	↑615%	2
	C3B10RF$_1$	Spl.	60	8*	NSD	3
	B6	Spl.	65[d]	6	↑30%	4
	CBA	Spl.	85[e]	5*	↑35%	4
	B10C3F$_1$	Spl.	60	35	↑160%	6
	B10C3F$_1$	Spl.	60	7	↑55%	7
Mixed lymph. rxn.	B10C3F$_1$	Spl.	50	7	↑100%	7
2. Antibody prod^n.	C3B10RF$_1$	Spl.	60	12*	NSD	3
	B/WF$_1$	Spl.	50	9	↑1200%	8
3. Prod^n. of IL-2	B/WF$_1$	Spl.	50	11	↑350%	5
	B6CBAF$_1$	PBL	60	33	↑250%	9
4. Response to IL-2	B/WF$_1$	Thy.	50	11	↑70%	5
5. T cell cytolysis	C3B10RF$_1$	Spl.	60	15*	↑30%	3
	B/WF$_1$	Spl.	50	9	↑230%	8
	B6CBAF$_1$	PBL	60	33	↑350%	9
6. NK cell cytolysis	C3B10RF$_1$	Spl.	50	30	↓300% (basal)	10
	C3B10RF$_1$	Spl.	50	24	NSD (poly I:C)	10

[a]Abbreviations: IL-2 = interleukin 2; Spl. = splenocyte; Thy = thymocyte; PBL = peripheral blood lymphocyte; NK = natural killer; prod^n. = production. Antibody prod^n. was assessed as the frequency of PFCs to SRBC.

[b]The most studied of the immune parameters is lymphocyte proliferation. Only a representative sampling of the mitogen-induced proliferation data is listed. Responses to B cell mitogens do not usually decline with age in rodents.

[c]"AL" indicates the percentage of the ad lib intake level at which the mice on DR were fed. "DUR" gives the duration of feeding in months. All diets used were PDs except for study #9. Most feeding started before 3 months of age except for studies #3 (12, 17 or 22 mo onsets tested [data in table for 12 mo onset]) and #4 (17 mo onset). "*" indicates that ADR was studied. In study #4, mice were underfed via an EOD regimen as described in Table 4.2 (footnote ^{e}, study #18).

TABLE 4.12
(Continued)

[d]The effect of DR relative to an ad lib fed control group (except for studies #1, 2, 6, 7 and 10 where controls were fed about 20% less than the ad lib level). Note that DR's effect was based on data reported for a given number of cells tested (e.g. the ^{3}H-TdR uptake of 1×10^5 lymphocytes/culture well after PHA stimulation). Not all workers see this as the best way to present immunologic data in DR rodents (e.g. Harrison et al. [1984] reported their findings only on a per spleen basis).

[e]References: (1) Weindruch et al. (1982c); (2) Weindruch et al. (1986); (3) Weindruch et al. (1982a); (4) Mann (1978); (5) Jung et al. (1982); (6) Cheney et al. (1983); (7) Weindruch et al. (1979); (8) Fernandes et al. (1978a); (9) Miller and Harrison (1985); (10) Weindruch et al. (1983).

actually *increase* immune responses (see Good et al. [1976] for a lucid review of this work).

Jose and Good (1971) observed that ad lib feeding of an 8 percent casein diet markedly lowered both BW gain and the serum activity of "blocking antibody" (which interferes with killing of tumor cells by lymphocytes) in rats injected with mouse tumors. Next, they studied immunity to several types of tumor cells in young mice fed for 10 weeks a diet reduced in either protein or in protein and calories (Jose & Good, 1973a). Specific antibody levels were low in sera from underfed mice, including both blocking and cytotoxic antibodies. In contrast, cell mediated killing increased with underfeeding. The authors suggested that a decrease in blocking antibody may permit greater T cell killing of tumor cells.

The nutritional basis for the effects on tumor immunity were further defined by feeding diets variably deficient in individual essential amino acids (Jose & Good, 1973b). A moderate decrease in any of seven amino acids produced the low tumor antibody/high tumor cytotoxicity observed previously.

Similar results were reported by Cooper et al. (1974) for mice fed ad lib on a short-term basis an 8 percent casein diet. Seven different immune responses were measured. These same investigators also studied immunity in underfed NZB female mice. They fed either Purina Mouse Chow™ (17% protein, 11% fat) or Purina Lab Chow™ (23% protein, 4.5% fat) to NZB mice beginning at time of weaning, and observed that the former diet hastened the onset of autoimmunity and the decline in immune response capacity (Fernandes et al., 1973). One recalls that for

NPDs like these the diet composition can vary and manufacturers typically provide only a guaranteed minimum formulation rather than actual levels of nutrients.

Next, PDs were used to study NZB mice (Fernandes et al., 1976a; see Table 2.5, #7). A 6 percent casein diet was compared to an isocaloric 22 percent diet, with equivalent group energy intakes adjusted to nearly the ad lib level. At 7 to 10 months of age, splenocytes from mice given the low protein diet showed higher age-sensitive immune responses. Those studied were plaque-forming cell (PFC) response to sheep red blood cells (SRBC), T cell killing of an allogeneic tumor, graft vs. host reaction, and PHA and ConA reactivities. The low protein diet delayed the onset of autoimmunity but did not halt the progression of the disease or prolong life.

Low protein diets do not always boost cellular immunity. In a long-term study testing mice aged 4, 12, 19 or 24 months, neither a 4 nor an 8 percent casein diet fed ad lib since weaning to Balb/c male mice influenced age-related declines in splenic PHA or ConA responses, or in antibody to injected SRBC (Stoltzner & Dorsey, 1980). One recalls also (Table 2.5, #12) that these diets did not increase LS.

Data on suppressor cell activity or numbers in DR animals are scant. Fernandes et al. (1978a) observed that spontaneous suppressor cell activity (measured as the capacity of spleen cells from DR or control mice to reduce the *in vitro* PFC response to SRBC of splenocytes from young mice) increased with aging in normally fed B/WF$_1$ females, but not in those on DR. In another study, Fernandes et al. (1976b) reported that young C3H mice on EDR for only 2 months showed greater antigen-induced splenic suppressor activity than did age-matched controls.

More recently, Fernandes' laboratory has published abstracts summarizing work on new disease models. The (NZB × BXSB) F$_1$ male mouse develops lymphoproliferative and coronary vascular diseases. Early-onset DR raised IL-2 production and increased the ratio of IgG/IgM PFC to SRBC for mice tested at 8 months of age (Bailey et al., 1983). In spontaneously hypertensive rats, either EDR or exercise lowered BW and blood pressure and raised splenic PHA and ConA responses for animals tested at 6 months of age (Rozek et al., 1983).

Our own first DR studies utilized B6 mice fed PDs (Walford et al., 1973/1974; Walford et al., 1975; Gerbase-DeLima et al., 1975). Diets and LSs of these mice were summarized in Table 2.5, #6. Splenocyte responses to either T- or B-cell mitogens (Figure 4.26) and to injected

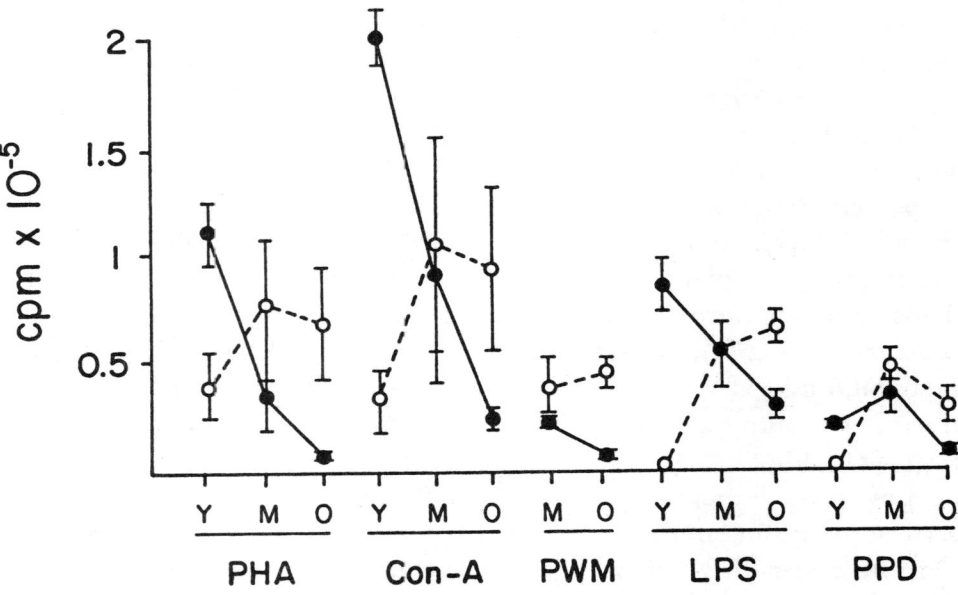

Figure 4.26. Mitogen-induced proliferation in spleen cells from young (Y = 4-8 month), middle-age (M = 13 month) and old (O = 25 month) B6 mice. o------o, restricted diet; •———•, control diet. Values are cpm ³H-thymidine. From Gerbase-DeLima et al. (1975).

SRBC were measured in these populations, as was the ability to reject an allogeneic skin graft. In young adulthood (4-8 months), the DR mice responded less vigorously in all tests. By mid-life (13 months), however, they outperformed the controls in all tests except skin allograft rejection, which did not differ between groups. Once acquired, the higher responses of DR mice were largely maintained. Overall, DR retarded immune system maturation but also kept it younger longer.

In further work, Cheney et al. (1983) explored immunologic aging in $B10C3F_1$ mice also being followed for LS (Table 2.5, #16) and tumor incidence (Table 3.6). Mitogen- or alloantigen-induced splenocyte proliferation was reported for mice on EDR and for controls. The results supported the prior finding that old EDR mice show more robust T cell proliferative responses than do age-matched controls; however, the immunologic advantage came quite early in life, so that this hybrid failed to show the early life immunosuppression seen in underfed female B6 mice. These comparative findings probably signify strain differences, and also indicate that the retardation of aging by DR cannot always be viewed as a simple maturational effect. Short-term (1-3 weeks) DR imposed on young B6 mice was found by others to depress PHA and ConA reactivity (Erickson et al., 1979a; Erickson et al., 1979b).

In most studies in our laboratory, the diets used were modelled after Ross' diet which yielded the greatest LSs. Our first results employing this diet were reported as part of a review (Weindruch et al., 1979). B10C3F$_1$ females were started on EDR (This was the cohort also used to study thymic involution.). In addition to the EDR population, 12 month old males were switched from eating a NPD ad lib since weaning to a gradually imposed ADR regimen (discussed below). Splenocyte responses to five T or B cell mitogens or to alloantigens were determined in the EDR group at ages between 6-7 weeks and 8 months. The responses to T cell but *not* to B cell mitogens increased by 60 percent with DR. Mixed lymphocyte reactivity doubled.

We next attempted to clarify the basis for higher T cell proliferative responses in splenocytes from C3B10RF$_1$ females on EDR (Weindruch et al., 1982c). This particular study did not test truly old subjects but rather young (5 month) to midadult (15 month) mice. We observed that:

(1) In six sets of studies, DR resulted in a 2- to 4-fold drop in numbers of nucleated cells per spleen and a 1- to 3-fold rise in splenic PHA-induced ^{3}H-TdR uptake. Responses to ConA or B cell mitogens were largely insensitive to DR.

(2) Surprisingly, despite cell yields from pooled peripheral lymph nodes being reduced by DR, the response of these cells to PHA was uninfluenced by DR.

(3) The higher maximal splenic PHA responses in DR mice could not be attributed to differences in kinetics (Figure 4.27) or mitogen concentrations. Spleen cells from DR mice displayed greater responses at both high and low culture densities (Figure 4.28). The higher PHA responses of DR mice were associated with 2-fold increases in both the proportion of PHA-stimulated blast cells (as judged microscopically) and in the proportion of splenic T cells (based on cytotoxicity and immunofluorescence). Neither synergy nor suppression was detected in PHA-stimulated mixed cultures of spleen cells for control and DR mice.

Thus, DR could raise spleen PHA responses by increasing the proportion of PHA-responsive T cells. Alternatively, DR might raise proportions of cells which secrete growth factors (e.g. IL-2 by Lyt-$1^+2^-3^-$ T helper cells which are preferentially activated by ConA), thereby causing several proliferative responses to increase. This latter possibility is argued against by DR's failure to significantly influence ConA reactivity in this study, although increases have often been reported (Table 4.12).

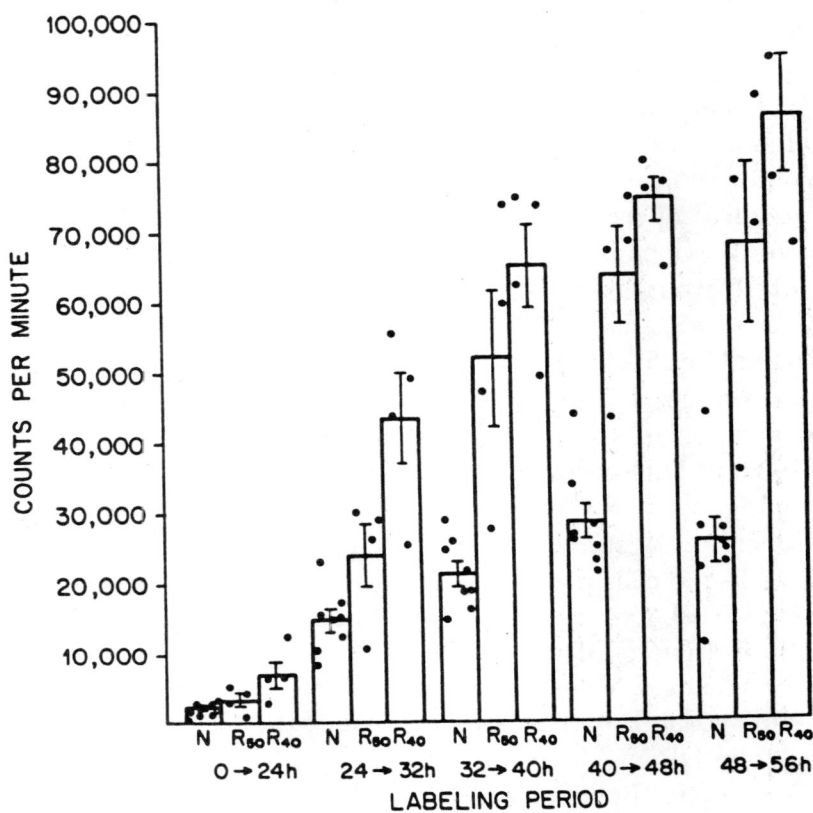

Figure 4.27. Kinetic study of PHA reactivity of spleen cells from 5-6 month old normally-fed (N = 85 kcal/week) and restricted (R_{50} = 50 kcal/week; R_{40} = 40 kcal/week) $C3B10RF_1$ mice. Values give mean ± SEM cpm of ^{3}H-thymidine for cultures labelled during different time periods. Adapted from Weindruch et al. (1982c).

In a later study (Weindruch et al., 1986) of $C3B10RF_1$ mice fed the same diets as above, *both* PHA and ConA responses fell with age, and both were increased by DR. In controls fed 85 kcal/week, PHA-induced ^{3}H-TdR uptake fell from 4400 cpm at 10 months to 700 cpm at 30 months of age, whereas in mice fed 40 kcal/week responses at these ages were 26,000 and 11,000 cpm respectively. For ConA-induced proliferation, control responses fell from 20,000 to 5000 cpm while DR mice averaged 57,000 and 32,000 cpm. The variability between studies in the effect of DR on ConA reactivity remains unclear.

The capacity of ConA-stimulated lymphocytes to produce IL-2 is raised by DR. This was first described in a preliminary way by Richardson and Cheung (1982) who studied two 19 month old Fischer 344 rats

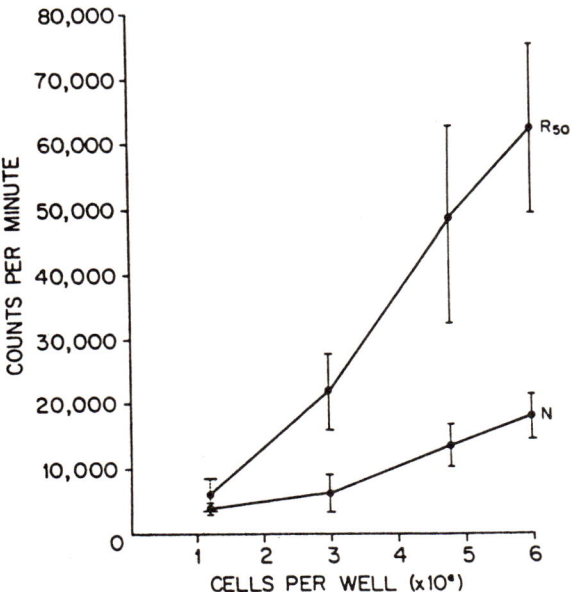

Figure 4.28. Cell dose-response study of splenocyte response (mean ± SEM ^{3}H-thymidine uptake) to PHA in 13-15 month old C3B10RF$_1$ mice fed either a normal (N = 85 kcal/week) or restricted (R$_{50}$ = 50 kcal/week) diet from 3 weeks of age. From Weindruch et al. (1982c).

fed 60 percent of ad lib since weaning, and two age-matched controls. They observed that DR increased ConA-induced IL-2 production and protein synthesis. Later work in B/WF$_1$ mice (see Table 4.12) confirmed the observation. In long-lived strains, and using a limiting dilution assay to measure frequencies of precursors to IL-2-secreting cells among peripheral blood lymphocytes, Miller and Harrison (1985) observed that the precursor cells fell in number with age, but less so in DR animals. Declines with age in the capacity of "old lymphocytes" to make and respond to IL-2 are now widely documented both in rodents and in humans (Thoman & Weigle, 1987).

How do these data on PHA and ConA responses fit with our preliminary finding that Lyt-1$^+$2$^-$3$^-$ proportions are raised by DR? In fact an increase in Lyt-1$^+$2$^-$3$^-$ cells accords nicely with the above data on IL-2 production, and could possibly potentiate proliferation induced by many stimuli. An age-related decline in IL-2 might explain the variety of T cell proliferative declines observed in old organisms. Prevention/correction of T helper cell losses may be a major mechanism whereby DR retards immunologic aging.

We also investigated natural killer (NK) cell activity in splenocytes from 2 to 33 month old EDR and control C3B10RF$_1$ mice (Weindruch et al., 1983). It is widely believed that NK cells provide one line of defense against tumor growth and metastasis. In contrast to our expectation of higher NK responses in DR mice (since they develop lymphomas less and later than do controls), DR animals showed much lower basal responses than did controls; however, after injection with poly I:C (an interferon-inducer which boosts NK activity) old DR mice displayed the NK cytolysis of young mice on either diet, and showed much higher responses than old controls (Figure 4.29). Also, DR mice showed increased *in vitro* generation of cytotoxic T lymphocytes to two murine tumors. The increased resistance of DR mice to cancer may reflect an NK system very responsive to induction signals, coupled with T cell killing more active than in controls.

Adult-onset DR also slows the pace of immunologic decline in mice from long-lived strains. Our first indication of this came from B10C3F$_1$ mice first restricted at 12 months of age (Weindruch et al., 1979). Restriction was gradually imposed and lasted for 4.5 months at which time the mice were killed to determine splenocyte proliferative responses. Adult-onset DR raised responses to PHA (by 122%) and ConA (by 70%), but did not influence mixed lymphocyte reactivity or B cell proliferation. Similarly, Mann (1978) observed that ADR (EOD feeding) imposed on 17 month old CBA mice increased splenic PHA and ConA responses.

We next studied immunosenescence in male C3B10RF$_1$ mice started on gradual ADR at 12, 17 or 22 months of age (Weindruch et al., 1982a; Table 4.12, #3). Body weights stabilized at 60 to 70 percent that of controls. Adult-onset DR decreased the numbers of nucleated cells per spleen and increased the percentages of T cells (by 72%). For mice restricted at these three ages and tested at various ages thereafter, splenic PHA responses were higher than for age-matched controls. Adult-onset DR sporadically raised spleen cell proliferation induced by ConA but affected neither splenic responses to B cell mitogens nor the PHA response of peripheral lymph node cells. In the splenic PFC response to SRBC, ADR and control mice differed more in response kinetics than in peak levels of PFCs. The cell mediated lymphocytotoxic response by spleen cells to an allogeneic tumor fell in ad lib fed mice by 30 percent between 6 and 28 months of age but responses of 28 month old mice on ADR since 12 months of age were as high as those of 6 month old controls (Table 4.13). These results point toward similar immunologic effects of ADR and EDR.

Dietary Restriction: Effects on Biological Parameters 195

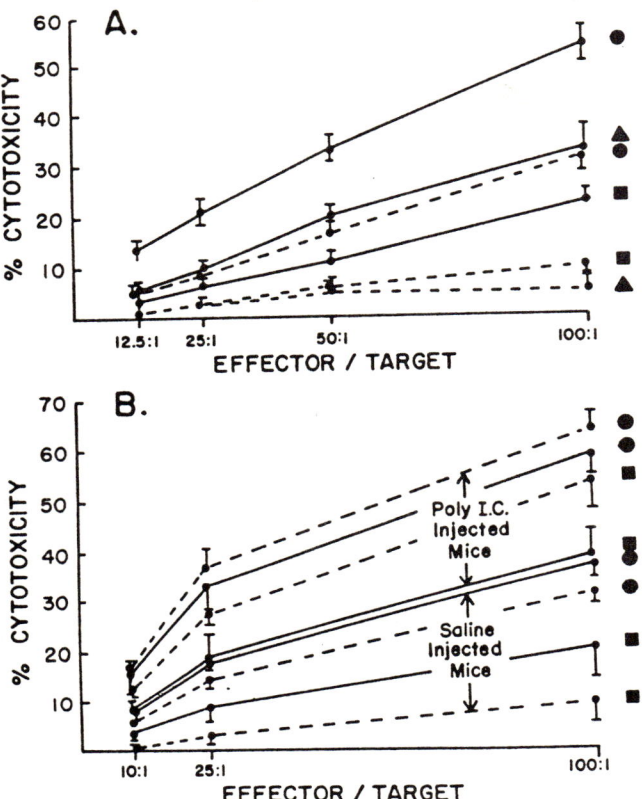

Figure 4.29. Natural killer (NK) cell response as affected by aging and EDR in female C3B10RF$_1$ mice. Values give percent specific lysis of YAC1 lymphoma cells in a ^{51}Cr release assay. Panel A gives basal responses whereas Panel B gives data for mice injected with poly I:C (an interferon inducer and NK response augmentor). *Diets:* Control (———); DR (-----). *Ages:* (●) = 3 months (Panel A) and 8 months (Panel B); (▲) = 15 months in both panels; (■) = 32 months (Panel A), 24 months (Panel B). From Weindruch et al. (1983).

TABLE 4.13
Influence of Age and ADR on T Cell Mediated Cytotoxicity in Mice[a]

		% lysis at effector/target ratio			
Group	Age (mo)	10:1	5:1	2.5:1	0.5:1
Old R$_{12}$	27	98 ± 3	87 ± 3	63 ± 4	27 ± 3
Old LC	27	78 ± 8	61 ± 10	40 ± 9	16 ± 4
Young LC	5	95 ± 2	90 ± 3	69 ± 6	30 ± 4

[a]Old R$_{12}$ = 27 month old mice on ADR from 12 months of age; Old LC = 27 month old mice fed Purina Lab Chow™ ad libitum since time of weaning; Young LC = young mice fed Purina Lab Chow™ ad libitum since time of weaning. Values are X ± SEM (n=5) percent specific lysis in a ^{51}Cr release assay after a 4 day *in vitro* sensitization with DBA/2 spleen cells. Target cells used were P815 mastocytoma cells. Adapted from Weindruch et al. (1982a).

The lymphocyte proliferation data for DR rodents overwhelmingly concerns nonspecific, polyclonal responses induced by plant lectins. An exception is a report (Christadoss et al., 1984) where 8 weeks of EDR (50% of ad lib) imposed on B6 mice reduced T-dependent lymphocyte proliferation to specific antigens (acetylcholine receptor, human hemoglobin) as well as the antibody response thereto. The difference was attributed to ". . . a defect in both macrophages and T cells in antigen processing, presentation, and/or proliferation."

To what extent are the immunologic effects of long-term DR attributable to energy restriction *per se*? This question seems most relevant to dietary fats (esp. linoleic acid) which can inhibit immune responses in mice (Erickson et al., 1983; Thomas & Erickson, 1985). In our earlier work we did not balance fat intake (both DR and controls at a 13.5% corn oil diet) so that the higher responses in DR mice could theoretically have been due to fat restriction; however, our most recent work (unpublished) utilized DR and control mice fed the same amount of fat, and the same basic results have obtained. Most likely, the immunologic outcomes of long-term, LS-prolonging DR derive mainly from energy restriction without overt nutrient deficiency, or what has been termed "undernutrition without malnutrition."

Autoimmunity

Influences of DR on autoimmunity have been examined mostly in short-lived, autoimmune-prone strains of mice. The extensive inhibition of autoimmune diseases by DR was detailed in Chapter 3. Serum parameters reflect this disease inhibition. In B/WF$_1$ mice, serum levels of anti-DNA antibody (Fernandes et al., 1978a) and immune complexes (Safai-Kutti et al., 1980) rise with age and both increases are blunted by DR.

Information on the impact of DR on autoimmunity in long-lived animal models is quite limited. Nandy studied serum levels of spontaneous brain reactive autoantibodies in female B6 mice on DR. When DR was imposed on 3 month old mice for 12 months, the appearance of these antibodies was largely prevented (Nandy, 1982). In contrast, 3 months of ADR imposed on 24 month old mice did not influence brain reactive autoantibody formation (Nandy, 1981). We determined serum immune complex levels in the B10C3F$_1$ mice subjected to ADR at 12 months of age. Other aspects of this population were described earlier (Table 2.6, #9). At 23 months of age, immune complex levels were 45 percent lower in sera from ADR mice compared to sera from controls (Weindruch et al., 1982b).

These scant data are consistent with the view that DR can suppress late-life increases in autoimmune phenomena.

Lymphoid Biochemistry

At time of writing, studies on biochemical alterations in immune system cells from animals on DR are only beginning to appear in print (now limited to meeting abstracts).

Richardson's group (Pahlvani et al., 1987) studied splenocytes from Fischer 344 rats on EDR (60% of ad lib). ConA-stimulated proliferation, protein synthesis, IL-2 production and IL-2 gene expression (mRNA levels) all fell with aging. These indexes were influenced by DR at 5 or 12 months of age; however, at 21 and 28 months, DR spleen cells exhibited higher values.

Working with the same DR rat model, Fernandes et al. (1987) reported that: (1) splenic oncogene mRNA expression as measured by cDNA:RNA hybridization was reduced by DR for v-bas, v-raf and v-src, with no major changes for c-myc and c-myb; (2) thymocytes from 6 month old DR rats contained much higher levels of oleic (18:1) and linoleic (18:2) acids than did controls while arachidonic acid (20:4) content was three-fold lower; and (3) splenic adherent and non-adherent cells from DR rats also contained much reduced levels of 20:4.

PHYSIOLOGIC PARAMETERS

A diverse lot of physiologic parameters have been explored in DR rodents. Certain indexes like metabolic rate and body temperature may prove germane to elucidating how DR retards aging and influences disease susceptibility. Studies on most other parameters provide still additional evidence that middle-aged or old DR animals are "younger" than age-matched controls.

Metabolic Rate

Explanations ascribing DR's actions to a lowering of metabolic rate are conceptually satisfying but not universally supported by available data. Some confusion exists regarding DR's effect on metabolic rate because of uncertainties of how to best express such data in animals, such as DR and control animals, which differ in body size and composition.

Metabolic rate has been assessed in three general ways in DR animals. One has been to calculate the lifetime energy intake (LEI) of the organism. Others have been to measure O_2 consumption (or occasionally heat production) of either the whole animal *in vivo* or its components (organs, tissues, homogenates, isolated mitochondria) *in vitro*. The basal metabolic rate (BMR) is usually defined as the rate of energy expenditure in a fasting subject who is completely relaxed in a thermoneutral environment. It comprises about 70 percent of a free-living animal's energy expenditure with the remainder accounted for by the thermic effects of exercise and food.

Insightfully reviewing "Metabolic adaptation to low intakes of energy and protein," Waterlow (1986) lists ways of adapting to a low energy intake. One may reduce BW, voluntary activity and/or involuntary activity. All of these would be expected to lower metabolic rate. A fourth strategy involves "true metabolic adaptations," which are poorly understood. Waterlow (1986) views BW loss as the most important adaptation.

Lifetime Energy Intake

Evaluation of DR's impact on LEI began with Sacher's (1977) analysis of data from two of Ross' studies (Ross, 1959 & 1969) of rats fed one of five different diets varying widely in energy intakes and resultant LSs. The main LEI calculations are these:

1. *Daily energy intake/g BW:* $\frac{\text{kcal/day}}{BW_{adult}} = \text{kcal}/(g \cdot \text{day})$
2. *LEI/g BW:* $\text{kcal}/(g \cdot \text{day}) \cdot \text{LS (in days)} = \text{kcal}/(g \cdot \text{LS})$
3. *LEI/whole animal:* $\text{LS (of animal)} \cdot \text{kcal/day} = \text{kcal}/(\text{animal} \cdot \text{LS})$

Sacher found that the LEI/g was nearly the same (100 kcal/g) among these groups (which however differed more than 4-fold in daily caloric intakes). He deduced that this near constancy indicated that DR prolongs LS by lowering the metabolic rate per gram of rat, allowing a longer time to reach a LS-limiting number of kcal/g. We believe that these calculations are marred by Sacher's combining data from two of Ross' studies in which differences existed between the populations. Also, Ross' data appear inappropriate for determining LEI, causing Sacher to make major, problematic assumptions.

Masoro's group described LEI data for Fischer 344 rats maintained on EDR. Sacher's findings could not be confirmed. Masoro et al. (1982)

found that kcal/(g · day) was not sensitive to DR whereas the LEI/g was increased by 45 percent by DR. Yu et al. (1985) reported similar findings (i.e. no effect on kcal/[g · day] but a 55 percent increase in kcal/[g · LS]) for another set of rats on EDR. Adult-onset DR (6 month onset) yielded a lesser increase (34%) in LEI/g. The LEI/whole rat, on the other hand, was *not* influenced by DR started at either age.

We (Weindruch et al., 1986) determined LEI in the mouse population described earlier (see *"Longevity."* and Table 2.5, #17, Chapter 2). The values used for all calculations appear in Table 4.14, and LEI estimates in Table 4.15. The daily energy intake/g was uninfluenced by all but the most severe DR which reduced this measure by 10 percent. Also in line with findings in the just-described rats was that LEI/g was increased 30 percent by DR (One recalls that the control rats were fed ad lib while our control mice were in fact on a slight DR regimen.). The rat and mouse data do differ when expressed as LEI/animal. We observed that control mice showed 30 to 55 percent greater values than DR mice. A side-by-side comparison of these rat and mouse findings is given in Table 4.16.

TABLE 4.14

Values Used in Lifetime Energy Intake (LEI) Calculations for Mice

Group[a]	kcal/day	$BW_{adult}(g)$[b]	Organ Wt. (g)[c]	Ave. LS (days)[d]
N/N_{85}	12.1	34.5	1.86	994
N/R_{50}	7.1	20.3	1.29	1286
R/R_{50}	7.1	20.1	--	1304
$N/R_{50lopro}$	7.1	20.0	1.21	1207
N/R_{40}	5.7	17.8	1.15	1371

[a]Group descriptions: N/N_{85}, fed normally before and after weaning, postweaning diet fed as 85 kcal/week (25% less than ad libitum); N/R_{50}, fed normally before weaning, restricted postweaning to 50 kcal/week; R/R_{50}, restricted in feeding level both before and after (50 kcal/week) weaning; $N/R_{50lopro}$, restricted after weaning to 50 kcal/week with a decrease with age in the protein content of the diet; N/R_{40}, restricted after weaning to 40 kcal/week.
[b]BW_{adult} = average of BWs at 5, 10, 15 and 20 months of age.
[c]Organ wt. = liver + kidney + spleen weights. The value given is the average for 10 and 30 month old mice.
[d]The average LSs for other mice fed these diets (see Table 2.5, #17) were used to calculate LEI per organ weight. For all other LEI values, individual LSs were used. From Weindruch et al. (1986).

TABLE 4.15

Effects of DR on Lifetime Energy Intake (LEI) in C3B1ORF$_1$ Mice[a]

Group[b]	kcal/(g•day)	kcal/(g•lifetime)	kcal/(mouse•lifetime)
N/N$_{85}$	0.365 ± .004[a]	354 ± 8[a]	12,080 ± 248[a]
N/R$_{50}$	0.356 ± .003[a]	455 ± 10[bc]	9,174 ± 284[bc]
R/R$_{50}$	0.355 ± .002[a]	464 ± 10[c]	9,312 ± 195[b]
N/R$_{50lopro}$	0.360 ± .004[a]	433 ± 10[b]	8,613 ± 202[c]
N/R$_{40}$	0.323 ± .003[b]	441 ± 8[bc]	7,833 ± 147[c]

[a]Values are mean ± SEM. The statistical significance of differences between means was evaluated by Duncan's Multiple Range Test which was applied when one-way analysis of variance indicated significant differences. Means in each column not sharing a common superscript letter ([a-c]) were significantly different ($p=0.05$). From Weindruch et al. (1986).

[b]Diet Groups: N/N$_{85}$, fed "normally" before and after weaning, postweaning diet fed as 85 kcal/week (25% less than ad libitum); N/R$_{50}$, fed normally before weaning, restricted postweaning to 50 kcal/week; R/R$_{50}$, restricted in feeding level both before and after (50 kcal/week) weaning; N/R$_{50lopro}$, restricted after weaning to 50 kcal/week with a decrease with age in the protein content of the diet; N/R$_{40}$, restricted after weaning to 40 kcal/week.

TABLE 4.16

Influence of DR on Lifetime Energy Intake (LEI) in Rats and Mice

	Rats[a]		Mice[b]	
	Control	DR	Control	DR
1. Average LS (months)	23	32	33	43
2. kcal/(g•day)	0.13	0.13	0.30	0.30
3. kcal/(g•LS)	92	134	330	400
4. kcal/(animal•LS)	40,000	40,000	12,000	9,000

[a]From Masoro et al. (1982). Calculation of kcal/(animal•LS) was made by us based on data presented in paper (similar findings reported later by Yu et al. [1985] from that laboratory).

[b]From Weindruch et al. (1986).

We also determined LEI per organ mass (Table 4.17). The liver, kidney and spleen weights for adult (10 month) and old (30 month) mice on each diet were added and used to calculate kcal/(organ weight • d) and kcal/(organ weight • LS) (using the average LSs from the LS study). DR clearly reduced the daily caloric input per organ weight; however, the LEI/organ mass was for these particular organs not much influenced by

TABLE 4.17

Lifetime Energy Intake Adjusted to Organ Weight (OW) in Mice[a]

Group[b]	OW (g)	kcal/(OW·d)	kcal/(OW·LS)
N/N$_{85}$	1.86	6.9 ± 0.4	6600
N/R$_{50}$	1.29	5.6 ± 0.1	7073
N/R$_{50lopro}$	1.21	6.1 ± 0.1	7097
N/R$_{40}$	1.15	4.9 ± 0.1	6772

[a]The OW values (=liver+kidney+spleen) were averages of measures from 10 and 30 month old mice on each diet. From Weindruch et al. (1986).

[b]Group Descriptions: N/N$_{85}$, fed normally before and after weaning, postweaning diet fed as 85 kcal/week (25% less than ad libitum); N/R$_{50}$, fed normally before weaning, restricted postweaning to 50 kcal/week; N/R$_{50lopro}$, restricted after weaning to 50 kcal/week with a decrease with age in the protein content of the diet; N/R$_{40}$, restricted after weaning to 40 kcal/week.

DR. Perhaps the number of kcals ingested per mass of critical organs over the lifetime varies little among animals whose LSs differ due to DR. The small deviation (<10%) in LEI/organ mass among the groups contrasts to large differences observed between DR and control mice in both LEI/g and LEI/mouse.

O$_2$ Consumption and Heat Production

Table 4.18 summarizes published data on metabolic rates in underfed rodents. The rates are expressed in three ways: per BW, per BW$^{0.75}$ ("metabolic BW" = MBW), and per whole animal. The BMR per MBW is most commonly reported (Many of the values in the Table were not in the original publications but have been calculated by us from the data reported for BW and MBW.). All but 3 of the 16 studies examined brief DR (<2 months) in rats (Mice have largely been ignored.). *One must distinguish between acute vs. chronic adaptations to DR!* This is well exemplified by data of an abstract by McGee and McCarter (1987): DR only lowered O$_2$ consumption per lean body mass of rats during the first 4 weeks and then the group differences vanished.

Heat production was measured in two older (1934, 1943) long-term (10-28 months) and two newer short-term (<1.4 months) studies. Long-term DR raised heat production per BW by 20 percent. It did not alter values per MBW. Whole animal heat production was 15 to 35 percent lower in DR animals. Increased heat generation by a non temperature-stressed animal seems a poor use of biological energy, which could otherwise be applied toward biosynthetic and repair processes.

TABLE 4.18

Effects of DR on Metabolic Rates in Rats and Mice

Parameter	Nature of DR[a]			Effect of DR per:[b]			Ref.[c]
	Diet	%AL[a]	DUR[a]	BW	MBW	Animal	
1. Heat production	PD	NR[a]	10	↑18%	-*	↓19%*	1
	NPD	70	27	↑21%	-*	↓15%*	2
	NPD	50	1.4	↑20%*	-	↓18%	3
	PD	53	1	↓10%*	↓15%	↓35%	4
2. O$_2$ consump.	PD[a]	70	1	↓33%*	↓35%	↓39%*	5
	NPD	50	0.4	↓7%*	↓8%	↓16%	6
	NPD	80	1.8	-	-	↓6%	7
	NPD	65	0.4	↓6%*	↓13%	↓27%*	8
	none	0	0.1	?	↓18%	?	9
	PD	50	1.8	↑30%*	-	↓27%*	10
	PD	40	0.4	-*	↓26%	↓49%*	11
	PD	50	1.8	-*	-	↓32%	12
	PD	50	1.8	-*	↓14%	↓42%*	13
	PD	60	4.6	↑9%	-	↓32%*	14
	NPD	50	1	-*	↓16%	↓38%*	15
	PD	60	0.7	↓11%*	↓15%	↓25%	16
	PD	50	25	-	-*	↓43%	17

[a]Except for study #3, all experiments involved rats. The DR probably started before 3 months of age in all studies but certain reports did not specify age of onset (only BW given). "% AL" is the % of the ad lib intake fed to the DR group. "DUR" is the duration of feeding in months. In study #1, rats were growth restricted by limiting the amount of a yeast supplement.

[b]"MBW" refers to metabolic BW ($=BW^{0.75}$ [but $BW^{0.56}$ was used in #11]) which is commonly used in analysis of physiologic indexes (like BMR) which vary with BW. An "*" indicates that the listed effect of DR was not reported but was calculated (and, in some cases, estimated) by us from the reported data. A "-" indicates no significant effect of DR. A "?" indicates that the value was neither reported nor estimable. In study #5 a low protein (5% casein) diet was fed.

[c]References: (1) Horst et al. (1934); (2) Will and McCay (1943); (3) Vander Tuig et al. (1979); (4) Forsum et al. (1981); (5) Khan and Bender (1979); (6) Boyle et al. (1981); (7) Gleeson et al. (1982); (8) Rothwell and Stock (1982a); (9) Rothwell et al. (1982a); (10) Mohan and Rao (1983); (11) Cox et al. (1984); (12) Mohan and Rao (1985b); (13) Mohan and Rao (1985a); (14) McCarter et al. (1985); (15) Hill et al. (1985); (16) Corbett et al. (1986); (17) Ichikawa and Fujita (1987).

Aside from two reports (Table 4.18, #14, 17), all O$_2$ consumption studies involved short-term DR. Thus, much is known about acute adaptational adjustments in metabolic rate soon after DR starts. The data indicate that O$_2$ consumption/BW is usually either unaffected or slightly lowered by short-term DR. The O$_2$ uptake/MBW typically is about 20 percent lower for such a DR group. A more substantial drop of 25 to 50 percent in the O_2 consumption/whole animal occurs. With longer-term DR, O_2 consumption/BW either rises slightly or is unchanged, while that per LBM was unchanged. Again, the whole DR rat uses much less total O_2 (32-43% in these two studies) than ad lib controls. The magnitude of this drop in O_2 consumption per DR rat approximated the extent of caloric restriction and LS prolongation with the DR regimen used in study #14.

If the rate of production of active oxygen molecules parallels rates of O_2 consumption, then whole body burdens of these potentially damaging substances should fall with DR, and underfed animals may have to deal with fewer damage-inducing molecules than do controls. The production of active oxygen species might also be expected to fall if increases in metabolic efficiency occur with DR (see *"Metabolic Efficiency and Energy Intake,"* Chapter 5). Because radical scavenging by catalase appears to be selectively upregulated with DR in mice (Koizumi et al., 1987a), it is possible that DR creates a situation where, relative to ad lib feeding, less active oxygen is made and what is made is rapidly detoxified.

Mitochondria

We know of but two studies on long-term DR's influences on mitochondrial numbers or functioning. These emphasized measuring O_2 consumption *in vitro* in the presence of substrate and were designed to provide information on coupling and the efficiency of phosphorylation (Tzagoloff, 1982 [p. 131-135]). O_2 uptake traces are shown in Figure 4.30 for respiration supported by glutamate and either stimulated by ADP (state 3 respiration rate) or uncoupled by dinitrophenol (DNP). State 4 respiration rate is that at which mitochondria oxidize substrates in the absence of a phosphate acceptor. Thus, phosphorylation does not occur in state 4 and in tightly coupled mitochondria this rate is low. The ratio of states 3 to 4 is designated the respiratory control index (RCI) and reflects the degree of coupling.

Tzagoloff (1982), in his book *Mitochondria* writes: "In poorly coupled or uncoupled mitochondria, state 4 respiration is high, and the RCI approaches values of 1. The dependence of substrate oxidation on the presence of a phosphate acceptor indicates that, in coupled mitochondria, electron transfer and ATP synthesis are geared to each other. Unless the energy released during electron transport is used in some energy-dependent process such as ATP synthesis or ion transport, oxidation of

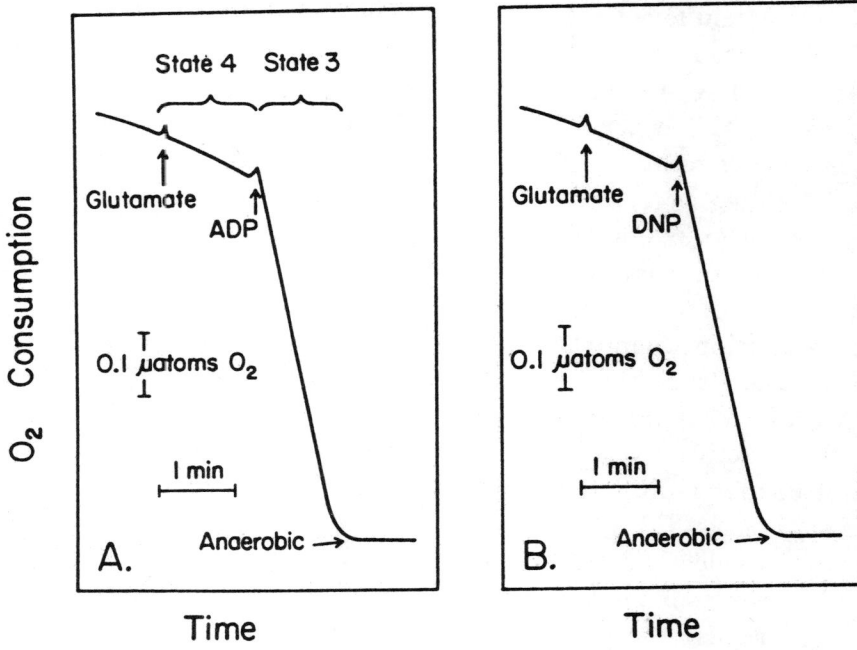

Figure 4.30. Stimulation of respiration by ADP (Panel A) or by dinitrophenol (Panel B). In each case the reaction mixture contained phosphate buffer, Mg^{2+}, and mitochondria. From Tzagoloff (1982), with permission.

substrate is limited. The true index of coupling, therefore, is the state 4 respiration which shows how readily the oxidative energy can be dissipated when it is not being utilized, and in perfectly coupled mitochondria, it might be expected that the rate would be zero."

The efficiency of phosphorylation can be estimated by calculating the ADP/O ratio during the burst of state 3 respiration after a small amount of ADP (all quickly consumed) is added. The ADP/O values approach 3 for NAD-linked substrates and 2 with succinate.

We examined DR's influences on liver and brain mitochondrial recovery and respiratory capacities using female $C3B10RF_1$ mice subjected to severe EDR for 2 to 5 months (Weindruch et al., 1980). When tested, the control mice weighed 30 g vs. 15 g for the DR group. Data on mitochondrial recovery are summarized in Tabel 4.19. Liver weight was 10 percent less for DR than for control mice. Total liver mitochondrial protein fell by 20 percent with DR. Mitochondrial protein content per wet weight was reduced 14 percent. As was shown in Table 4.2 (#13), liver cytochrome c oxidase activity per wet weight also fell (25%) with

TABLE 4.19

Influences of DR on Mitochondrial Recovery in Mice[a]

	Control	Restricted	Change in DR
1. Liver (n = 13)			
Wet weight, g	1.22 ± 0.06	1.10 ± 0.05	↓10%
Total mito. pro. (mg)	33.4 ± 1.5	26.6 ± 1.3	↓20%
Mito. pro./wet wt. (mg/g)	27.3 ± 1.1	23.4 ± 1.3	↓14%
2. Brain (n = 5)			
Wet weight, g	0.45 ± 0.01	0.39 ± 0.01	↓13%
Total mito. pro. (mg)	11.0 ± 0.4	10.4 ± 0.5	-
Mito. pro./wet wt. (mg/g)	24.7 ± 0.7	27.0 ± 0.9	-

[a]Data (mean ± SEM) are young, very severely restricted female C3B10RF$_1$ mice as reported in Weindruch et al. (1980). "Change in DR" gives the relative (%) effect of DR when statistically significant. Note that the 13% decrease in brain weight in the few mice studied is not typical of most DR findings which usually describe no decrease in brain weight. Abbreviations: mito. = mitochondrial; pro. = protein.

DR. No decrease in brain mitochondrial recovery was observed with DR despite brain weight falling about as much as did liver weight.

Table 4.20 shows data for liver mitochondrial respiration in mice from this same study. Preparations from DR mice generally revealed increased state 3 rates compared to controls, but with no differences in state 4 rates, for respiration supported by glutamate or pyruvate + malate. Thus the RCI was increased for these substrates. The DNP-uncoupled respiratory rate for pyruvate + malate rose with DR. These data suggest a larger effect of DR on the capacity to generate utilizable energy than on the coupling of utilizable energy for respiration supported by these substrates. The situation differed for β-hydroxybutyrate as substrate, which was oxidized at a slower rate by mitochondria from DR mice.

In contrast to the liver, brain mitochondrial respiration was not altered by DR.

Figure 4.31 shows electron micrographs of mitochondrial fractions isolated from livers of young DR and control C3B10RF$_1$ mice, and from ad lib-fed young (10 month) and old (25 month) B6 mice. Preparations from young mice showed less nonmitochondrial contaminants than those from old mice. Preparations from the DR mice appeared least contaminated and exhibited the largest mitochondria.

TABLE 4.20

Effects of DR on Liver Mitochondrial Respiration in Mice[a]

	State 4	State 3	2,4-DNP	RCI	ADP/O
1. Respiration per mitochondrial protein					
Glutamate (n=10)	-	-	-	↑17%	-
Malate+pyruvate (n=14)	-	↑31%	↑23%	↑34%	↑11%
Succinate+rotenone (n=10)	-	-	-	-	-
β-hydroxybutyrate (n=6)	-	↓21%	↓30%	↓21%	-
2. Respiration per unit of cytochrome c oxidase					
Glutamate (n=7)	-	-	-		
Malate+pyruvate (n=9)	-	↑45%	↑39%		
Succinate+rotenone (n=7)	-	-	-		
β-hydroxybutyrate (n=6)	-	-	↓17%		

[a]Adapted from Weindruch et al. (1980) to recap the magnitude of statistically significant effects of DR. Young mice were studied and the DR was rather severe. State 3 respiration rate is that stimulated by ADP. 2,4-Dinitrophenol (DNP) is an uncoupler which results in maximal rates of respiration. State 4 respiration rate is that at which mitochondria oxidize substrates in the absence of a phosphate acceptor (ADP). The ratio of states 3 to 4 is designated the respiratory control index (RCI) and reflects the degree of coupling. The efficiency of phosphorylation can be estimated by calculating the ADP/O ratio during the burst of state 3 respiration. The relative effects of DR on RCI and ADP/O values are the same by either (mitochondrial protein or cytochrome c oxidase) mode of expression.

A second long-term DR investigation involving mitochondrial measurements, that of Rumsey et al. (1987) (Table 4.2, #11), imposed either ADR (EOD feeding) or exercise on 10 month old male Fischer 344 rats. State 3 respiration rates were determined for liver and gastrocnemius muscle homogenates from 10, 18, 24 and 30 month old rats using pyruvate, octanoate, or glutamate (all shown in Figure 4.32) as substrate and for acetate and palmitoyl-l-carnitine.

In the liver, age did not reduce oxidative capacity in sedentary controls. Exercise had no consistent influence on liver substrate oxidation, whereas homogenates from DR livers displayed elevated oxidative capacities for all substrates. The authors proposed that the three 24 hour fasts per week which formed the basis of their DR regimen caused ". . . greater than normal levels of repetitive gluconeogenic activity to maintain plasma glucose levels. Energy expenditure for glucose synthesis (6 moles of ATP/mole of glucose) imposes what can be a substantial load on

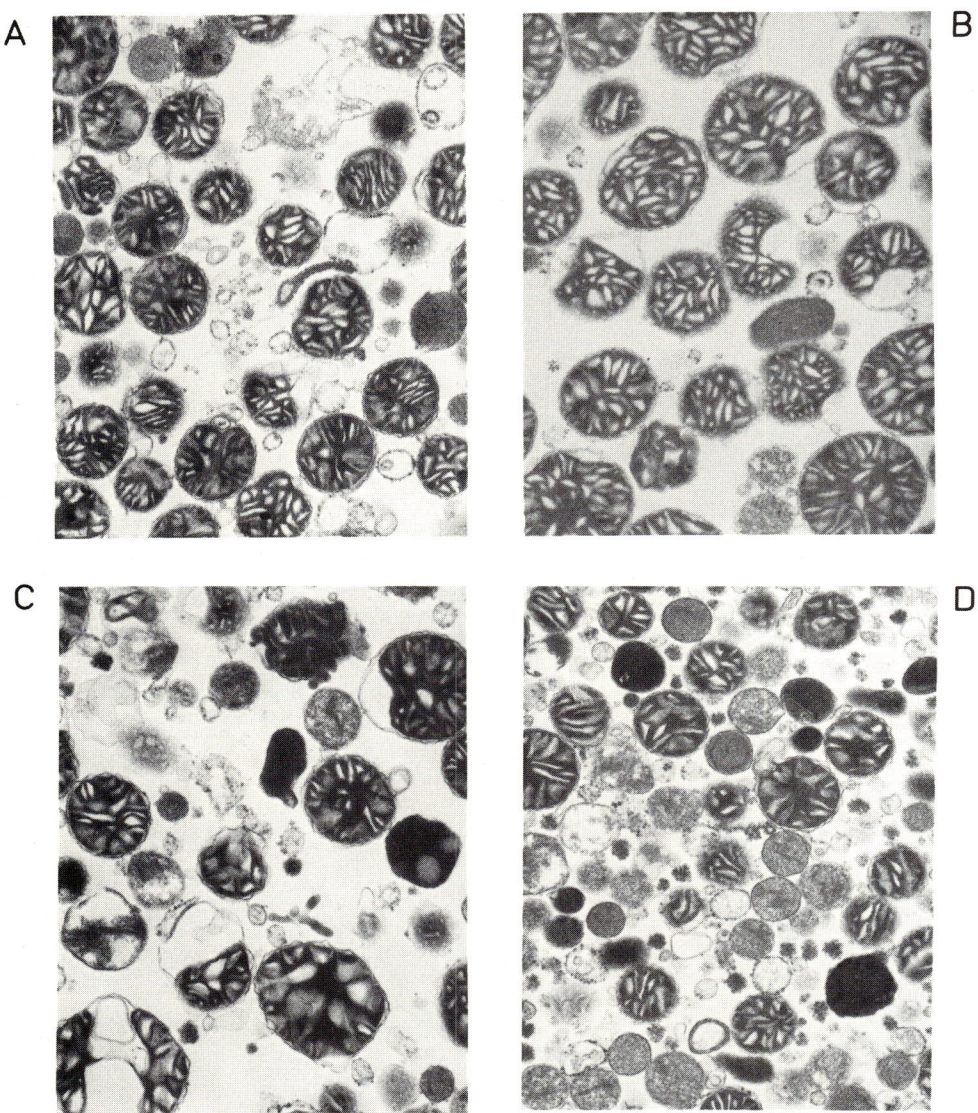

Figure 4.31. Electron micrographs (17,000x) of isolated liver mitochondrial fractions. A. Normally fed, young (5 month) $C3B10RF_1$ mouse; B. Diet restricted, young (5 month) $C3B10RF_1$ mouse; C. Normally fed, adult (12 month) B6 mouse; D. Normally fed, old (25 month) B6 mouse. From Weindruch et al. (1980).

the ATP generating pathways." They also suggested that (based also on enzymic data) the rats adapted to DR by increasing the number of respiratory assemblies in the liver.

In the gastrocnemius muscle, all five substrates were respired more slowly with advancing age. Exercise clearly opposed this decline at 24

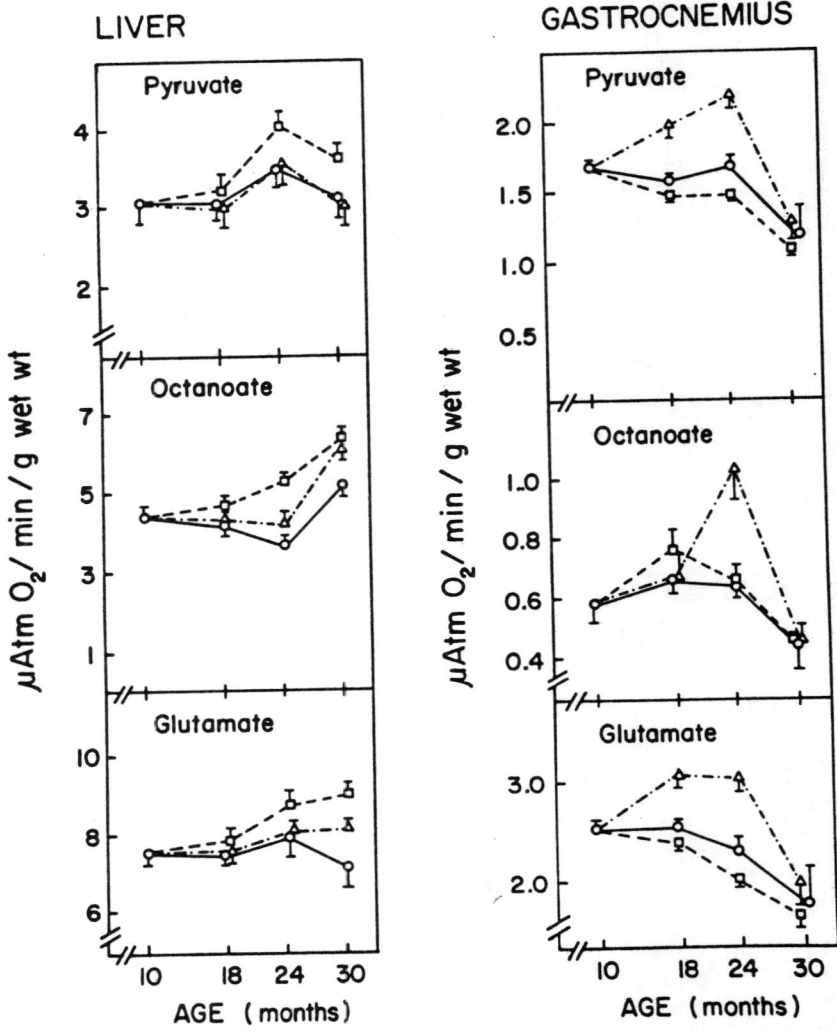

Figure 4.32. State 3 rates of O_2 utilization in liver and gastrocnemius homogenates from Fischer 344 rats. Three groups were started at 10 months of age: (o———o) = sedentary, ad lib fed controls; (△—•—△) = exercised, ad lib fed; (□-----□) = diet restricted. From Rumsey et al. (1987), with permission.

months but not at 30 months of age. The authors reported that compared to sedentary controls DR significantly reduced muscle respiration supported by pyruvate, glutamate and palmitoyl-l-carnitine; however, the changes were not large.

As repeatedly emphasized, short- vs. long-term DR, as well as DR with adequate nutrition ("true DR") vs. DR with malnutrition, can influence biological phenomena quite differently. Gold and Costello (1975) reported that imposition of very severe DR (25% of ad lib intake) imposed on young adult rats (BW, 275 g) for 1 week reduced BW by 45 percent, and lowered state 4 and DNP-uncoupled respiratory rates of mitochondria isolated from liver, heart or kidney. Solomon et al. (1984) found morphologic changes (enlargement, dense matrixes) in mitochondria 3 weeks after DR was started but not after 9 weeks.

Body Temperature

An association between severe undernutrition and low body temperatures in diverse human populations (e.g. during the Irish potato famine, World Wars I and II) has long been appreciated (Keys et al., 1950; McCance & Mount, 1960). Because body temperature reduction can increase LS in poikilotherms (Liu & Walford, 1972) and on thermodynamic grounds (Rosenberg et al., 1973) it is possible that DR's effect on aging might be at least in part so mediated.

The measurement of core body temperature in rats and mice has most often been done with a rectal probe. However, the stress accompanying the insertion of the probe may cause the subject's body temperature to rise. A better method for monitoring internal temperature is by telemetry from a small, surgically-implanted signalling device.

Hudson and Scott (1979) observed that laboratory mice are like many other small mammals in that under appropriate circumstances they can enter a state of daily torpor where — usually in the early morning hours — body temperature falls dramatically (by as much as 15°C) and approaches the ambient temperature (Figure 4.33). In their studies, torpor was only very rarely observed in ad lib fed mice but could be quickly induced by food restriction. Figure 4.34 reveals that O_2 consumption fell in the torpid mice. Torpor did not halt functionality. The cool mice were able to gather and ingest seeds at body temperatures of 24°C and behaved like normothermic mice at internal temperatures above 26°C.

Webb et al. (1982) further documented by telemetry the occurrence of torpor in lean and obese mice from various strains. Genetically obese (ob/ob) B6 mice differed from their genetically normal strainmates in becoming torpid even in the presence of food. The torpor was said to contribute to the high metabolic efficiency shown by this strain.

Evidence presented in Table 4.21 indicates that DR reduces the body temperature of mice but not of rats. The table does not cover DR in

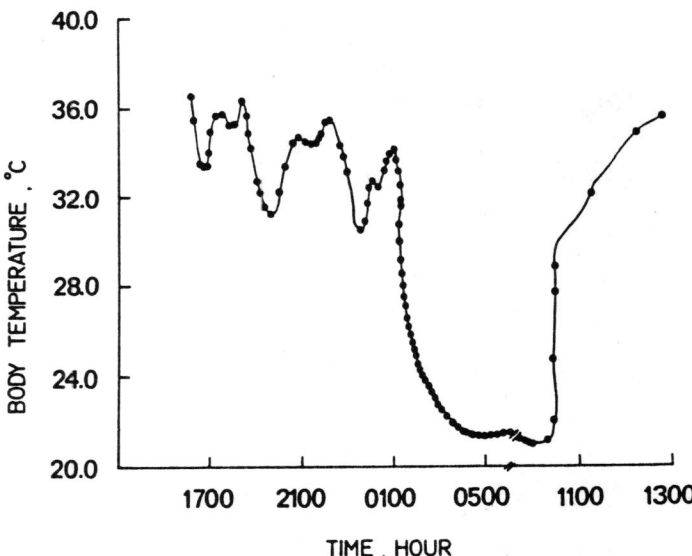

Figure 4.33. Body temperature of white mouse (*Mus musculus*) during a single episode of torpor. Temperature was measured via an implantable thermocouple. Redrawn from Hudson and Scott (1979), with permission.

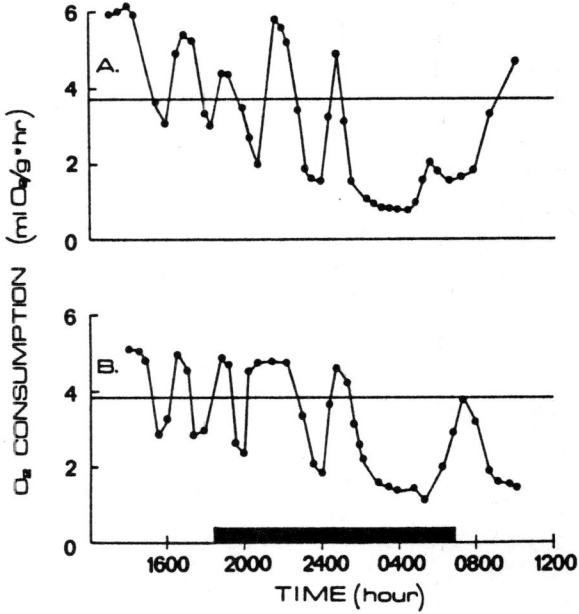

Figure 4.34. Records of O_2 consumption of two mice exhibiting torpor induced by food restriction. The ambient temperature was 20°C. The horizontal line in each recording is the resting O_2 consumption of that mouse. Mouse "A" was starved for an unstated period of time (The average time for 5 mice to become torpid after food was removed was 18 hours.). Mouse "B" was fed a restricted diet (2 g of millet/day). The solid rectangle at the bottom of the figure shows the dark period in the animal room. Adapted from Hudson and Scott (1979), with permission.

TABLE 4.21

Influences of Long-Term DR on the Internal Body Temperatures of Rats and Mice

Animal	Nature of DR[a]			Body Temp. (°C)[b]		Ref.[c]
	Diet	%AL[a]	DUR[a]	Control	DR	
1. Mice						
B6	PD[a]	90[a]	24	38.1	36.9	1
B10C3F$_1$	PD	50	5	38.0	35.8	2
B10C3F$_1$	PD	45	32	37.9	37.4	3
B6	NPD	80	20[a]	37.7	37.7	4
CD2F$_1$	NPD	75	24	37.7[b]	36.2[b]	5
2. Rats						
Sprague-Dawley	NPD	40	22	38.8[b]	38.7[b]	6

[a]Unless noted otherwise, DR started at or near the age of weaning. "%AL" is the % of the ad lib intake fed to the DR group. "DUR" is the duration of feeding in months. In study #1, the restricted mice were fed a 4% protein diet ad libitum (90% of the intake of a control diet) but BW was more severely lowered (by 37%) by this regimen. In #4, DR started at 6 months of age and was via EOD feeding (which increased average LS by 11%).

[b]In all studies except #5 (which used an implanted signalling device) body temperature was measured at ambient temperatures (21-24°) using a rectal probe. The difference between control and DR values was significant in studies #1, 2, 3, and 5. In #5, temperatures were telemetered and values listed above are overall means. The lowest hourly means were also reduced by DR (36.0 vs. 34.6°, see Fig. 4.35). In study #6, temperatures were measured around the clock. The values above are the peaks (which occurred at ~9PM). The trough values (36.6-37.0°C at ~7AM) also were not influenced by DR. In #4, baseline temperatures were not altered by DR but the ability to maintain body temperature at 10°C was lost with age in controls but less so in the DR group. Similarly, Segall and Timiras (1975) found that dietary tryptophan restriction of rats opposes age-related increases in recovery time to normal body temperature after being immersed in ice water for 3 minutes.

[c]References: (1) Leto et al. (1976b); (2) Weindruch et al. (1979); (3) Cheney et al. (1979); (4) Talan and Ingram (1985); (5) Nelson and Halburg (1986); (6) Volicer et al. (1984).

obese strains of rodents (see Himms-Hagen [1985a] for review). Both low protein diets fed ad lib and restricted feeding of adequate diets can reduce body temperature.

A study by Nelson and Halberg (1986, #5) is especially noteworthy because telemetry was used and 24 hour measurements were made (essential in view of the mouse's torpid tendencies). One recalls that DR (NPD at 75% of ad lib) carried out by giving a single meal during either early darkness, early light, or as six smaller meals during darkness all increased average and maximum LSs (see *"Longevity,"* Chapter 2). Figure 4.35 shows that all these DR regimens lowered internal body temperature. The extremely low temperatures of true torpor were not observed in this study.

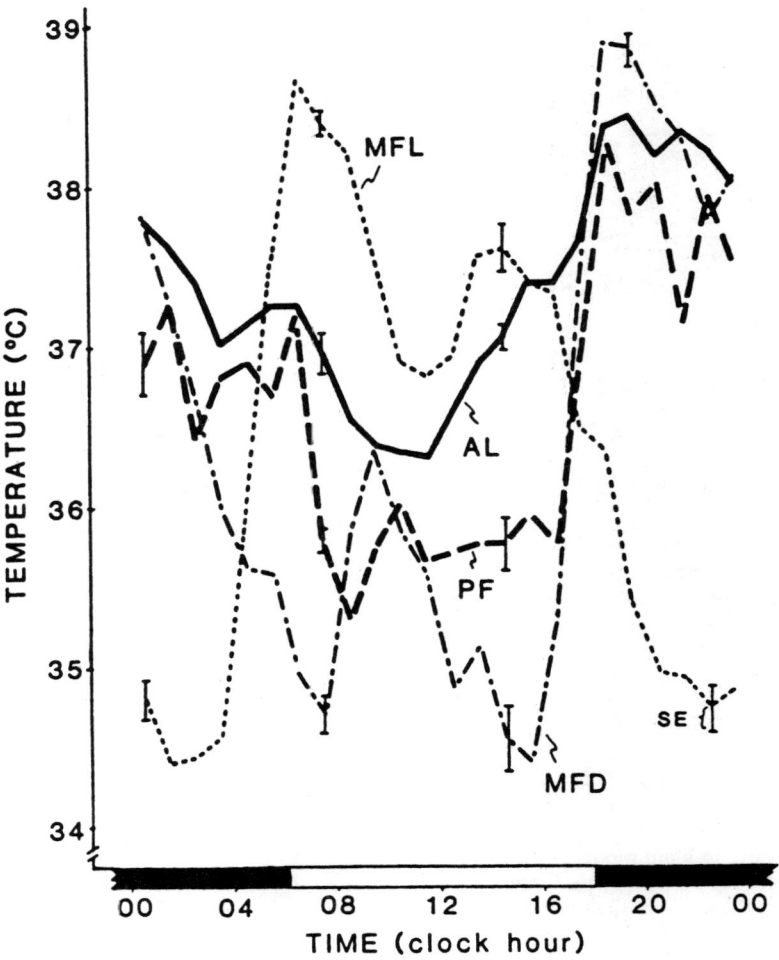

Figure 4.35. Day long patterns of telemetered temperatures in female CD2F$_1$ mice fed in four different ways. AL = ad libitum feeding. The other three groups were fed 75 percent of the ad libitum intake either as a single meal at the start of darkness (MFD = meal-fed dark) or at the onset of light (MFL = meal-fed light) or via six smaller meals aimed at approximating the feeding pattern of ad lib fed mice (PF = pattern-fed). From Nelson and Halberg (1986), with permission.

The report of Volicer et al. (1984) is the only study of body temperature in long-term underfed rats. Here the DR rats (Sprague-Dawley males) were fed enough of an NPD to maintain a BW of 300 g, one-third that reached by the ad lib fed controls. All rats were killed for study and LSs were not determined but the probable maximum LSs were said to be 34 months for controls and 48 months for the DR rats. This study provides evidence that internal body temperature reduction is not an essential component of DR's actions. Studies in other rat strains using proven DR regimens and telemetry are needed.

Thus, DR mice can enter torpor and reduce body temperature quite readily whereas DR rats apparently do not. The mouse's metabolic rate falls when torpor is first induced by DR. Whether or not mouse metabolic rates show daily periods of depression after months or years of DR is unknown.

Body Composition

Body composition was among the many physiologic parameters which Nolen (1972; Table 2.6, #6) measured in his important, broad study of DR begun at weaning or at 3 months of age. Data for rats fed 60 percent of ad lib from these ages and for ad lib controls are summarized in Table 4.22. Food restriction at either age reduced the level of body fat (especially striking in females) while raising the percentage compositions of body water, nitrogen, and ash. Calculating the actual whole body load of fat in 24 month old rats reveals large differences between control and DR animals: ad lib male, 195 g; DR male, 90 g; ad lib female, 256 g; DR female, 49 g.

TABLE 4.22

Effects of DR on Body Composition of Rats[a]

| Parameter | Diet | | | | | |
| | Ad Lib | | DR@1 month | | DR@3 months | |
	F	M	F	M	F	M
1. Total BW (g)	722	753	319	516	341	552
2. Evis. BW (g)	581	609	247	411	260	438
3. Body Composition (%):						
H_2O	42	49	56	53	56	51
Fat	44	32	20	22	21	25
Nitrogen	1.5	2.4	3.1	3.2	2.9	2.9
Ash	2.3	3.4	4.6	4.4	5.0	4.6

[a]Data are for 24 month old female (F) and male (M) rats fed 60 percent of the ad lib level starting at 1 or 3 months of age as described by Nolen (1972). Body composition is given as the percent of the eviscerated carcass weight.

Yu et al. (1982; see Table 2.4, #20) looked for possible correlations between longitudinally measured lean body mass (= total BW − total fat weight) and LS in Fischer 344 rats (San Antonio colony). (As Lesser et al. [1973] found in male Sprague-Dawley rats, lean body mass did not fall in any progressive way with advancing age, only with terminal disease.) The peak lean body mass for ad lib fed controls was 500 g; for DR rats, 300 g. A longer-lived subgroup of DR rats showed increasing lean body mass through 70 percent of their LSs (27 months), but decreasing lean body mass after 85 percent of their LSs. A longer-lived subgroup of ad lib rats showed a similar pattern (but 70% of their LS was only 18 months). Lean body mass did not fall in late life in the shorter-lived subgroups fed either diet. Because of the age when several rats were last tested prior to death, the study did not exclude the possibility that lean body mass might decline in some rats after 90 percent of their LSs.

In other studies involving rats and humans, muscle mass did not fall in late life. Holloszy's group reviewed this subject in a recent report (Garthwaite et al., 1986). In addition, they presented data from 6 month old male Long-Evans rats assigned to one of three groups: (1) sedentary controls fed an NPD ad libitum; (2) swimmers (5 sessions/week [3 hours/session!]); (3) DR (fed to maintain same BW as swimmers). The DR was mild (22 g/day, which represents only a 20% restriction), and quite long-term (to 28 months of age), but LS was not determined. Swimming caused a 9 percent increase in food intake. Body weight, lean BW, and the content of protein, fat, ash and water in the carcass were determined at 12, 18, 24 and (except for swimmers) 28 months. The results showed that lean BW and protein content fell progressively over these ages in sedentary controls. The exercise of swimming opposed these changes until 18 months of age. The main effect of mild DR was to reduce fat content by 40 percent relative to that of sedentary controls. But even lower levels of fat were found in the swimmers. Total lean BW was minimally affected by DR; however, DR rats lost proportionally less lean tissues than did sedentary controls. The DR opposed or prevented the following age-related changes in carcass composition observed in the sedentary controls from 12 to 28 months of age: 44 percent decrease in protein content, 43 percent increase in fat content, and 12 percent decrease in water content.

Harrison et al. (1984; Table 2.5, #18) imposed DR on genetically normal B6 mice (+/+) and on genetically-obese (ob/ob) B6 mice. In the +/+ mice, DR reduced the percent of body fat from 22 to 13 percent. In ob/ob mice, DR reduced body fat from 67 percent in ad lib to 48 percent in DR Mice. Even though LS was prolonged, the restricted ob/ob mice were much fatter than ad lib +/+ mice. Daily food intakes were 2 g for all DR mice, 3 g for +/+ controls, and 4 g for ob/ob controls.

Another way to view body composition is via organ weights. In a study of 24 month old EDR rats (60% of ad lib) and ad lib fed rats reported by Yu et al. (1985), EDR lowered organ weights by the following percentages: heart, 20; kidney, 31; lung, 14; and spleen, 55. Thyroid weight was reduced by 40 percent by EDR (Kalu et al., 1983b).

Many short-term underfeeding studies (e.g. Eisen & Leatherwood, 1978; Harris, 1980; Harris et al., 1986) have also investigated body composition. However, these fall outside the bounds of our emphasis here and will not be reviewed.

Muscle

Skeletal muscle has been studied in long-term DR animals. Almost all work has been limited to rats. In Masoro's colony, the mass of the gastrocnemius muscle of DR rats averaged 60 percent that of controls until 18 months of age when the fully-fed rats commenced to lose mass (Yu et al., 1982; Figure 4.36). At 25 months, muscle weight did not differ between groups but the DR group progressively lost mass thereafter. Gastrocnemius composition was also studied. Protein content fell with age in both groups. This fall was said not to be retarded by DR, although the value for the oldest (36 months) DR group was significantly (10%) higher than that recorded at 30 months. The collagen content per dry weight rose with age earlier in controls than in DR rats. Neither phospholipid nor cholesterol content changed with aging or DR.

McCarter et al. (1978) studied the lateral omohyoideus muscle (LOMO, a fast skeletal muscle) from 6 month old DR and control rats. Both LOMO mass and BW decreased by 40 percent with DR, while fiber diameter fell by 25 percent. The number of fibers per muscle as well as the length of the resting muscle were uninfluenced by DR, as were the mechanical properties of the muscle (e.g. maximum tension, contraction time), ultrastructure and histochemical staining patterns (NADH diaphorase, phosphorylase and ATPase). Furthermore, muscle mechanics were uninfluenced by DR in fast (LOMO) and slow (soleus) fibers (McCarter et al., 1983).

The above work was extended to include testing of LOMO from older rats and the measurement of resting O_2 consumption (McCarter et

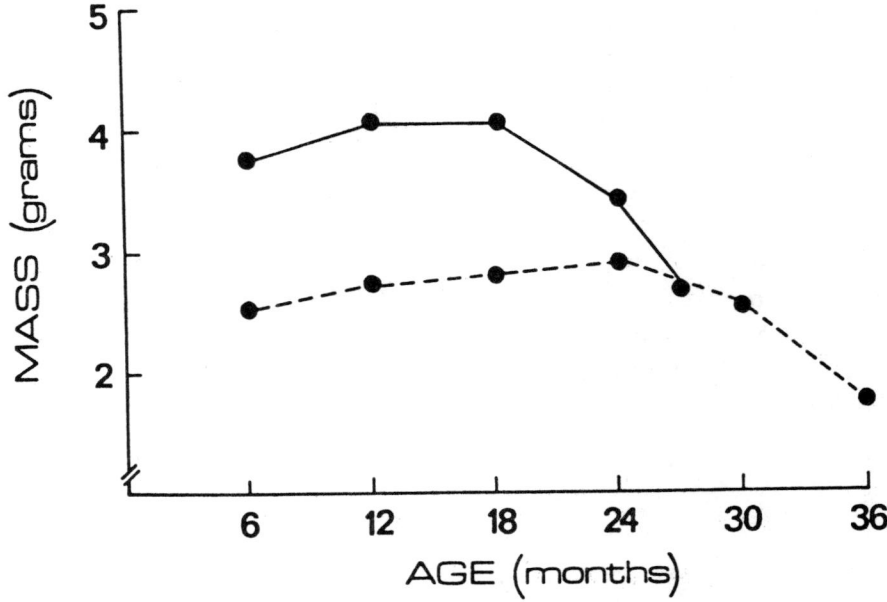

Figure 4.36. Gastrocnemius muscle mass in restricted (-----) and ad lib (———) fed male Fischer 344 rats. From Yu et al. (1982), with permission.

al., 1982). Figure 4.37 summarizes the effects of aging and DR on LOMO mass, fiber diameter, and fiber number per muscle. LOMO mass was reduced by DR but not by aging. (The authors suggest that the gastrocnemius muscle may lose mass with because of diminished use but that since the LOMO is constantly used, it loses no mass. Along these same lines, Park et al. [1982] reported that aging reduced the mass of the plantaris muscle but not of three other muscles.) Fiber diameter of LOMO was 25 percent lower in the DR rats until 24 months of age, when robust decreases in the diameter of fibers from the ad lib group occurred which all but erased the earlier differential. Very late life declines in fiber diameter in the DR group were present but mild. The number of fibers per muscle was not affected by DR but rose after 20 months of age in both groups, thereby preventing a loss in LOMO mass. Resting O_2 consumption per wet weight of LOMO decreased after 6 months of age quite strikingly in controls but not much in DR rats.

McCarter and McGee (1987) recently described the composition of LOMO and soleus muscles in relation to aging and DR. Contractile function was not influenced and composition was only weakly affected by age or diet. The main conclusion was that the factors investigated were probably not responsible for age-related losses in motor performance.

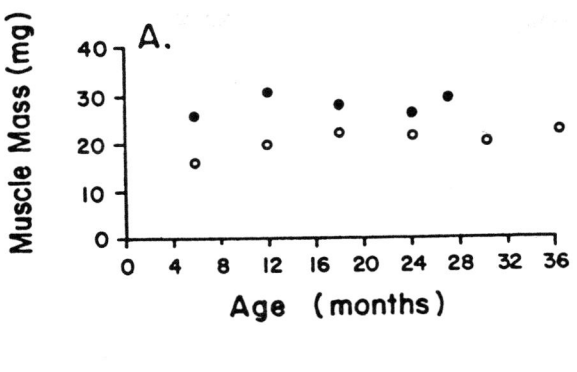
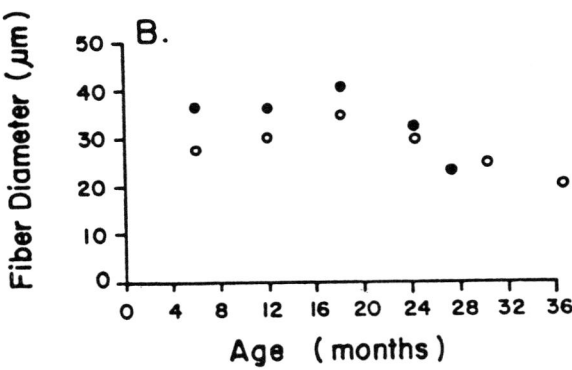
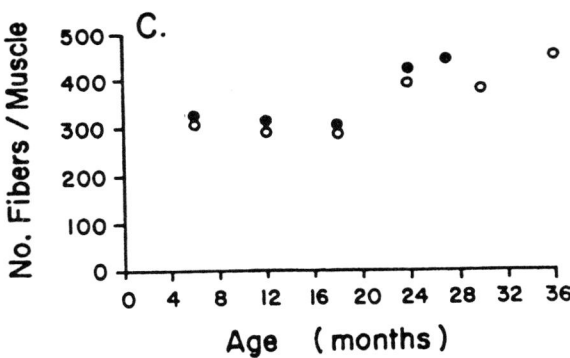

Figure 4.37. Lateral omohyoideus muscle mass (Panel A), fiber diameter (Panel B) and fiber number per muscle (Panel C) as influenced by aging and DR in male Fischer 344 rats. DR rats, (o); ad lib fed rats, (•). Adapted from McCarter et al. (1982), with permission.

Beyer et al. (1984) assessed the bioenergetic status of the gastrocnemius and quadriceps muscles from 25 month old male Sprague-Dawley rats subjected at 21 months of age either to exercise (treadmill running) or ADR (underfed to stabilize at same BW as exercised group [650 g vs. 750 g for controls]). An NPD was fed to all animals. Young (9 month old) sedentary controls were also studied. The main age-related changes seen in 9 vs. 25 month old sedentary controls were 30 percent decreases in: (1) state 3 oxidation rates for several substrates by gastrocnemius homogenates (but no age, exercise or DR effect on respiration by isolated mitochondria from the quadriceps), (2) flavin levels in the gastrocnemius and, (3) mitochondrial yield from the quadriceps. Exercise led to youthful (or hyperyouthful) values for all three age-sensitive indexes. Underfeeding was apparently detrimental, as these three age changes were either not improved or made worse by ADR. Perhaps imposing this fairly mild ADR regimen on somewhat elderly rats of a strain prone to obesity and short LSs when fed ad lib is simply "too little and too late."

Non-skeletal muscle physiology has been less studied in relation to DR. Investigating aortic smooth muscle function in DR rats, Herlihy and Yu (1980) noted that certain age-sensitive functional declines (isoproterenol-induced relaxation, tension development) were attenuated by DR. Spurgeon et al. (1983) published a conference abstract stating that EOD feeding of male Wistar rats resulted in cardiac atrophy but did not change cardiac muscle performance.

Many short-term underfeeding studies have examined muscle physiology. Hansen-Smith et al. (1977b) underfed young rats for 8-10 weeks (35% of ad lib intake). O_2 consumption (per dry weight) and mitochondrial appearance and distribution were determined in cardiac and red (high oxidative) and white (low oxidative) skeletal muscles. Dietary restriction without protein restriction did not influence these parameters, whereas DR achieved via a low protein diet lowered O_2 consumption and depleted mitochondria from the sarcolemma of white muscle. In another short term study, Hooper (1986) found that mice fed 70 percent of the ad lib level for 21 days showed lower muscle (biceps, tibialis anterior) weights, fiber length and numbers of sarcomeres per fiber.

Adipose Tissue

Bertrand et al. (1977) observed that 6 month old DR rats possessed 40 percent fewer and 25 percent smaller (average diameter) fat cells in epididymal and perirenal deposits than control rats. These data were contrary to the prevailing view that adipocyte numbers could not be influenced by post-weaning nutrition.

Dietary Restriction: Effects on Biological Parameters 219

The work was extended to encompass cross-sectional and longitudinal LS studies (Bertrand et al., 1980a). Total fat mass (perirenal, epididymal deposits) increased in both control and DR groups up to 70 percent of the LS, then fell (Figure 4.38) largely because of a drop in adipocyte size (not numbers) (Figure 4.39). At 6 months of age, perirenal deposits from DR rats contained 70 percent the number of adipocytes as were in control deposits. Average cell volume fell 50 percent with DR. At 30 months of age, cell number was halved in DR deposits but cell size was the same as in ad lib controls. As described previously (see *"Growth Rate, Body Weight and Lifespan,"* Chapter 2) this longitudinal study revealed a positive correlation in DR rats between LS and either peak absolute fat mass or peak percent body fat. Thus, a metabolically thrifty phenotype may accentuate DR's influences on the rate of aging.

In another report Bertrand et al. (1984) described fat cell numbers and volumes in these same depots for EDR, ADR and control rats fed as described previously (Table 2.4, #21). Again, fat cell numbers were influenced by caloric intake. Starting DR at 6 months of age did not alter

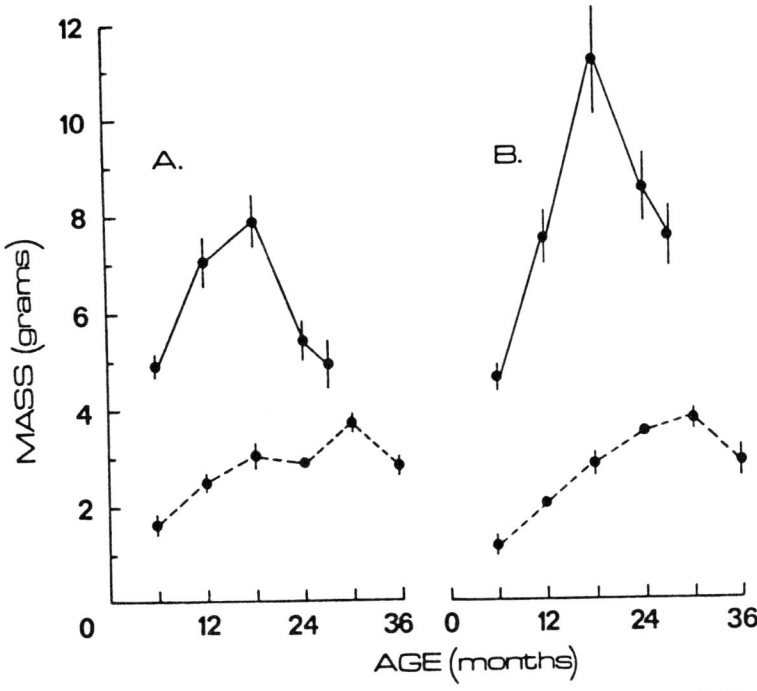

Figure 4.38. Influences of aging and DR on the mass of epididymal (Panel A) and perirenal (Panel B) fat depots of male Fischer 344 rats. DR rats, -----; ad lib fed rats, ———. From Bertrand et al. (1980a), with permission.

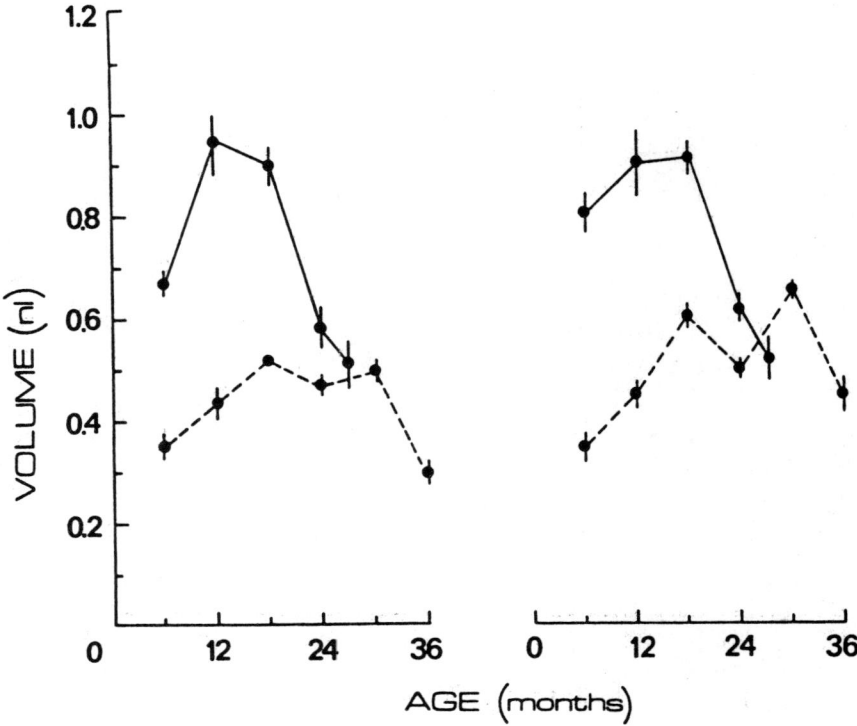

Figure 4.39. Influences of aging and DR on the average volume of adipocytes in epididymal (Panel A) and perirenal (Panel B) fat depots of male Fischer 344 rats. DR rats, -----; ad lib fed rats, ———. From Bertrand et al. (1980a), with permission.

epididymal fat cell numbers but did forestall the perirenal adipocyte hyperplasia which occurred in the control group between 6 and 18 months of age.

Lipid content and metabolism in Fischer 344 rats was studied by Panemangalore et al. (1986) (Table 4.2, #21). They subjected 3.5 and 16 month old male Fischer 344 rats either to a 4 month course of ad lib feeding or to 60 or 80 percent of ad lib feeding. The 60 percent regimen lowered epididymal fat pad weight by 45 percent in young rats and by 65 percent in the older rats such that the same pad weight (about 6 g) was reached by both groups. The older DR rats were more prone than younger rats to show reduced levels of free fatty acids in epididymal fat pads. Lipoprotein lipase activity was lowered more severely by DR in the older group. Late-onset DR was seen as leading to greater lipid mobilization than EDR. (For additional comments on fat metabolism in DR animals, see *"Insulin and Glucagon,"* this Chapter.)

Bone

Nolen (1972) studied the effect of long-term DR on femur lengths and weights. At 3 months of age, EDR rats possessed 10 percent shorter and 30 percent lighter femurs than ad lib controls. At 12 months of age, femur length in males was not influenced by DR, while actual weights were 30 percent lower in EDR rats than in controls. Femur weight was similarly reduced by EDR in 12 month old females. Starting DR at 3 months of age did not influence femur weight at 12 months. At 24 months of age the only significant difference attributable to DR was in the length of femurs in males, with values for the 3 month onset DR group being lower than those for the other groups; however, this result was deemphasized as attributable to a sampling bias. Between 12 and 24 months of age the EDR rats gained femur mass but the controls did not. Beauchene et al. (1982) state in a conference abstract that femurs of mature ad lib fed rats were 1 percent longer, 16 percent heavier and contained 20 percent more ash than those from DR rats. Thus, skeletal growth is retarded by DR but not as much as growth in most other tissues.

Kalu et al. (1984a) studied skeletal growth and senescence in Fischer 344 rats fed one of five dietary regimens. Both EDR (onset at 6 weeks) and ADR (onset at 6 months) were tested. Figure 4.40 shows the influences of aging and diet on five femur parameters. All five increased with age more rapidly in rats fed ad lib either a normal or moderately low (12.6%) protein diet than in DR rats. But only ad lib fed rats showed bone loss in late life (after 24 months). One notes that DR started at either age (and continued once started) led to similar outcomes. As discussed above, these findings may be causally related to DR's blunting of late-life increases in PTH. Histologic findings on the epiphyseal growthplate of the proximal tibia were also described. At 18 months of age the plates of ad lib fed rats were sealed off by bone, with no signs of growth. At the same age, the EDR group displayed active plates, which persisted up to 24 months of age. But growthplates of 18 month old rats started on ADR at 6 months of age resembled those of the age-matched ad lib fed rats.

Kalu et al. (1984b) determined femur strength in variously aged rats fed either ad libitum or on EDR. At 6, 12 and 24 months of age the femur strength to BW ratios were increased 55 to 95 percent by DR.

Calcitonin is the thyroid hormone that inhibits osteoclastic bone resorption and lowers plasma calcium. Both serum and thyroid calcitonin

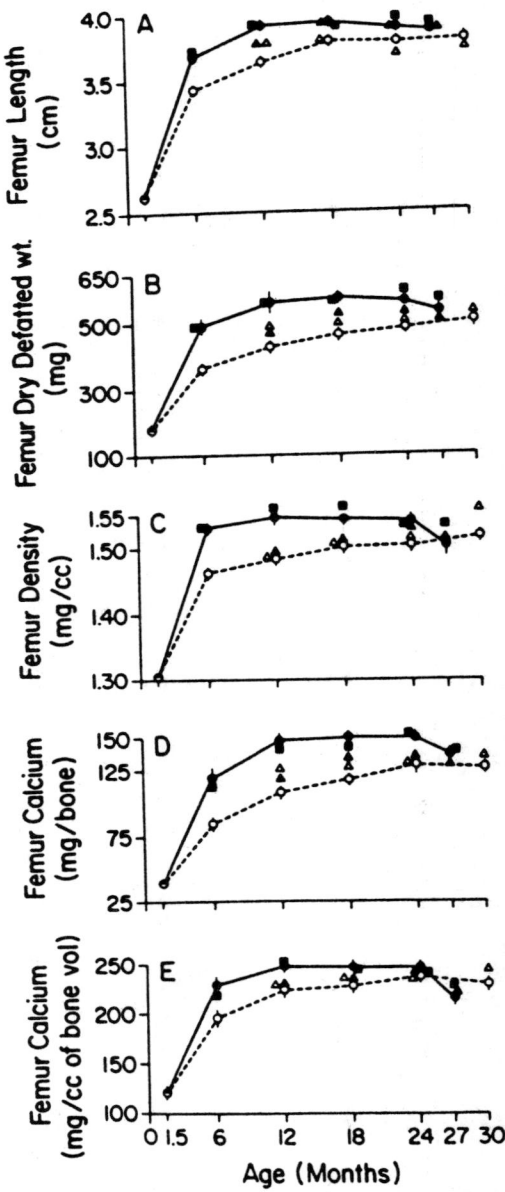

Figure 4.40. Effects of aging and diets on the femurs of male Fischer 344 rats. ● = ad lib (21% protein); ○ = EDR (60% of ad lib); ▲ = 60 percent of ad lib from 1.5 to 6 months and then fed ad lib; △ = 60 percent of ad lib starting at 6 months; ■ = ad lib (12.6% protein). From Kalu et al. (1984a), with permission.

increase markedly with age in fully-fed rats. However, this increase is far less in DR rats (Kalu et al., 1983b).

Thus, the work of Kalu and colleagues indicates that, for Fischer 344 rats, bone aging is substantially retarded by DR. It should be noted, however, that this strain of rat "dies young" of renal disease if fed ad lib and, as the authors discuss, this situation must impact on bone metabolism. In any case, the suitability of the rat as a model for bone aging in humans can be questioned.

A report by Lee et al. (1986) describes bone mineral content in male Fischer 344 rats subjected at 16 months of age to 4 months of ADR at 60 or 80 percent of ad lib. The primary focus of the investigators was not on DR but rather on pursuing an idea borne from their own clinical finding that osteoporotics who gained the most BW after 6 months of eating a calcium-enriched diet enjoyed the best gains in bone density. They hypothesized that energy restriction per se can lower bone mineral content. Their data on fairly small numbers (n = 5 − 7) of rats fed balanced intakes of minerals, protein, and vitamins do support this view (especially for the 60% of ad lib group) and generated the suggestion that a ". . . cautious approach is required when recommending energy intake reductions in weight control plans." However, sudden imposition of a 40 percent restriction regimen upon a late middle-age rat is a severe maneuver not representative of a good DR procedure. The most severely restricted rats lost 40 g of BW over the course of the study, while the other two groups averaged 50 and 80 g gains.

Reproductive Senescence

Most long-term DR work involving reproductive senescence has dealt with female rats on EDR regimens evaluated at various ages for cycling and/or fertility. Female mice have been less studied. Evidence for male reproductive senescence in rodents is unconvincing.

This area of inquiry began with Osbourne et al. (1917) who returned four food-restricted rats to ad lib feeding and allowed them to breed when 16 to 23 months old. Females who had never been restricted did not breed successfully at these ages, but all of the formerly underfed rats (the last at 31 months of age) bore multiple litters.

Evans and Bishop (1922) described cycling in rats maintained on 50 percent, 67 percent or "slightly" (% DR not stated, but BW at 12 months of age was 240 g vs. 320 g for ad lib controls) less than the ad lib intake from early life until 12 months of age. The 50 percent EDR group did not cycle. Only 8 of 10 rats cycled in the 67 percent EDR group, with an average age of onset of cyclicity of 7 months. Cycling commenced at less than 2 months for ad lib fed rats. Even the "slightly" restricted group showed a delay in the onset of cycling. When rats from this group and unrestricted littermates were followed for 7 months, the mildly restricted group averaged 7 cycles versus 25 for controls. The authors found it ". . . rather remarkable to see this abnormality in animals not greatly underweight—not more so than the lighter members of a large normal group on an adequate nutrition."

Two reports described cycling capacities in old rats from McCay's colony. Asdell and Crowell (1935) compared rats undergoing severe EDR (i.e. the rats being held at BWs of either 40 or 80 g until "signs of failure occurred," whereupon both groups were allowed to quickly gain 10 g) with ad lib fed controls. Most (71%) of the controls showed cornified vaginal smears during their lives. This was not seen in the DR rats. The difference was attributed to fewer ovulations in the DR rats. Surprisingly, some quite old rats (33 months) fed any of the diets cycled regularly, although this was more common in the DR groups. McCay et al. (1943) reported similar findings.

Berg (1960) found that 70 percent of a group of female EDR rats 25 months of age which had been fed at two-thirds of ad lib intake could bear litters, versus only 12 percent of an ad lib cohort aged 18 to 25 months.

Merry and Holehan have carefully studied long-term EDR's impact on cycling and breeding capacities in aging female rats (for review see Merry, 1986). One notes that their Sprague-Dawley rats were fed an NPD at half of the ad lib level, producing rats of BW around 300 g. The DR was far less severe than that used by McCay's group. Merry and Holehan (1979) reported that their DR rats still cycled and bred at ages when ad lib fed controls could not. For example, at 18 months of age only 9 percent of controls cycled vs. 61 percent of DR rats at 24 months. This same result obtained in a later study (Holehan & Merry, 1985b) which also found cycle length to rise sharply in controls after 13 months but not in DR rats through 25 months of study. As for fertility, controls were infertile by 15 months whereas 80 percent of a group of 17 month old DR rats bore litters. Eight of 32 very old (27-31 months) DR rats could breed.

Holehan and Merry (1985d) tested the capacities of control and DR rats of various ages and of DR rats switched to ad lib feeding (DR→AL) to bear and wean litters. Litter size (which fell with aging in controls) and overall fertility were reduced by DR. Again, DR animals could breed at ages when controls could not. Group DR→AL showed a rate of decline in litter size identical to that of controls and, irrespective of the mother's age (12, 18 or 24 months tested) when returned to full feeding, could breed for only 200 days and produce three litters.

Tryptophan restriction (which causes very severe DR) also delays reproductive aging as evidenced by rats remaining fertile at greater than 30 months of age with "young" ovarian histology (many ova and few corpora lutea) (Segall & Timiras, 1983).

Quigley et al. (1987) subjected 4 and 15 month old female rats to 50 percent ADR for 10 weeks and then fed all of them ad lib for 16 weeks. Vaginal smears indicated that: (1) initially all young rats cycled regularly while only 40 percent of the older ones cycled regularly or irregularly; (2) ADR at either age led to cessation of cycling; and, (3) upon refeeding, *all* rats resumed cycling which continued for about 2 months in the young rats and 1 month in the older rats.

Only a few studies have explored the effect of DR on reproductive aging in mice. Ball et al. (1947) found that female A strain mice fed two-thirds as many calories as controls were less fertile early in life (4-8 months old); but, after being switched to ad lib feeding at 8 months of age, were more fertile than controls over the next 4 months. Nelson et al. (1985) described estrous cyclicity and follicular reserves in B6 mice on mild DR (20% restriction) from 3.5 to 10.5 months of age and after return to ad lib feeding. Restricted mice were acyclic (largely in diestrus). When refed at 10.5 months, the "exDR" mice began to cycle regularly, whereas 80 percent of age matched, never-restricted controls were acyclic. At 12.5 months of age the follicular reserves of the DR mice were twice those of controls. The authors attributed the delayed loss of cycling in DR mice as due to a slowing of the rate of follicular depletion.

In a collaborative study with Patrick May and Caleb Finch, we are now examining cycling capacity in C3B10RF$_1$ mice on EDR (50% of ad lib intake). Vaginal smears show that these mice do not cycle. When EDR mice were switched to ad lib feeding either at 12 or 22 months of age, however, cycling rapidly ensued and lasted for a period of 10 to 12 months. These mice appear capable of going through about 70 estrous cycles. The cycles can be postponed to very advanced ages by EDR.

Other Physiologic Parameters

Harrison and Archer (1987a) described influences of EDR on LS (see Chapter 2, Table 2.5, #19) and a panel of age-sensitive physiologic parameters in B6CBAF$_1$, B6, and genetically obese (ob/ob) B6 mice. In B6CBAF$_1$ mice (where DR increased survival), the following measures stayed "younger longer" in EDR mice: tight wire clinging (a test of neuromuscular performance), open field movement (indicative of voluntary activity), urine concentration ability, tail collagen denaturation (Table 4.1), and hair regrowth rate. Wound healing was slower in DR mice. In B6 mice, DR did not improve survival but did lead to "younger" values for tight wire, tail tendon, and open field tests. Hair regrowth rates fell with DR, thereby standing in accord with shorter LSs

TABLE 4.23

Effects of DR on "Other" Physiologic Parameters in Rodents

Parameter[a]	Species	Nature of DR[b]			Effect of DR[c]	Ref.[d]
		Diet	%AL[b]	DUR[b]		
Kidney function[a]	rat	NPD	65	23	improved function	1
Thyroid calcitonin	rat	PD	60	LS	↓ calcitonin content	2
Intestinal absorption	mouse	PD	60	25	↑ absorption	3
Bile flow rate	rat	NR	60	23	↑ flow	4
Blood pressure	rat	PD	60	LS	None	5
	rat	NPD	35	25	None	6
Presbyacusis	mouse	NPD	NR	LS	↑ cochlear function	7
Corneal endothelial loss[a]	rat	PD	60	17	↓ endothelial loss	8
Pineal cell number	rat	NR	50	11	↑ cell number	9
Pineal O$_2$	rat	NR	50	11	↑ respiration	9
Cerebral cortex cells	rat	NPD	NR	45	↓ cell number[c]	10
Brain dendrites	rat	NPD	NR	29	↑ spine complexity	11

[a]Study #1 measured paraaminohippuric acid transport, proteinuria and lesions. In #3, the absorption of vitamin A was measured.

[b]"%AL" is the % of the ad lib intake fed to the DR group. "DUR" is the duration of feeding in months. NR, not reported.

[c]In #10, cell loss was observed for 47 month old DR rats compared to much younger rats on either diet.

[d]References: (1) Tucker et al. (1976); (2) Kalu et al. (1983b); (3) Hollander et al. (1986); (4) Tuchweber et al. (1987); (5) Yu et al. (1985); (6) Wyndham et al. (1983); (7) Henry (1986); (8) Nadakavukaren et al. (1987); (9) Walker et al. (1978); (10) Peters et al. (1987); (11) Mervis et al. (1984).

and making it the sole test predicting DR's differential effect on these two strains. In ob/ob B6 mice, LSs were increased by DR and most tests were improved relative to the performance shown by ad lib-fed ob/ob mice.

The influences of DR on diverse other physiologic phenomena are summarized in Table 4.23. Age-related changes in many kidney functions are opposed by DR. The age-related increase in thyroid content and concentration of calcitonin in rats is reduced by DR. In mice, vitamin A absorption by the small bowel was found to be increased by DR. Bile formation fell by 35 percent between 3.5 and 24 months of age in ad lib fed rats, was 20 percent higher in DR than ad lib rats at 3.5 months and did not drop through 24 months of age. Blood pressure rose with aging in one of two studies but was not influenced by DR in either study. Age changes in cochlear function were lessened by DR in one of two mouse strains. Corneal endothelial loss may occur widely with aging in rodents. This appears to be retarded by DR. The pineal gland retains greater cellularity in aging DR mice than in control mice. Area 17 in the cerebral cortex of a few extremely old DR rats contained less cells than were in this locale of much younger rats fed either diet. In the rat neocortex, the complexity of dendritic spines fell with age. This change was opposed by EDR, but not by a 5 month period of ADR beginning at 19 months of age.

LEARNING AND BEHAVIORAL PARAMETERS

Are rodents on DR intellectual geniuses or idiots? Does EDR interfere with brain development? Are age-dependent decrements in spontaneous activity or in motor skills influenced by DR? Recent reports provide some insight into these questions.

Because of the well-documented decrease with aging in the density of striatal dopamine receptors, Joseph et al. (1983) studied age-sensitive, striatally-mediated behavioral responses (e.g. sniffing, grooming, rotational behaviors) in 24 month old DR rats and in ad lib fed controls aged 6 or 24 months. The animals were challenged with dopaminergic agonists and cholinergic antagonists. One recalls that the Baltimore group reported (Levin et al., 1982; Roth et al., 1984) that DR (EOD feeding) lessens dopamine receptor loss. These biochemical findings seem translatable into behavioral ones, as some of the aging changes in the actions of ad lib rats did not occur in the old DR animals (Joseph et al., 1983).

Goodrick (1984) reported that EOD-fed, 22 month old rats from the NIA's Baltimore colony made fewer errors in a maze test than did age-matched controls. A complication in this study was the use of food as a motivator and the possibility of greater motivation in the DR group.

Brennan et al. (1985) state in a meeting abstract that either DR or dopamine added to a normal diet enhanced mouse behavioral performances (exploratory behavior, active avoidance, motor skills) followed longitudinally through 20 months of age. Idrobo et al. (1986) published an abstract maintaining that 12 months of DR of B6 mice resulted in faster and better maze learning, and in less neuronal lipofuscin in the hippocampus and frontal cortical neurons.

Mice from our colony were evaluated for psycho/physical function by Don Ingram at the NIA. These were adult (12 month) or aged (30 month) female $C3B10RF_1$ mice fed either control or EDR regimens. Soon after arriving in Baltimore, the adult and aged EDR mice were switched to the control regimen so that all mice ate the same diet for at least 10 weeks prior to testing. Age-related declines observed among control groups in tests of motor coordination (rotorod) and learning (complex maze) were prevented by DR (Ingram et al., 1987; Figure 4.41). Also, DR increased locomotor activity in a runwheel cage in mice of both ages but did not alter exploratory activity in a novel arena. These two activity assays were uninfluenced by age in both diet groups.

The greater wheel activity which we saw in our "former DR" mice (i.e. removed from DR for at least 16 weeks before being tested) also obtains for rodents still being maintained on an underfeeding regimen (Olewine et al., 1964; Goodrick et al., 1983a; Yu et al., 1985; Mohan & Rao, 1985a and 1985b). The extent to which higher activity of underfed rodents contributes to LS prolongation is unknown.

Campbell and Gaddy (1987) measured a variety of age-sensitive sensory and motor responses in Fischer 344 rats placed on ADR at 10 to 12 months of age. Feeding was EOD. Longevity was modestly increased (median LS of ad lib group was 26 months vs. 29 months for ADR rats). The ADR rats showed greater abilities in three motor tests: tight wire hang time, balancing on a beam, and descent time down a mesh pole. These responses declined with aging in all groups. Other tests such as the startle response to acoustic stimulation and its inhibition by visual or acoustic leads were impaired with aging but were not influenced by DR.

Maze performance was studied in EOD-fed male Sprague-Dawley rats by Beatty et al. (1987). Restriction was mild (20% reduction in BW) and from 3 to 21 months of age. The EOD feeding facilitated initial

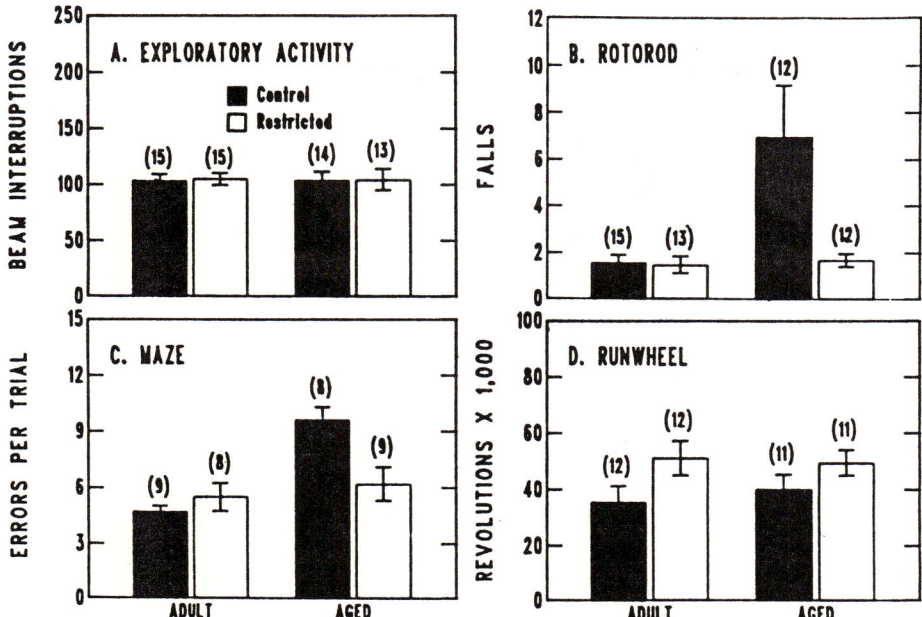

Figure 4.41. Age and diet comparisons of the behavioral performance of adult (12 months) and aged (32 months) C3B10RF$_1$ female mice. All data are mean ± SEM with sample sizes in parentheses. Exploratory activity (Panel A) is expressed as the number of light beam interruptions in a 10 minute period. Rotorod performance (Panel B) is shown as the number of falls during a 3 minute placement on a plastic rotating rod. Maze performance (Panel C) gives the number of errors per trial over 16 trials. Runwheel activity (Panel D) is presented as the number of wheel revolutions over a 72 hour placement in an activity-wheel cage. Adapted from Ingram et al. (1987).

adaptation to the maze but failed to retard age-related loss in the capacity for developing accurate spatial memory in the maze.

SUMMARY

This chapter reviews the rapidly expanding set of data on the biologic effects of long-term DR. Although information in many areas is limited, it appears that the vast majority of the age-sensitive parameters investigated in DR rodents are kept "younger longer" by the DR regimen, albeit a few (glucose secretion per volume of pancreas, startle responses, blood pressure) seem uninfluenced.

CHAPTER 5

MECHANISMS: HOW DOES DIETARY RESTRICTION RETARD AGING?

INTRODUCTION

SEVERAL recent reviews have discussed possible mechanisms whereby DR retards aging (Masoro, 1985b; Richardson, 1985; Holehan & Merry, 1986; Walford et al., 1987). Holehan and Merry (1986) incline to the view that an effect on "protein turnover, both directly and through amplification by adjustments in endocrine feedback, is the primary effect of underfeeding." Richardson (1985) holds a similar opinion. Masoro (1985b) casts a net so broad as to catch nearly all possible fish: "the total input of calories or nutrients per animal is the factor influencing the aging process . . . (and is) . . . probably coupled to the aging processes through endocrinic, intermediary metabolic or endocrine-metabolic events. Promising candidates for this coupling are: (1) the hypothalamic-pituitary system, (2) protein turnover and (3) free radical damage . . . (or) . . . a metabolic process yet to be considered."

Masoro (1985b) very properly suggests that some "old ideas" about how DR retards aging can now be discarded. The proposal by McCay et al. (1935) that DR extends LS by delaying maturation or, as suggested in several studies, by slowing the rate of growth and development during the early period of life has been disproven by the success of ADR experiments. The hypothesis of Berg and Simms (1960), reiterated by Young (1979), that a lack of excess body fat may be a major causal factor in the increased longevity associated with DR can also be discarded. In ad lib fed mice and rats there is no correlation between body fat and LS, and in DR rodents the heavier ones live longer (Bertrand et al., 1980a; Weindruch et al., 1986). Also, in studies by Holloszy and Smith (1986), ad lib-fed rats kept slim by exercise did not show an increased maximum LS, whereas sedentary rats maintained by DR at the same BW as the exercised ones did manifest such an increase.

Two main facts need to be kept in mind when considering DR's possible mode(s) of action:

(1) The first is the apparent *phylogenetic independence* of the effect. It is not simply a "rodent phenomenon"! Dietary restriction extends LS in all or nearly all species so far tested (The few exceptions seem to be special cases: see "STUDIES IN INVERTEBRATES," Chapter 2.), from animals as primitive as protozoans to others as complex as rodents. Does DR act via a common root mechanism in all these species? The accumulation of the age pigment lipofuscin, thought to be the end stage of free-radical-induced lipid peroxidation, is one of the most ubiquitous age-related changes in post-mitotic cells (Sohol & Allen, 1985). Dietary restriction decreases this accumulation in all species tested. Does this indicate a root mechanism? Must one discard DR's effect on the immune system as a fundamental mechanism because protozoa have no such system, yet are sensitive to DR's influence? Certainly the answer is yes, unless we differentiate between a potential universal cause of aging (the unifactorial approach: see "Mechanisms" in Chapter 1), multifactorial causalities, and simple "pacemakers" of aging. A "pacemaker" concerns pathogenesis rather than basic etiology, and is the means whereby a more fundamental or prior process leads to aging.

(2) The second main fact to be kept in mind is that *only energy restriction retards aging in mammals*. So long as the calorie level be not decreased, maximum LS has not been prolonged beyond the characteristic limit of the species by alterations limited to protein, fat, carbohydrate, or mineral content of the diet (Stunkard, 1983; Yu et al., 1984b; Iwasaki et al., 1988a, b). Even in short-lived strains, it is restriction of total calorie intake (from whatever source) that exerts an overriding influence on LS (Kubo et al., 1984b; Johnson et al., 1986).

The fact that incidences of a number of diseases can be substantially altered by variation in both type and quantity of certain dietary variables independently of a calorie effect, without influencing maximum LS, merely underscores that disease is distinct from aging. Reducing protein intake may retard the development of chronic nephropathy in rats, or renal disease in autoimmune strains of mice, but will not substantially affect species-specific maximum LS nor the age-related deterioration of other physiologic systems (Yu et al., 1984b; Fernandes, 1987).

In our own published studies, the protein, vitamin, and mineral intake of DR and control animals has been kept as equivalent (isonutrient) as possible, with the carbohydrate (sucrose and cornstarch, or in ongoing studies, glucose and cornstarch) content being the main variable (Weindruch & Walford, 1982; Cheney et al., 1983; Weindruch et al., 1986). Unpublished studies from our laboratory indicate that balancing the fat intake of DR and control mice did not alter DR's effect on aging.

In addition to the two main facts listed above, it is important also to keep in mind the existence of age-sensitive but DR-resistant parameters. These may have little to do with basic aging, even if they change with age, or they may be responsible for the fact that DR animals do not live even longer. Table 5.1 lists a number of these parameters.

TABLE 5.1
Age-Sensitive But DR-Resistant Parameters[a]

Parameter	Change with Age	Reference[b]
Circulating TSH (thyrotropin)	↓	1
Insulin secretion (islets in vitro)	↓	2
Insulin secretion (per vol of islet)	↓	3
Antilipolytic effect of insulin	↓	4
Oxidative damage products in urine	↑	5
Blood pressure	↑	6
Forskolin-stim. adenylate cyclase activ.	↓	7
Protein synthetic activity in brain	↓	8
β-oxidation in liver	↓	9

[a]Certain of these findings require repetition using DR regimens proven to extend maximum LS.
[b]References: (1) Sarkar et al. (1982); (2) Reaven and Reaven (1981b); (3) Reaven et al. (1983a); (4) DiGirolamo et al. (1984); (5) Saul et al. (1987); (6) Yu et al. (1985); (7) Scarpace and Yu (1987); (8) Sparks et al. (1983); (9) Rumsey et al. (1987).

We conclude this introduction by emphasizing that *future work aimed at elucidating the mechanism(s) behind DR's effect must not just show by ever more sophisticated means that DR animals are functionally younger.* There is a tendency to reason that because the immune response is "younger" in DR animals, and that the immune system seems involved in aging, that DR acts via the immune system. Or that because protein synthesis is sometimes greater (= functionally "younger") in DR animals, the mechanism of DR's action is to increase protein synthesis. But this "increase" in protein synthesis may merely mean that the animal has been kept functionally "younger" by some other, non-protein-synthesis mechanism, and of course younger animals do possess better protein synthesis than older ones.[1]

To elucidate the mechanism(s) whereby DR retards aging and extends LS is no easy task, especially in view of the present level of understanding on the etiology of aging. However, with the above caveats in mind, we shall now discuss what seem the most likely possibilities. While these will be discussed under seven headings or categories, the categories are obviously interrelated, and comments pertinent to one will sometimes be found in another. To avoid endless speculative digressions, we shall in most instances limit our discussion to phenomena which have already been investigated, at least to some degree, by means of the DR paradigm.

EVOLUTIONARY PERSPECTIVE

Totter's Hypothesis

Totter (1985) proposed that energy to maintain temperature as well as reproduction are "the main sources of oxygen radicals that may be the direct cause of aging," and that the energy expended for gathering food and resisting predation, i.e., most voluntary muscular actions, does not contribute to aging. When food is scarce, energy is diverted from basal metabolism and reproduction into muscular work, leading to an increased LS potential. The reverse process occurs when food becomes abundant. (According to Totter [1985], even some human populations show evidence of such an adaptation to differences in food supply.) A

---

[1]This point can be further illustrated by current DR work. At the 1988 FASEB meeting a session on DR was comprised of 10 talks on new findings in rodents. Fischer 344 rats were used in 8 of these. Age-related changes which stayed younger longer in old DR animals included: a decrease in the amount of kidney microsomal and mitochondrial membranes and the ratio of unsaturated: saturated fatty acids therein; increases in liver lipofuscin, serum prolactin and splenocyte Ig+ and Ia+ cells; decreased splenocyte lymphokine (IL-2, IL-3) production and mitogen-induced proliferation; decreased hepatic gene ($\alpha 2\mu$-globulin, SOD, catalase) expression; increased hepatic gene expression of the androgen-repressible SMP-2 locus; and decreased renal and hepatic UV-induced DNA repair. Thus the list of aging changes which are sensitive to DR lengthens, broadens and becomes more molecular; however, underlying mechanisms remain unclear.

8-02-89

111 Giltner Hall

Physiology

31-1063

1

The Retardation of Aging and Disease by Dietary Restriction

Drs. Weindruch and Walford

Charles C. Thomas
Springfield, IL

Dr. Joseph Meites

direct correlation between metabolic rates and reproductive output has also been claimed in comparisons between different mammalian species of the same body sizes (Lewin, 1982).

Without necessarily subscribing to Totter's acceptance of the free radical theory of aging, we believe that a number of observations about the effects of DR upon reproductive fitness, metabolism, the neuroimmune system, and other matters can be subsumed under such an evolutionary perspective.

It makes good evolutionary sense not to have babies when food is scarce, to divert reproductive energy to personal survival, and to outlive the time of scarcity. It makes additional sense, in terms of evolution, if DR were to have a rejuvenating effect on the reproductive apparatus after food again became available, and indeed Quigley et al. (1987) have found that a 10 week period of 50 percent DR, followed by ad lib feeding, will cause young rats to cease and then begin estrous cycling, and older rats who had ceased to cycle (i.e., before institution of DR) to recommence cycling. In another study (Nelson et al., 1985) mice on DR became acyclic and lost follicles more slowly with age; however, when switched to an ad lib food intake, older mice commenced cycling at an age when control mice had become acyclic.

As we shall see in the following section, there is evidence in humans for an age-related decline in oxygen consumption by skeletal muscle, but not by nonmuscle tissue (Tzankoff & Norris, 1978), so that energy shifts between the two might well influence aging in relation to the available food supply. The reproductive system clearly influences the immune system, by neuroendocrine feedback mechanisms (Grossman, 1985), and immunologic aging is retarded by DR. One can thus make an intriguing case for an evolutionary multisystem adaptational interpretation of DR's effect.

An evolutionary approach does not teach us the basic mechanism(s) whereby DR retards aging, but may allow an ordering of observations that makes sense of what otherwise would seem a scattered set of data. Thus, the effects of DR may not be simply a collection of biological curiosities but may embody a selected adaptive response to food scarcity, a very basic environmental challenge.

Sacher's Equations

Sacher inquired: Do variations in maximum LSs of species have anatomical or physiological correlates? He first studied 63 homeothermic mammalian species and found a linear relationship between the logarithm of maximum LS and the logarithms of brain weight (log BrWt) and body weight (log BdyWt) (Sacher, 1959):

$$\log LS = 0.64 \log BrWt - 0.23 \log BdyWt + 1.035$$

About 85 percent of the variance in LSs among the 63 species was accounted for by this equation.

Next, he expanded the number of species to 85 and added both resting metabolic rate (MR, in watts/g) and body temperature (T_b) to the regression calculation (Sacher, 1976). These two new variables improved the accuracy of predicting LS for a species according to the following best-fit regression:

$$\log LS = 0.62 \log BrWt - 0.41 \log BdyWt - 0.52 \log MR + 0.03 T_b + 0.90$$

Thus, LS was positively correlated to brain weight and body temperature, and negatively to body weight and metabolic rate. When separate regressions were done of log LS on log BrWt or log BdyWt, LS was found to increase with increases in BrWt or BdyWt. The negative coefficient for log BdyWt in the multiple regression means that when BrWt is fixed, LS decreases as BdyWt increases.

Sacher (1976) defined $K_c = (BrWt \times BdyWt)^{-2/3}$ as an Index of Cephalization (having dimensions of information density/unit area) and $K_m = MR_s \times 10^{-0.05 T_b}$ as a metabolic factor (MR_s is the metabolic rate for constant BW) and arrived at this relationship:

$$LS = 8 K_c^{0.6} K_m^{-0.5}$$

Thus, among mammals, there is a strong positive association between LS and K_c, whereas the metabolic factor MR_{BW} is inversely related to LS.

For animals on DR, K_c should increase (because BdyWt falls to a far greater extent than does BrWt) and K_m should either fall or be unchanged. We calculate that K_c increases for DR mice in our colony by 40 to 80 percent (depending on the regimen). Thus, Sacher's best interspecies LS predictors apply nicely to the DR case of intraspecies LS disparity.

These interspecies correlations provide support for a metabolic component in aging. We next consider the possibility that dietary energy restriction influences aging by affecting energy metabolism.

ENERGY METABOLISM

Background

The fundamental requirement for all DR regimens which extend species-specific maximum LS is restriction of *energy intake*. This clearly suggests that major energy-producing and -consuming metabolic processes, as well as processes which detoxify noxious byproducts of energy metabolism, merit close attention in considering DR's underlying mechanisms. We shall focus here on four non-mutually exclusive possibilities, namely, that DR acts by: (1) *lowering the metabolic rate* at some important but as yet unappreciated level (e.g. per whole animal or per total mass of internal organs) or locale (e.g. per brain or per physiologic "sensing center" within the neuroendocrine system); (2) *increasing metabolic efficiency;* (3) *decreasing heat and free radical production,* with decreased damage to mitochondria and/or other sites; and (4) *increasing detoxification* of metabolically generated active oxygen.

To evaluate the possibility that dietary energy restriction retards the rate of aging via effects on energy metabolism requires that further, multifaceted background information be discussed.

Age Changes in Normal Metabolism

Metabolic Rate. It is essential to consider the individual tissues which together comprise whole animal O_2 consumption values. Table 5.2 gives relative O_2 consumption values for various organs for humans at rest and at heavy work. Overall O_2 consumption rises 8-fold with heavy work as under this circumstance skeletal and cardiac muscle comprise about 90 percent (vs. 40% at rest) of the total energy expenditure.

That muscle mitochondria dominate the total mitochondrial profile of rats is illustrated in Figure 5.1. According to Else and Hulbert (1985), the summated internal organ (i.e., non-muscle) mitochondrial membrane surface area comprises only 18 percent of the whole (i.e., non-muscle plus muscle). The authors found that the total tissue mitochondrial surface area for rats averaged 460 m^2 (which is slightly larger than the size of a basketball court!). Also, among six species of small mammals varying in BW from 20 to 2000 g, species BW and mitochondrial membrane surface area per ml of tissue were inversely related. As Sacher's equations indicate, low BW mammalian species (with high mitochondrial volume densities) exhibit higher metabolic rates and shorter LSs.

TABLE 5.2

Relative O_2 Consumption Values in Different Human Tissues at Rest and During Heavy Work[a]

Tissue	At Rest	Heavy Work
Skeletal muscles	0.30	6.95 (86%)
Abdominal organs	0.25	0.24 (3%)
Brain	0.20	0.20 (3%)
Heart	0.11	0.40 (5%)
Kidneys	0.07	0.07 (1%)
Others	0.07	0.14 (2%)
Sum	1.00	8.00

[a]Data are adapted from Hochachka and Guppy (1987). The value at rest is set at 1.00. The actual V_{O_2} at rest is about 0.17 nmol min^{-1} kg^{-1}. The number in parenthesis gives the percent of the total O_2 consumption performed by that organ during heavy work.

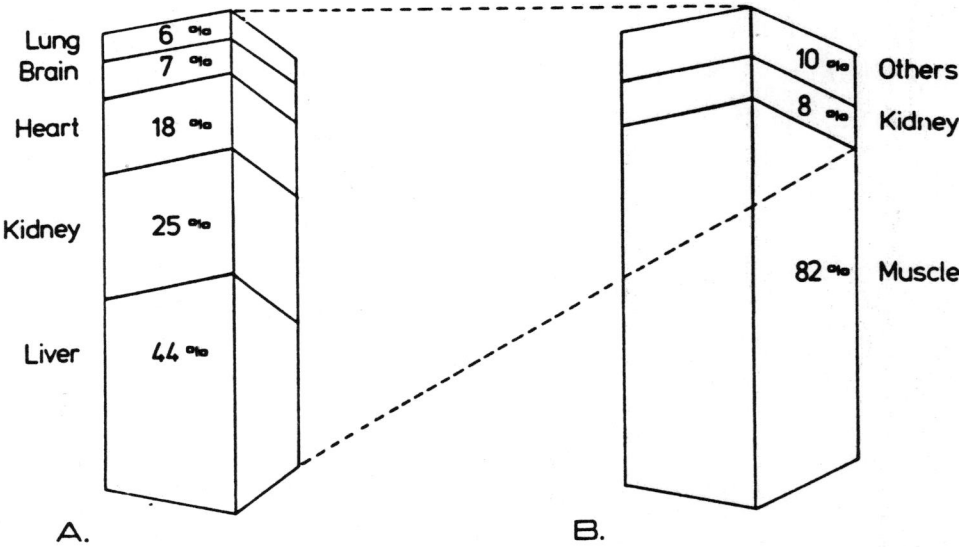

Figure 5.1. Comparison of mitochondrial membrane surface areas of internal organs (Block A, skeletal muscle not included) and total tissues (Block B, skeletal muscle included) in rats. Adapted from Else and Hulbert (1985).

Tzankoff & Norris (1978) distinguished between non-muscle vs. muscle metabolism. Whole body O_2 consumption was measured five or more times in 355 adult (30-90 years) men over an average period of 11 years. Whole body O_2 consumption fell steadily and impressively with aging (by 3.7%/decade); however, at advanced ages, O_2 consumption of nonmuscle tissue rose. This rise was associated with diseases (cancer, cardiovascular), which can increase metabolic demands. The fall with age in O_2 consumption by muscle was due to the loss of muscle mass. In 30 year olds the nonmuscle component used 38 percent of the whole body O_2 uptake, whereas after 80 years of age nonmuscle O_2 uptake was 53 percent of the total.

This late-life, disease-associated increase in nonmuscle metabolic rate is of interest in view of Totter's hypothesis (see "EVOLUTIONARY PERSPECTIVE," this Chapter) that nonmuscle O_2 consumption is more damaging to the organism than is muscle metabolism. Also providing evidence that muscle or muscle metabolism are not much involved in aging is the repeated finding that exercise does not much affect maximum LS or rate of aging.

Mitochondria. Figure 5.2 provides an overview of mitochondrial ATP generation. Panel A shows the sites of the main processes and the directions where intermediates must move for NADH to eventually donate electrons to the respiratory chain in the inner membrane (Panel B). Protons are then driven through the ATP synthase protein complex (Panel C) where ATP is made. Quite recently an anion-conducting channel was discovered in the inner membrane which moves hydroxide ions out from the matrix and uncouples the system (discussed by Selwyn, 1987).

What factors are the most important physiologic controllers of electron flux through the mitochondrial respiratory chain? In reviewing this complex subject, Brand and Murphy (1987) discuss a number of the most significant stimulators (ADP, NADH, Ca^{++}) and inhibitors (long-chain fatty acyl-CoA [an inhibitor of the adenine nucleotide carrier], fatty acids [which, as discussed below, act as uncouplers]) of respiration. Hormonal variation (T_3 is best studied.) may change the kinetics of oxidative phosphorylation by altering the concentration of individual proteins, or by changing their properties. Brand and Murphy (1987) view the respiratory stimulation induced by Ca^{++} and T_3 as primarily due to activation of dehydrogenases. They did not discuss dietary caloric intake.

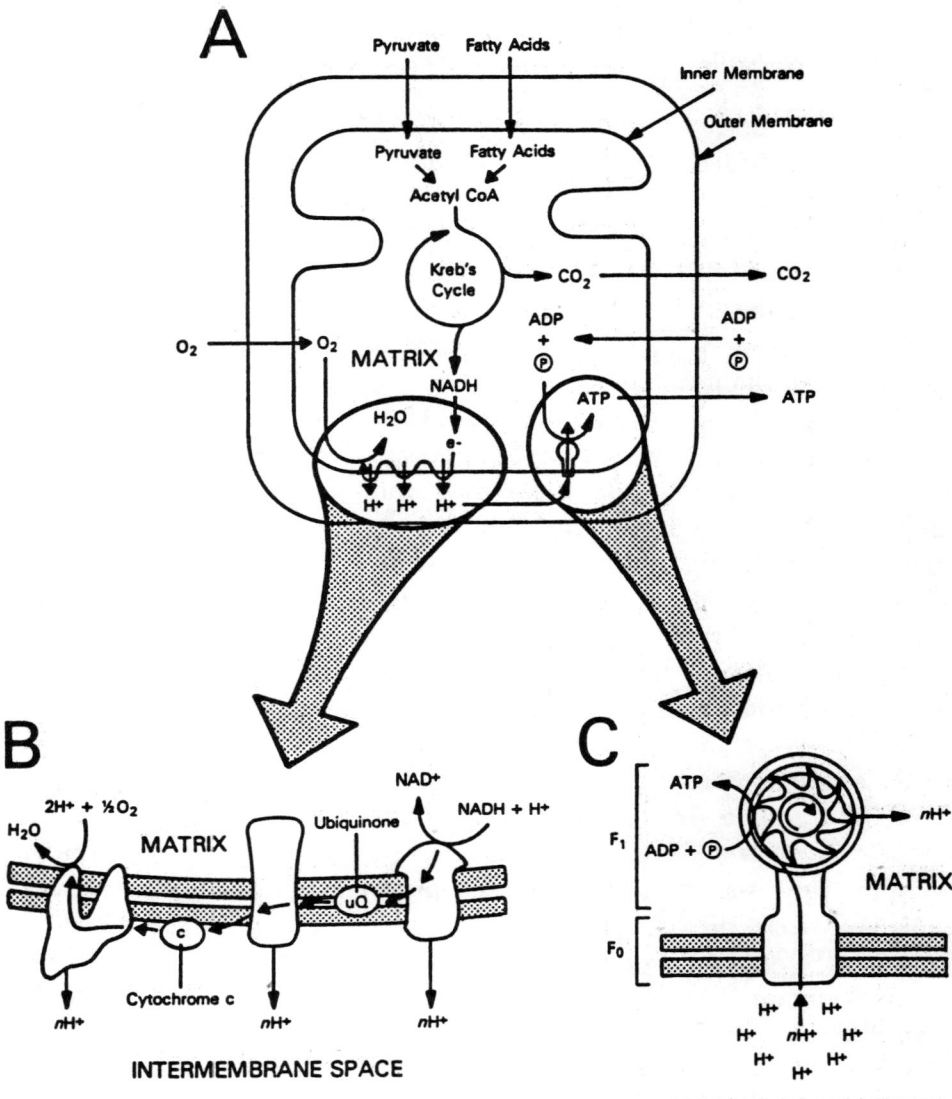

Figure 5.2. Overview of mitochondrial ATP generation. Panel A shows that pyruvate and fatty acids are converted into acetyl coenzyme A, the raw material for the citric acid cycle. This cycle produces NADH which supplies the respiratory chain of the inner mitochondrial membrane with two electrons per NADH molecule. The respiratory chain (Panel B) is comprised of three major enzyme complexes inserted into the membrane with a defined orientation so that protons are pumped from the matrix to the intermembrane space. The path of electron flow is: NADH → NADH dehydrogenase complex → ubiquinone → b-c_1 complex → cytochrome c → cytochrome oxidase complex → O_2. As a high energy electron is passed along the electron transport chain to lower energies, protons are pumped out from the matrix at three energy-conserving sites. These protons

Reported age-dependent mitochondrial changes are outlined in Table 5.3. Age-related declines in mitochondrial numbers and/or recovery are both morphologic (electron microscopy) and chemical lower mitochondrial DNA and protein recoveries; lower cytochrome c oxidase specific activity). Some evidence points toward lower substrate-stimulated *in vitro* oxygen uptake by "old mitochondria" in the presence of ADP (state 3 rate), but not after ADP has been used up (state 4 rate). Certain mitochondrial enzyme activities and transport rates also decline with age. Some of these phenomena may be causally linked to chemical changes in mitochondrial membranes (altered lipid composition, increased peroxidation, less fluid membranes). Heart mitochondria from old rats have been found to produce O_2 radicals at a rate 25 percent higher than young mitochondria. Low intramitochondrial water content may occur in old organisms. Many of these observations require confirmation.

In reviewing relations between aging and mitochondria, Hansford (1983) challenged the notion that mitochodria are the cell's "Achilles heel" on these grounds: (1) mitochondria turn over in all tissues (including post-mitotic tissues), and turnover rates do not appear to change with age; (2) there is little evidence for aberrant mitochondrial protein synthesis with age; and, (3) mitochondrial energy generation does not appear greatly compromised with aging.

An alternative scenario needs to be considered: because mitochondria are turned over, these oxidative "internal combustion engines" could "burn out" at a defined rate, and their continual replacement provides an endless source of active oxygen which can attack other critical parts of cells (especially post-mitotic cells which do not turn over). The failure to find damaged mitochondria in old animals does not mean that this organelle is not playing an etiologic role in aging.

Free Radicals and Aging

Harman (1956) first proposed that aging results from damage to important molecules caused by free radicals generated in the course of normal metabolism. Membrane molecules were originally emphasized.

---

create an electrochemical gradient (nH^+) across the inner membrane, driving protons through the ATP synthase protein complex and into the matrix. The ATP synthase (Panel C) is a large (MW of $\sim 5 \times 10^5$) complex of 9 polypeptides ($\alpha_3, \beta_3, \tau, \delta, \epsilon$) which uses the energy of the proton gradient to make ATP from ADP and Pi in the matrix. This unusual subunit stoichiometry holds for ATPases from animals, bacteria and chloroplasts. Redrawn from figures in Alberts et al. (1983).

TABLE 5.3
Mitochondrial Changes in Old Compared to Young Mammals[a]

Age-Related Change	Tissue	Refs.[b]
1. ↓ in # or in recovery	brain, liv, hrt	1-5, 21
2. ↓ state 3 O_2 uptake[c]	brain, liv, hrt	6-9
3. ↓ enzyme activities	hrt, skel musc	10, 11
4. ↓ uptake rate for:		
a. glutamate	brain	12
b. pyruvate	brain	13
c. calcium	brain, hrt	14, 15, 24
d. adenine nucleotides	hrt	16, 23
5. ↓ calcium efflux	brain	25
6. ↓ protein synthesis	liv	17, 18
7. ↓ memb fluidity	liv, hrt	11, 19
8. ↓ memb phospholipid; ↑ memb cholesterol	liv	19
9. ↑ O_2 radical production	hrt	20
10. ↓ water content	liv, hrt	22

[a]Age-related change #1 was studied in four species (human, monkey, rat, mouse). All other studies were on rats. Abbreviations: liv = liver; hrt = heart; memb = membrane; mit = mitochondria; skel musc = skeletal muscle; # = number of mitochondria.

[b]References: (1) Tauchi and Sato (1968); (2) Herbener (1976); (3) Stocco and Hufson (1978); (4) Burns et al. (1979); (5) Vorbeck et al. (1982a); (6) Weinbach and Garbus (1959); (7) Chen et al. (1972); (8) Hansford (1978); (9) Chiu and Richardson (1980); (10) Hansford and Castro (1982a); (11) Nohl (1979); (12) Vitorica et al. (1985); (13) Deshmukh and Patel (1982); (14) Hansford and Castro (1982b); (15) Leslie et al. (1985); (16) Nohl and Kramer (1980); (17) Marcus et al. (1982a); (18) Marcus et al. (1982b); (19) Vorbeck et al. (1982b); (20) Nohl and Hegner (1978); (21) Harmon et al. (1987); (22) von Zglinicki and Bimmler (1987); (23) Nohl (1982); (24) Vitorica and Satrustegui (1986a); (25) Vitorica and Satrustegui (1986b).

[c]Decreases reported for mitochondrial O_2 utilization are limited to certain substrates and tissues. Study #19 was on rat brain mitochondria and age-related differences were largely confined to synaptosomal mitochondria.

More recently, Harman (1983 & 1986) and several others (e.g., Fleming et al., 1982; Miquel & Fleming, 1986; von Zglinicki, 1987) have emphasized mitochondria as possible sites of free radical damage, proposing that these organelles acting as sources of active oxygen, promote their own disarray and destruction. The main agents of damage are thought to be derived from O_2 as it is reduced to H_2O during energy-producing oxidative metabolism. Free radical damage could cause oxidative changes in cell and organelle membranes and in long-lived molecules (e.g. collagen, elastin, DNA [both nuclear and mitochondrial], and chromosomal proteins), accumulation of lipofuscin and ceroid via oxidative polymerization reactions, and mucopolysaccharide breakdown (Harman, 1981).

Today's free radical theory is conceptually linked to older views on metabolic rate and LS. Rubner (1908) reported an inverse correlation between the LSs of domestic animals and their LEI per unit BW. The LEI was about 200 kcal/g for horses, cows, dogs, cats and guinea pigs but 800 kcal/g for humans. (The inverse relationship between species LS and daily caloric intake [cal/[g • day]] based on newer data was shown in Figure 1.7.) Studying the LS of *Drosophila* living at different temperatures, and finding that LS was inversely related to metabolic rate, Pearl (1928) suggested that LS was determined by the exhaustion of a vital substance consumed at a rate proportional to the BMR. He proposed the "rate-of-living" theory.

The free radical theory of aging has gained some popularity over the last decade as it has become more likely that active oxygen species play important roles in normal physiology and pathophysiology. However, there are very knowledgeable dissenters who believe free radicals cause disease (e.g. cancer, emphysema) but not basic aging (Pryor, 1987).

A metabolic interpretation of DR's effects on aging requires that a possible role for free radicals be carefully considered. Pertinent to this consideration is some understanding of mitochondrial energy coupling, free radical generation, and free radical neutralization.

Energy Coupling in Mitochondria. The chemical basis of coupling is being actively investigated (see recent summaries by Lane et al., 1986 and Pedersen & Carafoli, 1987). The focus is on proton translocation and precisely how proton gradients drive the synthesis of ATP at the ATP synthase complex (see Figure 5.2). The F_0 moiety is membrane bound and serves as a proton pore transmitting energy from the proton gradient into the F_1 piece where the catalytic site resides within the F_1-β subunit. A protein (known as OSCP) appears to bind F_0 to F_1 and be critically involved in energy transduction between the two regions. Dithiols may be important in coupling. The catalytic site in F_1-β probably involves a flexible loop which closes over the magnesium-dependent binding site of ATP. A lysine and several carboxyl residues are leading candidates for interacting with protons.

We predict that future studies will establish that the energetic efficiency of mitochondrial ATP production is subject to profound genetic variation and physiologic regulation, and that DR increases this efficiency. If coupling is loose, more energy is lost as heat and (perhaps) as free radicals, with less trapped in the high energy bond of ATP. Tight coupling would accord with high metabolic efficiency (i.e. a "thrifty" phenotype) while loose coupling would lower the efficiency of ATP production while making much heat (a "burner"). Our prediction is supported by several observations:

(1) *E. coli* mutants with single amino acid substitutions in mitochondrial ATP synthase show 70 percent reductions in the conversion of energy into ATP (Cox et al., 1987).

(2) Mitochondria from brown adipose tissue are uncoupled normally. They contain a unique protein (MW of 33,000) which can short-circuit the respiratory chain via a proton conductance pathway, and generate heat (reviewed by Ricquier & Bouillaud, 1986). Noradrenaline increases heat production in brown adipose tissue, probably by controlling the rate of synthesis of the uncoupling protein via communication with β-receptors on brown fat cells. Perhaps other inter- and intra-tissue variations occur in mitochondrial efficiency. Might DR lead to decreases in the level or activity of energy-wasting uncoupling proteins? Do other molecules exist which increase coupling efficiency?

(3) The P/O ratios found in textbooks are 3 for NADH oxidation, 2 for succinate oxidation, and 1 if electrons are fed to the chain at cytochrome c. Such integer values for this indicator of the efficiency of phosphorylation have been questioned as newer evidence points toward non-integral coupling stoichiometries for oxidative phosphorylation (Ferguson, 1986). Thus, understanding of the efficiency of oxidative phosphorylation is still developing.

Gunter and Jensen (1986) estimated the efficiencies of the component steps of oxidative phosphorylation assuming that the product of the efficiencies of the steps is equal to that of the entire process. As diagrammed in Figure 5.3, they defined two efficiency terms: ηog, the efficiency of use of substrate energy in generating a proton gradient, and ηgp, the efficiency of use of gradient energy in phosphorylation. Because these two terms can be experimentally measured (Jensen et al., 1986), it would be of extreme interest to evaluate DR's influence thereon.

(4) There is evidence that the degree of coupling of oxidative phosphorylation in rat liver is subject to physiologic regulation. Klug et al. (1984) found that exhaustive exercise partially uncoupled succinate-stimulated respiration by isolated rat liver mitochondria. This effect was rapidly reversed upon adding an albumin-containing solution, thereby suggesting that an increase in plasma free fatty acid levels with exercise may have uncoupled the mitochondria without permanently damaging

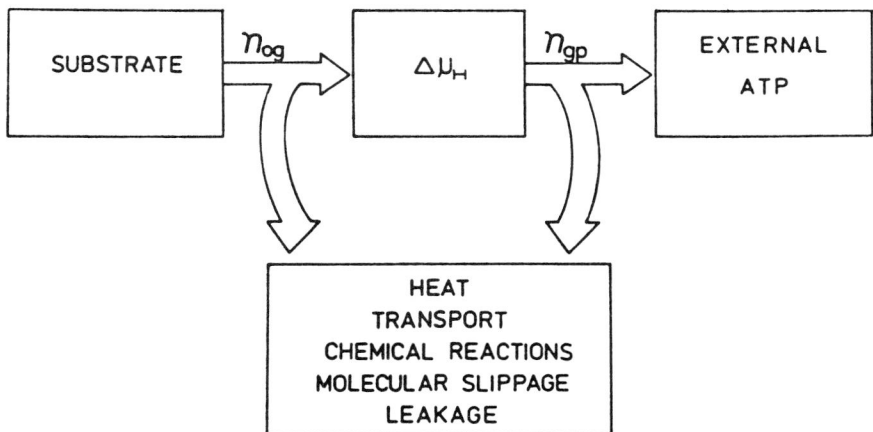

Figure 5.3. Schematic diagram of energy usage during oxidative phosphorylation. The term ηog is the efficiency of use of substrate energy in generating an electrochemical proton gradient ($\Delta \mu_H$). ηog is the fraction of the energy released by substrate oxidation that can be accounted for within the proton gradient. The term ηgp is the efficiency of use of gradient energy in phosphorylation and is the fraction of the energy in the proton gradient which is recovered as energy in ATP. The main ways by which energy is lost are indicated. Adapted from Gunter and Jensen (1986).

them. Soboll and Stucki (1985) found that coupling in perfused livers fell with fasting. Coupling was also reduced when fatty acids were added, leading to the suggestion that "fatty acids could act as metabolic regulators of the degree of coupling, enabling the cell to optimize efficiency of oxidative phosphorylation under different metabolic regimes."

Based on the general tendency for long-term DR to reduce the tissue levels of several lipids (see *"Lipid Content,"* Chapter 4), the possibility exists that mitochondria from rodents on DR are more tightly coupled than are those from controls. If so, this would be yet another instance where long-term DR produces an effect opposite that of fasting.

Free Radical Production in Mitochondria. Do mitochondria produce free radicals *in vivo* during normal metabolism and, if so, do these radicals inflict the sorts of damage predicted by the free radical theory of aging? Evidence for these occurrences is inconclusive.

There are several reports of respiring mitochondria producing free radicals. Loschen et al. (1973) observed that respiring but uncoupled rat heart mitochondria produced H_2O_2 (possibly at phosphorylation site II) and that superoxide radicals (O_2^-) are precursors of H_2O_2 in membrane fragments of beef heart mitochondria (Loschen et al., 1974). The latter observation was confirmed by Cadenas et al. (1977). Nohl and Jordan (1986) suggested that cytochrome b566 is involved in mitochondrial O_2^-

formation. Most recently, Nohl (1987) found a new and potent NADH-requiring O_2^- generator in rat heart mitochondria (but not in liver mitochondria) which is not involved in energy-yielding respiration. The radicals formed by this system are released into the cytosol.

Aging may increase the mitochondrial production of O_2^-. Nohl and Hegner (1978) detected an age-related increase of some 30 percent in O_2^- production by intact rat heart mitochondria (Table 5.3). About 80 percent of the O_2^- was converted into H_2O_2 by SOD, with the remainder leaving the mitochondria. Peroxidative changes in membrane lipids paralleled concentrations of O_2^-.

The chemistry of oxygen radical release by the respiratory chain and the possible influence of aging thereon were reviewed by Nohl (1986). Radical release was deemed due to transfer of electrons out of sequence, and "a direct relationship between changes in the steady state of ubisemiquinone populations and generation rates of O_2^-" was emphasized. A redox loop was proposed involving ubiquinone (coenzyme Q10), ubisemiquinone (reduced ubiquinone), and cytochromes b-562 and b-566. The loop would carry out normal electron transport and proton translocation while forming activated oxygen species. Nohl hypothesized that age-related increases in the peroxidation of inner membrane phospholipids causes increases in the membrane's hydrophilic properties, and creates thermodynamic conditions favoring destabilization of ubisemiquinones by autoxidation.

There exists a very small gerontologic literature on ubiquinone. According to Beyer et al. (1985) the levels of ubiquinone fall dramatically in late life in rat cardiac and skeletal muscles. The authors, like Nohl, argue that ubiquinone plays a central role in energy conservation during oxidative phosphorylation. Injection of 22 month old mice with ubiquinone partially restored the primary antibody response to SRBC (Bliznakov, 1978).

Much evidence suggests that free radicals, whether from mitochondria or elsewhere, inflict significant biological damage (see Cerutti, 1985; Fridovich, 1986; Johnson et al., 1986). However, there are uncertainties over which radicals are potentially most damaging (Youngman, 1984) and even whether or not free radical reactions *cause* or sometimes merely *accompany* tissue damage (Halliwell & Grootveld, 1987). Free radicals have never been quantified in animals on DR.

Free Radical Neutralization. What is the basis for the huge LS differences among mammals? Does a mouse age 30 times faster than a human because it has 30 times more (or more active) "death genes" or a much faster BMR, or is the difference due to mice being deficient or inefficient in repair and protective processes? Based on known mutation rates, Sacher (1975) and Cutler (1975) have estimated that the rapid increase in LS as hominids evolved was due to changes in quite a small part of the genome (<0.5%). Also not requiring a large part of the genome are some 70 loci estimated by Martin (1978) to control major phenotypic aspects of aging. It is critical to know if these influential genes cause self-destruction or health maintenance.

Cutler has written extensively (e.g. Cutler, 1976, 1982, 1985a) on this issue, formulating a "Longevity Determinant Gene Hypothesis": aging is a dysdifferentiative process caused by the side effects of normal development and metabolism. Differences in species LS are assumed to be the result of species differences in opposing these causes of aging. Cutler (1985a) wrote: "The longevity of a species is consequently determined largely by quantitative differences in the expression of a common set of anti-aging genes acting against a common set of aging processes." Only a few changes in regulatory genes are seen to be required to uniformly lower the aging rate of the entire organism.

Genes which govern active oxygen detoxification are good candidates for being determinants of longevity potential. Thus, the SOD enzymes which convert O_2^- into H_2O_2 (i.e. $2 O_2^- + 2 H^+ \rightarrow H_2O_2 + O_2$) and catalases which remove H_2O_2 (i.e. $2 H_2O_2 \rightarrow 2 H_2O + O_2$) have received much attention. As emphasized in Chapter 4 (see "Enzymes and Metabolites"), catalase deserves special attention as its activity in liver and kidney falls with aging (Ross, 1969; Baird & Samis, 1971; Baird et al., 1974; Baird & Massie, 1976; Haining & Legan, 1973; Imre & Juhasz, 1987) and it is strongly and selectively raised by DR in mice (Koizumi et al., 1987a). Brain catalase activity also reportedly falls with age in rats but mostly during the first 4 months of life (Scarpa et al., 1987).

Cutler and colleagues have measured activities or levels of several antioxidants in species of diverse LS (see *"Dietary Restriction and Between-Species/Within-Species Comparisons,"* Chapter 1 and Table 1.5). The main findings are:

(1) For cytoplasmic SOD (SOD-1, which contains Cu and Zn) in liver and brain, the ratio of SOD-1 activity:metabolic rate of the tissue or whole animal increased with increasing maximum LS (Talmasoff et al., 1980). Data were normalized in this way based on the view that the degree of protection a tissue possesses against radicals is related to the concentration of antioxidants per rate of oxygen metabolism.

(2) The other form of SOD is mitochondrial (SOD-2, which contains Mn). The ratio of SOD-2:total SOD activity in the brains of primates increases with species LS and is much higher than that in rodents, suggesting that higher levels of mitochondrial defense may be associated with the evolution of longevity (Cutler, 1984a).

(3) Other antioxidants whose levels in brain and serum expressed per metabolic rate show a positive correlation with species maximum LS are urate (Cutler, 1984b) and carotenoids (Cutler, 1984c).

(4) The peroxide-producing potential of brain and kidney appear inversely related to species LS (Cutler, 1985b).

(5) On the other hand, ascorbate levels did not correlate with species LS, while liver glutathione level and catalase activity correlated negatively (Cutler, 1985a). Cutler dismisses these negative tests of his hypothesis by assuming ascorbate, glutathione and catalase not to be important in aging. Glutathione level (Hazelton & Lang, 1980) and catalase activity (see "Enzymes and Metabolites" in Chapter 4, the preceding page, and *"Increased Free Radical Neutralization by DR,"* this Chapter) do both decline after middle-age in rodent tissues.

Certain genes for the SOD enzymes have been mapped. Two such genes are reportedly linked to the mouse MHC on chromosome #17. One regulates SOD-1 activity (Novak et al., 1980) whereas the other appears to be the structural gene for SOD-2 (Szymura et al., 1981). Renal catalase activity is also influenced by MHC-linked genes (Hoffman & Grieshbar, 1976). The close proximity of the MHC to genes involved in important antioxidant defenses underscores the possibility that a very small fraction of the genome may strongly influence longevity potential (Walford, 1987).

Metabolic Efficiency

Metabolic efficiency can be viewed from the standpoints of energy generation and usage. The *efficiency of energy generation* can be thought of as the fraction of the energy content of ingested foods actually absorbed and trapped in a biologically useful form (ATP). The *efficiency of energy usage* can be viewed also as the percentage of trapped energy used for essential physiologic functions, versus that wasted as heat generation, or in maintaining the tissues of an obese animal, or in other non-essential ways. Figure 5.4 illustrates energy flow in an animal.

It is possible that a major part of DR's effects in retarding aging is due to an increase in the efficiency of energy generation and/or use. The

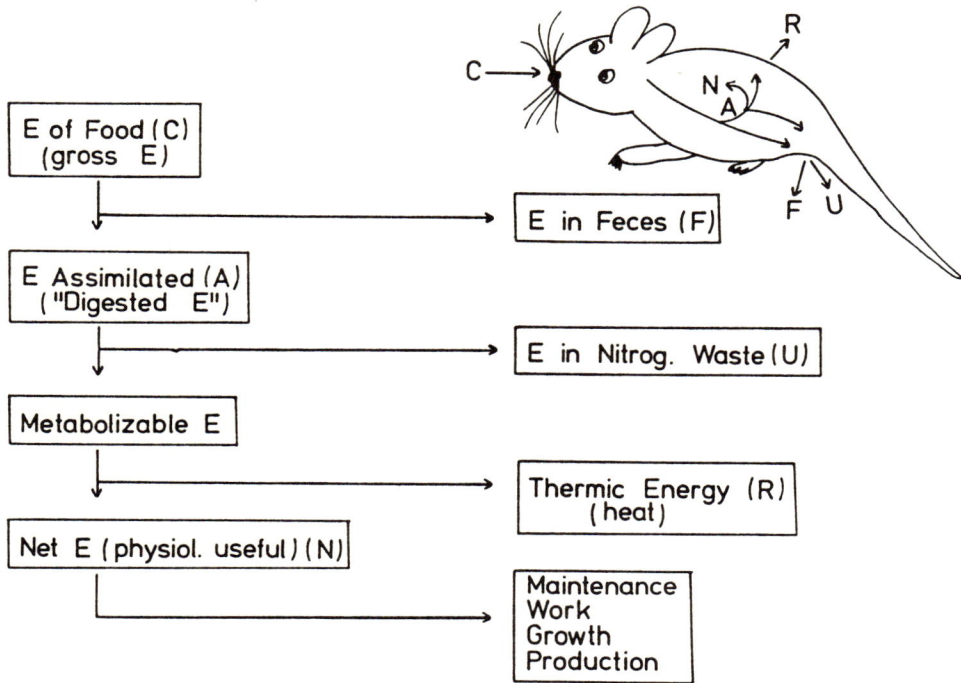

Figure 5.4. The fate of energy (E) in the body. Thermic energy (R) includes work-induced thermogenesis, thermoregulatory thermogenesis, and diet-induced thermogenesis. Adapted from Brafield and Llewyllyn, 1982.

consideration of this problem by researchers of energy metabolism, especially by those interested in metabolic efficiency (e.g. the basis of energy coupling during ATP formation, cellular energy costs and budgets, thermogenesis, futile cycles) would seem timely. Good discussions of metabolic efficiency are those of Stock and Rothwell (1982) and Sims and Danforth (1987).

A high metabolic efficiency is not always good for an organism and may only prove beneficial when energy intake is restricted (e.g., in the spiny mouse [Wise, 1977a]). With ad lib feeding, high metabolic efficiency was associated with the shortest LSs in Ross' self-selection study (Ross et al., 1985), which contrasts with our finding for DR mice (Weindruch et al., 1986), and for DR rats (Bertrand et al., 1980a), where thrifty individuals tended to live longest. In genetically obese rodents, the combination of metabolic thrift and ad lib feeding is detrimental but, as discussed, the ob/ob mouse can live a very long life if subjected to DR (Harrison et al., 1984; see Table 2.5, #18). Thus, in the case of ob/ob mice, thrifty animals have the potential to be quite long-lived but only when the diseases associated with obesity are prevented by DR.

What is the basis for the extreme metabolic thrift of genetically obese rodents? Defective brown adipose thermogenesis appears to be a major factor, and two types of flaws are apparent in these animals (reviewed by James & Trayhurn, 1981; Himms-Hagen, 1985a). The brown adipose tissue of ob/ob and db/db mice fails to respond to norepinephrine despite central control mechanisms being intact. Such mice cannot respond strongly to cold or diet by induction of thermogenesis. Subnormal body temperatures have been repeatedly observed in obese mice. The fa/fa rat and rodents made obese via hypothalamic lesions show a different defect, one allowing thermogenesis to occur in response to cold exposure but not to diet. Here the defect is a central one. The response to cold is thought to be preserved via direct sympathetic innervation to brown adipose tissue.

Other factors which may contribute to increased metabolic thrift in ob/ob mice are reductions in: Na^+/K^+-ATPase levels in skeletal muscle (Rosmos, 1981), motor activity (Dauncy, 1986), and adipsin (a serine protease homolog) levels in adipose tissue and blood (Flier et al., 1987).

The liver has been implicated in diet-induced thermogenesis. Berry et al. (1985) observed that hepatocytes from rats overeating a "cafeteria diet" showed greater heat production and lower metabolic efficiency than hepatocytes from rats eating a standard diet. They suggested that overfeeding led to an increased operation of the futile glycerophosphate shuttle in hepatocytes, resulting in heat but not work.

Much energy in animals is used to pump ions. Milligan and McBride (1985) estimated that more than 20 percent of the energy used by tissues (liver, muscle, duodenal epithelium) from domestic ruminants went toward pumping Na^+ and K^+ across the plasma membrane. In overfed sheep this value rose. In starved sheep it fell. The investigators estimated that the energy cost of Ca^{++} transport in resting skeletal muscle was less than 10 percent of the total energy expenditure, a figure that is ". . . rather small, but not inconsequential, at rest, and would markedly increase with activity." Calcium is an important metabolic regulator (reviewed by Carafoli & Penniston, 1985). Because intracellular calcium concentrations in most cells are very low (about 10^{-4} times that in blood), relatively few Ca^{++} ions must be moved within the cell to regulate an enzyme (i.e. Ca^{++} is an energy-efficient regulator).

In $C3B10RF_1$ mice of both sexes we have regularly observed surprisingly large mouse-to-mouse variations in BW responses to a given level of DR (unpublished findings). The effect is most overt in mice fed about 15 percent below the average adult ad lib level, so that it is common to see in most cohorts some 40 to 45 g adult mice not eating all the food they are fed as well as 30 to 35 g animals who leave no food. These behavioral differences could not be attributed to litter size and are especially curious in view of the genetic homogeneity of the mice studied. We predict that in a large group of $C3B10RF_1$ mice fed an amount of food eaten by all (say 70% of ad lib), a significant "metabolic heterogeneity" will result. If so, this will allow the exploration of physiologic differences and aging rates of the most efficient ("thrifty") and inefficient ("burners") animals. Our predictions of physiologic status and of an inverse relationship between metabolic efficiency and the rate of aging in such groups are summarized in Table 5.4.

TABLE 5.4

Predicted Differences Between Metabolically Efficient ("Thrifty") and Inefficient ("Burners") Individuals

Parameter	Prediction for:	"Thrifty"	"Burners"
1. Life Span		Longer	Shorter
2. Body Weight		Higher	Lower
3. O_2 Consumption/MBW		Lower	Higher
4. Body Temperature		Lower	Higher
5. Biomarkers		Younger	Older
6. Free Radical Production		Lower	Higher

[a]Predictions are for a large population (say 100 or more) of $C3B10RF_1$ mice fed a restricted amount of food such that all food is consumed. The "thrifty" group would be comprised of the 20 animals with the highest BWs while the "burners" would be the 20 lowest BW mice. The other 60 percent of the mice would be expected to show intermediate characteristics. MBW is metabolic BW.

Dietary Restriction and Energy Metabolism

Metabolic Arrest and the Control of Biological Time, a book by Hochachka and Guppy (1987) on the uses and mechanisms of metabolic arrest and slowdown in animals is pertinent to our inquiry. The authors argue (based on their work and that of others [e.g. Lindstedt & Calder, 1981]) that *biological time is extended when metabolic rate is reduced in animals by torpor, hibernation, estivation or by freezing in insects.* Data supporting their view comes also from Lyman (1981) who reported that among hamsters who hibernated from 0-33 percent of their lives, the maximum LS was generally longer in animals that hibernated longer.

Hochachka and Guppy (1987) cite two "primary and necessarily coupled processes" that must occur with metabolic slowdown: (1) suppression of oxidative and anaerobic paths of ATP production, and (2) reduction in the rates of ATP-requiring processes (especially those [e.g. Na/K pump] which maintain a cellular environment distinct from the external one). Activation of a third set of processes — those which protect intracellular structures — is also associated with metabolic slowdown. These three changes of hypometabolism closely resemble our favored energy-based explanations of DR's effects on aging. Hochachka and Guppy (1987) remark: "Some capacity for latent life may exist in all of us; what is more, it may be good for us."

Dietary Restriction and Metabolic Rate

In discussing the finding that metabolic rate falls in humans undergoing various forms of weight loss (but see also "EVIDENCE AND CONJECTURE AGAINST THE PROPOSITION" and "Energy Requirements," Chapter 6), Bray and Fisler (1985) propose five mechanisms which may underlie this adaptation. These are reductions of: T_3 concentration, sympathetic nervous system activity, futile cycles (= a cycle in which ATP is used to form a phosphorylated product which is then dephosphorylated with the energy once in the ATP molecule thereby lost), protein turnover, and Na^+/K^+ pump activity. Waterlow (1986) posits another mechanism: because humans show a relative preservation of slow-twitch muscle fibers after severe energy restriction or hypothyroidism, efficiency could increase because slow-twitch fibers can develop more mechanical force per ATP used than fast-twitch fibers. All of these adjustments would be expected to lower the rate at which ATP is used (and thus the rate at which it must be generated) and clearly warrant study in the DR model.

Usually, when the $T_3:T_4$ ratio decreases, BMR decreases. This happens with quick BW loss (see Chapter 6 [Table 6.1]). If DR lowers the $T_3:T_4$ ratio (and the data suggest this to be the case), one might expect that BMR would be reduced.

On the contrary, the very limited data for long-term DR regimens suggest that BMR per lean BW may not fall (see "Metabolic Rate," Chapter 4). The finding by McCarter et al. (1985) that O_2 consumption per lean BW of rat is unaltered by long-term DR seems to us inadequate grounds on which to abandon metabolic rate reduction as possibly contributing to DR's effects. One must ask how closely O_2 consumption by the intact animal estimates actual rates of oxidative metabolism. What percent of the total O_2 consumed is used for mitochondrial energy metabolism versus O_2 used otherwise (e.g. mixed function oxidase pathways, various oxygenases)? Smith et al. (1983) state that in liver the non-energy metabolism component can be one-third of the total O_2 consumption. Clearly, O_2 consumption is lower per whole DR animal by a large amount (about 30%, Table 4.18). One recalls that DR strongly reduces the weight of most organs or tissues (e.g. lymphoid tissue, liver, muscle, fat) but not that of the brain. Thus, the brain's relative contribution to the total metabolic rate is likely higher in the DR rodent. A higher relative metabolic contribution by the brain fits well with Sacher's K_c term being increased by DR.

To better evaluate the nature of DR's influence on the rate of oxidative metabolism, it appears essential that nonmuscle and muscle components be individually considered, and that oxidative metabolism be more directly measured than is possible via whole animal O_2 consumption. Also systems analysis-based approaches may be quite useful in determining the importance of factors thought to control metabolic rate (see Brand & Murphy, 1987).

Metabolic Efficiency and Energy Intake

Young, growing rodents on short-term DR are "thriftier" with the limited energy resources they ingest than are free-eating controls. For example, Lee and Lucia (1961) imposed energy restriction on young, growing (200 g) rats, and attempted to keep them at this BW for a 48 day period. At the onset, a daily food intake of 10 g was required. This fell to 6 g by the 48th day. The authors suggest that adaptation to energy restriction may work ". . . through pathways which influence the efficiency of energy yields from the diet." These same paths may be fundamentally involved in the retardation of aging by DR.

Other studies have measured energy utilization in young rodents on short-term DR. These include:

(1) Young Wistar rats fed half of the ad lib level for 8 weeks used a lower fraction of the total energy intake for tissue deposition, leaving more available for BMR, activity and maintenance (Mohan & Rao, 1983; Table 5.5). The O_2 consumption per MBW was not altered by DR (see Table 4.18, #10).

TABLE 5.5

Energy Intake and Use in Female Wistar Rats Under Ad Lib and DR Conditions[a]

Parameter	Ad Lib	DR	Eff. of DR
1. E intake (kcal/8 wk)	1643 ± 96	817 ± 49	↓50%
2. E for BMR (kcal/8 wk)	741 ± 59	605 ± 27	↓18%
3. E for tissue dep. (kcal)	345 ± 55	98 ± 28	↓72%
4. % of total E intake deposited	22 ± 2	12 ± 4	↓45%
5. % of total E intake remaining[b]	78 ± 2	88 ± 4	↑13%

[a] Values are means ± SEM (n = 5) for rats started on the diets very early in life (BWs averaged 43 g at onset) and fed for 8 weeks. Abbreviations; E, energy; dep., deposition; maint., maintenance. Adapted from Mohan and Rao (1983).

[b] The "% total E intake remaining" is (E intake − E deposited)/E intake and gives the percent of ingested energy remaining for BMR, activity and maintenance.

(2) Hill et al. (1985) subjected young (325 g) male Wistar rats to one of a variety of underfeeding regimens and then sought to maintain BW at a constant level for at least 18 days. A reduction in the amount of energy needed for maintenance occurred in proportion to the amount of BW lost, and continued to fall even when BW was maintained. This reduction in energy requirements was viewed as largely due to decreases in metabolic rate (see Table 4.18, #15). Also, ad lib fed rats showed a large thermic effect of food while rats on DR did not.

(3) In a study where 3 month old (250 g) female Wistar rats were fed 40 percent of the ad lib intake for 32 days and then fed to maintain the new BW for another 50 days, Hill et al. (1986) again observed that DR increases energy conservation but, when compared to the earlier study on males, gender differences were apparent. Females preserved lean body mass more than did males by utilizing relatively more fat for energy needs. The authors suggested that females would lose less BW for a given decrease in carcass energy because fat has a higher caloric density than lean body mass. They also reported a rapid and major decline (of about 60%) in the mass of interscapular brown adipose tissue from rats on DR.

Not only are rodents metabolically thriftier when on DR, but an increased efficiency of food use follows a return to normal feeding, as demonstrated by a study by Boyle et al. (1978). The food intake of young (375 g) male Sprague-Dawley rats fed an NPD ad lib between 8 PM and

8 AM was measured. The rats were then subjected to a 6 week course of either one of two levels of DR, or continued to be fed ad lib at night. The BWs of the two DR groups fell to 92 and 81 percent of the initial level, while control BWs remained stable. For the next week all rats were fed an amount of food equal to what they ate just before the three diet groups were formed, but adjusted for the change that had just occurred in metabolic mass (i.e. initial food intake/$BW^{0.75}$). The most severely restricted group gained 30 g of BW on 140 g of food, the group on milder DR gained 21 g on 154 g of food, and the controls gained an average of only 2 g after eating 156 g of food.

Metabolic efficiency is also influenced by the quality of the diet. As discussed earlier (see *"Importance of Restriction of Dietary Energy vs. Fat . . .,"* Chapter 3), high fat diets are used more efficiently than are low fat ones. This effect is thought to be due in part to the need to synthesize fat from carbohydrate when low fat diets are fed (Boissonneault et al., 1986). Donato and Hegsted (1985) found that sucrose and protein each contribute 3.9 kcal/g of energy to the bodies of growing rats (very close to the Atwater value of 4 kcal/g), whereas dietary fat conferred 11.1 kcal/g (i.e., 23% greater than the expected value of 9 kcal/g). The energy cost of fat deposition in rats was only 60 percent that of protein (Pullar and Webster, 1977). Quite probably the severity of caloric restriction tolerable by animals could be increased by feeding high fat diets. Whether this would further increase LS in animals on DR is worthy of study. These various findings also underscore the crudeness of LEI as an index of metabolic rate because *what* (not just how much) is eaten affects metabolism.

Our view of metabolic efficiency and of DR's effects on aging contrasts with that emerging to explain disease inhibition observed after feeding the steroid DHEA (a major adrenal product with no clear biological role). Adding DHEA to the diet at the 0.2-0.6 percent level has retarded the onset or progression of breast cancer in A^{vy}/a mice (Schwartz, 1979), chemically induced tumors (Pashko et al., 1985; Moore et al., 1986), renal disease in B/WF_1 mice (Lucas et al., 1985), and diabetes in mutant mice (Coleman et al., 1984) and rats (Gansler et al., 1985). In most of these studies DHEA was found to prevent obesity but not to lower food intake. A caveat here is that ad lib feeding of DHEA-containing diets has been found in other studies to reduce food intake (Nyce et al., 1984; Weindruch et al., 1984) perhaps because DHEA-containing diets are unpalatable (Gosnell, 1987). It is critical to separate effects of DHEA from those of DR.

The metabolic effects of DHEA and DR appear very different: DHEA increases liver weight and peroxisomal β-oxidation (which leads to increased uncoupled respiration and heat production) (Leighton et al., 1987). This "caloric wasting" is presumed to underlie DHEA's anti-obesity effect. We suspect that DHEA (like exercise) acts by preventing obesity, resulting in less and later diseases, but that it will not increase the maximum LS in an already long-lived strain (the crucial experiment needed to evaluate DHEA's effect on aging).

Decreased Free Radical Production by DR as a Mechanism

The hypothesis that DR decreases free radical production by either or both of two metabolic effects (↓ rate, ↑ efficiency) is supported by increasing amounts of indirect evidence (see *"Lipid Peroxidation and Lipofuscin,"* Chapter 4) but on nothing approaching direct proof. This hypothesis needs further investigation.

Increased Free Radical Neutralization by DR as a Mechanism

Observing no effect of DR on activities of SOD and glutathione peroxidase, we suggested that the increase in hepatic catalase in restricted mice may represent a selective upregulation event which is both distinctive and significant (see discussion in Koizumi et al., 1987a). Diabetes, a high fat or a vitamin-E deficient diet, or induction of peroxisomal proliferation can increase liver peroxisomal β oxidation, H_2O_2 production and catalase activity. None of these initiating conditions were ongoing in the DR mice we studied.

Catalase activity is known to be high in liver and kidney and low in brain and cardiac and skeletal muscle.[2] Catalase is a tetrameric enzyme with a total molecular weight of about 240,000. Mammalian liver catalase exists in multiple forms (e.g., 4 in mice) believed to originate from epigenetic changes (sulfhydryl oxidation, carbohydrate attachment, and partial proteolysis) (reviewed by Masters et al., 1986). The intracellular location of rat liver catalase remains a matter of some controversy, with the earlier view that all catalase resides in peroxisomes being displaced by the belief that most of the cell's catalase activity is free in the cytosol (Fukami & Flatmark, 1986; Masters et al., 1986). Because we observed

---

[2] Baird and Samis (1971) point out that the catalase-poor tissues are the ones prone to accumulate large amounts of lipofuscin with age.

that liver β oxidation was either unchanged or perhaps even lowered by DR, it is likely that non-peroxisomal catalase provides the higher activity in the livers of DR animals. Whether this catalase is free, is mitochondrial, or is otherwise contained needs to be examined, as does the possibility that DR selectively alters a particular subtype of catalase.

As noted in Chapter 4 (see "Enzymes and Metabolites"), catalase and NADPH are intimately associated. Kirkman and Gaetani (1984) found that each tetrameric catalase molecule from human RBC or bovine liver could bind four molecules of NADPH. When these catalases were exposed to H_2O_2, physiologic levels of NADPH could prevent and reverse the accumulation of an inactive form of catalase (compound II) (Kirkman et al., 1987). Perhaps DR could influence the ratio of active:inactive catalase by mechanisms related to NADPH levels (see Table 4.2, #1, 2) or by altering catalase gene expression. Catalase and other protective enzymes can also be inactivated by O_2^- (Fridovich, 1986). Thus, diminished O_2^- production could be a cause of increased catalase activity in rodents on DR, acting by feed-forward controller mechanisms (see Walford et al., 1983 for comments on feed-forward control).

The gerontologic literature on catalase is sparse. It consists largely of the aforementioned age-related declines in liver and kidney catalase activities. However, certain other observations may aid in evaluating the significance of DR's effects on catalase.

(1) Injecting rodents with aminotriazole destroys existing liver and kidney catalase molecules but does not inhibit synthesis. Baird and Samis (1971) observed that livers and kidneys from B6 mice injected with aminotriazole showed an age-related loss in ability to restore catalase activity. About half of a group of 32 month old mice were unable to renew catalase activity in the first 24 hours after injection, whereas all 10 and 21 month old mice were able to do so. Haining and Legan (1973) conducted a very similar experiment on Fischer 344 rats ranging in age from 6 weeks to 30 months, but attempted to determine rates of degradation and synthesis of catalase. The rate of synthesis fell in late life in both kidney and liver. The degradation rate fell in late life in liver only. In both studies, basal catalase activities underwent substantial late-life decreases in liver and kidney.

(2) Imre and Juhasz (1987) added H_2O_2 to the drinking water of 14 and 27 month old BALB/c mice for a two month period and then measured liver activities of catalase and SOD in 8000 × g supernatants.

Old mice exposed to this oxidative stress were unable to increase catalase activity whereas young mice did show significant induction. In untreated animals, catalase activity fell with age by 60 percent, while SOD was unchanged. Thus, both basal and inducible activities of liver catalase declined after middle age in mice. Whether or not DR influences the ability of animals to deal with oxidative stress remains unexplored.

(3) In heart mitochondria, activities of catalase and glutathione peroxidase were 40-60 percent higher in 24 month than in 3 month old rats, whereas SOD did not change with age (Nohl & Hegner, 1979). Clearly this age-related increase in heart mitochondrial catalase activity is opposite to the decreases reported for less purified preparations from liver and kidney of older animals.

(4) Vitorica et al. (1984) observed that catalase activity in rat brain is largely associated with the outer mitochondrial membrane, and shows no major changes with aging.

How important is catalase activity to an organism? Even bacteria have defense mechanisms to deal with oxidative stress. Accoring to Morgan et al. (1986), treatment of *Salmonella typhimurium* with H_2O_2 induces the synthesis of 30 proteins, and catalase is one of these. The expression of mRNA by the catalase gene (katG) was positively regulated by another locus (oxyR). Thus, regulated gene systems capable of dealing with active oxygen appear to be a fundamental part of aerobic life.

Scott et al. (1987) transformed *Escherichia coli* with multiple copies of the SOD gene, thereby creating an organism with more than 10 times the normal SOD activity but with normal activities of all other oxidant defenders. These bacteria were *more* sensitive to oxidative stress, accumulating more H_2O_2 and not surviving the stress as well as wild types. Scott et al. (1987) suggested that the product of SOD (H_2O_2) must be at least as toxic as the substrate (O_2^-), a finding which points toward catalase as being a crucial protective enzyme. Also, antioxidant defenses need to be in balance for optimal resistance.

Other evidence indicates that catalase and DNA repair systems have distinct protective roles against H_2O_2, a molecule which appears to carry out its lethal effect on *E. coli* via the production of DNA damage (Yonei et al., 1987). One might predict on the basis of end products that an increase in catalase activity is "better" for an organism than is higher SOD activity. It would be of interest to determine the impact of a selective 50 percent increase in catalase activity (like that rendered by DR) on the capacity of bacteria to combat oxygen toxicity.

Catalase may also be important in opposing the development of lens cataracts. Aminotriazole fed to rabbits caused 2- to 3-fold increases in H_2O_2 levels in aqueous and vitreous eye humors and lead to the development of cataracts (Bhuyan & Bhuyan, 1978). Catalase activity falls with age in rabbit eye tissues which border the anterior chamber, and when H_2O_2 was injected into the anterior chamber, eyes from young rabbits cleared the H_2O_2 more rapidly than did older eyes (Csukas & Green, 1987). Compared to normal human lenses, cataractous lenses show low activities of catalase, SOD and glutathione peroxidase along with high amounts of H_2O_2 and lipid peroxides (Bhuyan et al., 1986). Perhaps DR's ability to retard the loss of lens τ-crystallins with aging (Leveille et al., 1984: see Figure 4.20) reflects a catalase-mediated lowering of oxidative changes in lens proteins.

Catalase may also be involved in the control of physiologic processes. According to Wolin & Burke (1987), guanylate cyclase in extracts of bovine pulmonary arteries is activated either by compound I of catalase (Compound I is a catalase-oxygen intermediate between native catalase and the inactive compound II.) or a mediator generated by compound II. These authors suggest that the formation of H_2O_2 may accurately reflect oxygen tension and that guanylate cyclase activation by catalase ". . . could be involved in coupling the sensing of oxygen tension to the regulation of physiological processes such as vascular relaxation." Could the involvement of catalase in physiological regulation be a broad one?

Acatalasemia has been observed in humans and mice. Takahara (1952) first described human acatalasemia as featuring low erythrocyte catalase activity and oral ulcers but not long-term health problems. Acatalasemic mouse strains have been bred and catalase activity varies by tissue, with most strains showing erythrocyte, kidney and liver catalase activities of about 10, 60 and 90 percent of normal levels (Feinstein, 1970). The genetic defect underlying the tissue-specific reductions in catalase activity in acatalasemic mice does not alter expression of the catalase structural gene or the stability of its mRNA but rather affects translation and/or catalase turnover (Shaffer et al., 1987). Actalasemic mice on C3H and B6 backgrounds fed a diet containing 1 percent aminotriazole are not long-lived (mean LSs of about 7-10 months) (Feinstein et al., 1978a & 1978b). We are unaware of any reports on the longevity and disease patterns of normally-fed acatalasemic mice.

In sum, catalase is an enzyme with fascinating proven and possible actions. A selective, large, DR-induced increase in catalase activity provides a way for DR to more efficiently neutralize free radicals. Whether or not DR's effects on catalase occur in extra-hepatic tissues needs to be determined.

Other Possibilities

It would be unwise to ignore metabolic effects unrelated to free radicals. For example, an increased metabolic efficiency could trigger a neuroendocrine shift and retard aging via Totter's evolutionary explanation. The key point is that it is not essential to tie energy metabolism to a damage theory.

BODY TEMPERATURE

Poikilotherms

In poikilotherms there is no question but that over a broad range maintenance at a lower temperature leads to a longer LS. The situation in invertebrates has been reviewed thoroughly by Sohol and Allen (1985) and Balin and Allen (1986). Life span can be substantially prolonged and the slope of the Gompertz plot altered so as to indicate true retardation of aging in these species. In invertebrates at least, the LS effect of temperature lowering has been attributed, on rather convincing evidence, to metabolic rate reduction.

Temperature effects on LS and immune and biochemical processes in poikilothermic vertebrates were reviewed by Liu and Walford (1972). Life span can be substantially prolonged, for example in annual fish, by a 3 to 5°C temperature decrement. Sacher (1977) interpreted these data to indicate deceleration of the process of aging. The positive effect of lower temperature on LS in annual fish is most manifest if instituted during the last half of life (Liu & Walford, 1975; Liu et al., 1975). There is some evidence for a similar effect in rotifers (Fanestil & Barrows, 1965). It is important to realize that in both invertebrates and poikilothermic vertebrates, as well as in homeotherms, metabolic processes may vary disproportionately at different temperatures, and in the intact animal lower temperature does not simply mean a "turning down" of all biochemical processes (Liu & Walford, 1972; Sohol & Allen, 1985).

Homeotherms

A diet low in protein but not planned to be energy restricted (i.e., isocaloric and ad lib: nevertheless, the "low protein" mice consumed 10 percent less food than their "higher protein" partners) was noted by Leto et al. (1976b) to lead to a decrease in BW and body temperature in female mice, and to some increase in LS, although not beyond that characteristic for the species.

We were the first to document a significant decrease in internal body temperature in mice on an actual DR regimen that led to an increased species-specific maximum LS. The DR/control temperature differences, recorded via rectal thermometer in mid-morning, ranged from 2.5°C to 1.2°C respectively in our two studies (Weindruch et al., 1979; Cheney et al., 1983: see Table 4.21).

In a study in which body temperature of mice restricted to 75 percent of ad libitum intake was continuously measured via implanted telemetering devices, and in which maximum LS was clearly prolonged, Nelson and Halberg (1987) noted an average difference of about 1.5°C between DR and control mice and a much wider circadian temperature amplitude in the DR mice. Turturro and Hart (cited by Kahn [1987]) have made similar observations.

Still further studies indicate that, in the mouse, restricted energy intake may be associated with reduced body temperature not only in normal mice but to an even greater measure in the genetically obese ob/ob mouse (Dubuc et al., 1985; Himms-Hagen, 1985a), and in a number of rodent species adapted to live in hot arid environments (James & Trayhurn, 1981). To what extent, if any, can the observed increases in LS induced by DR be attributed to a temperature differential?

Contrary to mice, rats may not lower their body temperature or experience torpor when energy intake is restricted (Volicer at al., 1984; Himms-Hagen, 1985a). If this holds true, it would be strong evidence against a primary temperature effect as DR's mode of action. In our view, therefore, current evidence does not support the concept that a lowered internal body temperature plays a major role in the LS extension induced by DR in mammals. Nevertheless, some observations about the effects of ambient temperature on metabolic rates, thermogenesis, and LS may allow insight into the question of DR's mechanism(s).

Rats fed ad lib and kept throughout life at an environmental temperature of 34°C exhibited 1.3°C higher rectal temperatures, and higher rates of metabolism, but 59 day longer LSs (p < .05) than controls maintained at thermoneutrality of 28°C (Kibler & Johnson, 1966). In this same study a DR group at 28°C lived 138 days longer than the ad lib 28°C group (p < .01), and 80 days longer than a 34°C group which had the same average food intake (p < .05). A 28°C ad lib subgroup with lower rectal temperature did not live longer than a 28°C ad lib subgroup with higher temperature, but a 34°C ad lib subgroup with lower rectal temperature lived 101 days longer than the 34°C ad lib subgroup with higher rectal temperature (p < .01).

At the other side of the ambient temperature scale, metabolic rate of normal or lean mice kept at 20°C is twice that of mice kept at 34°C (Cawthorne, 1982). The increase in metabolic rate is maintained, at least in part, by non-shivering thermogenesis, the sites of which probably include both brown fat and red muscle (Cawthorne, 1982). Data on their comparative LSs are not available.

If there were no significant LS difference between 20°C and 34°C mice, such would go along with our surmise (see "EVOLUTIONARY PERSPECTIVE" and "ENERGY METABOLISM," this Chapter) that in terms of metabolic rate and aging, and among lean body mass constituents, the contributions of muscle and nonmuscle tissue should be considered separately. Along these lines, evidence suggests that the liver may be implicated in dietary-induced thermogenesis, as contrasted to non-shivering or cold-induced thermogenesis (Cawthorne, 1982). The fact that decreased food intake (i.e., less dietary-induced thermogenesis) increased LS would fit very nicely here, and tends to reinforce the concept that energy expenditure in the liver and other vital organs may be more relevant to LS and the rate of aging than energy expenditure in skeletal muscle.

Since both normal and genetically obese ob/ob mice decrease food intake by about one-third when kept at a thermoneutral ambient temperature (33°C), it would be interesting to know if energy restriction of a rather extreme degree could be tolerated at this ambient temperature, and whether this would yield an exceptionally great LS prolongation. We predict that it would not, providing that the homeotherms's response to temperature shifts does in fact primarily involves muscle rather than nonmuscle vital organ tissue.

Admittedly we tread a poorly understood area, as can be illustrated by the data in Figure 1.2 (Chapter 1), where the left panel shows the survival times of 100-day old fasting rats kept at different environmental temperatures, and the right panel the relative BW loss by time of death of these same rats. One might expect that at lower temperatures the rats would die sooner because their body substance was used up faster to maintain body temperature, and that at all temperatures death should occur when the BW had decreased to a given percentage of the initial value. But this was not the case. At 20°C the rats died when they had lost only 34 percent of BW, whereas at 30°C they were able to lose 44 percent of initial BW before death.

Reports in the Russian literature maintain that the temperature of thermoneutrality for full-fed rats is 28°C, for DR rats[3] 24-25°C, and that for full-fed rats oxygen consumption and respiratory and cardiac rates are 15 to 40 percent lower at 28°C than at 20°C (Arshavsky, 1979; Frolkis, 1982). At 28°C these same rates are 30-70 percent *higher* for DR rats than for controls, but at 20°C the indices are 33 percent *lower* for DR rats than for controls.

It is difficult to know how the above temperature variables impact upon attempts to evaluate effects of DR on energy metabolism. We shall emphasize, in a discussion of the relation between BW and LS (see "EVIDENCE AND CONJECTURE AGAINST THE PROPOSITION," Chapter 6), our view that it is *hazardous to extrapolate from ad libitum fed populations as to how DR animals will respond*. We believe the same holds with regard to temperature variables. Ambient temperature effects on DR animals may be other than an extrapolation from ad libitum animals. This is clearly the case, for example, with the ob/ob mouse (Trayhurn & James, 1978; Coleman, 1985). Also, species of rodents such as the spiny mouse, the white-footed deer mouse *(Peromyscus)* and others from warm dry regions, which have adapted to minimizing calorie requirements and which show anomalous thermoregulation (Wise, 1977a & b), may require special care in testing DR's effects. A positive effect may only be demonstrable at certain environmental temperatures. This area merits exploration.

PROTEIN SYNTHESIS, DNA, CHROMATIN, GENE EXPRESSION, DNA REPAIR

The subjects subsumed under the above heading are interrelated in terms both of aging theories and experimental evidence which concerns age-related and DR-related changes.

---

[3]Unfortunately in the translation summary of this literature available to us, that of Frolkis (1982), the word "starvation" seems to be used interchangeably with LS-prolonging DR. But we believe from the context that long-term DR is intended.

A comprehensive review of protein synthesis and degradation in relation to aging in many animal species was published by Makrides (1983). Later reviews include those of Reff (1985) and Richardson (1985). Richardson and Cheung (1982) proposed that a loss with age in the ability to synthesize new proteins and respond to stimuli which involve the necessity for enzyme induction, linked to a fall in protein turnover, may be instrumental in aging.

Considerable evidence exists for: (1) a delay in the time required for induction of some enzymes in older animals (Adelman, 1975) and, (2) a fall in protein synthesis with age in most organs (but not in skeletal muscle or lung) in both invertebrates and mammals (Richardson, 1985; Richardson et al., 1985; Reff, 1985), although there seem to be different age-related rates of fall if *in vitro* are contrasted with *in vivo* measurements (Bailey & Webster, 1984). The decreased synthesis may be based on changes in gene structure or expression or on irregularities in translational control (Gabius et al., 1983; Richardson et al., 1983 & 1985). A fall in activity of Elongation Factor-1 (EF-1), which comprises 3 to 11 percent of the total protein content of eukaryotic cells (one of the major proteins of the cell, therefore) may be particularly involved (Webster & Webster, 1983).

Several theories of aging focus on DNA and the chromatin complex. Some of these (e.g. Yielding, 1974; Smith, 1976) can be considered as modernized versions of the somatic mutation theory (Failla, 1958; Szilard, 1959; Curtis, 1963). They postulate loss of DNA integrity as a cause of aging. Evidence for age-related changes in DNA include increased chromosomal aberrations and strand breaks in cells from old organisms (reviewed by Tice & Setlow, 1985). Other approaches implicate age changes in the chromatin complex, for example the accumulation of cross links (reviewed by Tice & Setlow, 1985). Work from our laboratory indicates that an increase in chromatin compactness occurs with age and is due at least in part to an increased number of disulfide bonds in the non-histone chromatin proteins, presumably inhibiting transcription at the affected regions of the genome (Tas & Walford, 1982a).

A role for DNA repair in influencing LS was first clearly suggested by the work of Hart and Setlow (1974) which demonstrated a linear correlation between the log of LS and the ability of fibroblasts from different species (e.g., shrew, mouse, cow, elephant, human) to carry out excision repair of UV-induced damage. A similar correlation was also reported for lens epithelial cells from six mammalian species (Treton &

Courtois, 1982). In our laboratory, Hall et al. (1984) showed that the correlation also obtained between different primate species, and for lymphocytes as well as fibroblasts. The subject has been ably reviewed and interpreted by Tice and Setlow (1985), and by Hanawalt (1987). With regard to the possibility of a decline in DNA repair with age, the weight of evidence is against it (Tice & Setlow, 1985; Hanawalt, 1987) except probably for lymphocytes (Lambert et al., 1979; Licastro & Walford, 1985), but there are dissenting reports. Plesko and Richardson (1984) reported a decline in the ability of hepatocytes isolated from the rat liver to repair UV-induced DNA injury.

A rather abundant literature has developed about each of the above areas. Our brief synopsis here is meant only to serve as background for those (relatively few) DR studies which have addressed these phenomena. Much more intensive investigations of DR in relation thereto are called for.

Protein Synthesis

Except for a few dissenting voices (Barrows & Kokkonen, 1982), evidence suggests that in most organs (skeletal muscles and lung perhaps excepting) DR leads to an increase in protein synthesis, degradation and turnover compared to age-matched fully fed controls. This obtains for cells in vitro, in cell free systems, and in studies of whole body protein, and has been proposed to reflect a fundamental mechanism for DR's influence (Richardson, 1985; Richardson et al., 1985; Lewis et al., 1985; Holehan & Merry, 1986). We find this hypothesis attractive but possibly an oversimplification. In its present form it raises two problems.

First, since protein synthesis and turnover decline with age, and as DR animals are functionally "younger" than age-matched controls, they might indeed be expected to display a higher rate of protein synthesis and turnover than age-matched controls. Protein synthesis and turnover might thus simply be considered biomarkers of aging. Despite its attractiveness on theoretical grounds, the increased synthesis and turnover can no more be taken as causative than any other biomarker, for example the even more impressive (quantitatively) increased immune response capacity in DR rodents compared to controls. In fact the delayed age-related peaks in certain enzyme activities illustrated by Barrows and Kokkonen (1982) for DR animals somewhat resemble the age-related shifts in peak humoral antibody response for DR animals noted by Walford et al. (1973/74), and could reflect a common biochemical basis.

Priestly and Robertson (1973) observed that in mice selected over 20 generations for high and low BWs, animals from the low BW strains showed increased protein synthesis and turnover. If protein synthesis were a primary factor in LS extension in DR mice, one might expect enhanced maximum LSs in these genetically selected smaller mouse strains. Data on this critical point are unfortunately not available.

It seems more likely to us that a selective upregulation in synthesis of one or several critical proteins, such as EF-1, might be a causative factor in DR's retardation of aging, and that the general increase in synthesis of other proteins is simply a biomarker phenomenon. Supporting the thesis for a primacy role for EF-1 is the finding that with normal aging in *Drosophila* a significant decrease supervenes in synthesis of EF-1 just prior to the age when overall protein synthesis drops most sharply (Webster & Webster, 1983). In mice and rats Vargas and Casteneda (1981) reported parallel exponential declines with age of both EF-1 activity and protein synthesis. Gabius et al. (1983) noted a marked decrease in rat liver and kidney with age of two steps in peptide chain elongation: the EF-1 dependent binding of aminoacyl-tRNA to ribosomes, and the peptide bond formation.

A recent study from our laboratory (Koizumi et al., 1987a) (see "Enzymes and Metabolites," Chapter 4) lends further support to the idea of a *selective up*regulation of protein synthesis under DR conditions, in that DR animals were found to have elevated activities of catalase but not of SOD or of several other enzymes in the liver. However, an alternate explanation for the increase in catalase activity might be that more NADPH is available in DR animals to rejuvenate spent catalase (see *"Increased Free Radical Neutralization by DR,"* this Chapter).

The second problem about a postulated overall increase in protein synthesis/turnover as primary cause for DR's effects is related to energetics. Twenty to fifty percent of the BMR may be due to the energy requirements for protein synthesis (Garrow, 1978; Bray & Fisler, 1985). According to Stock and Rothwell (1982), some 23 percent of the BMR or 17 percent of maintenance metabolic rate goes for protein synthesis, and if the dietary induced thermogenesis needed for food assimilation be added thereto, these figures become 37 and 27 percent respectively. An *increased* protein synthesis in DR animals becomes somewhat difficult to reconcile with the sharply decreased energy availability in these same animals, although on a lean body mass basis, there may be no decrease. Or there may be an increase in efficiency of utilization of available energy, and this shift and its mechanism could be the fundamental mechanism behind DR.

It is worth remembering that an increase in synthesis of a protein may reflect not necessarily increased gene expression in the form of more mRNA, but the working of translational control (initiation) factors, the unmasking of mRNA, and binding of mRNA to ribosomes (Clemens, 1987). This area has not been explored in DR animals.

DNA and Chromatin

Whereas Nikitin (1979) reported that in DR rodents[4] there occurs a decreased activity of RNA polymerase A and B, the review of Richardson et al. (1985) concluded that the activities of RNA polymerases were probably not responsible for age-related drops in transcription, and that changes in chromatin itself are likely contributing to transcriptional declines. Although age-related alterations in chromatin have been documented (Tas & Walford, 1982a & b; Khilobock et al., 1983; Zongza & Mathias, 1979), there are no reorts on the effect of DR on chromatin and the chromatin DNA complex, except again for that of Nikitin (1979), who reported a decrease in nonhistone chromatin proteins, phospholipids, and free phosphate groups of DNA in DR animals.

Although DR has not been much investigated in relation to chromatin, evidence does exist that dietary variables such as the ratios of fat and protein may induce alterations in the higher order structure of chromatin, as reflected in sensitivity to digestion by micrococcal nuclease and DNAse I (Castro & Sevall, 1980; Castro et al., 1986). Chromatin from neuronal or microglial populations of older animals appears less digestible by micrococcal nuclease than chromatin from young animals (Berkowitz et al., 1983). And chromatin from older animals (Tas & Walford, 1982b) or from late passage fibroblasts in culture (Dell-Orco & Whittle, 1982) appears less digestible by DNAse I than chromatin from young animals or early passage cells. This area clearly merits investigation in terms of DR.

Recent studies suggest that the chemical attachment of glucose to proteins or nucleic acids without the aid of enzymes, i.e., a process of nonenzymatic glycosylation, may culminate in the formation of irreversible cross-links between adjacent molecules (Cerami et al., 1987). Glucose may alter conformation of proteins or nucleic acids so that

---
[4]See footnote #3, this chapter.

unexposed SH groups are susceptible to combine with adjacent SH groups to form disulfide bonds. (Disulfide bond formation does appear increased in aging in some tissues [Tas et al., 1980; Tas & Walford, 1982a].) The eye lens develops both glycosylated and disulfide cross-links with age (Cerami et al., 1987). Glycosylation may inactivate enzymes, such as SOD (Arai et al., 1987). On the basis of an age-related increase in glycosylation of osteocalcin (the matrix protein of bone), it has been suggested that glycosylation may play a role in the pathogenesis of senile osteoporosis (Gundberg et al., 1986). Much of the pathology of diabetes may be secondary to the development of glycosylation cross-links (Cerami et al., 1987). In this regard it is noteworthy that Reaven et al. (1983a & b) have shown that many (not all) of the age-related changes in certain aspects of glucose metabolism related to insulin secretion and metabolism are very responsive to energy restriction induced by feeding a very high fiber diet on an ad lib basis. But the effects of DR on glycosylation per se have not yet been investigated.

Gene Expression

Richardson (1985) claimed that an age-related decline in gene expression may be a universal phenomenon in higher organisms. This is mainly an inference from the fact that protein synthesis generally declines with age, which may represent decline in gene expression. Direct measurements, for example of mRNA levels for specific gene products in relation to aging, are not plentiful, although some do exist (Richardson et al., 1985; Crew et al., 1987), and the transcription of total RNA indeed declines with age as shown in a number of studies (reviewed by Lindell, 1982, and by Richardson et al., 1985). Table 5.6 lists studies in which the levels of specific mRNA species or their activities have been measured as a function of age. As noted, some did not change and some decreased. The values are basal levels. But although malic enzyme and tyrosine aminotransferase mRNAs did not change with age, the *induction* of these mRNAs did decrease substantially with age.

The above studies, including those involving induction, do support the idea of age-specific defects in gene expression. It has been suggested, therefore, that DR may act by enhancing gene expression (Cheney et al., 1980; Lindell, 1982). Lindell (1982) hypothesized that DR is a physiological "stress" that enhances gene expression, and that this enhanced expression is a significant factor in the maintenance of cellular homeostasis in an organism as it ages. The hypothesis is at some variance with

TABLE 5.6

Studies in Which the Activities or Levels of Specific mRNAs Have Been Measured as a Function of Age[a]

mRNA species	Organism	Tissue	Sex	Ages	Assay system	Change
Cytochrome P450LM$_2$	Rabbit	Liver	M	50-800 d	Translation	↓
Malic enzyme	Rat	Liver	M	1.5 and 10 mo	Translation	None
Tyr. aminotransferase	Rat	Liver	M	10 and 24 mo	cDNA probe	None
Trytophan oxygenase	Rat	Liver	M	10 and 24 mo	cDNA probe	None
$\alpha_{2\mu}$-Globulin	Rat	Liver	M	2.5-30 mo	cDNA probe	↓
EF-1	Drosophila	Body	-	0-21 d	Translation	↓
GH, Prolactin	Mouse	Pituitary	M	3,12,27 mo	cDNA probe	↓
α-tubulin	Mouse	Pituitary	M	3,12,27 mo	cDNA probe	None

[a]Abbreviations: Tyr. = tyrosine; EF-1 = elongation factor-1; GH = growth hormone. The translation assays were cell free. For references see Richardson et al. (1985) and Crew et al. (1987). Adapted from these sources.

Barrows' earlier speculation (Barrows, 1972), based on his now contested findings that DR is associated with reduced protein synthesis, or that DR works by decreasing use of the genetic code (a variation perhaps of the wear-and-tear hypothesis), or with Johnson's suggestion (Johnson, 1986) that DR works by retarding certain aspects of the genetic expression of programmed senescence. Richardson et al. (1987) presented evidence that in hepatocytes isolated from rats, DR substantially increased the synthesis, mRNA levels, and transcription of $\alpha_{2\mu}$-globulin, considered a "senescence marker protein."

Our view of this area is as follows. If aging is regulated not by changes along the whole genome, but by a small number of genes or gene systems, which is in fact the prevailing view (Walford, 1974, 1987; Sacher, 1975; Cutler, 1975, 1982; Martin, 1978), it seems more likely in terms of a gene expression theory of DR's action that the primary effect would be on these critical genes or gene systems, and that any increased expression of other genes and gene products would be secondary "biomarker" effects, i.e., the animals are "functionally" younger and therefore these secondary genes are better expressed. Good candidates for primary genes or gene systems are, we believe, the major histocompatibility complex (see below under "IMMUNOLOGIC INTERPRETATION"), genes which segregate with coat color in mice on the 4th chromosome (Yunis et al., 1984) and which may relate to DNA repair (Genes for DNA repair are also on the 4th chromosome.), genes encoding enzymes which protect cells from oxidative damage (Cutler, 1982, 1984a), and the gene(s) responsible for EF-1 (Webster & Webster, 1984). As maintained in earlier sections, the study by Koizumi et al. (1987a) may support the idea of a DR-driven selective upregulation of gene expression.

In long-lived rodent strains the levels of several, physiologically useful mRNAs are increased by DR (Richardson et al., 1985 & 1987). In short-lived strains on DR the levels of expression of a number of oncogenes have been found to be diminished (Khare et al., 1986). Admittedly different gene systems were being dealt with, and the findings could indicate either general strain-specific traits linking levels of gene expression, rates of aging, and DR, or else upregulation of some whole categories of genes, down-regulation of others, by DR. We suspect the latter.

DNA Repair

As noted in the introductory part of this section, a number of observations have suggested that DNA repair phenomena are important in aging. In this regard the close parallel between age-related decrease in DNA repair and decline in transcription in liver noted by Plesko and Richardson (1984) is intriguing (Figure 5.5).

Studies by Licastro et al. (1986), using UDS in splenocytes, indicated an increase in DNA repair in DR animals compared to age-matched controls. Weraarchakul and Richardson (1988) observed a 30 percent increase in UDS following UV-induced damage to liver and kidney cells from DR compared to ad lib fed rats. Measuring levels of O^6-methylguanine acceptor protein in tissues of rats, Woodhead et al. (1985) found no difference with either age or DR in ability to remove alkylation products from DNA. It should be noted, however, that repair of alkylation products such as this *cannot* be measured by UDS or by repair replication. These three studies, therefore, are not directly at odds. Preliminary studies in Ames' laboratory (Saul et al., 1987), in which levels of oxidative DNA damage products were measured in urine, but using only a small number of animals on 0, 15, and 30 percent DR, did not reveal any decrease in DNA damage products in DR animals.

In view of the results with UDS and DR (Licastro et al., 1986, 1988), it will be important to see if repair of the DNA lesions induced by

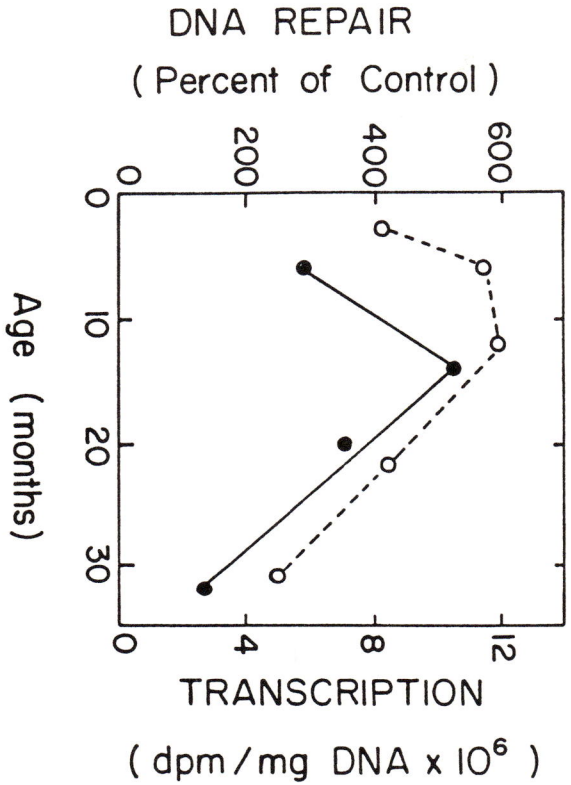

Figure 5.5. Effect of age on repair of UV-induced DNA damage (•) and on transcription (o) in hepatocytes of rats. From Plesko and Richardson (1984), with permission.

N-acetoxyacetylamino-fluorene (AAAF) (lesions mimic UV damage, induce long patch repair, and repair of which decreases with age) is also increased by DR. Studies on this are in progress in our laboratory.

Again we believe that *selective up*regulation either of certain forms of DNA repair, or repair of certain sites of DNA damage (obviously those sites which contain the genes or gene systems most concerned with aging) are what DR might preferentially influence as its primary method of increasing maximum LS. A combination of DNA repair methodology and molecular genetic techniques are probably necessary to make this assessment. Hanawalt (1987) has reviewed site-specific repair of DNA lesions. Since the MHC is thought to show the highest mutation rate of any mammalian gene system (reviewed by Walford, 1987), it would seem a site worthy of investigation in terms of DR and site-specific DNA repair.

NEUROENDOCRINE INTERPRETATION

In this and the following section, on the immune system, we discuss DR data as it relates to the idea that in highly organized animals cellular function and survival and therefore possibly aging depend largely on the *extracellular* homeostatic and integrative mechanisms provided by the neuroendocrine, immune, and intercellular communicating systems. This approach is different from being wholly preoccupied with events at the cellular-molecular level in the different organ systems, as in the preceding section.

The place for genomic expression and molecular mechanisms in aging may be not general but specific, and in the "command cells" of the homeostatic and integrative systems of the body (Meites et al., 1987). General age-related structural changes in the brain, such as neuronal loss in selected cortical areas, a decline in dendritic spine density, and shrinkage of the dendritic arbor, as well as other changes, are reviewed by Duara et al. (1985). Partial reversal of cholinergic cell body atrophy and improvement of retention of spatial memory in old rats by intracerebral infusion of nerve growth factor may indeed suggest an extracellular mechanism for aging in this system (Fischer et al., 1987), as does the fact that neurons can regenerate, and that survival of neurons is at least in part dependent on numerous endocrine and secretory materials (Lockshin, 1987).

Timiras (1983) distinguished between cellular-molecular theories of aging (free radicals, lipid peroxidation, membrane changes, altered gene expression, defective protein synthesis, DNA repair) and neuroendocrine theories, adding that in terms of the latter, aging must depend more on interrelations between hormonal and neural signals than on isolated endocrine reactions. The finding by Kelley et al. (1986) that implantation of GH-secreting pituitary adenoma cells into old rats regenerated thymic tissue *in situ* and reversed age-related losses in cellular immunity was interpreted to suggest that the lymphoid cells in aged animals are not inherently defective, a conclusion at least partly at variance with the views of many immunogerontologists (Makinodan et al., 1987a & b; Miller, 1987; Schwab & Weksler, 1987). As Meites et al. (1987) have emphasized, there is a much better chance of interfering with aging if extracellular homeostatic integrative processes are primarily involved.

The notion that the brain houses pacemakers (clocks) which regulate aging processes is attractive but far from proven. Several theories of aging are based on neuroendocrine phenomena (e.g., Dilman, 1976;

Everitt, 1973; Finch, 1976; Landfield, 1978), whereby age-related changes in higher regulatory systems are hypothesized to affect other systems lower in the regulatory pathway, and/or where peripheral endocrine factors influence the rate of aging of (parts of) the brain. Feed-back loops turn out to be loop-the-loops. Nevertheless, after carefully reviewing endocrine changes of aging, Cole (1982) concluded that, despite a number of clear-cut alterations, a coherent picture awaits the results of future work. Recent comprehensive reviews are those of Finch and Landfield (1985), Strong (1985), Gregerman (1986), and Meites et al. (1987).

Hypothalamus-Pituitary Axis

Most neuroendocrine theories of aging are particularly concerned with the hypothalamus-pituitary axis. Hypothalamic neurotransmitters (norepinephrine, dopamine, serotonin, acetylcholine) are believed to participate in the regulation of hypothalamic releasing and inhibitory factors, which in turn control pituitary hormone output. Alterations with aging in the pulsatile release of pituitary hormones appear at least partly caused by changes in hypothalamic neurosecretion and may exemplify "old clocks" not keeping good time (Finch & Landfield, 1985).

Frolkis (1976) argued that individual components of the hypothalamus may age at different rates, leading to irregularities of function. And Dilman (1976) hypothesized that due to intrinsic changes of aging the hypothalamus becomes less sensitive to negative feedback suppression by estrogens, corticoids, and glucose. To the extent that any such decreased sensitivity could be due to receptor loss, it is interesting to recall that DR may be associated with decreased receptor loss, as manifested in DR animals by better age-related retention of behavioral responses mediated by the neostriatum (Joseph et al., 1983), or by direct measurement (Roth et al., 1984).

Some evidence suggests that with aging the pituitary may secrete a senescence-promoting substance, a so-called "death hormone" (Denckla, 1974; Bolla, 1982). Hypophysectomized rodents (treated with an appropriate hormone replacement regimen) show certain features of decelerated aging: less cross linking of collagen (Olsen & Everitt, 1965; Everitt et al., 1983), less proteinuria and kidney disease (Everitt & Cavanaugh, 1965), reduced late-life disease incidence, and increased maximum LS (but not increased beyond the species-specific limit, only beyond the strain limit and hence in our view not a "true" increase in maximum LS) (Everitt et al., 1980 & 1983).

It has also been reported that Hx retards age-related decreases in: (1) the ability of rats to reject allografts (Bilder & Denckla, 1977), (2) rat liver nuclear RNA synthesis (Bolla & Denckla, 1979), (3) minimal O_2 consumption (Denckla, 1974), (4) regrowth of hair after shaving in mice (Harrison et al., 1982), and (5) mouse thymus size and ratios of cortex-medullary areas, and T-dependent immunity (Harrison et al., 1982). These and other outcomes of long-term Hx with hormonal replacement are shown in Table 5.7.

TABLE 5.7

Effect of Long-Term Hypophysectomy with Hormone Replacement on Changes in Physiological and Biochemical Parameters in Aging Rodents[a]

Parameter	Age Change	Activity Level in Old Hxed Rats
Minimal O_2 consumption	↓	younger
VO_2 max	↓	younger
Carbon clearance	↓	younger
Kidney morphology	pathologic changes	age change delayed
T_3 receptors	no change	no change
Antibodies to SRBC	↓	younger
Vascular relaxation	↓	younger
Total RNA synthesis	↓	younger
Initiation of RNA synth.	↓	younger
Liver aldolase synth.	↓	younger
Number of oocytes	↓	younger
Ovarian interstitial cells	various changes	changes retarded
Splenic PHA response	↓	younger

[a]The effect of hypophysectomy (Hx) gives the comparable activity level of 18–24 mo old Hxed rats compared to age-matched controls. For original references see Bolla (1982), Aschheim (1983), and Harrison et al. (1982). Adapted from these sources.

Another interpretation of these phenomena besides postulating the secretion of an actual "death hormone" is that with age the pituitary may secrete a higher percentage of "prohormones," which occupy the target receptors and thereby act like a "death hormone" (Segall, 1979). For example, in old rodents GH may circulate as a higher molecular weight species (Sonntag et al., 1983).

Because several outcomes of long-term DR may also follow Hx, including great loss in splenic weight, anestrus in (some) female rodent species, and retardation of features of aging in immune tissues, collagen, skeletal muscle, kidneys, heart, bones, and reproductive systems (Meites et al., 1987), it has been suggested that DR induces a pseudo-Hx, and that therein lies its effect on aging. This view is discussed in depth by Everitt and Porter (1976). A decreased secretion of pituitary hormones does appear to follow long-term DR. Effects of long-term Hx with hormone replacement on reproductive senescence are shown in Table 5.8.

There are a number of problems, however, with such an exclusive "pituitary theory" as interpretation of DR's mechanism. Number one is that Hxed animals, even though they show features of greater youthfulness, do not enjoy an extended species-specific maximum LS, and in fact in mice average and maximum longevities may be reduced (Harrison et al., 1982). The "excuse' of the pituitary proponents for this lack in LS extension is that the hormonal replacement regimen for Hxed rodents is imperfect. Ultimately this is no more acceptable than the "excuse" of the free radical theorists for the fact that feeding antioxidants has not been shown so far to increase maximum LS, which excuse is (among others) that exogenous antioxidants may not penetrate to the site(s) of free radical production, or that the body readjusts the activities of its free radical production or removal systems to maintain original homeostasis, with no net gain in scavenging capacity.

A second problem with the pituitary theory is that not all effects shown by DR which seem pertinent to aging are necessarily found in Hxed animals. Clearly, GH is decreased following Hx whereas in *long-term* DR (as opposed to short-term food restriction or fasting, in which GH is definitely decreased) it is not at all clear that GH levels are actually diminished (see *"Growth Hormone and Somatomedins."* Chapter 4). Furthermore, while basal levels of most pituitary hormones might be diminished in DR, the pulsatile release of GH (Gregerman, 1986), on which we have no information at all in the DR situation, could be normal or greater than normal. Such would correspond to the observation that in severe fasting the decrease in pituitary hormones is largely secondary to a decrease in release of those hypothalamic hormones which control pituitary function: the pituitary cells themselves are neither injured nor unresponsive (Campbell et al., 1977).

A third and quite serious complication with an exclusive pituitary theory for DR's effect is that ad-lib-fed Hxed rats consume only 30 to 50 percent as much food as controls (Everitt & Porter, 1976); therefore it seems equally tenable to presume that Hx induces spontaneous DR which then affects aging, rather then that DR exerts its effect by causing a "dietary Hx." An important question here is, *if* Hx induces DR and if therein lies its rejuvenescence effect, why do the animals still not exceed the maximum LS? An attempt to countermand this variable was made by Everitt et al. (1983) by limiting a control Hxed population to the same food intake as the ad lib fed but Hxed rats. Collagen aging was somewhat slower in the latter group, but LSs were about the same, and in fact did not exceed the species-specific LS. A further complication derives from the important study of Harrison et al. (1982) which reported that Hxed mice, while weighing 24 percent less than controls, consumed 18 percent more food than controls, and had, as noted, a shorter survival.

Reproductive Senescence and the Hypothalamus

A reciprocal relationship clearly exists between the ovaries and hypothalamic involvement in reproductive senescence. Table 5.8 from Aschheim (1983) shows the long-term effects of ovariectomy or early Hx upon a number of features of reproductive senescence.

Chronic administration of estrogens to young female rats may damage dopamine-containing neurons in the arcuate nucleus and the medial basal hypothalamic area (Everitt, 1976; Meites et al., 1987). Ovariectomy will retard certain morphologic aging changes in the arcuate nucleus (Finch & Mobbs, 1983). Giving ethinyl-estradiol or a progesterone-estrogen mixture will desensitize the hypothalamus to estrogen and delay reproductive aging (Aschheim, 1983). When ovariectomy at 6 or 12 months of age is followed at 24-27 months by grafting of a young *or* old ovary, cycling is restored (Aschheim, 1983).

Female reproductive senescence (reviewed by Finch et al., 1984, and Finch & Landfield, 1985) is ovary-dependent, can be slowed by ovariectomy, and is accelerated by estradiol treatment. The hypothalamus can trigger non-cycling rats to cycle again (transiently). Ovaries in old animals can be induced to function by electrical stimulation of the preoptic area of the brain, by giving drugs which increase the catecholamine content of the hypothalamus, by injecting gonadotropins or gonatropin-releasing hormone, or by transplanting old ovaries to a young animal (Meites et al., 1987).

A major contributor to reproductive decline thus lies in faults within the hypothalamus, as opposed to or in addition to events within the ovary (Meites et al., 1987). Age-related reduction in hypothalamic

TABLE 5.8
Long-Term Effects of Early Hypophysectomy (Hx) or
Ovariectomy (Ovx) in Aging Rats[a]

Age at operation	Time elapsed	Results	Interpretation
26 d (Hx)	7-24 mo	Proliferation of ovarian epithelial cords; thickening of basement membranes	Intrinsic aging of these ovarian structures
26 d (Hx)	>11 mo	Intramitochondrial inclusions in ovarian interstitial cells after hormone stimulation	Intrinsic aging seen only after stimulation
40 d (Hx)	12-13 mo	+ young pituitary graft: resumption of cycles	Suspended aging during Hx
6 or 12 mo (Ovx)	21 or 12 mo	+ old or young ovarian graft: resumption of cycles	Suspended aging during Ovx
60 d (Ovx)	22 mo	Castration levels and pulsatile fluctuations of LH, not maintained; LH responses to hormones maintained	No aging of pituitary sensitivity
45 d (Ovx)	12 mo	Decrease of prolactin secretion *in vitro*, stimulation by estrodiol, & inhibition by dopamine *in vitro*, all maintained	Intrinsic pituitary aging? No aging of pituitary sensitivity

[a]For original references see Aschheim (1983). Adapted from Aschheim (1983).

catecholamines, including norepinephrine, may be instrumental in this decline. Norepinephrine arises normally in the preoptic area just prior to ovulation, and L-DOPA, which increases brain catecholamines, can reinitiate estrus cycles (Finch, 1979; Meites et al., 1987). However, the limited number of ovarian follicles appears to act as a pacemaker for reproductive senescence while interacting with neuroendocrine aging changes. The loop-the-loop is not final.

The fact that DR greatly delays the time of reproductive senescence (Holehan & Merry, 1986) but at least in some species (mice more so than rats) renders the animals less fertile during the DR period, on the whole supports the idea of hypothalamic aging mechanisms. In rats, cyclicity on DR persists well beyond the age of control animals who have ceased to cycle (Merry & Holehan, 1979), while DR mice cease entirely to cycle but the cycling can be reinstituted in late life by refeeding (see "Reproductive Senescence," Chapter 4). Indeed, DR mice refed nomally beginning at 240 days of age subsequently produced 13 times as many litters as age-matched controls (Ball et al., 1947). In older rats a 10 week period of DR followed by ad libitum feeding will reinitiate cycling (Quigley & Meites, 1987). These findings also lend support to an evolutionary interpretation of DR's mechanism (see "EVOLUTIONARY PERSPECTIVE," this Chapter).

The interplay between hypothalamus (and pituitary) and the gonads, in which age changes in one leads to age-changes in the other but in which it is difficult to decide which (if either) comes first, is a good example of the quandary of neuroendocrine aging. It illustrates why studies of reproductive senescence, which at first sight may seem of rather secondary interest with respect to "true" senescence, remains a fertile field for aging research, and why Finch's group, for example, has concentrated so heavily on studying this area. Therefore, the fact that DR so markedly influences reproductive senescence assumes additional interest. The missing element, of course, is that DR *also* increases maximum LS, whereas no other of the several means to alter reproductive senescence shows this added organismal effect.

Nevertheless, following Totter's hypothesis, but excluding his enchantment with the free radical theory, we suggest the possibility that DR might act primarily by delaying reproductive senescence, with secondary effects on the neuroendocrine system leading to LS extension. If this be the pathway, than we predict that DR might be less effective in gonadectomized rodents. This could be tested.

Glucocorticoid and Neuroendocrine Cascades

A hypothesis originally from Landfield (1978) (see also Finch & Landfield, 1985), that glucocorticoids may modulate hippocampal aging, is supported by the particular susceptibility of the hippocampus to early and severe morphologic aging changes, and by the apparent restriction of this neuronal loss to cells with corticosterone receptors. Sapolsky et al. (1986) have recently extended this hypothesis to propose a glucocorticoid cascade involving aging as in part a stress response. They envisage a feed-forward cascade whereby stress leads to corticosterone hypersecretion, which eventually causes neuronal cell loss in the hippocampus, the function of which cells is to inhibit corticosterone hypersecretion. Again a loop-the-loop, in which the gradual neuronal loss renders the inhibition less and less effective, resulting in hyperadrenocorticism! Hyperadrenocorticism is known to cause a decrease in the immune response, muscle atrophy, osteoporosis, arteriosclerosis, diabetes and other features of aging.

Unfortunately only scant evidence is available pertinent to the possible effect of long-term DR on the hippocampal adrenal axis (but see Figure 4.9). Likewise there is no evidence available about the effect of long-term DR on levels of another steroid hormone, DHEA. Higher levels of DHEA, the most abundant circulating steroid hormone in humans, have recently been reported to be associated with decreased mortality from any cause, and the DHEA level can be augmented by weight loss such as being on an 800-1000 kcal/day diet (Hendrikx et al., 1968) (But also by smoking [Barrett-Connor et al., 1986]!).

Figure 5.6 illustrates two hypotheses of neural-endocrine interactions during aging, Finch's neuroendocrine cascade, and the hippocampal-glucocorticoid hypothesis of Landfield, including the above-mentioned Sapolsky modification. Whereas many of the hormones depicted in Figure 5.6 are affected by DR, as detailed in Chapter 4, a clearcut picture in terms of mechanisms does not emerge. For one thing, lack of understanding of the basic neuroendocrine control of pituitary ACTH secretion has made it difficult to relate changes in neuroendocrine function to age alterations in the hypothalamic-pituitary-adrenal axis (Reigle, 1983). Nesterenko et al. (1977) did report that DR inhibited age-related decreases in functional indexes of this axis.

Neuroendocrine-Immune Interactions

The possibility exists that changes in calcium distribution, transport, and binding may be involved not only in many features of aging in the brain (see review by Gibson & Peterson, 1987, and commentaries thereon in the same journal), but in the immune system (Miller, 1987). In this regard it is important to recall that the age-related increases in PTH and calcitonin are mitigated by DR (see "Neuroendocrine" section in Chapter 4).

Whereas the potential importance of neuroendocrine-immune interactions to be instrumental in aging can be illustrated by the observa-

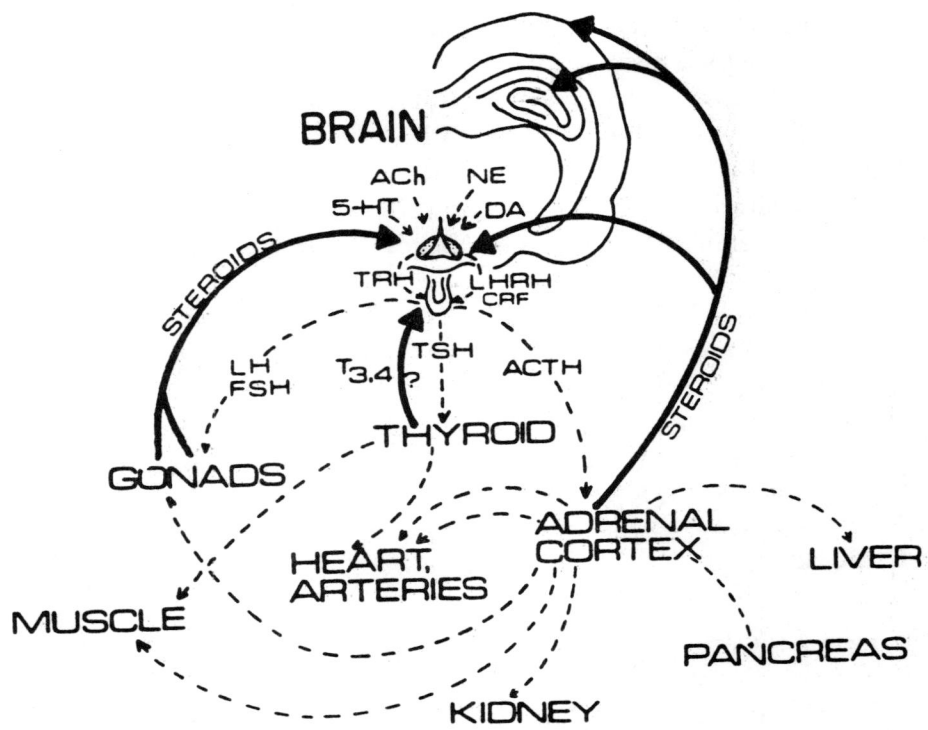

Figure 5.6. Representation of two hypotheses of neuroendocrine interactions during aging: the neuroendocrine cascade hypothesis of Finch (1976) and the hypothesis that endocrine factors may lead to brain cell damage (Landfield, 1978). Neuroendocrine regulatory alterations (cascade) (----->); endocrine modulation (destruction of brain cells) (——>). Adapted from Finch and Landfield (1985).

tion of a permanent decrease of plasma thyroxine in neonatally thymectomized mice, or the ability of thymosin fraction 5 to stimulate secretion of LHRH *in vitro* from hypothalamic fragments (Finch & Landfield, 1985), or the effect of GH on immune function (Sonntag et al., 1983), as well as other studies reviewed by Fabris (1986), there are to our knowledge no DR studies of the area of neuroendocrine-immune interactions.

Conclusion

It seems clear that neuroendocrine and neuroendocrine-immune phenomena may contribute fundamentally to the mechanism whereby DR retards aging, but the available information, while tantalizing, is insufficient and too disconnected to allow a clear formulation of possibilities.

IMMUNOLOGIC INTERPRETATION

Aging, Immune Function and MHC-Related Functions

We propose that aging in each cell system most prominently involves those aspects of the cells which concern their differentiated function, or whatever special function is revealed with greatest clarity in that cell system. In this sense it is not surprising that some types of stem cells may not age (Harrison et al., 1978; Harrison et al., 1987: but see Hirokawa et al., 1986 for a contrary view).

In any case, according to this proposal, to study age-related changes in mitochondria and/or actin filaments, one might select muscle tissue. Neurons accentuate the cytoskeleton and plasma membrane, considering respectively their long cell bodies and the highly specialized generation of electrical or chemical signaling. Cells of the immune system accentuate the phenomenon of proliferative response to a specific stimulus, of fine-tuned recognition of suface patterns, and reactive responses characteristic of the cell subsets. The opportunity to test for a system's most accentuated complex function(s) in relation to aging is arguably more available for the immune than for other systems. And some systems may age at a rapider rate than others (immune system vs. skeletal muscle, as a possible example).

One of the most widely documented and severe physiologic decrements of aging mammals is in fact immunosenescence, which is accompanied at the organismal level by an increased susceptibility to infection, disorders of autoimmunity, immune complex disease, amyloidosis, cancer, and other maladies in which immune dysfunction may play a part. Longer LSs have been claimed for mice selected for high-responder status to SRBC and Salmonella flagellar antigens, while selection for NK cell activity showed no such correlation (Covelli et al., 1984). Reviews of immunosenescence from the standpoints of pathology, biochemistry, and immunologic function of the system may be found in Walford et al. (1981b), Hausman and Weksler, 1985; Tollefsbol and Cohen (1986), and Siskind (1987) respectively, and in the excellent and timely book edited by Goidl (1987).

The original immunologic theory of aging (Walford, 1962, 1969) proposed that aging in mammals is due to decline in immune response capacity associated with failure in homeostatic mechanisms for maintaining tolerance to self, with the consequent rise of autoimmunity, and that aging is a kind of self-destruct process analogous to a chronic graft-versus-host reaction. It was considered initially more a pathogenetic than an etiologic theory. However, to the extent that these changes may be related to the major histocompatibility complex (MHC, see following section), or to a programmed thymic involution (Burnet, 1970; Weksler, 1981), the theory may be considered etiologic, in the latter case because thymic aging would affect not only T cell immunity but through thymic hormones also activities of the neuroendocrine system (Fabris et al., 1983; Piantanelli et al., 1985). Also in terms of an etiologic theory, it is noteworthy that in B6-A/J allophenic mice the total LS of the mice seems directly related to the percentage of peripheral blood lymphocytes derived from the longer-lived partner strain (B6), as based on H-2 typing (Warner et al., 1985).

The immunologic theory has been extended by the demonstration that the MHC, which in large part regulates the immune system, influences maximum LS, age-specific incidence of neoplasia, the rate of immunologic aging, (Meredith & Walford, 1977; Smith & Walford, 1977; Walford, 1987), and serves also to gather under one "genetic umbrella" a number of non-immune phenomena of aging, including aspects of DNA-repair, free radical damage, reproductive senescence (Lerner et al., 1988), and mixed function oxidases (Koizumi et al., 1987b; Walford, 1987). And programmed senescence has recently been shown to be MHC-influenced in protochordates (Harp et al., 1988)!

Dietary Restriction, Immune Function, and the MHC

First, it is clear that DR extends LS in animals which have no immune system, at least in the ordinary sense of the word, although a surprising number of invertebrate species do manifest features of cellular recognition, reaction, and memory (Cooper, 1982). To be inclusive, one would have to extend the meaning of "immune system" to encompass these phenomena, or speculate that the mammalian immune system derives from phylogenetically older systems such as the free radical scavenging systems (Walford, 1981), which may well be involved in aging. Immune function and immunosenescence are in this concept "evolved" features of a very old regulatory system.

Many more age-related changes have been documented in the immune system than studied by the DR paradigm. Nevertheless, it is clear, as detailed in Chapter 4, that DR exerts a profound influence upon immunosenescence. This fact is consistent with the thesis that in mammals

DR extends LS primarily or in part via immune system effects and/or perhaps by modulating MHC gene expression. For example, DR appears to modulate expression of the H-2-linked gene responsible for serum gp70 production in mice (Izui et al., 1981; Maruyama & Lindstrom, 1983). Such modulation would include immune genes as an easily measurable hallmark of expression of MHC-linked genes.

However, the evidence is equally consistent with the thesis that as part of the life extension induced by DR the immune system is kept "younger" longer by a mechanism whose ultimate origin lies elsewhere. In keeping with this latter surmise is the fact that non-DR mechanisms which at least in part "rejuvenate" the immune system have not been shown to extend maximum LS, including grafts of newborn or infant thymuses to older animals (Hirokawa & Makinodan, 1975) and injection of normal adult mice with thymic hormone (Hiramoto et al., 1987); however, even these negative experiments can be countered by the argument that only one of the multifactors of aging is being corrected (see *"Uni- and Multifactorial Aging,"* Chapter 1). While DR inhibits early thymus structural involution (Weindruch & Suffin, 1980), it does not appear to affect the early, mid- or late-life levels of thymosin $\alpha 1$ (Weindruch et al., 1988).

Available evidence allows some discussion of the above complexities with reference to DR's impact on aging and immunity in long- and short-lived mouse strains, the role of extrinsic and intrinsic factors in immunosenescence, age-related biochemical changes in immune system cells, and MHC-related but basically non-immune phenomena.

Long-Lived Strains

In long-lived strains virtually all aspects of age-related changes in the immune system thus far tested are substantially retarded by DR. Immunosenescence is most marked for cellular immunity, and DR affects this the most. Production of and sensitivity to IL-2 are decreased by age, and these are retarded or reversed by DR. Evidence exists that intrinsic defects in lymphocytes from old animals impede their response to mitogens (Tollefsbol & Cohen, 1986; Makinodan et al., 1987; Schwab & Weksler, 1987). Old lymphocytes display reduced protein synthesis and turnover following mitogenic stimulation, and this change can be ameliorated by DR (see sections on protein synthesis, Chapter 4 and this Chapter). Alterations in cyclic nucleotides occur with age in lymphocytes (Tam & Walford, 1980; Tollefsbol & Cohen, 1986) and preliminary evidence indicates that these can be retarded by DR (Walford et al., 1981a).

Mitogen-stimulated lymphocytes from older animals display an impaired glycolytic flux. Tollefsbol et al. (1981) showed that induction of 11 glycolytic enzymes in human lymphocytes by PHA stimulation decreased by 48 percent between the ages of 21 and 75 years. Agreeing with Tollefsbol and Cohen (1986), we suspect that pathways of glycolysis may be key factors in the faulty metabolism of proliferative cell populations of aged animals. Unfortunately, no data on the possible effects of DR on glycolytic pathways in lymphocytes are available as yet. Faulty calcium metabolism may be particularly important in lymphocyte proliferative declines with aging (Miller, 1987), but again no DR data are available.

If the superoxide ion and oxygen metabolites are in part a source of immune-complex mediated tissue damage in late life (Schwartz, 1985), DR might in part ameliorate age-related immune effects by inhibiting development of these agents.

Short-Lived Strains

In general, DR studies in short-lived strains parallel the above, but with some additions and/or differences. In B/WF$_1$ mice, DR enormously prolongs LS and retards immunosenescence and autoimmune disease. However, a low protein diet may delay autoimmunity, decrease the rate of thymic involution, inhibit the development of splenomegaly, and slow down the rate of development of age-related immunodeficiency, but will *not* change ultimate survival if the calorie intake is not lowered (Fernandes et al., 1976c; Fernandes, 1987). In short-lived autoimmune strains a high sucrose ad lib diet or DR may both increase the PFC response of mice to SRBC in vitro, and the cell-mediated cytotoxic response generated by in vitro exposure to allogeneic antigen, but only DR affects LS (Kubo et al., 1984b).

It thus appears that nutrients other than calories may affect the immune status and disease patterns of the various autoimmune strains while having no or at least much less effect on survival than calorie restriction. These findings suggest either that immune dysfunction is involved neither etiologically nor pathogenetically in aging, or else that special problems with short-lived strains render interpretation confusing.

MHC-Influenced But Non-Immune Phenomena

The effect of DR on certain MHC-influenced but non-immune phenomena may be significant. This area has been considered an extension of the original immunologic theory of aging (Walford, 1987). Levels of SOD and catalase are at least in part regulated by genes linked to the MHC (see *"Free Radical Neutralization,"* this Chapter). The effect of DR on these free radical scavenging enzymes has been discussed earlier (see *"Increased Free Radical Neutralization by DR,"* this Chapter). Thereto may be added the observation that in mice the MHC influences induction of xanthine oxidase activity by poly IC, and that elevated xanthine oxidase activity is associated with increased lipid peroxidation (Koizumi et al., 1986c). Age-related increases in lipid peroxidation in livers of rats and mice are reduced by DR (see *"Lipid Peroxidation and Lipofuscin,"* Chapter 4).

Evidence exists for an influence of the MHC on DNA repair (for review see Walford, 1987), and studies to date have indicated that DR may influence this parameter in spleen and liver cells (see "DNA Repair," this Chapter).

Activities of some of the mixed function oxidases (cytochrome p-450 enzymes) seem related to aging, either inversely in between-species comparisons (Schwartz, 1975), or directly within different inbred strains of mice (Nebert et al., 1984). There are many of these enzymes and their activities in the liver have been reported to decline with age in rats (Hawcroft et al., 1982; Sun et al., 1986), and in mice to decline in some instances (Schmucker, 1985), but not in others (Hawcroft et al., 1982; Koizumi et al., 1987b). To make matters more complex, they may decline with age in the liver but increase in other tissues (Sun & Strobel, 1986).

Recent studies of congenic mice indicated that the H-2 system influences basal and induced levels of some mixed function oxidases (Koizumi et al., 1986b & 1987b). However, we did not find DR in mice to exert any effect on either basal or induced activity levels of several mixed function oxidases, including aryl hydrocarbon hydroxylase (Koizumi et al., 1987b), which is one of the enzymes influenced by H-2. On the other hand, Sachan and Das (1982) noted that in rats, short-term 50 percent DR increased the activities of aniline hydroxylase and p-nitrobenzoate reductase. If mixed function oxidases in fact play a role in oxidation reactions leading to accumulation of altered enzymes with aging, via H_2O_2 production (Oliver et al., 1987), and possibly to DNA strand breakage by a similar pathway (Cantoni et al., 1987), DR might in part exert its effect by upregulation of free radical scavengers to prevent the damage. Short-term DR (70 days) has indeed been shown to decrease the percentage of altered heat-labile enzymes (in this instance, of two aminoacyl-tRNA synthetases) in elderly mice (Takahashi & Goto, 1987). Orchestration of some of these effects by a common genetic system, the MHC, remains a distinct possibility.

Conclusion

No clearcut picture emerges from the above various studies of possible interrelations of DR, aging, the mixed function oxidases, free radical scavengers and the MHC, but further work is clearly indicated.

THE BASAL/INDUCED ACTIVITY HYPOTHESIS

Johnson et al. (1986) suggested that DR may exert its influence preferentially at the stage of initiation of cell replication. We have proposed that DR may act in part by retarding the basal turnover rate of proliferative or potentially proliferative cell populations (e.g., by lengthening the G_1 period), at the same time enhancing the proliferative as well perhaps as other responses to an inductive stimulus (Walford et al., 1987). Such a condition would have the dual benefits of retarding programmatic or deteriorative aging while increasing adaptability to environmental stimuli, and would accord with the observation that DR animals are both long-lived and have increased resistance to disease. Prior studies in our laboratory on NK cells support such a concept (Weindruch et al., 1983). We found diminished NK cell activity in unstimulated DR mice, but increased activity after stimulation, compared to controls (see "Immune Response Capacities" in Chapter 4).

Other scattered observations may support our view. In rodents, protein synthesis was found to decrease only slightly with age in resting lymphocytes, but on mitogen stimulation a dramatic decrease was observed (Cheung et al., 1983). It is well known that DR sharply increases mitogen-induced T cell proliferation. In rodents subjected to long-term DR, mitotic indices of pineal gland cells (Walker et al., 1978) and hamster cheek pouch cells (Andreou & Morgan, 1981) were found to be decreased. Short-term DR in mice down to about half of ad libitum intake reduced the mitotic indices of epidermal cells by 75 percent (Bullough & Ebling, 1952). Koga and Kimura (1978, 1979, 1980) reported that relatively short-term DR (60% of ad libitum intake) decreased the poliferative pool size and mitotic activity in crypts of the small intestine (Nevertheless, DR increases the ability of the small intestine to absorb vitamin A [Hollander et al., 1986] while opposing age-increases in crypt cellularity [Heller et al., 1987].). When mice are subjected to intermittent feeding for a period of weeks, the recovery of their hemopoietic system following irradiation is enhanced, with expansion of the pool size at time of irradiation, and more intensive proliferation after irradiation (Kozubik et al., 1985). The peripheral blood of short-lived autoimmune strains of mice on DR shows about a 50 percent reduction in white blood cell count (Kubo et al., 1984b).

In ongoing work with long-lived strains under DR, we have observed not only a reduced total white blood cell count, but a relative lymphopenia. Data are shown in Table 5.9. Spleens are comparatively more reduced in size in DR animals than most other organs (Weindruch et al., 1986). Note that these seemingly lymphocyte-poor DR animals can mount strong immune responses and are more resistant to develop spontaneous tumors than controls.

TABLE 5.9

Influence of Dietary Restriction Upon White Blood Cell and Differential Counts in Female Mice of a Long-Lived Strain[a]

Diet	Age	Total WBC/mm^3	Neutrophils (%)	Lymphocytes (%)
Control	9 mo	2017 ± 380	24 ± 2	70 ± 2
	22 mo	1991 ± 338	30 ± 3	65 ± 3
Restricted	14 mo	950 ± 262	48 ± 5	49 ± 5
	22 mo	1070 ± 160	69 ± 7	31 ± 6

[a]Data are our unpublished observations in C3B10RF$_1$ female mice fed control (about 80% of ad lib intake) and DR (about 50% of ad lib intake) regimens.

When fibroblasts in tissue culture are placed under conditions in which no division occurs but cell maintenance is adequate, and are then returned to normal conditions, they go on to achieve the same number of total doublings. Even if refed only once every several weeks, they reach the same replicative LS (Cristofalo, 1983). Thus, cells measure sequential molecular events, not chronologic time. But the LS of the whole animal measures chronologic time! We postulate that a decrease in the basal (i.e., non-induced) rate of proliferative turnover will prolong organismal time (= LS) without actually altering the sequential molecular events involved in aging. The Hayflick phenomenon can thus be married to the DR model.

While the data are not entirely clearcut, prior studies in holometabolous insects suggest that DR extends LS during the larval (proliferative) stages but not during the adult (post-mitotic) stage (see "STUDIES IN INVERTEBRATES," Chapter 2, plus Everitt & Porter, 1976). To the extent that this observation is supported by further study, it accords with our view towards proliferative systems as being prime mover(s) in DR's effect on aging in general, and therefore towards their being major components in mammalian aging, as we now know it. Amelioration of these proliferative systems changes might then shift the driving force of mortality in a longer-living population towards changes in non-proliferative systems. Dietary restriction does affect these systems, for example the age-related loss of corneal cells, which are post-mitotic (Nadakavukaren et al., 1987) but the extent of its influence is not yet well delineated.

Implicit in a basal/induced proliferation hypothesis is the concept that while aging changes may well occur in post-mitotic cells, these are less clearcut—for example in the liver (Popper, 1987), skeletal muscle (McCarter & McGee, 1987), or even brain (Mann, 1987), and/or less immediately connectable to reduced organismal survival, than changes in proliferative cell populations. Thus, in a multifactorial aging complex, proliferative systems come first, and it is in these that DR is particularly effective.

To put the matter another way, the downswing in the current rectangularized survival curves of mammalian populations under laboratory conditions reflects, on a pathenogenic (not necessarily etiologic) level, failure of proliferative cell systems. If this is in part prevented, as by DR, the downswing of the expanded survival curve may to a greater degree than at present reflect failure on a pathogenetic level of post-mitotic systems.[5]

---

[5]Indeed Peters et al. (1987) reported that while DR increased LS in rats, the very old LS-extended DR animals sustained a loss of neurons in area 17 of the cerebral cortex. Unfortunately, the DR regimen consisted simply of giving a smaller amount of the same diet. It is quite possible that this could extend LS by its effect on proliferative systems but be of marginal nutritional value, and detrimental to certain other cell systems. Studies of this nature which do not use isonutrient diets are in our view seriously flawed.

A corollary to the above would be that if aging could be substantially retarded by manipulation of proliferative cell populations, disease problems associated with post-mitotic cell aging could become more manifest in a longer-living population. Jut as we have seen a striking shift in human disease patterns from 1869 to 1970 (Walford, 1983, one might anticipate the possibility of another shift to neurological and musculoskeletal diseases in populations in whom maximum LS had been greatly extended.

SYSTEMS ANALYSIS

So far in this chapter we have more or less limited our purview to theories of aging about which pertinent DR data are available. In the present section we must relax this criterion. There has been as yet very little in the way of a "systems analysis" treatment of aging to serve as background. Implicit in the idea of systems analysis, however, is the concept that new properties "emerge" from the interactive combination of parts, that the whole is more than the sum of the parts when there are complex interactions. This basically non-reductionist approach to biology does not fit well with current paradigms, but an excellent in-depth example of its scope may be found in H.T. Odum's book, *Systems Ecology, An Introduction* (Odum, 1983) (The animal body can also be viewed as an ecological system.), and the recent book edited by Yates (1987), *Self-Organizing Systems, The Emergence of Order*. Prior gerontological papers that deal at least partly with a systems approach are those of Still (1969), Wright and Davison (1980), Rosen (1981), Walford et al. (1983), Walford (1986a), and Hibbs and Walford (1988).

Implicit in systems analysis of the aging process is the idea that aging and certain other aspects of biology (development, for instance) cannot ultimately be explained by means of a reductionist approach. Aging may involve interdependent changes dictated by complex reactions between organs, cells, cellular components, and communication systems in which the driving force is the relation between events rather than the events themselves. As the cumulative failure of many components within a multicellular organism, aging cannot be explained by simple models such as free radical damage, or the metaphor of "programmed senescence," and it may be insufficient or an oversimplification to invoke the action of genes as being primarily responsible for controlling variation in LS. As there is merely reductionist faith but no hard evidence that "gene expression" is the main type of cellular activity controlling the rate of aging (a corollary of the "gene is God" school of biology), so explanations of aging must be sought at a level of complexity and/or integration that is much greater than the interplay of genes. According to this view, aging is a "multi-rate-limiting-events-process" (Wright & Davison, 1980). Like a fractal surface, it in fact has a higher dimension than the sum of its parts (Mandelbrot, 1982; Rucker, 1987).

One guiding postulate of a systems analysis of aging might be that for evolutionary reasons species survival takes preference over individual survival. It is gratifying to note that this postulate derives from a nutritional experiment, that of Ross and Bras (1974), which we have elsewhere designated "the parable of Ross' rats" (Walford, 1986a). Given free choice of food types, rats will so select as to maximize growth rate, body size, and (probably) fecundity, to the eventual detriment of individual health and longevity.

A second postulate might be what has elsewhere been termed "hierarchical homeostasis" (Walford et al., 1983), which means that within each system or subsystem there exists a hierarchy of requirements for homeostasis. For example, at the whole organism level one of the highest requirements is to maintain brain oxygenation. We know that other systems will readjust and even be largely compromised to sustain this end. At another level, a prime requirement might be to maintain a constant energy charge within the cell (Walford & Tam, 1981). However, as DNA damage progresses and requires repair, it appears that the pool of NAD^+ may be depleted (Licastro & Walford, 1986), which could lead in turn to depletion of ATP and cell death. If so, then DNA integrity can be assumed to take precedence over energy charge. At another level, a prime requirement might be to avoid anti-self destructive immune reactivity (Rather than react against myself I won't react against anything; hence the immunodeficiency of aging.). Hierarchical homeostasis, or what components of a subsystem are preserved at the expense of others, could be assumed to result from evolutionary selection.

If aging is multifactorial (see *"Uni and Multifactorial Aging,"* Chapter 1), the various factors may correspond to or reflect, as a first approximation, the major current theories of aging: the DNA damage/repair theory, the immunologic theory, the free radical theory, and others. While these factors may individually affect aging and survival, they clearly also interact with each other.

One approach to a systems analysis of aging, that of Hibbs and Walford (1988), attempts to consider the interactive factors in a manner that derives from analysis of coupled systems, and may be summarized as follows:

A coupled system is one in which the output of one system (e.g., that regulating DNA damage and repair) affects the behavior of another, and vice versa. For example, DNA damage affects immune function. Altered immune function (e.g., allowing the development of autoimmunity) may lead to accumulating DNA damage. Now if X = a measure of the state of health of system X (e.g., where X equals the level of unrepaired DNA damage), and Y = the state of health of system Y (e.g., the functional capacity of the immune response), and t = the passage of time after an injury, then, as a simple example, suppose these two equations govern the changes in X and Y under normal circumstances:

$$(1) \quad \frac{dX}{dt} + kX = aY$$

$$(2) \quad \frac{dY}{dt} + jY = bX$$

where $\frac{1}{k}$ = the time for X to recover to a level equal to $\frac{1}{e}$ (where e = the natural logarithm) of the magnitude of the original displacement of X if a = 0 (Panel A1, Figure 5.7), and, in a similar manner, $\frac{1}{j}$ = the time for

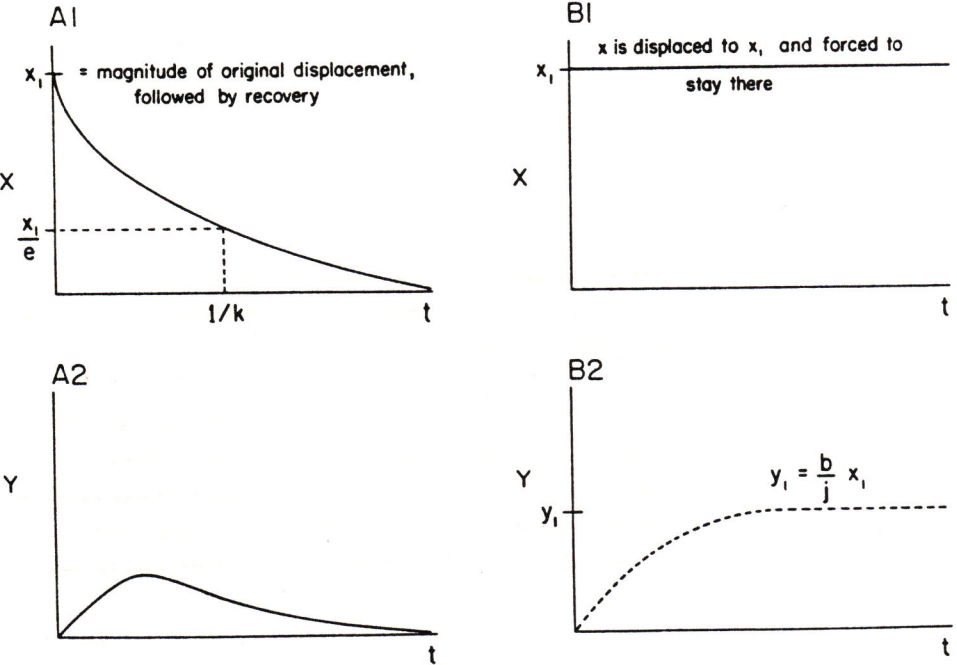

Figure 5.7. Illustrative derivation of recovery constants (k in Panel A1), and coupling constants (b in Panel B2). Adapted from Hibbs and Walford (1988).

Y to recover to a level equal to $\frac{1}{e}$ of the magnitude of an original displacement of Y if b = 0. Constants k and j are thus inverses of the recovery times. They are called "recovery constants," or (in physics) "decay constants."

Now in equations (1) and (2), a and b are the "coupling constants." A coupling constant can be defined as follows. If X is displaced to X_1 and forced to stay there (Panel B1, Figure 5.7), then Y rises to a new equilibrium level of $\frac{b}{j}X_1$, and visa versa for a. Thus a and b are defined, and can be determined by experimental manipulation of the systems. For example, if a constant level of unrepaired DNA damage can be for a while maintained (Panel B1, Figure 5.7), and the immune response shifts to a different level, then one could determine b for the immune system in this interaction (Panel B2, Figure 5.7). Notice that it is not necessary to know the *pathway* whereby DNA damage leads to immune system alteration. The pathway may be considered as a "black box."

The solution of equations (1) and (2) can be expressed as follows:

$$(3) \quad X = e^{-\tau t}(Ae^{\alpha t} + Be^{-\alpha t})$$

$$(4) \quad Y = e^{-\tau t} b \left(\frac{Ae^{\alpha t}}{\alpha + j - \tau} - \frac{Be^{-\alpha t}}{\alpha - j + \tau} \right)$$

where A, B, are constants depending on the initial conditions, and α and τ are constants depending on j, k, a and b as follows:

$$\tau = \frac{j + k}{2} \quad \text{and} \quad \alpha = \sqrt{\left(\frac{j + k}{2}\right)^2 + (ad - jk)}$$

Next suppose that at time = 0, one of the variables, say X, is displaced from its equilibrium value. As time passes, Y will be affected via the coupling of X into the equation for Y (Eq. 2). If $\alpha < \tau$, then both variables will eventually return to zero, their equilibrium positions. X will follow a path similar to (but not identical with) that illustrated in A1 of Figure 5.7, and Y will follow a path like that of A2 of Figure 5.7. This course of events requires that jk > ad. If, on the other hand $\alpha > \tau$, then the values of both variables will diverge exponentially in response to any disturbance of either one. This would occur if jk < ad.

To connect the above type of analysis more directly to concepts about aging, we note that for most forms of biologic injury, the recovery time in fact does tend to grow longer with increasing age. As the recovery time lengthens, j and k become smaller. Nevertheless, *without coupling*, each system would eventually recover. With coupling present, however, there is a critical value for recovery times. In our simple example, these critical times might be labeled $\frac{1}{j_c}$ and $\frac{1}{k_c}$, where $j_c k_c = ad$, i.e. the critical recovery times depend on the coupling constants. (Note: we assume that the change in recovery times is so slow compared to the recovery times themselves, e.g. a matter of years compared to a matter of hours, days, or weeks, that we can neglect $\frac{dj}{dt}$ and $\frac{dk}{dt}$ in equations [1] and [2]).

It is also generally observed that with aging the level of damage or change from which a system is able to recover decreases. This phenomenon might be explained by an age-related change in the coupling constants, a and b. Finally, it is interesting to note that long term changes in recovery times, such as k and j in this example, can be shown to be related to the exponential growth of mortality rates in populations (Hibbs & Walford, 1988).

The above represents a simplified systems analysis approach applied to aging. To go forward: (1) more than two interacting systems would have to be permitted in the analysis, (2) more complicated differential equations would need to be considered, and (3) experiments would have to be conducted to observe the responses of two or more systems to input disturbances, whereby the coupling constants could be derived. Dietary restriction does in fact represent such an input disturbance. Most major factors underlying the different theories of aging appear to be altered by DR, which therefore may be assumed to alter the coupling constants. As a next step following determination of the coupling constants, methods to determine recovery times, which are *characteristics of the individual systems,* could be established. This "top-down" approach may be useful where one cannot easily uncouple the separate systems to conduct a typical reductionist analysis ("bottoms-up" approach), and where pathways are highly complex.

CONCLUSION AND INTERPRETATION

It remains to unify as much as possible the various points brought out in this chapter, and to present our current hypothesis about how DR affects aging. This involves a synthesis of the possibilities. It may also allow some insight into the aging process itself, a good thing since one studies DR primarily as a "model" system for investigating aging. Our synthesis is as follows:

Aging is a multifactorial process albeit with interaction between the various systems or factors, and can be broadly divided into aging of proliferative and non-proliferative systems, and into intrinsic cellular and extrinsically-caused aging events. A portion at least of the latter can be viewed as "programmed" events. All these impact upon one another, and can be viewed as coupled systems. The intrinsic cellular events are at least in part secondary to accumulating, unrepaired cellular damage caused by free radicals, glycosylation, or other processes acting in mitochondria and on membranes and DNA or chromatin.

Long-term dietary restriction of energy evokes an evolutionarily selected adaptive response whose main site of impact upon aging is at the level of proliferative systems. This adaptation involves a selective upregulation in repair and protective processes, an increased metabolic efficiency, a decreased production of damaging agents, and is accompanied by signals to the neuroendocrine network, particularly the hypothalamus. The signals may come from the release of transmitter substances, or the failure to release such substances, or by immune system, gonadal or other cells to make appropriate adjustments, for example in reproductive matters, to survive the time of energy restriction. As part of this survival adjustment, the neuroendocrine response may also involve glucoregulatory, thyroid, adrenal and sympathetic nervous system pathways. Intrinsic cellular aging events in non-proliferative systems do occur, but are less involved in the actual mortality (including maximum LS statistics) of fully fed populations than are intrinsic events in proliferative systems or extrinsic (programmed) events, but may become more important as causes of mortality in long-living calorically restricted populations. Beyond the adaptive DR response there remain a basic "program" for aging, the nature of which may not ultimately be accessible to a reductionist analysis.

CHAPTER 6

PROSPECTS FOR RETARDING HUMAN AGING BY DIETARY RESTRICTION

INTRODUCTION

EVIDENCE presented in the preceding chapters allows us to conclude firmly that in a variety of species, representing at least five different orders of animals, DR extends the maximum LS characteristic for the species. In rodents at least (other species have not been closely studied), DR also markedly decreases susceptibility to most diseases, and keeps the biomarker pattern "younger" longer. For some diseases, DR may exert not only a preventative but a therapeutic effect.

What is the probability that some or all of these effects would accrue in humans on an appropriate DR regimen? Can DR extend maximum human LS beyond its present limit of 110 to 115 years, with retention during most of that time of youthful or middle-aged vigor? Trying to answer these questions involves giving a judgement on the basis of imperfect evidence, and thrusts one into the polemical world of preventive medicine. But since, for example, The Gerontological Society of America has in the recent past sponsored two scheduled public debates on this subject (Schneider, 1985; Chesky & Zakeri, 1987), it seems appropriate and even required that we state our own views.

One may adopt various postures towards the question of human applicability. Pertinent evidence stems from two sources: animal experiments, which are extensive, and human epidemiologic data plus studies from related fields which may allow inferences to be drawn as to what effects DR might have in humans. The attitude that evidence must be "conclusive" before any human recommendations can be made for such a dietary goal is in our view simply evasive. For example, Ed Schneider, former Deputy Director of the National Institute on Aging, who is in fact a booster for DR studies in animals, has several times taken the public position, "I can tell you dietary restriction will work in rodents. I can't tell you it will work in humans." This not uncommon response simply avoids confronting the question of probabilities, and implies that recommendations about anti-aging regimens require a certainty that is not insisted upon for other preventative or therapeutic medical measures.

PROOF AND PROBABILITY IN MEDICAL PRACTICE

Let us illustrate the above thesis. The Council on Foods and Nutrition of the American Medical Association stated in 1962, ". . . there is not sufficient information available at the present time to warrant a change in the American diet aimed at preventing heart disease in the general population" (Darby, 1962). The Intersociety Commission for Heart Disease Resources (1970) recommended substantial dietary modification for preventing heart disease, but in 1971 the Task Force on Arteriosclerosis of the National Heart, Lung and Blood Institute (Arteriosclerosis, NHLBI Report, 1971) was unwilling to champion *any* substantial dietary modification for this purpose. In 1977 the Select Committee on Nutrition and Human Needs of the U.S. Senate recommended major alterations in diet to combat arteriosclerosis. In 1980 the Food and Nutrition Board of the National Research Council (Food and Nutrition Board, 1980a) was unwilling to recommend much at all in the way of nutritional changes, whereas in the same year and *on the same body of data* a committee of the American Heart Association (1980) advised life-long adoption of an altered diet. More recently the Council for Agricultural Science and Technology (1986), considering possible relationships between diet and coronary disease, would go no farther than saying, "Adequate daily intake of foods containing essential nutrients and reduced energy seems like a reasonable approach."

A number of other consensus reports could be cited showing a considerable spread of views, but the point hardly needs belaboring. In the past quarter century, prestigious panels of experts have argued for substantial changes in the food habits of Americans, and equally prestigious panels have maintained that the information is not adequate to support such recommendations. Indeed not until 1984 did the American Cancer

Society officially acknowledge the probable role of diet in promoting or preventing cancer.

MacGregor (1983) argues against a too rigorous position, represented by the views of some of the above committees, that "any alteration of diet, however unnatural or abnormal our present day diet may be, must be justified by careful scientific trials." To quote Stallone (1983) on the same issue, "To fail to promote dietary change is as firmly a public policy decision as to promote a change, for a primary characteristic of public policy is that a neutral position, such as deciding to wait for scientific clarification, is not truly neutral." A potential effect of this non-neutrality can be illustrated by Figure 6.1. If diet has in all probability such a marked influence on cancer susceptibility as indicated in the figure, to wait until this probability is formally proven by well-controlled experiments means consigning hundreds of thousands of people to cancer deaths in order to maintain a certain rigor of method.

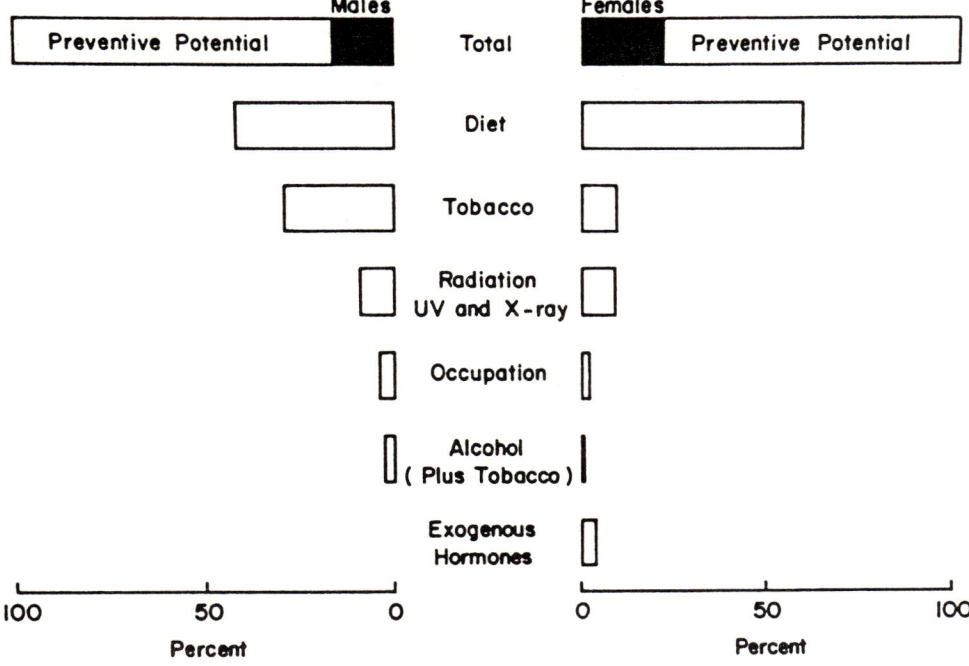

Figure 6.1. Environmental factors and cancer. Only 10-20 percent of cancers are primarily determined by genetic influences, as shown by the solid portion of the topmost horizontal bar. The rest are principally due to environmental effects, among which diet appears to be the most important. Adapted from Gori (1979).

Hegsted's astute remarks in his W.O. Atwater Memorial Lecture in 1985 are directly to the point, ". . . cancer (may) appear as many as 20 to 25 years after exposure. If dietary influences have a similar lag period, the possibilities of experimentally demonstrating presumably protective effects of diet become remote indeed." And again from Hegsted, "For many national health problems, the kind of clear-cut experimental evidence that everyone desires will not and cannot be produced anytime in the near future" (Hegsted, 1985). And to quote Al Meyerhoff, spokesman for the Natural Resources Defense Council, ". . . you've failed as a public health agency if you have to count bodies before you take action" (cited by Marshall, 1987).

The above conflicting views exemplify the fact that medicine has frequently and throughout its history chosen or been forced to recommend (or not recommend) procedures on the basis merely of probability or inferential evidence, or even on what one might designate an "educated guess." For instance, from about 1930 to 1960, and based largely on the "rate of living" theory of aging (for review, see Masoro, 1985b), and the related "General Adaptation Syndrome" of Selye, medical communities in the United States and Europe adopted an ultra-conservative attitude toward any exercise more vigorous than walking. Exercise was thought to cause the body to "wear out" more rapidly, to be "stressed." Medicine now holds the opposite view. For both these views, hard evidence is rather skimpy. The on-again off-again judgement of whether lowering blood cholesterol through diet and drugs might eliminate a significant share of the 500,000 yearly fatal heart attacks in the U.S. is another case in point. The modern shift in opinion about the dangers, or more recently the benefits of complex carbohydrates in diabetes represents a similar case of basing medical practice on judgement in the absence of unequivocal evidence.

A still further example: while evidence *within* rather than *between* populations for a role of excess sodium intake in the genesis of hypertension is hard to come by—and indeed *within* population data have been interpreted to favor not so much an excess of sodium as a deficiency of calcium (McCarron et al., 1982)—nevertheless on the basis of overall epidemiologic and clinical evidence in humans, and a small amount of experimental animal data, the American Heart Association, the American Medical Association, and the National Academy of Sciences have all recommended a decrease in salt intake for the general population.

Many additional examples of recommendations given on the basis of inferential or probability evidence can be cited, and indeed from throughout the entire history of medicine.

Vaccination for small pox and the provision of clean water and drainage in Europe in the 19th century were undertaken without hard evidence as to their benefits (MacGregor, 1983). Semmelweiss introduced sterile techniques into obstetrical delivery many years before the germ theory of disease was promulgated by Pasteur.

Not only preventive medicine but choice of therapy itself is often based on no better than consensus or probability evidence. The use of radical mastectomy as treatment for breast cancer on the old assumption that cancer spreads in concentric circles is a case in point (Rovner, 1987). The use of drugs (some of them toxic) to treat ventricular arrhythmias on the hypothesis (largely incorrect) that such arrhythmias represent an independent predictor of sudden cardiac death is another (Surawicz, 1987). Innumerable examples could be cited.

In the absence of experimental proof, medical practice is often based on judgement, judgement about matters not firmly established but which cannot or ought not be ignored. It is in part for this reason that medicine has been described as both an "art" and a science: the "art" of making right guesses on the basis of probability evidence, and ultimately and hopefully the "science" of hard-core biology.

PROFESSIONAL "AGEISM"

In the medical community one observes a strong tendency to subject recommendations about anti-aging measures to criteria which are much more demanding than those acceptable for other medical measures, i.e., no "art," only "science" is allowed. One is apt to read such pronunciamentos as "There is no unequivocal evidence that such diets (i.e., DR) influence the aging process in humans," without at first realizing that there is also no "unequivocal evidence" that lowering average blood cholesterol levels will affect susceptibility to arteriosclerosis, or decreasing fat intake the susceptibility to cancer, or that exercise has broad health benefits. In fact there is no "unequivocal evidence" for a sizeable portion of what modern orthodox medicine confidently prescribes, and for psychotherapy almost none. In our view, therefore, the tendency to demand "unequivocal evidence" before recommending regimens which may affect the rate of aging represents a sort of "ageism" (Walford, 1983) on the part of the biomedical profession.[1]

We shall now discuss evidence and conjecture supporting the proposition that DR, if properly carried out, would with a high order of probability, extend maximum human LS. A discussion of the contrary view follows.

EVIDENCE AND CONJECTURE IN FAVOR OF THE PROPOSITION

Are the Animal Data Translatable to Humans?

Small-scale phenomena sometimes are not translatable, but large-scale phenomena generally *are* translatable across mammalian species barriers. For example, man and other primates do not synthesize their own vitamin C. Rats and mice do. To translate the results of feeding experiments with vitamin C from rodent to man would be hazardous. Another example: when added to the diet, orotic acid induces hypocholesterolemia in rats, hypercholesterolemia in mice, and normocholesterolemia in hamsters and guinea pigs (Harden & Robinson, 1984).

In contrast to the above, large-scale phenomena seem for the most part translatable. The general operation of the immune system, the

---

[1] A personal anecdote illustrates the degree of irrationality that one may encounter when the question is posed, "Is it probable that DR will retard aging in humans, as it does in lower animals?" At the annual meeting of the Gerontological Society of America in New Orleans in 1985 one of us (RLW) participated in a public debate on this question. Later that same day RLW was chairman of a non-DR session which began with the projector bulb achieving its maximum LS, necessitating that RLW (as Chairman) had to ad lib for 5 minutes until the bulb was replaced. He inquired, "Most of you were at the debate this morning. How many were convinced that DR will very likely retard human aging, and how many think it will not?" The show of hands was about equally divided. But it was immediately apparent that most of the obese gerontologists thought DR would not work in humans, while most slim ones thought it would. That a group of sophisticated gerontologists, having just heard a debate on the subject, would still vote with their stomachs suggests that objective thinking is rare when life extension strategies are discussed.

Sociological gerontologists have their own form of "ageism," which in this context has been defined as having two components, (1) negative attitudes based on age-related stereotyping, and (2) distorted perception in the service of maintaining this stereotype (Kimmel, 1987). At the symposium "Life Extension and Ethical Considerations" held at the 1987 meeting of the Gerontological Society of America (Chesky & Zakeri, 1987: see also the report on this symposium in Washington Post, HEALTH section, Nov. 24, 1987), few of the invited sociogerontologist speakers were able to escape the vision of a Struldbrugian society (extension of maximum LS *without* retardation of aging) if LS is extended, even though such a projection is probably a biological impossibility. This attitude represents the type (2) component of "sociological ageism."

nature of DNA repair, the functioning of the neuroendocrine network — while details may differ, these phenomena appear quite similar among mammalian species. Growth, development, and aging probably proceed by similar or identical mechanisms in most mammals, and nutritional modulation of these can be classified as a large-scale phenomenon. As such, one would expect DR effects to be translatable. In his analysis of the evolutionary significance of the apparent relation between LS, reproductive fitness, and food supply (see "EVOLUTIONARY PERSPECTIVE," Chapter 5), Totter (1985) found no difference between human and other mammalian populations.

It is a fundamental tenet justifying animal experimentation that most findings in animals are relevant to and applicable to humans. Of course this is not always true, but usually it is. Dietary restriction retards aging in many different invertebrate species, in fish including both laboratory (Comfort, 1963; Walford, 1983) and wild populations (Reimers, 1979), and in rodents (as this book abundantly describes). Pilot studies (including average but not maximum LS observations) have shown positive effects in cattle (Pinney et al., 1972). In short, with few exceptions which can be viewed as special cases (see "STUDIES IN INVERTEBRATES," Chapter 2), DR extends maximum LS in all of the many species so far tested and across wide phylogenetic barriers. This does not prove it would do so in humans or other primates, but surely it allows us to presume, with a substantial order of probability, that it would. To be unwilling to make even a presumption to that effect (Rothstein, 1986) is close to saying that more than 50 years of animal experimentation on the subject (since McCay's 1935 report) are irrelevant to human application, which is not far from being an antivivisectionist position (Walford, 1986b).

Human Studies

Although sophisticated studies of the effects of long-term consumption of a calorically restricted but high quality diet on the health and LS of humans or other primates have not yet been done, a moderate amount of pertinent human data do in fact exist.

The Okinawan Population Isolate

The dietary intake of the population isolate on Okinawa approximates a low calorie/high quality regimen. The Okinawan data has been carefully scrutinized by Kagawa (1978). Accurate legal birth records have been kept in Japan since 1872. These indicate that the incidence of centenarians on Okinawa is 2 to 40 times that of any other Japanese island. The older data on longevity have been confirmed by a report issued in September 1987 by the Ministry of Welfare and Health in Koseisho. In Japan, a large scale accurate survey on nutritional intake has also been conducted by the Ministry of Health and Welfare, since 1946. Every year, data are collected from randomly chosen households in hundreds of districts in Japan by detailed personal interviews and direct weighing of the foods eaten during a period of three consecutive days.

The total energy consumed by school children in Okinawa (1300 kcal) is only 62 percent of the "recommended intake" for Japan. The intake of sugar is only about 25 percent of the average for Japan; of cereals, 75 percent; of green-yellow vegetables, 300 percent; and of meats (mainly fish), 200 percent that of the Japanese average. Total protein and lipid intake are about the same as, but energy intake for adults is about 20 percent less than, the national average. The average heights and weights on Okinawa are less than on mainland Japan. Death rates from cerebral vascular disease, malignancy and heart disease in Okinawa are only 59 percent, 69 percent, and 59 percent respectively of those averaged over the rest of Japan. In the last decade the total death rate of people 60-64 years of age was only 1280 in Okinawa but 2181 per 100,000 elsewhere in Japan.

Okinawa thus presents a longevous population, somewhat foreshortened in stature, with a substantially lower incidence of late life diseases. Kagawa (1978) comments: "Caloric restriction at a young age, provided that nutrients are balanced, is reported to cause both slow growth and longevity. In Okinawa, along with nutrition, the warm climate, hard continuous work, and genetic factors must be taken into account."

Recent studies by Takata et al. (1987) on the HLA distribution in different age brackets in Okinawans revealed an increased frequency of DR1 and a decrease in DRw9 in individuals over 90 years of age, suggesting a resistance to autoimmunity or immune deficiency syndromes in this older group. Since the HLA distributions of Okinawans in general is not different from that of main-island Japanese, the finding does not indicate that Okinawan longevity reflects a population-specific genetic trait, but perhaps that the general improvement of health and nutritionally retarded aging allows a genetic factor common to many populations to become manifest in this one. The role of the MHC (HLA in man, H-2 in mice) in regulating aging has been discussed in depth elsewhere (Walford, 1987).

Vallejo's Experiment

An experiment carried out by Vallejo (1957) and favorably cited by Stunkard (1976) represents the only example of a controlled DR study in humans. Healthy subjects over 65 years of age living in a religious institution for the aged received on the odd days in each month for three years a diet containing 2,300 calories per day, with 50 g protein and 40 g fat; and on even days, one liter of milk plus 500 g of fresh fruit. Such a diet is of good quality but not top-notch nutritionally. Sixty elderly persons in the same institution served as controls and were fed the 2,300 kcal diet every day. Over a period of 3 years of observation the DR subjects spent 123 days in the infirmary; the control subjects, 219 days ($p < 0.001$). Six of the DR subjects died, 13 of the control group (not statistically significant). The average age of both populations at time of initiation of the experiment was 72 years.

Anorexia Nervosa

Patients with anorexia nervosa often eat a good-quality diet, albeit in amounts leading to slow starvation (one egg a day, for example, nothing else!). Typically they restrict their intake of fat and carbohydrates but allow themselves relatively more protein in vegetables and low-fat cheeses. They undergo drastic BW loss but with considerably less comparative *mal*nutrition than seen in semistarved individuals from famine or poverty areas (Ayers et al., 1984; Casper, 1986).

Clinically, anorexics do surprisingly well despite their growing emaciation. They may reach BMIs as low as 15-16, yet remain symptom free and very active (Ayers et al., 1984; Waterlow, 1986). Far from being lethargic, they are typically hyperenergized. Serious problems do not generally occur until 30 to 40 percent of BW has been lost (Pertshuk et al., 1982). Despite an extremely low calcium intake, *post-pubertal* anorexic subjects do not experience an automatic increase in PTH levels, nor do they necessarily resorb calcium from bones (Ricotti et al., 1984). In this regard they almost exactly mimic the situation found in DR rats by Kalu et al. (1984a & b). On the other hand, patients with severe anorexia of early *teenage* onset may show significant osteopenia (Ayers et al., 1984). In part this could be due to delay in the steroid-mediated pubertal increase in cortical thickness, i.e., what might be anticipated on a DR regimen.

During the early stages of anorexia, the patients show if anything a normal (Bowers & Eckert, 1978) or even *increased* resistance to infection, and immune responses equal to or even *higher* than control values (Golla et al., 1981; Pertshuk et al., 1982). Responses of lymphocytes to the mitogens PHA and Con-A may be significantly elevated above control values (Golla et al., 1981). This same phenomenon of heightened immune response capacities is of course characteristic of DR rodents. Paradoxically, this pattern of heightened immune response to a stimulus may be accompanied by a basal (i.e., unstimulated) state of leukopenia with relative lymphopenia in both anorexic humans and DR rodents (Bowers & Eckert, 1978; Pertshuk et al., 1982; Tables 4.10 and 5.9).

Long-Term Dietary Studies

Long-term (3-9 months) very low-calorie, (usually around 400 kcal/day), supplemented diets have been investigated in the treatment of obesity and of diabetes (Carmena et al., 1984; Hughes et al.,1984; Zimmerman et al., 1984; Howard, 1985). While these are much more hypocaloric than are typical life-extending DR regimens, and would lead to outright caloric starvation if continued indefinitely, they tend to yield metabolic effects in humans resembling those seen in rodents on DR, including an improved insulin response and regulation of blood sugar. Furthermore, on a 500 kcal per day intake with 50 g protein, humans may show slightly greater protein synthesis and turnover than on a 2000 kcal per day 75 g protein diet (Genuth, 1985). This is quite reminiscent of the situation in DR rodents (see sections on protein synthesis in Chapters 4 and 5).

Like other animals, the human adapts to long-term, low-calorie regimens, but in this regard has not been well studied. It is important to realize that one can infer very little from short term experiments as to long-term effects. For example, 1 week on a 500-750 kcal per day diet led to a 20 percent *decrease* in endurance (exercise time to exhaustion), but 6 weeks on this same intake led to a 55 percent *increase* in endurance (Horton, 1982: Phinney, 1985), with a decrease in the oxygen cost of exercise, i.e., an improved exercise efficiency.

The oft-cited Minnesota study by Keys et al. (1950), involving 32 conscientious objectors not long after World War II, may clarify one essential point. On a 1,600 kcal per day diet for 6 months, the subjects lost an average of 25 percent of BW. They were listless and apathetic. However, the diet used, constructed to resemble the semi-famine intake of a number of European countries immediately after World War II, consisted largely of cabbage, turnips, whole-wheat bread, cereals and potatoes with only token amounts of meat and dairy products. Thus the subjects received not merely a low calorie but a *malnutrition* diet. This is quite unlike what is sought in rational human weight loss, or in the best rodent DR regimens. It is worth noting that poor Indian laborers work well and are symptom free with a Body Mass Index (BMI = wt(kg)/ht(m)^2) of 15-16, no greater than Keys' semistarved subjects, and with a body fat content of 6 percent (Waterlow, 1986). Despite the undoubtedly malnourishing state of their diet, they have achieved a long-term adaptation at least to the energy differential.

Other Dietary Studies

Fasting has been reported to favorably affect human rheumatoid arthritis, an autoimmune disease (Skoldstam and Lindstrom, 1979). Correspondingly, DR is known to exert a highly favorable effect on diverse autoimmune diseases in mice (see *"Studies With Mice" and "Short-Lived Strains,"* Chapter 3).

Hypotheses linking fat intake to cancer of the breast and certain other organs are based largely on cross-country comparisons. Caloric reduction clearly decreases cancer risk in animals, and nutritionists are coming to realize that it also does so in humans, and to a considerable degree (Albanes, 1987a, b). This constitutes yet an additional factor favoring the "translatability" of the DR effect. Moreover, to quote Pariza (1987), "Current hypotheses on the diet/cancer link that focus on specific nutrients (e.g. fat) as cancer risk factors for humans are not supported strongly or consistently by epidemiologic data." Stemmermann et al. (1984) proposed that the balance among energy consumption, retention, and expenditure might represent a common underlying factor.

Thus it may be calories, instead of or in addition to fat, that makes the difference (Pariza, 1986; Kolata, 1987). A caloric effect would accord better with the animal evidence. In mice DR markedly reduces the incidence of breast cancer (see Table 3.4), and in carcinogen-induced mammary cancer in rats modest caloric restriction will almost completely override the tumor enhancing effect of a high fat intake (see Table 3.13 and Figure 3.8).

While not a DR study, the report by Borkan et al. (1986), which included measurements of vital capacity in relation to weight change among 1396 men followed longitudinally for 15 years, is of great interest. Vital capacity appears to be an excellent biomarker of aging in humans, and seems independent of environmental influences such as physical fitness (Walford, 1986a). It's age-related rate of fall showed some degree of inverse correlation with BW gain.

Comment on Human Studies

Thus humans in various weight loss situations, especially if chronic, and providing the quality of the intake is good, display certain physiologic changes like animals on LS-extending DR. There may also be differences, however, and one can clearly emphasize either the similarities or differences. The difficulty with such comparisons is that the human data usually entail rather rapid BW loss and/or that the human diet has not been carefully controlled as to quality.

Nevertheless, to the extent that the data permit, Table 6.1 compares physiologic changes in humans on regular BW loss programs, humans on fasting or semi-starvation regimens, and anorexic humans, with mice and rats on quick weight loss regimes (usually starvation), and mice and rats on long-term DR. Among the similarities, and noting that insulin resistance is increased in diabetes mellitus (Rosenthal et al., 1982), a disease showing many features of accelerated aging (Monnier et al., 1984), we note that insulin resistance is increased in normal human aging (Rowe et al., 1983) but decreased by caloric restriction both in humans (Hughes et al., 1984) and in rodents (Reaven et al., 1983a). It seems also that caloric restriction has little or no effect on islet cell function in either humans or rodents. Many other human/rodent similarities are evident from the table.

We conclude from the inherent probability of translatability to humans of numerous almost uniformly positive animal studies, coupled with the fact that diverse (albeit limited) human studies do point in the same direction, that DR will with a high order of probability retard the rate of aging and extend maximum LS in humans.

EVIDENCE AND CONJECTURE AGAINST THE PROPOSITION

Actuarial Analyses

Using insurance company data from a number of studies, Andres (1980, 1981) and Keys (1980) concluded that the heaviest and thinnest individuals in the population had the shortest survival, while those slightly over the "ideal body weight" at mid-life or later survived longest.

TABLE 6.1
Comparative Findings in Humans on Reduced-Intake Weight Loss Programs, Fasting or Semi-Starvation or "Very Low Calorie" Diets, and Anorexic Humans, with Fasting and Long-Term Calorically Restricted Rodents[a]

Parameter	Humans			Rodents (m = mice, r = rats)	
	Reduced Intake, moderate (15% below norm)	Fasting, Semi-Starvation or "Very Low Calorie" Diet (<800 kcal)	Anorexics	Fasting or Very Short-Term DR	DR
Hormonal					
Thyroid related					
T3 in serum	↔ or ↓(1)	↓↓(2-7,8); ↓, then ↔(9); CHO sensitive(8)	↓↓(5,10-12)	↓↓(r13-16); ↔(r17,18)	↓(r19,20,21); ↔(22)
T3 resp. to TRF		↓(7)	↔(5)		↓(r19)
T4	↔(1)	↓(5); ↔(3,4,6,8)	↔(10,11,23)	↓(r13)	↓(r19)
TSH in serum	↔(1)	↔(3,5,6)↓(8)	↔(10,11,23)	↓↓(r13,24)	↔(m29)
peak TSH resp. to TRH		↓(5,7,9);↑then ↔(8)	↔but delayed(11)	↓(r13,24)	
Other Hormonal and Related Factors					
Growth hormone in serum		↑(25);↑↑then ↔(5,26)	↑↑(10,11,27); ↔(23)	↓(r24);↑(r28)	↓(r19); ↔(m29)
Prolactin		↔(5),↓(8)	↔(10,12)	↓(r24)	↓(m29)
resp. to TRH		↓(5)	↓&delayed(11)	↓(r24)	↓(m29,r30)
FSH	↓(11)	↓(31)	↓↓(10,11,32); ↔(12)	↓then ↔(r24)	↓(r19)
resp. to LHRH	↔but delayed(11)	↓(33)	↔but delayed(11)	↓(r24)	
LH	↔(11)	↔(31)	↓↓(5,10,11,23)	↓↓(r24)	↑(r30)
resp. to LHRH	↑(11)	↓(33)	↓(5); ↔but delayed(11)	↓(24)	
Insulin in plasma		↓(25,31,34)	↓(35)		
Fasting blood sugar	↓(38)	↓(25,31,34)	↓(27,35,39)	↓(r38)	↓(r36,37)
Insulin resistance	↓(38)	↓(40)[b]	↓(35)	↓(r38)	↓(r37)
Plasma norepinephrine			↓(35,39,20)		↓(r36)[b]
Cortisol	(urinary) ↔(1)	(plasma)↑(8)	↑(39)		↑(r20)
Cardiovascular					
Heart rate			↓(39)	↓(rabbit,41)	

Table 6.1 (continued)

Parameter	Humans Reduced Intake, moderate (15% below norm)	Humans Fasting, Semi-Starvation or "Very Low Calorie" Diet (<800 kcal)	Anorexics	Rodents (m=mice, r=rats) Fasting or Very Short-Term DR	Rodents (m=mice, r=rats) DR
Blood pressure			↓(39)	↓(r42)	--(r66)
Cardiac symp. nervous system activity	↓(43)			↓(r42)	
BMR: whole animal	↓then--(44)	↓(45,46)	↓(11,39)	↓(Tbl. 4.18)	↓(Tbl. 4.18)
per LBM or BMI	↓(47)	↓↓, then↓or--(2)	--(11,47)	↓(Tbl. 4.18)	--(r19,48)
Internal body temperature				↓↓(m50)	↓(m51,52)
Protein synthesis, turnover		--or↓(53)			
Heart				↓(r54)	↑(r55,19)
Skeletal muscle				↓(r54)	↓(r55,19)
Liver				↓(r56)	↑(r57)
Immune system					
Antibody response	↓(58)		--or sl. ↓(32)		↑(m59)
T-cell mitogen resp.	↑(58)	↓(60)	↑↑(61) or ↓(60)		↑↑(m51)
WBC pattern			leucopenia w/relative lymphopenia (21,62-65)		leucopenia w/relative lymphopenia (Table 5.9)

[a]References: (1) Garrel et al. (1984); (2) Barrows and Snook (1987); (3) Merimee and Fineberg (1976); (4) Vagenakis (1977); (5) Carlson et al. (1977); (6) Sherwin (1985); (7) Burman et al. (1980); (8) Jung et al. (1980); (9) O'Brian et al. (1980); (10) Vigersky et al. (1977); (11) Vigersky and Loriaux (1977); (12) Ayers et al. (1984); (13) Harris et al. (1978); (14) Schussler and Orlando (1978); (15) Rothwell et al. (1982a); (16) Cox et al. (1984); (17) Glass et al. (1978); (18) Rothwell and Stock (1982b); (19) Holehan and Merry (1986); (20) Nikitin (1979); (21) Merry and Holehan (1985a); (22) Snyder and Wostmann (1987); Snyder and Pollard (1982); (23) Brown et al. (1977); (24) Campbell et al. (1977); (25) Cahill et al. (1966); (26) Palmbland et al. (1977); (27) Casper et al. (1977); (28) Holehan (1984); (29) Sarkar et al. (1982); (30) Merry and Holehan (1981); (31) Cahill et al. (1973); (32) Smith (1978); (33) Warren et al. (1975); (34) Saudek and Felig (1976); (35) Zuniga-Guajardo et al. (1987); (36) Reaven et al. (1983a & b); (37) Reaven and Reaven (1981b); (38) Landsberg and Young (1981); (39) Casper (1986); (40) Hughes et al. (1984); (41) Reyman and Schmidt (1979); (42) Einhorn et al. (1982); (43) Chebotarev et al. (1976); (44) Garrow (1986); (45) Sherwin (1985); (46) Keys et al. (1950); (47) Waterlow (1986); (48) Masoro et al. (1982); (49) Wimpfheimer et al. (1979); (50) Webb et al. (1980); (51) Weindruch et al. (1982c); (52) Cheney et al. (1983); (53) Genuth (1985); (54) Curfman et al. (1980); (55) Goldspink et al. (1987); (56) Howard et al. (1986); (57) Richardson (1985); (58) Good et al. (1981); (59) Walford et al. (1973/4); (60) Cason et al. (1986); (61) Golla et al. (1981); (62) Young and Scrimshaw (1971); (63) Carryer et al. (1959); (64) Bowers and Eckert (1978); (65) Pertshuk et al. (1982); (66) Yu et al. (1985).

[b]Interestingly, in both of these studies, islet cell function was not affected by dietary restriction.

Andres' analyses are reflected in the curves of Figure 6.2, which represent reinterpretations of earlier studies, but also accord with Metropolitan Life data published in 1983. Mortality was lowest at 10 percent to 25 percent above average BW. The data of Figure 6.2 suggest that subsequent mortality after age 65-74 may have been least for mildly underweight persons, but that at all lower ages persons about 10 percent to 15 percent above average weight experienced the lowest mortality.

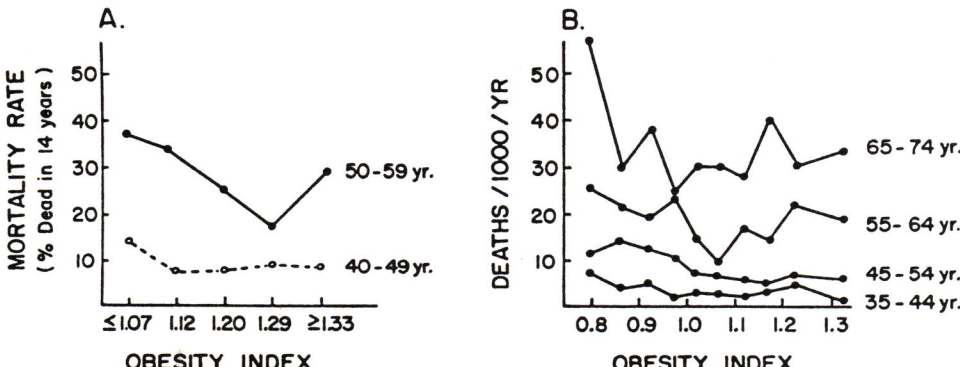

Figure 6.2. Two large-scale, long-term studies of the relation between obesity and subsequent death rates. Obesity index of 1.0 represents average weight for an individual's height and age group. In panel A, from the Chicago Peoples' Gas Co. Study, death rates are the percent who died in the 14 years after the obesity indexes were determined. In panel B, from the Framingham study, death rates are expressed as the number dying within the next year, per 1,000 of population. In both panels the age groups are those at the start of the studies. Adapted from Andres (1980).

An analysis of the Framingham data by Hubert et al. (1983) did not seem to square with 1983 Metropolitan Life "desirable weight" tables, and indicated that among the 5209 men and women of the original Framingham cohort followed for 26 years the minimal mortality occurred at the previously published, i.e., 1959, levels of desirable weight. Nevertheless, analyzing these same Framingham data, Andres (1980) as we have seen (Fig. 6.2) located the highest mortality rates among the leanest people in most age groups.

What are we to make of these various data, these conflicting views? First of all, the trend of the data do not seem in doubt (Stunkard, 1983). Recent general population data indicate that underweight persons experience higher mortality, slightly overweight persons the lowest. But the underlying question remains, what does this mean biologically?

The "heavier is better" thesis has been advanced as evidence against the applicability of DR to humans (Rothstein, 1986; Andres, 1980 & 1981). We have responded to this elsewhere in some detail (Walford, 1986b). A contrary analyses is also given by Stunkard (1983).

In essence there are two major objections to the "heavier is better" thesis, which incidentally represents only a minority view among obesity experts (Rhoads & Kagan, 1983; Simopoulos & van Itallie, 1984; Manson et al., 1987; Chernoff, 1987).

The first concerns the actual data. Stunkard (1983) concluded that most of the mortality data are not adequately controlled for smoking: for example, in the Framingham study (Castelli, 1982) the proportion of smokers in the overweight group was 55 percent, as opposed to 80 percent in the underweight group. Increased mortality in the underweight group might reflect smoking habits rather than leanness per se. Waterlow (1986) pointed out that any increases in mortality with BMI less than 19 may well be an artifact of western societies, and does not necessarily obtain elsewhere. A recent reevaluation of the various published mortality data from Western sources by Manson et al. (1987) found three major biases: failure to control for smoking, inappropriate control of biologic effects of obesity (e.g., hypertension, hyperglycemia), and failure to control for low BWs due to subclinical disease. Allowing for these biases, it was concluded that minimum human mortality occurs at relative weights *at least 10 percent below* the U.S. average. Also, a recent careful analysis of data from the Normative Aging Study, started in 1961, showed that men who had lost 10 percent of their initial weight at time of entry into the study enjoyed the least age-related increase in coronary risk factors (Borkan et al., 1986).

Second objection: even if the Andres and Keys "heavier-is-better" thesis were correct for the general population, it might be quite irrelevant to the subject of caloric restriction. *The Andres/Keys data do not involve caloric intake!*

We may recall the study by Harrison et al. (1984) (Table 2.5, #18) which compared LSs of normal and genetically obese mice of B6 strain derivation. The ranges of the maximum 10th decile LSs of the mice were as follows: unrestricted genetically obese mice, 776-893 days; unrestricted normal mice, 954-976 days; restricted normal mice, 1,089-1,287 days; restricted genetically obese mice, 1,209-1,307 days: yet the "restricted obese" mice were of the same BW as unrestricted normal mice. If inbred strains of mice which are genetically highly obese, slightly obese, of normal weight, or slender are calorically restricted, they *all* live longer. It is quite possible that a similar situation would obtain in humans, and the initial "heavier-is-better" subgroup would live still longer if on DR, since individual BW correlates as much with genetic background as with actual food intake in humans.

Indeed, in populations of *fully fed* mice followed throughout life, we found no correlation between adult BW and LS (Weindruch et al., 1986), wherefrom one might have predicted that DR would not extend mouse LS either. But of course that would have been incorrect! It is probably wrong to use data from an ad lib population to try to predict survival of a DR population, in any species and including humans.

A number of additional objections to the "heavier-is-better" thesis may be found in Walford (1986a).

Masoro's Objections

Objections voiced by Masoro to the proposition that DR will prolong the human LS include the following:

(1) If a McCay-type DR regimen would extend maximum human LS, someone in history should have done it by happenstance and lived to exceed the recognized maximum human LS (Masoro, cited by Bennett, 1984). We find this a weak argument for several reasons. There are in fact claims of extravagant LS in history (Walford, 1983) but in the absence of vital statistics, no one accepts them. The argument thus becomes self-fulfilling. Also, since even today only one person in 50,000 to 100,000 lives to be 105 or more years of age, well over 100,000 persons would have to be "by happenstance" on DR for one or more to break the ordinary maximum LS barrier. Since the diet must not be too low in essential nutrients, only calories, this seems unlikely. In fact, Masoro (personnel communications) no longer favors the "someone ought to have stumbled onto it by chance" argument.

A corollary to the above is this argument: if DR would work in humans, one ought to be able to see evidence of it among currently long-lived populations (e.g. Swedes, Japanese and others) where substantial differences exist in environment and types of food eaten, yet the life expectancies are about the same. This corollary is wholly beside the point because these populations are nowhere near a DR regimen, and it is *energy* restriction, not type of diet, be it fish, fowl, whale, or corn, that retards aging. And the one population which seems substantially energy restricted, the Okinawans, may well have extended survival, as noted above.

(2) To quote other Masoro objections (Masoro, cited by Jacobson, 1986), "The rodent is metabolically a different animal than man," and "If all you have is rodent data, then you really have an open question. . ." The first objection here seems odd to the extent that it may refer to metabolic rates, in view of the fact that Masoro's own laboratory and has measured metabolic rates in DR and control rats and concluded that DR does not extend LS via a metabolic rate effect (Masoro, 1985b). Moreover, unicellular organisms are, one may contend, metabolically different than insects, which are different from worms, and worms from fish, and fish from rodents, yet DR works in all these species, so that one might facetiously conclude therefrom that humans should respond to DR the same as rodents *because* they are metabolically different.

As to the second quotation cited above, the DR effect is phylogenetically independent, and it is not at all true that "all you have is rodent data."

In claiming that the rodent is metabolically different from humans, Masoro apparently means to contrast the finding by his group (McCarter et al., 1985) that the oxygen consumption per lean body mass in DR rats is not less than in controls, with the observation that in fasting humans or in humans undergoing fairly rapid and extensive weight loss (for example, in the semi-starvation study by Keys et al., 1950), metabolic rate is decreased. On a 15 day fast, for example, the O_2 consumption of humans was decreased (Apfelbaum et al., 1971). The counterargument here is that one cannot legitimately compare DR rodents with relatively quick weight-loss humans. It must be quick weight-loss rodents with quick weight-loss humans, and here *both show decreased metabolic rates* (Table 6.1): or DR rodents with DR humans, and the latter are not readily available.

What scant data are in fact available suggest that, when expressed per lean body mass, DR humans might *not* have metabolic rates or oxygen consumption much less than fully fed humans. In one study (Garrow, 1986), obese women who had reduced and stayed reduced did not have a lower BMR than people of the same (lower-weight) body composition who had not lost weight, even though during the initial stage of reduction, their BMR was lower. An important study by Geissler et al. (1987) showed that the "calculated" BMR was the same for the long-term post-obese as for the lean, even though at all levels of activity the post-obese expended less energy and had a lower energy intake. This paper does on the whole suggest some differences between rodents and humans in the metabolic rate response to DR (and/or that further work is needed in rodents), although obese humans, like ob/ob and other mice, may have special metabolic characteristics (see Wise, 1977a; and James & Trayhurn, 1981). On 4 to 6 months of a very calorically low diet (429 kcal/day), Barrows and Snook (1987) found a 20 percent decrease in regular metabolic rate, but only a 7 percent drop when this was expressed per lean body mass. Even in the study by Keys et al. (1950), whereas a 1,600 kcal/day diet for 6 months led to a 30 percent drop in BMR, the decrease "per unit of active tissue" was only 10 percent. And in anorexia nervosa, with its great but usually long-term weight loss the metabolic rate "per cell mass" may not be different from normal (Ljungren et al., 1961). In some studies of severe anorexics the BMR was 80 percent of normal, but in others no decrease per kg of BW was found (Waterlow, 1986).

In short, none of Masoro's so far expressed objections seriously challenge the concept that DR ought to retard aging in humans, and the metabolic rate argument might well end by turning upon its maker.

The "differences" argument might also be made in the reverse direction. Dieting or fasting humans decrease gluconeogenesis and adapt their energy requirements to the long-term use of ketoacids derived from fatty tissues (Cahill et al., 1973). Rats similarly develop ketosis but deplete their body fat by 3-4 days, whereupon gluconeogenesis progressively increases. Unlike humans, they cannot survive prolonged starvation. Because of this greater adaptability, the severity of DR needed for a positive effect might be less critical in the human.

As a further development of the argument that "rodents and humans are different," it seems obvious that any difference that might induce one to predict failure of DR to work in humans ought to be relevant to the question. Rats have tails, humans don't. That's an irrelevant difference in terms of DR. It behooves those making this argument to conceptualize a difference that seems relevant, perhaps even a phenomenon that is similar in all lower animals (since DR works in all of them, special cases excepting, as noted in Chapter 2) but different in humans, if one presumes that DR will not work in humans. Disease differences are not relevant, as it is agreed generally that DR does not extend LS simply by influencing disease susceptibility, but strikes at fundamental biologic aging. Certainly, DR extends LS in different inbred strains and species of rodents whose disease patterns are widely different.

Other Arguments

An argument advanced by Comfort (1985) is "that mice and rats in the wild are annuals, and they may have a special device which enables them to overwinter by postponing their aging when their food supply is low, whereas humans already have a long period of latency introduced in their childhood. So probably the whole life cycle in primates, with this long latency period, is different in its control mechanism from what it would be in other mammals." This speculation is again a wholly rodent-oriented argument, and simply disregards the fact that the effects of DR seem, at least so far, to be phylogenetically independent.

Richard Cutler (personal communication) has argued that because all species tested for the effects of DR are short-lived, the mechanism of DR may be to "up-regulate something," and that perhaps in long-lived species this something has already been upregulated. It is difficult to form a firm opinion on this speculation, which does require, however, that DR work in short-lived bird species, not in long, in short-lived primate species (like marmosets) not in long (as humans), in short-lived fish species (like annual fish [Walford, 1983]) or guppies (Comfort, 1963) but not in long (like trout). But apparently DR does work in trout (Reimers, 1979)!

The above reflects what we regard as reasonable albeit probably incorrect conjectures against a DR effect on maximum LS in humans. In addition, a number of arguments against DR's applicability to humans have been put forward which largely reflect the non-familiarity of the authors with the relevant literature.

In their 1981 book "Vitality and Aging," Fries and Crapo (1981) avoid the human applicability argument by denying even that DR will increase maximum LS in laboratory animals, maintaining that it merely restores rodent LSs to what is "natural" for the species. We have treated this argument elsewhere (Walford, 1985). Suffice it to say that these authors, writing in 1979-1981, review no DR literature later than 1961 — a remarkable feat of oversight in view of the wealth of pertinent literature published subsequent to that date.

A parallel argument has been advanced by Munro (1981), to the effect that a large component of the life extension induced by DR may be secondary to a later occurrence and lower incidence of lethal diseases, rather than true retardation of aging. It should be unnecessary to point out at this juncture that significant extension of *maximum* LS can probably not be obtained merely by preventing disease, and that a later occurrence of specific diseases, being a good biomarker, would in fact support an age-retarding effect.

Harper (1982) advanced the argument against human applicability that "the research done so far has been with rodents which have a prolonged growth period, one that extends well beyond the time of sexual maturity." Again the persistent failure to see that DR experiments have not been limited to rodents! Even with regard to rodents, a prolonged (but asymptotic) growth curve obtains with rats but less so with mice and hamsters. And DR extends maximum LS in mice even if begun at one year of age, or even later (see *"Adulthood-Onset Dietary Restriction (ADR),"* Chapter 2), well beyond the period when growth has ceased entirely in this species. Finally, while human growth ceases a few years after sexual maturity, the time-span from birth to maturity is, in relation to total LS, much longer than for nearly any other species, leading Sacher (1977) to speculate that DR beginning in childhood in humans might in fact extend LS even more than in rodents.

Morrison (1983) asserts, as evidence against human applicability, that in underdeveloped countries or other situations where people are underfed, there is no increase in longevity. This argument is wholly untenable in view of the fact that such underfed populations are also *mal*nourished: their calorie restriction is usually accompanied by inadequate vitamin, mineral, and protein intake. Morrison (1983) writes also that "natural experiments do not show any signs of altering . . . the maximum potential life span." But in fact there are no appropriate "natural experiments" corresponding to the "undernutrition without malnutrition" regimen of DR rodents, with the possible exception of the Okinawans, whose survivorship data do in fact support extension of human LS by DR.

Both Morrison (1983) and Harper (1982) have maintained that in terms of possible human application, DR (in animals) gives a high infant mortality, stunted growth, impaired structural and functional development, and a greater susceptibility to bacterial and parasitic diseases, and such that surviving animals are highly selected. High infant mortality occurred sometimes in early experiments in this field, not currently. Stunting of growth does occur but only if DR is begun in childhood, not in adulthood. None of the other assertions by these authors have ever been a significant feature of DR, and are certainly not found at all in modern experiments.

In conclusion, there is no evidence against DR's ability to retard aging and extend LS in humans that cannot be readily countered. There is a fair amount of speculation that DR might not work in humans, much of it ill-informed and naive.

LEVEL OF RESTRICTION AND METHODOLOGY APPROPRIATE FOR A HUMAN STUDY

We shall not discuss here whether DR in humans would be socially or psychologically desirable. This point has been addressed in some detail elsewhere (Walford, 1983), and will be touched on later in this chapter. Here we are solely concerned with the biology of potential human application: at what age to begin, how rapidly to proceed, how much weight loss to induce, maintenance levels, the nature of a suitable diet for such a goal, potential dangers, and potential benefits besides actual life extension.

When to Begin

DR should not be recommended for humans during childhood, in view of the growth retardation routinely seen in rodents under DR, and the (less likely) risk that childhood mortality might be increased even though the survivors might enjoy greatly extended LSs. While DR is not "starvation," it is to be emphasized that the ability of an adult to survive prolonged starvation (50-60 days without supplements, and 100-200 days or even longer with vitamin and mineral supplementation) is not shared by children (Young & Scrimshaw, 1971). Children would presumably be more susceptible than adults to any negative effects of substantial restriction of energy intake. Note once more, that the so-called "experiments of nature" (famine, poverty, etc.) involving underfed children almost always involve *mal*nutrition.

An excellent example in mice of the difference between LS-prolonging DR (calorie restriction only) and "malnutrition" concerns the thymus. Extremely susceptible to "malnutrition," the thymus in malnourished animals undergoes profound involution, with corticomedullary involution and loss of lymphocytes, followed by degeneration and loss of Hassall's corpuscles. By contrast, "undernutrition" confined to energy restriction can actually inhibit thymic involution (Weindruch & Suffin, 1980; Good et al., 1982).

Restriction beginning at about 20 years of age in humans would, in our view, be free of the potential childhood drawbacks, yet afford the greatest extension of LS consistent with safety. It may never be too late to obtain some benefit. The data of Vallejo on a human population of average age 72 was referred to (Vallejo, 1955). Ingram has obtained a modest but significant increase in LS in mice commencing DR at 24 months of age in a strain with an average life expectancy of 26 months (Ingram, cited by Zoler, 1984).

But the time in life to begin also depends on the goal. If the goal be to determine whether DR (or any other intervention technique) will retard human aging, a biomarker program must be included. Most of the potential human biomarkers change only mildly up to mid-life, then begin fairly rapid alterations. Skin elasticity is a good example. Dietary restriction or other life-extension programs might be appropriately tested in humans by starting with a cohort averaging 40 to 45 years of age.

Rapidity of Weight Loss

Early investigators were unsuccessful in obtaining extended survival beginning DR in adulthood in rodents: the animals were introduced to a DR regimen too suddenly, and/or the restriction was too severe. Working with a naturally long-lived mouse strain, we found, however, that if two decrements in calorie intake were instituted over a 2 month period, dropping gradually to about 60 percent of the initial intake, life extension could be obtained beginning at 12 months of age (Weindruch & Walford, 1982). With regard to severity of restriction, Ross (1972) found that in rats restricted since young adulthood the longest lives were obtained with an adult intake of 6 g/day; if DR started later, 8 g/day gave greatest survival; if DR began still later, 10 g/day was optimal. Thus for ADR there may be an age-related range of greatest effectiveness. One assumes from Ross's data that the level of DR and rapidity of weight loss should be less severe if DR is instituted at an older age in humans.

How Much Weight Loss

Experiments with genetically very obese, (ob/ob) mice (Harrison et al., 1984), genetically mildly obese mice such as our own C3B10RF$_1$, hybrid strain (Weindruch et al., 1986), or relatively slender mice such as the B/WF$_1$ strain (Fernandes et al., 1976a) or the B6 strain (Weindruch & Walford, 1982) show that all live longer if subjected to DR. However, the ob/ob mice are now only mildly to moderately obese, and the other strains have lost weight proportionately. It is not percent of body fat that seems important, but the BW of the animals in relation to the genetic make-up of the strain. In humans, this would presumably correspond to the "set-point" of the individual.

The concept of an equilibrium "set point" argues that the body defends a particular weight by shifting the energy efficiency of the metabolic machine (Bradley, 1982; Stunkard, 1982). Each individual has a particular set-point determined by genetic endowment plus his or her early feeding history. The response to decreased caloric intake is to increase efficiency; and to increase caloric intake, to decrease the metabolic efficiency. Thereby BW is maintained.

It is well known that in any group of 20 or more subjects of about the same size, food intake can vary as much as two-fold without significant alterations in BW (Durnin et al., 1973; Apfelbaum, 1978). Humans can adapt to widely different intakes of energy with maintenance of BW (Dubos, 1972; Apfelbaum, 1978). Studies in a number of countries indicate that some people can be healthy and active on energy intakes which would be regarded by U.S. standards as quite inadequate (Durnin et al., 1978; Trusswell, 1978; Edmundson, 1979).

It is possible that individuals with a "thrifty genotype" are more able to survive under conditions where the food supply is poor, and that natural selection of such genotypes has taken place over many generations. But adaptation might be equally operative. It explains the results of animal and human studies (Cawthorne, 1982; Rothwell & Stock, 1981), which point to adaptive processes which reduce metabolic rate and protect against excessive breakdown of lean body mass, an effect seen in thin as well as obese individuals. Nor is there any obvious detriment to such adaptation. During World War II the population of Switzerland lost BW, but the mortality remained unchanged, and social performance actually increased (Apfelbaum, 1978).

To judge from the rodent literature, any degree of sustained BW loss below the genetic set-point of the individual might yield survival benefits in terms of maximum as well as average LS. Subject to the caveat suggested by Ross' data cited above, the degree of extension would increase progressively as the caloric intake was lowered, so long as the nutrient intake remained high. In rodents a limit is reached at a level of about 70 percent restriction, below which the animals die of gradual caloric starvation.

One would presume, therefore, that in humans a total BW loss of about 10-25 percent below the personal set-point would be a reasonable goal in terms of a positive effect on aging without being too excessive to threaten health. While depending on the actual starting weight of the individual, i.e., thin to average to obese, a 25 percent BW loss approaches but does not enter a fullblown anorexic status, which of course should be avoided.

The set point for individuals whose BW has been stable since ages 20-30 is precisely that BW. For those who have gradually gained BW with age, the appropriate set point in terms of a DR regimen is uncertain. In rats the capacity for thermogenesis is lost by 6.5 months of age (Rothwell & Stock, 1983). A similar phenomenon might in part underlie the human tendency to gain BW with age. For such as these, we suggest the target "set-point" would be their weight at 20-30 years of age.

Energy Requirements

The recommended energy intake for a U.S. male age 23 to 50 years and weighing 154 pounds, height 5'10" has been given by the Committee on Dietary Allowances of the Food and Nutrition Board as 2,700 kcal, (range = 2,300-3,100) (Food and Nutrition Board, 1980b). Calloway and Zanni (1980) found the BMRs of 63-77 year old healthy men to be 1,600 kcal/day, and the energy intake to maintain their BW to be 2,500 kcal/day. These recommendations and measurements reflect the idea that similar adults possess similar energy requirements when engaged in similar activities. But this concept requires considerable modification.

Two studies by Edmundson (1977, 1979) describe metabolic differences among 54 Javanese peasant farmers. A great variation in energy intake (from 1,500 to 3,800 kcal/day) was noted between individuals who were showing the same energy expenditure, as judged by work output, and who did not differ from one another in average height or BW. The average BMR of the high intake group was twice that of the low intake group, and the output per unit of energy intake of the 10 individuals with the lowest intake was fully 80 percent higher than that of 10 subjects with the highest energy intake. Edmundson (1977) concluded that compensatory mechanisms must exist such as higher metabolic efficiency, lower BMRs, or greater physical fitness, to enable those on a low energy intake to produce more work per unit of intake than those on a high intake. Later, Edmundson (1979) measured BMR and the energy cost of standardized work—peddling a bicycle at a certain speed—in five high- and six low-intake individuals. Although the individuals were of equal size, the high intake group consumed 2,400 kcal/day, the low intake group 1,500 kcal/day, in performing the same amount of standardized work. It should be stated that findings contrary to Edmundson's have been reported, and there may in fact be a drop of about 10 percent in BMR in persons habitually low in energy intake (for review, see Waterlow, 1986).

Besides variation between individuals, temporal variation in energy metabolism may exist in the same individual. Sukhatme and Margen (1982) have argued cogently that the energy requirement of an individual can vary over a wide range across time, a variation accomplished through an autoregulatory adjustment of the efficiency of metabolism. Thus, a particular individual's energy requirement may vary even though body composition and physical activity remain the same, and he or she can adapt to energy intakes perhaps 30 percent lower or higher than customary, without change in BW or activity. Studies of non-obese humans subjected to alternating two-weekly periods of 3,000 kcal/day versus 500 kcal/day support this interpretation (Lammert & Hansen, 1982).

Despite the above evidence of individual variation in calorie requirements, studies of cohorts on carefully monitored and fairly extended periods of moderately low calorie intake may allow an estimate of what energy intake level would constitute DR in humans. In an early study by Benedict et al. (1919), young men (N = 25) were fed less than 2,000 kcal/day for four months. Following a loss of about 10 percent of BW, they showed a decrease in total metabolism as the most prominent feature, a drop in blood pressure from the prestudy value of 145/80 to 90/70, and a fall in pulse pressure. In functional tests they displayed a decrease in reaction time and in the acoustical threshold for pitch discrimination (hence, improvements!), and no change in intellectual performance. On the negative side, these subjects experienced a general malaise and loss of bodily power as measured by work tests. They could be maintained without further BW loss on about 2,000 kcal/day.

An extensive study of "semistarvation" was reported by Keys and coworkers (Keys et al., 1950; Taylor & Keys, 1950). Thirty-two conscientious objectors were fed 1,600 kcal/day for 24 weeks via a diet which was not highly nourishing, consisting of about 55 g protein, 27 g fat, and daily riboflavin and vitamin A at only half the RDA. The subjects lost much BW in less than 6 months, then leveled off to a maintenance level of about 75 percent of their initial BW. Thus, in the face of a 55 percent reduction of what had been their normal calorie intake, the subjects were able to maintain calorie balance, but at a BW reduced by 25 percent. Body fat declined from an initial average value of 13-14 percent to 6 percent by 12 weeks and 4 percent by 24 weeks. Basal metabolic rate dropped by 20-32 percent by the 24th week. Although serum proteins remained within normal ranges, the subjects developed "famine edema" and suffered a marked loss of strength and endurance, were apathetic and depressed. When at the end of the 24 week period, the intake was raised to 2,000 kcal/day, the subjects did not gain BW. At 2,400 kcal, however, they began to gain BW.

Fed a 1,000 kcal/day nutrient dense diet for 20 weeks, subjects in a study by Weinseir et al. (1985) lost 12 percent of BW at a rate of about 1 kg/week. Fat was lost but muscle mass maintained, and there was no deterioration in any of a number of measured parameters of nutritional status. A comparison of post-obese women stabilized at normal BW, compared to lean controls, revealed that at all levels of activity the post-obese expended less energy and had a lower energy intake, about 1,300 vs. 2,000 kcal/day (Geissler et al., 1987).

The above studies suggest that since individual variation in energy metabolism is quite wide, calorie intake must be individualized to induce the gradual BW loss which is associated with LS extension in adult rodents. However, it seems probable that for a U.S. population, a daily intake of around 1,800 to 2,000 kcals should induce the very gradual BW loss which we surmise to be the best procedure. The average person can probably adapt over time and at a reduced BW to about an 1,800 kcal/day diet, without continued BW loss (Apfelbaum, 1978). The symptoms of lethargy, apathy, and listlessness observed in the studies of Benedict et al. (1919) and Keys et al. (1950) probably reflected less a calorie undernutrition than essential nutrient deficits.

Essential Nutrients

The "safe" level of nitrogen requirements for balance has been estimated to be about 0.6 g protein/kg/day for men (Zannie et al., 1979). The Dietary Allowances Committee of the National Academy of Sciences recommended a daily allowance of 0.8 g protein/kg/day.

In rats, potential biomarkers of aging values were improved by periodic fasting so long as vitamins were given during the fast periods whereas fasting without vitamin supplementation shifted the values towards an older age (Konoplya et al., 1984). By contrast, under conditions of total fasting in rats, addition of salts and vitamins to the fluid ingested did not affect the time of death (Kleiber, 1975), once more underscoring the difference between short-term and long-term DR. In humans, however, vitamin/mineral supplementation will indeed prolong survival of a totally fasting individual (Thomson et al., 1966).

Although humans can apparently adapt to widely different levels of nutrients (Some native South American populations, for example, maintain calcium balance with 200-300 mg/day, in contrast to the 600-800 or more mg required in young U.S. males [Shock, 1982].), it seems obvious that all "essential nutrients" and probably all those in the "safe and adequate" category should be present in appropriate amounts in any DR regimen for humans. This is not easy to achieve on, say, a 1,500 kcal/day basis (Mareschi et al., 1984). Surveying via "brute force" computer techniques up to 10,000 different, random, 1,500 kcal/day or lower combinations of high quality foods selected from the recognized food categories, one of us found that only rarely would a combination have RDA or larger amounts of *all* essential nutrients (Walford, 1983). Those nutrients in low supply were, in order of scarcity: zinc, vitamin E, copper, magnesium, iron, niacin, vitamin B12, pantothenic acid, calcium, riboflavin, folacin, vitamin A, vitamin B6, thiamine, and vitamin C.

Summary of Dietary Recommendations

We recommend a suitable "undernutrition without malnutrition" regimen for humans as containing 0.8 to 1.0 g protein/kg of BW, no more than about 0.4 to 0.6 g fat/kg of BW, and enough complex carbohydrates to reach the level of calories desired. For a 70 kg individual on a 2,000 calorie diet, this calculates out to 11-14 percent of calories derived from protein, 13-19 percent from fat, the remaining 1,400 calories from carbohydrates. Either the foods must be carefully selected or the diet supplemented so that intake approaches the RDA for all essential nutrients, at whatever calorie level is found to achieve slow BW loss towards a maintenance level. Combinations of foods which fulfill these criteria, at a 1,500 calorie level or lower and without supplementation have been described elsewhere (Walford, 1986a).

As to appetite and satiety, these depend very much on diet make-up. In one study (Lissner et al., 1987), unrestricted consumption of a palatable diet in which 15-20 percent of calories were derived from fat was associated with an intake of calories 13-26 percent less than that consumed by the same subjects when the percentage of calories from fat was 30-50 percent. In another study (Duncan et al., 1983) subjects were allowed to eat to satiety over a 5 day period, with equal acceptance ratings of the diets, satiety was reached on a *nutrient-dense, energy-non-dense* diet at a mean daily calorie intake half that of a diet high in *energy* density (1,570 vs. 3,000 kcal).

The nutrient density composition of any diet has a marked influence on BW and fat gain, due apparently to effects of macronutrients on energy efficiency (Rothwell & Stock, 1987). Clearly in rats, diets of unbalanced nutrients composition, the so-called "cafeteria diets," in which animals are offered a variety of palatable food items to choose from, lead to much greater energy consumption and increased heat production, energy expenditure, lower energy efficiency and sometimes (but often not) excess BW gain compared to controls (Rothwell et al., 1982b; Rothwell & Stock, 1982b & 1983; Nutrition Rev., 11 Nov. 1985; Ismail et al., 1986). In rodents, variations in food intake are more strongly determined by the type of diet, whereas variations in energy efficiencies are more strongly determined by genetics (Ismail et al., 1986). Rodents may increase energy intake by 30-50 percent without gaining BW, due to increased thermogenesis.

POTENTIAL DANGERS AND/OR DISADVANTAGES OF DR FOR HUMANS

Morrison's view (Morrison, 1983) that significant life extension can only be achieved by DR if the regimen is begun in early childhood, and that such is associated with a high infant mortality rate, even though the survivors have extended LSs, is simply incorrect for modern methodology. Even in the older literature the increased infant mortality only began at 50 percent restriction (Ross, 1978) and only reached a severe stage at 30 percent of ad libitum intake (Ross, 1976). Also, in many studies the test animals were simply fed less of the same mixture given ad libitum to controls, and thus might be malnourished as well as calorically restricted. Infant animals, as we have seen, are much more susceptible to a nutritionally marginal, restricted diet.

Too rapid weight loss, even beginning in adulthood, might be dangerous. Also, as noted previously (Ross, 1972), with ADR, the older the rat the less severe the DR to achieve maximum extension from that age forward. The precise calorie level in relation to age group in humans can only be surmised.

On very long term, low energy intake, even if carefully selected, the possibility of low-grade malnutrition exists. Even at its calorie level of over 3,000 kcal/day, the average American diet is at best borderline as indicated by the following findings:

(1) In the USDA's National Food Consumption Survey of 7,500 families (Swan, 1983), about half were judged deficient in one or more important nutrients, especially calcium, vitamins A and C, iron, thiamine, and riboflavin.

(2) Americans frequently consume less than the 2-3 mg of copper regarded as the RDA, and even less than the 1-2 mg regarded as the minimum daily need (Klevay et al., 1979; Mertz, 1982; Mayer & Goldberg, 1983).

(3) According to a survey by Walker and Page (1975), the daily vitamin B6 intake provided by meals served in 50 American colleges was 1.4 mg/person, with a range of 0.6 to 2.9: over 80 percent of the colleges were below the RDA of 2.0 mg.

(4) In a survey of 1,150 college students, less than 25 percent were found to have a "good dietary history," 75 percent did not have what was regarded as adequate nutrition, and 54 percent were currently dieting or had done so in the past (Marrale et al., 1986).

(5) An extensive 10 state survey of 86,353 persons divided into seven cohorts according to eating patterns, revealed that no cohort had less then 40 percent of individuals with clinical symptoms and/or 20 percent with biochemical abnormalities that might be attributed to nutritional deficiency (Schwerin et al., 1981).

(5) Fleming (1982) reported that vitamin C, vitamin A, and niacin intakes were less than 66 percent of the RDA in over 25 percent of elderly subjects in over 50 percent of the studies reviewed.

While the significance of the various above survey data can be overinterpreted, clearly to simply decrease calorie consumption of the average American diet as a putative DR regimen, without change in food quality, could lead on a longterm basis to serious malnutrition.

Depending on the severity of the caloric restriction, DR in humans might lead to a decline in fecundity while the individuals were on the regimen. Mice on 40-50 percent restriction cease to cycle, although rats are much more resistant to this effect (see *"Growth, Puberty Onset and Health."* in Chapter 2 and "Reproductive Senescence," Chapter 4). In rats restricted from early in life, puberty may be considerably delayed; however, the onset of infertility (menopause) is also greatly delayed. The lowered fertility of DR rodents is promptly reversed when they are placed on full feeding. Indeed, most DR rodents can produce young when nearly all animals of a fully fed control population have aged and died.

How these results would translate for human females on DR is unknown. Effects of DR on cycling could depend on the percent body fat, rather than amount of BW lost. The situation may be analogous to that of female athletes who, when their body fat falls substantially below the 15 percent level, tend to become anovulatory and amenorrheic. Menses return if BW is regained. Anorexics may become amenorrheic upon loss of 10-15 percent of normal weight for their height (a loss of about 30% of body fat) (Frisch, 1977). Dietary restriction might in fact be made to act as a birth-control measure, at the same time prolonging the time of the child-bearing age. This could be a blessing or a curse, depending on the viewpoint of the individual.

Theoretically a prolonged anovulatory state, if accompanied by a reduction of estrogen output, might increase the risk of osteoporosis later in life. In fact, however in rats, DR actually *decreases* senile bone loss, perhaps due to suppression of the otherwise age-related increase in PTH (Kalu et al., 1983a; 1984a & b). Human vegetarians are *less* prone to osteoporosis than omnivores, even though their calcium intake is lower (Ellis et al., 1972). Calcitonin, the thyroid hormone that inhibits osteoclastic bone resorption, increases quite dramatically with age in rats (But decreases with age in humans!), and DR inhibits this rise in rats (Kalu et al., 1983b). Thus if DR were to cause a still further decrease in calcitonin with age in humans, it might potentiate osteoporosis. However, if DR in fact shifts the parameters of bone metabolism towards a younger age, as it does with most of the body's machinery, it might lower blood calcitonin in rats and raise it in humans. In any case, the status of bone metabolism should be followed carefully in human DR studies.

A final problem concerns possible effects of DR on the incidence of certain tumors. While DR studies in rodents have confirmed a striking decrease in the total tumor incidence, a few studies have reported increased frequencies of some tumor types (Mostly, however, this is *not* the case [Albanes, 1987a].) In the most unfavorable studies in the literature on this alarming possibility (Ross & Bras, 1973; Ross, 1976), DR rats displayed only half the total tumor incidence of controls (e.g., fewer reticulum cell sarcomas, chromophobe adenomas, adenomas of islets of Langerhans, bladder papillomas), but an increase in skin carcinomas.

However, skin carcinoma was an infrequent tumor in both groups (see Table 3.3). And the age of onset of skin cancer was delayed in DR animals, the first cancer occurring in them at an age when *all* those in control animals had become manifest. And one notes that in these studies the DR was not only life-long but exceedingly severe, down to 30 percent of ad libitum intake and probably bordering on or crossing the malnutrition threshold for essential nutrients. These tumor data are not typical of less severely restricted animals, including those from the same laboratory (Ross, 1978).

POTENTIAL BENEFITS OF DR BESIDES LS EXTENSION

A carefully engineered, low-calorie, high quality food intake, with gradual weight loss, may be expected to yield a number of health benefits even if LS is not extended. Failure in LS extension might occur either because the animal work really is not applicable to man, or because it proves impractical or too difficult to adopt a sufficient degree of restriction. But other benefits of a DR regimen might still be observed.

Evidence is accumulating that the alleged beneficial effects of low fat intake on tumor incidence (Cohen, 1987) may really mostly be due to the fact that low fat diets are also low calorie diets (Albanes, 1987b; Pariza, 1987). The evidence for these effects derives from human as well as animal studies, and is therefore irrespective of whether DR retards aging in man. And, extrapolating from rodent data, the calorie reduction need not be drastic. Reviewing the literature, Albanes (1987b) concluded that a mild reduction in caloric intake of 16 percent led to an overall tumor incidence reduction in rodents of 40 percent. Albanes' analyses (1987a, b) of the growing literature on the relation between total calories and tumorigenesis in rodents and its independence from dietary fat, reported an absence of an overall effect (or at most minimal effect) of dietary fat on spontaneous and induced tumorigenesis in mice. Any influence of dietary fat on cancer might stem largely from its effect on the efficiency of dietary energy utilization (Boissonneault et al., 1986). Thus, "net energy" may be somewhat different than actual calorie intake, and vary with the percent of fat in the diet, involving a complex interaction involving energy intake, energy retention, and body size (Boissonneault et al., 1986).

During World War II in northern Europe, where average calorie intake was sometimes as low as 700-800 kcal/day, there occurred fewer new cases than expected of hypertension, heart disease, gout, and diabetes (Itallie & Hirsch, 1979). A recent study of the dietary habits of 1,462 Swedish women reported that the 12 year incidence of myocardial infarction was inversely correlated to energy intake, and that this correlation was independent of age, smoking habits, serum cholesterol, serum triglycerides, diabetes, systolic blood pressure, physical activity, and relation between amounts of fat, protein, and carbohydrate in the diet (Lapidus et al., 1986). An 800 kcal/day diet, admittedly much lower than an appropriate DR regimen for humans, leads to a decrease in serum cholesterol and triglycerides, blood pressure, fasting blood sugar in diabetics, but does not alter blood HDL levels (Howard, 1985).

It is worth repeating that *longitudinal* data analyzed by Borkan et al. (1986) indicated that BW change proved a significant predictor of long-term alterations in risk factors for coronary disease. Excepting fasting glucose, changes over time in these factors were more strongly related to change in BW than to the general level of adiposity reflected in the initial BWs of the subjects. (This would strengthen our recommendation that being below "set-point" is more important than what the "set point" actually may be.). And men who in the course of the study lost 10 percent or more of their initial BW enjoyed the least age-related change in all eight risk factors (Borkan et al., 1986), again precisely in line with our DR recommendations.

Albeit less evidence is available, in humans and also in animals it is quite possible that DR would exert not only a preventive but an actual therapeutic effect on certain diseases. Clearly this is true for maturity-onset diabetes, in which judicious energy restriction and considerable BW loss may render the human diabetic non-diabetic by existing tests (Davidson, 1976; Atkinson et al., 1985). The incidence of maturity onset diabetes increases from 0.1 percent of persons less than 20 years of age to about 15 percent in those over 60, and data suggest that most of these are precipitated by excessive caloric intake (Davidson, 1976). Diabetic rats are greatly benefited by a severely restricted diet, on the basis of which it has been suggested that insulin-dependent obese diabetics should reduce their energy intake (Krishnamachar & Canolty, 1985). Indeed a good case can be made for the thesis that the diabetic genotype has persisted because it has survival advantages under conditions of low food intake, and that the overt diabetic syndrome can be prevented by food scarcity (Wise, 1977a; Rotter & Diamond, 1987).

Dietary restriction might well be beneficial in hypertension (Tuck, 1985; Carman, 1985). There is also some evidence that symptoms of arthritis and especially rheumatoid arthritis may be bettered by food restriction (Skoldstam & Lindstrom, 1979; Moment, 1980; Carman, 1985). The remarkable effects of DR on rats with the genetic syndrome of obesity, renal disease, hypertension and vascular disease (see "Dietary Restriction Started in Adulthood (ADR)," Chapter 3) suggests that DR might be tried in the more serious and difficult-to-manage hyperlipidemias of humans.

Restriction of energy intake in 5 month-old B/WF_1 mice (i.e., at an age when autoimmunity and early renal lesions are established in many of the mice) clearly retards the progression of immunologic abnormalities and renal disease, and survival is improved (Friend et al., 1978). From results of mouse studies carried out by Robert Good and his associates (see Kubo et al., 1984a; Johnson et al., 1986), one may surmise that energy restriction may exert an extraordinarily beneficial effect on other auto-immune diseases. And while most reports on anti-tumor effects of low energy intake concern prevention, evidence also exists (partly in humans, more abundantly in rodents) for therapeutic effects (Albanes, 1987b).

The recent observation by Quigley et al. (1987) that if female rats of an age when only 41 percent are still undergoing estrous cycling are placed on a 10 week DR regimen, during which none will cycle, then allowed to feed ad libitum, 100 percent will resume and continue cycling, suggests that DR might have some application in cases of human infertility.

We suggest that DR may provide substantial health benefits even if maximum LS were not prolonged. It is in fact the most important common denominator of preventive and perhaps even therapeutic dietary measures in relation to a variety of human diseases.

SOCIAL EFFECTS OF LS EXTENSION

The question here applies not only to DR but to any successful life extension method. How will it affect society? This depends first of all on the simplicity of the method. Presumably, DR would not be adopted by an entire population, even if it were proven to be successful. According to Morrison (1983), "There are obvious and justified reasons why such Draconian regimes would be politically and socially unacceptable." We find such remarks a curious example of the "ageism" that afflicts even the biomedical community on the subject of increasing maximum human LS. Why not "politically" acceptable? If a subgroup of individuals elects to follow a 1,500 calorie high-quality diet, is that "politically" unacceptable? Or socially? One can readily think of numerous far more bizarre customs which are accepted within Western societies.

What would be the social effects of successful extension of maximum LS? The subject has been discussed elsewhere in some detail (Walford, 1983). To our knowledge only two rigorous pertinent studies have examined this question: that of Gori and Richter (1978) concerning curve-squaring technologies (cure or prevention of more and more diseases but leaving maximum LS fixed, i.e., no retardation in aging rate), and that of Kotlikoff (1982) concerning span-extending technologies (retardation of aging and extension of maximum LS).

It might well be difficult or impossible to cure what Brody and Schneider (1986) have classified as age-dependent diseases, meaning those which show a progressive increase with normal aging and may be considered as intimately connected or secondary to the aging process. Just as there has been a marked shift in the top 10 killer diseases from 1860 to today (Walford, 1983), one might expect a further shift with a curve-squaring technology, possibly with neurological and musculoskeletal diseases emerging as the new major mortality/morbidity agents. The only way around this dilemma might be retardation of aging, with postponement of these seemingly inevitable maladies.

In any case, a comparison of curve-squaring and span-extending technologies suggests that further cure of diseases without retardation of aging has large-scale negative economic implications (Gori & Richter, 1978), whereas retardation of aging has the reverse potential, and may prove highly beneficial to society (Kotlikoff, 1982). Recently, the Population Reference Bureau (1984) in Washington, D.C., has reached the same conclusion.

It is of interest that governmental census predictions, limited always to the curve-squaring, forecast that by the year 2050 the percent of persons over 65 years of age will be double what it is today. C.P. Snow in his book "The Physicists" (1981) tells that in 1933 Einstein, Niels Bohr, and Lord Rutherford all predicted that mankind would never get power from the atom. So much for the fallibility of experts! It seems extremely foolish to make long-term predictions of population structure without considering the scenario of a span-extending technology. The fact that none of the professional futurologists, Herman Kahn, Paul Ehrlich, Alvin Toffler have considered extended LSs as possible features of their future worlds again illustrates the habit of "ageism" that inhibits thinking on this subject, even though life extension is a clear and historic goal of applied gerontology, possibly not far off, and will have profound social implications (Walford, 1983).

RESEARCH NEEDS AND RECOMMENDATIONS FOR HUMAN STUDIES

The following areas require emphasis with regard to application of DR to humans: development of a reliable human biomarker battery, decision as to suitable test populations, and some degree of social planning or forethought as to effects on society of a breakthrough in life extension, either by DR or other methodologies.

Biomarkers of Aging

In animals with a relatively short LS, such as rodents, mean and maximum LS data can indicate whether an attempt to retard aging has succeeded. In longer lived animals, such as humans, assessment via survival curves is less practical, demanding a 40 year or longer experiment (i.e. about 50% of the average LS of the ad lib fed investigator). Biomarkers which might be able to tell in, say, 5 years, whether the aging rate is being altered are therefore needed to test intervention strategies in humans. At first sight easy (so many functions do measurably change with age), the biomarker problem is complex conceptually, mathematically, and physiologically.

Most past attempts to set up biomarker tests in humans have assumed, usually without fully questioning the assumption, that some as yet unascertained factor or process causes progressive aging of all systems, that a unitary "rate of aging" exists, and therefore that some equation indicating an overall "index of aging" might be devised. But with regard to psychological testing at least, Poon (1980) suggests that finding an overall index of "functional age" may be a false hope: "Within any one individual, different functional capacities change at different rates with age, and the rate for any one functional capacity differs between one individual and another. Moreover, changes of capacity that limit performance of a task making one set of demands may not do so for another task making different demands."

This "index of aging" approach has also been criticized by Costa and McCrae (1980a & b) who point out that one cannot predict one set of age-related variables from other sets, i.e., rates of aging do not covary across systems. Skin collagen aging cannot be predicted from immunologic aging data. In addition, the distribution of scores around the mean at any age may be due as much to differences in initial levels, or presence or absence of an age-related illness, as to any hypothetical rate of aging. Most so-called "biomarkers" do not predict survival. These comments are well put, but the authors' conclusion, i.e., that "measures of biological or functional age are useless" is in our view faulty. It confuses the complexity of the problem, particularly as it relates to humans, with concepts about aging. It applies much less strongly to multifactorial than to unifactorial approaches to aging (see *"Uni- and Multi-Factorial Aging,"* Chapter 1).

Influences on survival are genetic, environmental, and the interaction between the two. In our view an ideal animal strain for studying "pure aging" would be one whose survival curve is rectangular under laboratory conditions and crosses zero at the maximum LS span point for that species. Under such conditions, and with such a strain, unifactorial and multifactorial causality might be indistinguishable in terms of biomarker tests, and aging of connective tissue, for example, would be predictable from immunologic markers as both would reach their respective "levels of lethality" at the same time.

It is deviation from this ideal perspective which creates nonconcordance among groups of biomarker tests. Those animal strains which even under optimal laboratory conditions do not reach the maximum LS for the species create genetic problems of variance among biomarkers, as illustrated in the studies of Meredith and Walford (1977). And of course outbred strains would show an accentuation of this variance. Humans are both genetically heterogeneous and are not under optimal, or even uniform environmental conditions. This situation renders human biomarker studies, particularly cross-sectional studies, extremely difficult to evaluate.

Mathematical problems in biomarker testing are in large part a reflection of the above conceptual problems. Multiple linear regression analysis, which has been most often used for human biomarkers (Furukawa et al., 1975; Marmorston et al., 1975; Voitenko & Tokar, 1984) reflects a unitary aging rate theory. It yields good correlations with age using average values for groups of subjects, but not on an individual basis (Conard et al., 1966). In the Normative Aging Study, instead of a single prominent factor, 20 specific factors were found to change with age, but did not show the covariance that would be expected of a unitary rate of aging (Costa & McCrae, 1980b).

In an extensive consideration of biomarkers, Ludwig and Smoke (1980) concluded that "Age related changes progress at widely different rates. The range is so wide that a relatively small number of rapidly progressing changes kills before a majority of slowly progressing ones becomes clinically significant." This statement implies but does not quite spell out the concept of multifactorial aging.

In multifactorial aging, groups of factors ought to be found which move together in relation to aging (immune biomarkers, for example), with some groups independent of the others, except in long-lived strains, where a greater degree of interdependence might be expected. Under this scenario one might investigate factors in humans that change with age, and seek to group them by means of correlation coefficients, or factorial analysis (Clarke, 1960). The groups might change with age, but one group would not necessarily correlate with another.

Factorial analysis of 23 biomarkers was employed by Hofecker et al. (1980) and Skalicky et al. (1980) to estimate functional age in rats. Six sets of mutually correlated variables were defined, representing sets of independent processes, five of which correlated with the natural logarithm of chronologic age. But the groups showed little correlation with each other!

We predict that such seemingly independent sets would be found characteristically in short-lived rodent strains, but that inter-correlation between the sets would be greater in long-lived strains. In short-lived strains also, and in individual humans, certain sets would have enhanced predictive value for subsequent longevity. Only in this way, at present, can we make conceptual sense out of the array of published biomarker data.

The sample size is also a critical issue in assessing biomarkers (Schlesselman, 1973; Overall, 1987). This includes the size of the study population at each age group, frequency of measurements, and the length of time over which the study must be continued. For longitudinal analysis using the Wechsler Adult Intelligence Scale as biomarker, the sample sizes required to detect changes on intervention studies of 1 to 3 years is very large (Overall, 1987), albeit only about a tenth as large for a 3 year as for a 1 year study, and perhaps of a more manageable size for a 5 year study. In practice, and using the Hamburg-Wechsler Intelligence Test for Adults, over a 3 year period a population size of 148 individuals was sufficient to show a significant decrease in test time, but no improvement in other aspects of performance (Koberle & Spiegel, 1984).

The third consideration beyond concept and mathematics concerns physiologic variables related to the biomarker tests themselves, as applied to humans, and how potential biomarkers might conform to the general criteria laid down in Chapter 1.

Additionally, many biomarkers useful for rodents cannot be tested easily or at all in humans, as a biopsy would be required, or even sacrifice of the animal. Rodents have another advantage in that their lifetime environment can be kept constant. There are no cohort differences in education or occupational history among experimental rodent populations, as there are in humans.

But certain advantages do accrue to using humans for biomarker studies. A major one is that much more is known about human than rodent diseases so that confusion over the impact of disease on a biomarker versus that of an intrinsic aging effect can be more readily avoided. Also, many potential biomarkers can be tested readily in humans but only difficultly or not at all in rodents, for example those involving visual accommodation, hearing, psychological testing, and pulmonary vital capacity.

It is not our purpose here to conduct a general survey of human biomarkers of aging. An excellent historical review of studies dating as far back as Helmholtz may be found in Morgan (1986). Major studies or reviews of the modern era would include those of Hollingsworth et al. (1965), Conard et al. (1966), Comfort (1969 & 1972), Bourliere (1970), Suominan et al. (1980), Heikkinen (1982), Schneider et al. (1982), Borkan (1983 & 1986), Dean (1986), Morgan (1986), and others. Studies have included pulmonary function, especially vital capacity (Hollingsworth et al., 1965; Bourliere, 1970; Tobin as cited by Barrows [1981]); forced expiratory volume (Borkan & Norris, 1980); breath holding time (Voitenko & Tokar, 1984); cardiovascular function (Suominen et al., 1980; Gerstenblith, 1982), including maximum oxygen consumption (Suominen et al., 1980; Gerstenblith, 1982; Regelson, 1983; Bruce, 1984;) and systolic blood pressure (Hollingsworth et al., 1965; Morgan, 1986); renal function (Rowe et al., 1976); immunologic function (Mackay, 1972; Hallgren et al., 1973; Hallgren & Yunis, 1981; Roberts-Thompson et al., 1974; Weksler & Hutteroth, 1974; Weksler, 1982), hormonal parameters (Marmorston et al., 1975) including levels of DHEA (Orentreich et al., 1984; Barrett-Connor et al., 1986) and of thymic hormones (Goldstein, et al., 1983); glucose tolerance (Andres, 1972; Barrows, 1981; DeFronzo et al., 1981; DeFronzo, 1982); different chemical determinations including blood fats and cholesterol (Hollingsworth et al., 1965; Marmorston et al., 1975; Borkan & Norris, 1980), serum albumin and globulin (Hollingsworth et al., 1965; Borkan & Norris, 1980), adenosine deaminase, urinary osteocalcin, gamma-carboxyglutamic acid (Regelson, 1983); physiologic parameters such as greying of hair (Hollingsworth et al., 1965), skin elasticity (Hollingsworth et al., 1965), wound healing (Regelson, 1983), hand grip strength (Bourliere, 1970; Potvin et al., 1980); sensory tests including pupil size (Sekuler, 1982), visual acuity (Hollingsworth et al., 1965; Borkan & Norris, 1980; Sekuler, 1982), visual accommodation (Bourliere, 1970; Sekuler, 1982), and depth perception (Corso, 1982); and tests for auditory function, vibratory tests, balance and psychomotor and cognitive function (Jalavisto, 1965; Potvin et al., 1980; Salthouse, 1982; Petros et al., 1983; Rabbitt, 1983).

Those potential biomarkers which are most influenced by physical fitness may be less useful, as meaningful comparisons would have to be limited to cohorts at equal levels of physical fitness, or in longitudinal studies to individuals who maintain a constant level of fitness over the period of study.

Those biomarkers would seem most suitable which tend to predict subsequent mortality, so long as they are not simply disease-susceptibility markers (e.g., high blood cholesterol might predict earlier cardiac death, but this is not necessarily accelerated aging). Candidates for biomarkers of aging in humans include vital capacity, probably the best predictor in humans of later overall mortality (Kannel & Hubert, 1982), maximum work rate (Borkan & Norris, 1980), suppressor cell response (Hallgren & Yunis, 1981), the presence of autoantibodies (Mackay, 1972), delayed-type hypersensitivity (Roberts-Thompson et al., 1974), serum albumin and globulin levels (Borkan & Norris, 1980), reaction time and tapping time (Borkan & Norris, 1980), and hearing threshold at a fixed frequency (Corso, 1982).

It is clear from the above that the biomarker field, while replete with data, is extremely confused. We recommend the establishing of periodic

Biomarkers of Aging Workshops, modelled on the justly famous International Histocompatibility Workshops, out of which developed much of modern immunology. Initially these Workshops might include actual testing by a number of laboratories of biomarkers on cohorts from the same restricted and normally fed rodent populations of different ages, including in some instances non-lethal tests, with data therefrom to be correlated with subsequent mortality, to be presented at the following workshop. The subjecting of these data to statistical analyses by a panel of experts, with appraisal of different statistical approaches, and issuance of a joint report would be guiding and instructive. Similar treatment of available data from ongoing human studies such as the Baltimore Longitudinal Study, the Framingham Study, and the Veterans Normative Study would also provide valuable information. Advantage should also be taken of the abundant physiologic data available on the U.S. astronauts, most of whom have continued to be fully tested after their service period has ended, and on into their mature years.

Primate Populations

Demonstration of LS prolongation and suitable biomarker changes in primates would make the jump to human application more certain of success and of acceptance. Such a project has recently been started by investigator's from the NIA with squirrel monkeys (Maximum LS about 25 years) and rhesus monkeys (maximum LS 40 years) being fed about 70 percent of the ad lib level. The biomarkers selected should include, as much as feasible, those which have been shown to be dramatically influenced by DR in rodent studies, as well as biomarkers which might be most suitably measured in nonhuman primates. A potential problem is that optimum nutrient requirements for nonhuman primates are less known than for either humans or rodents.

Testing of Human Cohorts

Aside from problems of motivation and compliance, and in view of the high probability that DR would work the same in humans as in other mammals, we see no reason not to recommend DR for humans, provided only that the diet be suitably engineered. A 1,500 to 2,000 kcal daily intake will in most instances induce gradual weight loss in men, and if it includes RDA amounts of all essential nutrients, can hardly be regarded as a dangerous program, or indeed as other than an extremely healthy program. Women would on the average require somewhat fewer calories.

Besides the possibility of decelerated aging, gradually induced DR ought to exert a preventive influence on various diseases, including arteriosclerosis/autoimmune disease, diabetes mellitus, and cancer. A high degree of motivation might be found in those individuals with a genetic or environmentally induced propensity towards one of these diseases. Also, the discovery of new drugs which safely control appetite would obviously make a DR regimen more easily followed by humans.

Social Planning

Whereas by DR or other means, gerontology may well be approaching the possibility of significant retardation of the aging process, virtually no social thought or planning has gone into this eventuality. Even if the possibility of success in the foreseeable future—and the future is often surprising—were small, the social implications of a long-living society are so great (Walford, 1983) as to merit much forethought (Chesky & Zakeri, 1987). The subject would obviously require a separate treatment, well beyond the scope of our present inquiry.

SUMMARY

The effect of DR in extending the maximum LSs of animals appears thus far to be phylogenetically independent. This alone is enough to make the probability that it would do so in humans a strong one. While such a regimen has not been carefully tested in any primate species, a small amount of direct and a substantial amount of indirect or inferential evidence in humans support the suggestions derived from the combined animal data. No sound arguments against an effect of DR in human or primate LS exist.

The overall probability that DR will retard human aging, and exert wide-spread favorable effects on health and function, is as great as the probabilities of efficacy of many preventative and therapeutic measures which orthodox medicine currently recommends. There is no compelling reason to demand a much higher level of evidence before recommending an anti-aging regimen than for other medical regimens, particularly preventive ones. We thus regard DR as an ethical option for human use, on existing evidence, under the appropriate conditions. We have outlined the principal features of such a regimen. Research needs and recommendations are discussed, with emphasis on further development of human biomarkers of aging.

Significant extension of maximum LS, the classical goal of gerontology, will create a new society, radically different than the present one, and in our view with many advantages. In any case, it behooves us to anticipate to some degree the nature of these changes, and how they may be turned to advantage in the conduct of our lives.

BIBLIOGRAPHY

Adelman, R.C.: Disruptions in enzyme regulation during aging. In Parke, D.V. (Ed.): *Enzyme Induction.* New York, Plenum Press, 1975, pp. 303-311.

Albanes, D.: Total calories, body weight, and tumor incidence in mice. *Cancer Res, 47*:1987, 1987a.

Albanes, D.: Caloric intake, body weight, and cancer: a review. *Nutr Cancer, 9*:199, 1987b.

Alberts, B., Bray, D., Lewis, J., Raff, M., Roberts, K., and Watson, J.D. *Molecular Biology of the Cell.* New York, Garland, 1983.

American Heart Association: Risk factor and coronary disease. Dallas, American Heart Association, 1980.

American Institute of Nutrition: Ad Hoc Committee on Standards for Nutritional Studies. Report of the Committee. *J Nutr, 107*:1340, 1977.

Andreou, K.K., and Morgan, P.R.: Effect of dietary restriction on induced hamster cheek pouch carcinogenesis. *Arch Oral Biol, 26*:525, 1981.

Andres, R.: Aging and carbohydrate metabolism. In: *Symposia of the Swedish Nutrition Foundation. X, Nutrition in Old Age.* Upsala, Almguist & Wiksell, 1972, pp. 24-31.

Andres, R.: Influence of obesity on longevity in the aged. In Borek, C., Fenoglio, C.M., and King, D.W. (Eds.): *Aging, Cancer and Cell membranes.* New York, Thieme-Stratton, 1980, pp. 238-246.

Andres, R.: Aging, diabetes, and obesity: standards of normality. *Mt Sinai J Med, 48*:489, 1981.

Apfelbaum, M.: Adaptation to changes in caloric intake. *Prog Food Nutr Sci, 2*:543, 1978.

Apfelbaum, M., Bostarron, J., and Lacatis, D.: Effect of caloric restriction and excessive caloric intake on energy expenditure. *Am J Clin Nutr, 24*:1405, 1971.

Arai, K., Iizuka, S., Tada, Y., Oikawa, K., and Taniguchi, N.: Increase in the glycosylated form of erythrocyte Cu-Zn-superoxide dismutase in diabetes and close association of the nonenzymatic glycosylation with the enzyme activity. *Biochim Biophys Acta, 924*:292, 1987.

Armario, A., Montero, J.L., and Jolin, T. Chronic food restriction and the circadian rhythms of pituitary-adrenal hormones, growth hormone and thyroid-stimulating hormone. *Ann Nutr Metab, 31*:81, 1987.

Arshavsky, I.A.: Mechanisms which determine the life span of rats that develop under the conditions of a limited calorie diet from the standpoint of the non-entropy theory of ontogenesis. In Chebotarev, D.F. (Ed.): *Gerontology and Geriatrics, Life Prolongation: Prognosis, Mechanisms, Controls.* Kiev, Institute of Gerontology, 1979, pp. 135-140 (in Russian) (cited by Frolkis, 1982).

Arteriosclerosis: A report by the NHLBI Task Force on Arteriosclerosis. Washington D.C. DHEW Publ. #(NIH) 78-1526, 1971, pp. 72-219.

Aschheim, P.: Relation of neuroendocrine system to reproductive decline in female rats. In Meites, J. (Ed.): *Neuroendocrinology of Aging.* New York, Plenum Press, 1983, pp. 73-101.

Asdell, S.A., and Crowell, M.F.: The effect of retarded growth upon the sexual development of rats. *J Nutr, 10*:13, 1935.

Atkinson, R.L., Berke, L.K., Kaiser, D.L., and Pohl, S.L.: Effects of very low calorie diets on glucose tolerance and diabetes mellitus in obese humans. In Blackburn, G.L., and Bray, G.A. (Eds.): *Management of Obesity by Severe Caloric Restriction.* Littleton, Mass, PSG Publishing Co., Inc., 1985, pp. 279-280.

Austad, S.N.: Life extension by dietary restriction in the bowl and doily spider, *Frontinella pyramitela. Exp Gerontol* (submitted).

Ayers, J.W.T., Gidwani, G.P., Schmidt, I.M.V., and Gross, M.: Osteopenia in hypoestrogenic young women with anorexia nervosa. *Fertil Steril, 41*:224, 1984.

Bafitis, H., and Sargent, F.: Human physiological adaptibility through the life sequence. *J Gerontol, 32*:404, 1977.

Bailey, P.J., and Webster, G.C.: Lowered rates of protein synthesis by mitochondria isolated by organisms of increasing age. *Mech Ageing Dev, 24*:233, 1984.

Bailey, R., Pigg, M., Talal, N., and Fernandes, G.: Influence of food restriction on IgG/IgM plaque forming cell (PFC) ratio of (NZB × BXSB)F$_1$ mice prone to develop coronary vascular disease. *Fed Proc, 42*:1205, 1983.

Baird, M.B., and Samis, H.V., Jr.: Regulation of catalase activity in mice of different ages. *Gerontology, 17*:105, 1971.

Baird, M.B., and Massie, H.R.: Subcellular distribution of renal and hepatic catalase activity in senescent rodents. *Exp Gerontol., 11*:167, 1976.

Baird, M.B., Zimmerman, J.A., Massie, H.R., and Samis, H.V.: Response of liver and kidney catalase to α-p-chlorophenoxyisobutyrate (Clofibrate) in C57Bl/6J male mice of different ages. *Gerontologia, 20*:169, 1974.

Balazs, E.A. (1977): Intercellular matrix of connective tissue. In Finch, C.E. and Hayflick, L. (Eds.): *Handbook of the Biology of Aging.* New York, Van Nostrand Reinhold, 1977, pp. 222-240.

Balin, A.K.: Testing the free radical theory of aging. In Adelman, R.C. and Roth, G.S. (Eds.): *Testing the Theories of Aging.* Boca Raton, CRC Press, 1982, pp. 137-182.

Balin, A.K., and Allen, R.G.: Mechanisms of biologic aging. *Dermatol Clin, 4*:347, 1986.

Ball, S.S., Weindruch, R. and Walford, R.L.: Antioxidants and the immune process. In: *Free Radicals, Aging and Degenerative Disease,* edited by J.E. Johnson, R. Walford, D. Harman and J. Miquel. Liss, NY, pp. 427-456, 1986.

Ball, Z., Barnes, R., and Visscher, M.: The effects of dietary caloric restriction on maturity and senescence, with particular reference to fertility and longevity. *Am J Physiol, 150*:511, 1947.

Barnett, E.V., Chia, D., Knutson, D., Van Lancker, J.L., Cheney, K.E., Weindruch, R.H. and Walford, R.L.: SLE, an accelerated form of aging. In: *Immunological Aspects of Aging,* edited by D. Segre and L. Smith. Dekker, NY, 1981, pp. 467-477.

Barrett-Connor, E., Khaw, K., and Yen, S.S.C.: A prospective study of dehydroepiandrosterone sulfate, mortality, and cardiovascular disease. *New Eng J Med, 315*:1519, 1986.

Barrows, C.H.: Nutrition, aging, and genetic program. *Am J Clin Nutr, 25*:829, 1972.

Barrows, C.H.: The effect of age on physiological functions. In: *Aging and the Geochemical Environment.* National Academy of Sciences Press, Wash. D.C., pp. 20-24, 1981.

Barrows, C.H., Jr., and Roeder, L.M.: The effect of reduced dietary intake on enzymatic activities and life span of rats. *J Gerontol, 20*:69, 1965.

Barrows, C.H., and Kokkonen, G.: The effect of various dietary restricted regimes on biochemical variables in the mouse. *Growth, 42*:71, 1978.

Barrows, C.H., and Kokkonen, G.C.: Dietary restriction and life extension—biological mechanisms. In Moment, G.B. (Ed.): *Nutritional Approaches to Aging Research.* Boca Raton, CRC Press, 1982, pp. 219-243.

Barrows, C.H., and Kokkonen, G.C.: Nutrition and aging: Human and animal laboratory studies. In Ordy, J.M., Harman, D., and Alfin-Slater, R. (Eds.): *Nutrition in Gerontology.* New York, Raven Press, 1984, pp. 279-322.

Barrows, C.H., and Kokkonen, G.: The effect of age and diet on biochemical characteristics of the tissues of mice. *Age, 8*:101, 1985.

Barrows, C.H., and Kokkonen, G.: The effect of age and diet on the cellular protein synthesis of liver of male mice. *Age, 10*:54, 1987.

Barrows, C.H., Roeder, L.M., and Fanestil, D.D.: The effects of restriction of total dietary intake and protein intake, and of fasting interval on the biochemical composition of rat tissue. *J Gerontol, 20*:374, 1965.

Barrows, K., and Snook, J.T.: Effect of a high-protein, very-low caloric diet on resting metabolism, thyroid hormones, and energy expenditure of obese middle-aged women. *Am J Clin Nutr, 45*:391, 1987.

Batory, G., Onody, C., Gyodi, E., Nemeskeri, J., & Petranyi, G.G.: HLA and T-lymphocyte function in old age. *Human Immunol, 7*:187, 1983.

Beach, R.S., Gershwin, M.E., and Hurley, L.S.: Dietary zinc modulation of Moloney sarcoma virus oncogenesis. *Cancer Res, 41*:552, 1981a.

Beach, R.S., Gershwin, M.E., Hurley, L.S.: Nutritional factors and autoimmunity. I. Immunopathology of zinc deprivation in New Zealand mice. *J Immunol, 126*:1999, 1981b.

Beach, R.S., Gershwin, M.E., and Hurley, L.S.: Nutritional factors and autoimmunity. II. Prolongation of survival in zinc-deprived NZB/W mice. *J Immunol, 128*:308, 1982.

Beatty, W.W., Clouse, B.A., and Bierley, R.A.: Effects of long-term restricted feeding on radial maze performance by aged rats. *Neurobiol Aging, 8*:325, 1987.

Beauchene, R.E., Bales, C.W., Smith, C.A., Tucker, S.M., and Mason, R.L.: The effect of feed restriction on body composition and longevity of rats. *Physiologist, 22*:8a, 1979.

Beauchene, R.E., Hendrix, M.J., Bales, C.W., and Davis, T.A.: Effect of age and protein and caloric restriction on bone composition of male rats. *Fed Proc, 41*:464, 1982.

Beauchene, R.E., Bales, C.W., Bragg, C.S., Hawkins, S.T., and Mason, R.L.: Effect of age of initiation of feed restriction on growth, body composition, and longevity of rats. *J Gerontol, 41*:13, 1986.

Bell, R.G., and Hazell, L.A.: The influence of dietary protein insufficiency on the murine thymus. Evidence for an intrathymic pool of progenitor cells capable of thymus regeneration after severe atrophy. *Aust J Exp Biol Med Sci, 55*:571, 1977.

Bell, R.G., Hazell, L.A., and Price, P.: Influence of dietary protein restriction on immune competence. II. Effect on lymphoid tissue. *Clin Exp Immunol, 26*:314, 1976.

Bellamy, D. Long-term action of prednisolone phosphate on a strain of short-lived mice. *Exp Gerontol, 3*:327, 1968.

Benedict, F.G., Miles, W.E., Roth, P., and Smith, H.M.: Human vitality and efficiency under prolonged restricted diet. *Carnegie Inst Wash Publ,* #280, 1919.

Bennett, W.: Gurus of longevity. *Am Health,* May 1984, p. 85.

Berg, B.N.: Nutrition and longevity in the rat. I. Food intake in relation to size, health and fertility. *J Nutr, 71*:242, 1960.

Berg, B.N.: Pathology and aging. In Everitt, A.V., and Burgess, J.A. (Eds.): *Hypothalamus, Pituitary and Aging.* Springfield, Charles C Thomas, 1976, pp. 43-67.

Berg, B.N., and Simms, H.S.: Nutrition and longevity in the rat. II. Longevity and onset of disease. *J Nutr, 71*:255, 1960.

Berg, B.N., and Simms, H.S.: Nutrition and longevity in the rat. III. Food restriction beyond 800 days. *J Nutr, 74*:23, 1961.

Berg, B.N., Wolf, A., and Simms, H.S.: Nutrition and longevity in the rat. IV. Food restriction and the radiculoneuropathy of aging rats. *J Nutr, 77*:439, 1962.

Berkowitz, E.M., Sanborn, A.C., and Vaughan, D.W.: Chromatin structure in neuronal and neuroglial cell nuclei as a function of age. *J Neurochem, 41*:516, 1983.

Berry, M.N., Clark, D.G., Grivell, A.R., and Wallace, P.G.: The contribution of hepatic metabolism to diet-induced thermogenesis. *Metabolism, 34*:141, 1985.

Berry, R.J., Jakobson, M.E., and Triggs, G.S.: Survival in wild living mice. *Mammal Rev, 3*:46, 1973.

Bertrand, H.A.: Nutrition-aging interactions: life-prolonging action of food restriction. In Rothstein, M. (Ed.): *Review of Biological Research in Aging,* Vol. 1. New York, Alan R. Liss, Inc., 1983, pp. 359-378.

Bertrand, H.A., Masoro, E.J., and Yu, B.P.: Post-weaning food restriction reduces adipose cellularity. *Nature, 266*:62, 1977.

Bertrand, H.A., Lynd, F.T., Masoro, E.J., and Yu, B.P.: Changes in adipose mass and cellularity through the adult life of rats fed ad libitum or a life-prolonging restricted diet. *J Gerontol, 35*:827, 1980a.

Bertrand, H.A., Masoro, E.J., and Yu, B.P.: Maintenance of glucagon-promoted lipolysis in adipocytes by food restriction. *Endocrinology, 107*:591, 1980b.

Bertrand, H.A., Stacy, C., Masoro, E.J., Yu, B.P., Murata, I., and Maeda, H.: Plasticity of fat cell number, *J Nutr, 114*:127, 1984.

Bertrand, H.A., Anderson, W.R., Masoro, E.J., and Yu, B.P.: Action of food restriction on age-related changes in adipocyte lipolysis. *J Gerontol, 42*:666, 1987.

Beth, M., Berger, M.R., Aksoy, M., and Schmahl, D.: Comparison between the effects of dietary fat level and of calorie intake on methylnitrosourea-induced mammary carcinogenesis in female SD rats. *Int J Cancer, 39*:737, 1987.

Beyer, R.E., Starnes, J.W., Edington, D.W., Lipton, R.J., Compton, R.E., III, and Kwasman, M.A.: Exercise-induced reversal of age-related declines of oxidative reactions, mitochondrial yield, and flavins in skeletal muscle of the rat. *Mech Ageing Dev, 24*:309, 1984.

Beyer, R.E., Burnett, B., Cartwright, K.J., Edington, D.W., Falzon, M.J., Kreitman, K.R., Kuhn, T.W., Ramp, B.J., Rhee, S.Y.S., Rosenwasser, M.J., Stein, M., An, L.C.: Tissue coenzyme Q (ubiquinone) and protein concentrations over the life span of the laboratory rat. *Mech Ageing Dev, 32*:267, 1985.

Bhuyan, K.C., and Bhuyan, D.K.: Superoxide dismutase of the eye. Relative functions of superoxide dismutase and catalase in protecting the ocular lens from oxidative damage. *Biochim Biophys Acta, 542*:28, 1978.

Bhuyan, K.C., Bhuyan, D.K., and Podos, S.M.: Lipid peroxidation in cataract of the human. *Life Sci, 38*:1463, 1986.

Bilder, G.E., and Denckla, W.D.: Restoration of ability to reject xenografts and clear carbon after hypophysectomy of adult rats. *Mech Ageing Dev, 6*:153, 1977.

Birchenall-Sparks, M.C., Roberts, M.S., Staecker, J., Hardwick, J.P., and Richardson, A.: Effect of dietary restriction on liver protein synthesis in rats. *J Nutr, 115*:944, 1985.

Birt, D.F., Higgenbotham, S.M., Patil, K., and Pour, P.: Nutritional effects on the lifespan of Syrian hamsters. *Age, 5*:11, 1982a.

Birt, D.F., Baker, P.Y., and Hruza, D.S.: Nutritional evaluations of three dietary levels of lactalbumin throughout the lifespan of two generations of Syrian hamsters. *J Nutr, 112*:2151, 1982b.

Bischoff, F., and Long, M.L.: The influence of calories per se upon the growth of sarcoma 180. *Am J Cancer, 32*:418, 1938.

Bischoff, F., Long, M.L., and Maxwell, L.C.: Influence of caloric intake upon the growth of sarcoma 180. *Am J Cancer, 24*:549, 1935.

Blackett, A.D., and Hall, D.A.: The effects of vitamin E on mouse fitness and survival. *Gerontology, 27*:133, 1981.

Blank, J.L., and Desjardins, C.: Food restriction alters pituitary-testicular function. *Fed Proc, 42*:977, 1983.

Bliznakov, E.G.: Immunological senescence in mice and its reversal by coenzyme Q10. *Mech Ageing Dev, 7*:189, 1978.

Blum, J.W., Schnyder, W., Kunz, P.L., Blom, A.K., Bickel, H., and Schurch, A.: Reduced and compensatory growth: endocrine and metabolic changes during food restriction and refeeding in steers. *J Nutr, 115*:417, 1985.

Boersma, W.J.A., Steinmeier, F.A., and Haaijman, J.J.: Age-related changes in the relative numbers of Thy-1- and Lyt-2-bearing peripheral blood lymphocytes in mice: a longitudinal approach. *Cell Immunol, 93*:417, 1985.

Boissonneault, G.A., Elson, C.E., and Pariza, M.W.: Net energy effects of dietary fat on chemically induced mammary carcinogenesis in F344 rats. *JNCI, 76*:335, 1986.

Bolla, R.I.: Hormonal regulation of molecular events during aging. *Life Sci, 31*:615, 1982.

Bolla, R., and Denckla, W.D.: Effect of hypophysectomy on liver nuclear ribonucleic acid synthesis in aging rats. *Biochem J, 184*:669, 1979.

Borkan, G.A.: Factors in clinical aging: variation in rates of aging. In Regelson, W., and Sinex, F.M. (Eds.): *Intervention in the Aging Process. Part A: Quantitation, Epidemiology, and Clinical Research.* New York, Liss, 1983, pp. 99-112.

Borkan, G.A.: Biological age assessments in adulthood. In Bittles, A.H., and Collins, K.J. (Eds.): *The Biology of Human Aging.* Cambridge, Cambridge University Press, 1986, pp. 81-93.

Borkan, G.S., and Norris, A.H.: Assessment of biological age using a profile of physical parameters. *J Gerontol, 35*:177, 1980.

Borkan, G.A., Sparrow, D., Wisniewski, C., and Vokonas, P.S.: Body weight and coronary disease risk: patterns of risk factor change associated with long-term weight change. *Am J Epidemiol, 124*:410, 1986.

Bouille, C., and Assenmacher, I.: Effects of starvation on adrenal cortical function in the rabbit. *Endocrinology, 87*:1390, 1970.

Bouliere, F.: World Health Organization, *Public Health Paper, #37,* 1970.

Boutwell, R.K., Brush, M.K., and Rusch, H.P.: Some physiological effects associated with chronic caloric restriction. *Am J Physiol, 154*:517, 1948.

Boutwell, R.K., Brush, M.K., and Rusch, H.P.: The stimulating effect of dietary fat on carcinogenesis. *Cancer Res, 9*:741, 1949.

Bowers, T.K., and Eckert, E.: Leukopenia in anorexia nervosa. *Arch Intern Med, 138*:1520, 1978.

Boyd, E.M.: *Protein Deficiency and Pesticide Toxicity.* Springfield, Charles C Thomas, 1972, pp. 127-143.

Boyle, P.C., Storlien, L.H., and Keesey, R.E.: Increased efficiency of food utilization following weight loss. *Physiol Behav, 21*:261, 1978.

Boyle, P.C., Storlien, H., Harper, A.E., and Keesey, R.E.: Oxygen consumption and locomotor activity during restricted feeding and realimentation. *Am J Physiol, 241*:R392, 1981.

Bradley, P.J.: Is obesity an advantageous adaptation? *Int J Obes, 6*:43, 1982.

Brafield, A.E., and Llewyllyn, M.J.: *Animal Energetics.* Glasgow, Blackie, 1982.

Brand, M.D., and Murphy, M.P.: Control of electron flux through the respiratory chain in mitochondria and cells. *Biol Rev, 62*:141, 1987.

Bray, G.A., and Fisler, J.S.: Integration of energy intake and expenditures: the autonomic and adrenal hypothesis. In Muller, E.E., MacLeod, R.M., and Frohman, L.A. (Eds.): *Neuroendocrine Perspectives.* New York, Elsevier Science Publishers, 1985, pp. 219-242.

Brennan, M.J., Randt, C.T., Samuels, S., and Quartermain, D.: Longitudinal analysis of the behavioral effects of prolongevity diets. *XIIIth Intl Congr Gerontol* (Book of Abstracts). 1985, p. 355.

Brody, J.A., and Schneider, E.L.: Diseases and disorders of aging: an hypothesis. *J Chronic Dis, 39*:871, 1986.

Bronson, F.H.: Puberty in female rats: relative effect of exercise and food restriction. *Am J Physiol, 252*:R140, 1987.

Brown, G.M., Garfinkel, P.E., Jeuniewie, N., Moldofsky, A., and Stacer, H.C.: Endocrine profiles in anorexia nervosa. In Vigersky, R.A. (Ed.): *Anorexia Nervosa*. New York, Raven Press, 1977, pp. 123-125.

Brown, J.G., Bates, P.C., Holliday, M.A., and Millward, J.: Thyroid hormones and muscle protein turnover. *Biochem J, 194*:771, 1981.

Bruce, R.A.: Exercise, functional aerobic capacity, and aging—another viewpoint. *Med Sci Sports Exerc, 16*:8, 1984.

Bullough, W.S., and Ebling, F.J.: Cell replacement in the epidermis and sebaceous glands of the mouse. *J Anat, 86*:29, 1952.

Burch, R.E., and Hahn, H.K.J.: The effect of aging on rat tissue content of moisture, protein, zinc, copper and manganese with partial food deprivation. II. Middle stages of aging. *Age, 5*:80, 1982.

Burman, K.D., Lukes, Y., Wright, F.D., and Wartofsky, L.: Reduction in hepatic triiodothyronine binding capacity induced by fasting. *Endocrinology, 101*:1331, 1977.

Burman, K.D., Smallridge, R.C., Osburne, R., Dimond, R.C., Whorton, N.E., Kesler, P., and Wartofsky, L.: Nature of suppressed TSH secretion during undernutrition: effect of fasting and refeeding on TSH responses to prolonged TRH infusions. *Metabolism, 29*:46, 1980.

Burnet, F.M.: An immunological approach to aging. *Lancet, 2*:358, 1970.

Burns, E.M., Kruckerberg, T.W., Comerford, L.E., and Buschmann, M.T.: Thinning of capillary walls and declining numbers of endothelial mitochondria in the cerebral cortex. *J Gerontol, 34*:642, 1979.

Cadenas, E., Boveris, A., Ragan, C.I., and Stoppani, A.O.M.: Production of superoxide radicals and hydrogen peroxide by NADH-ubiquinone reductase and ubiquinol-cytochrome c reductase from beef-heart mitochondria. *Arch Biochem Biophys, 180*:248, 1977.

Cahill, G.F., Herrera, M.G., Morgan, A.D., Soeldner, J.D., Steinke, J., Levy, P.L., Reichard, G.A., Jr., and Kipnis, D.M.: Hormone-fuel interrelationships during fasting. *J Clin Invest, 45*:1751, 1966.

Cahill, G.F., Aoki, T.T., and Ruderman, N.B.: Ketosis (The Jeremiah Metzger Lecture). *Trans Am Clin Climatol Assoc, 80*:184, 1973.

Calloway, D.H., and Zanni, E.: Energy requirements and energy expenditure of elderly men. *Am J Clin Nutr, 33*:2088, 1980.

Campbell, B.A., and Gaddy, J.R. Rate of aging and dietary restriction: Sensory and motor function in the Fischer 344 rat. *J Gerontol, 42*:154, 1987.

Campbell, G.A., Kurcz, M., Marshall, S., and Meites, J.: Effects of starvation in rats on serum levels of follicle stimulating hormone, leutinizing hormone, thyrotropin, growth hormone and prolactin; response to LH-releasing hormone and thyrotropin-releasing hormone. *Endocrinology, 100*:580, 1977.

Cantoni, O., Murray, D., and Meyn, R.E.: Induction and repair of DNA single-strand breaks in EM9 mutant CHO cells treated with hydrogen peroxide. *Chem Biol Interact, 63*:29, 1987.

Carafoli, E., and Penniston, J.T.: The calcium signal. *Sci Am, 253*:70, 1985.

Carlson, A.J., and Hoelzel, F.: Apparent prolongation of the life span of rats by intermittent fasting. *J Nutr, 31*:363, 1946.

Carlson, H.E., Drenick, E.J., Chopra, I.J., and Herschman, J.M.: Alterations in basal and TRH stimulated serum levels of thyrotropin, prolactin and thyroid hormones in starved obese men. *J Clin Endocrinol Metab, 45*:707, 1977.

Carman, J.M.: An analysis of user experience with a very low calorie diet. In Blackburn, G.L., and Bray, G.A. (Eds.): *Management of Obesity by Severe Caloric Restriction*. Littleton, Mass., 1985, pp. 33-49.

Carmena, R., Ascaso, J., Tebar, J., Soriano, J.: Changes in high-density lipoproteins after body weight reduction in obese women. *Intl J Obes, 8*:135, 1984.

Carr, C.J., King, J.T., and Visscher, M.B.: Delay of senescence infertility by dietary restriction. *Fed Proc, 8*:22, 1949.

Carryer, H.M., Berkman, J.M., and Masen, H.L.: Relative lymphocytoses in anorexia nervosa. *Mayo Clinic Proc, 34*:426, 1959.

Cason, J., Ainley, C.C., Wolstencroft, R.A., Norton, K.R., and Thompson, R.P.: Cell-mediated immunity in anorexia nervosa. *Clin Exp Immunol, 64*:370, 1986.

Casper, R.C.: The pathophysiology of anorexia nervosa and bulimia nervosa. *Ann Rev Nutr, 6*:299, 1986.

Casper, R.C., Davis, J.M., and Pandey, G.N.: The effect of the nutritional status and weight changes on hypothalmic function tests in anorexia nervosa. In Vigersky, R.A. (Ed.): *Anorexia Nervosa*. New York, Raven Press, 1977, pp. 134-147.

Castelli, W.P. Cited by *Wall Street Journal*, Dec. 1, 1982, p. 32.

Castro, C.E., and Sevall, J.S.: Alteration of higher order structure of rat liver chromatin by dietary composition. *J Nutr, 110*:105, 1980.

Castro, C.E., Armstrong-Major, J., and Ramirez, M.E.: Diet-mediated alteration of chromatin structure. *Fed Proc, 45*:2394, 1986.

Cawthorne, M.A.: Metabolic aspects of obesity. *Mol Aspects Med, 5*:293, 1982.

Cerami, A., Vlassara, H., and Brownlee, M.: Glucose and aging. *Sci Am, 256*:90, 1987.

Cerutti, P.A.: Prooxidant states and tumor promotion. *Science, 227*:375, 1985.

Chandra, R.K., Heresi, G., and Au, B.: Serum thymic factor activity in deficiencies of calories, zinc, vitamin A and pyridoxine. *Clin Exp Immunol, 42*:332, 1980.

Chebotarev, D.F., Frolkis, V.V., and Grigorov, Iu. G.: Nutrition and state of health of older persons during physiologic aging. *Vopr Pitan, Nov-Dec*:22, 1976.

Chen, J.C., Warshaw, J.B., and Sanadi, D.R.: Regulation of mitochondrial respiration in senescence. *J Cell Physiol, 80*:141, 1972.

Cheney, K.E., Liu, R.K., Smith, G.S., Leung, R.E., Mickey, M.R., and Walford, R.L.: Survival and disease patterns in C57BL/6J mice subjected to undernutrition. *Exp Gerontol, 15*:237, 1980.

Cheney, K.E., Liu, R.K., Smith, G.S., Meredith, P.J., Mickey, M.R., and Walford, R.L.: The effect of dietary restriction of varying duration on survival, tumor patterns, immune function, and body temperature in B10C3F$_1$ mice. *J Gerontol, 38*:420, 1983.

Cherkin, A.: Letter to the editor. *Age, 2*:51, 1979.

Chernoff, R.: Aging and nutrition. *Nutr Today, 22*:4, 1987.

Chesky, J., and Zakeri, Z. (Symposium organizers): Life extension and ethical considerations—the perspective of the biologist. *Gerontologist, 27*:59A, 1987.

Cheung, H.T., Twu, J.S., and Richardson, A.: Mechanism of the age-related decline in lymphocyte proliferation: role of Il-2-production and protein synthesis. *Exp Gerontol, 18*:451, 1983.

Chipalkatti, S., De, A.K., and Aiyar, A.S.: Effect of diet restriction on some biochemical parameters related to aging in mice. *J Nutr, 113*:944, 1983.

Chiu, Y.J.D., and Richardson, A.: Effect of age on the function of mitochondria isolated from brain and heart tissue. *Exp Gerontol, 15*:511, 1980.

Chowers, I., Einat, R., and Feldman, S.: Effects of starvation on levels of corticotrophin releasing factor, corticotrophin and plasma corticosterone in rats. *Acta Endocrinol, 61*:687, 1969.

Christadoss, P., Talal, N., Lindstrom, J., and Fernandes, G.: Suppression of cellular and humoral immunity to T-dependent antigens by calorie restriction. *Cell Immunol, 88*:1, 1984.

Chvapil, M., and Hruza, Z.: The influence of aging and undernutrition on chemical contractility and relaxation of collagen fibres in rats. *Gerontologia, 3*:241, 1959.

Chvapil, M., and Holeckova, E.: Lowered structural stability of collagenous fibres induced by intermittent feeding and fasting in the rat. *Physiol Bohemoslov, 11*:505, 1962.

Clapp, N.K., Satterfield, L.C., and Bowles, N.D.: Effects of the antioxidant butylated hydroxytoluene (BHT) on mortality in BALB/c mice. *J Gerontol, 34*:497, 1979.

Clarke, J.: The aging dimension: a factorial analysis of individual differences with age on psychological and physiological measurements. *J Gerontol, 15*:183, 1960.

Cleary, M.P., Muller, S., and Lanza-Jacoby, S.: Effects of long-term moderate food restriction on growth, serum factors, lipogenic enzymes and adipocyte glucose metabolism in lean and obese zucker rats. *J Nutr, 117*:355, 1987.

Clemens, M.: Translational control, developments in development. *Nature, 330*:699, 1987.

Cohen, L.A.: Diet and cancer. *Sci Am, 257*:42, 1987.

Cohn, C., and Joseph, D.: Effects of caloric intake and feeding frequency on carbohydrate metabolism of the rat. *J Nutr, 100*:78, 1970.

Cole, G.M., Segall, P.E., and Timiras, P.S.: Hormones during aging. In Vernadakis, A., and Timiras, P.S. (Eds.): *Hormones in Development and Aging.* New York, Spectrum Publications, 1982, pp. 477-550.

Coleman, D.L.: Increased metabolic efficiency in obese mutant mice. *Int J Obes, 2*:69, 1985.

Coleman, D.L., Schwizer, R.W., and Leiter, E.H.: Effect of genetic background on the therapeutic effects of dehydroepiandrosterone (DHEA) in diabetes-obesity mutants and in aged normal mice. *Diabetes, 33*:26, 1984.

Comfort, A.: Nutrition and longevity in animals. *Proc Nutr Soc, 19*:125, 1960.

Comfort, A.: Effect of delayed and resumed growth on the longevity of a fish (*Lebistes reticulatus,* Peters) in captivity. *Gerontologia, 8*:150, 1963.

Comfort, A.: Test battery to measure aging-rate in man. *Lancet, ii*:1411, 1969.

Comfort, A.: Measuring the human aging rate. *Mech Ageing Dev, 1*:101, 1972.

Comfort, A.: *The Biology of Senescence.* New York, Elsevier, 1979.

Comfort, A.: Living all your life. In Woodhead, A.D., Blackett, A.D., and Hollaender, A. (Eds.): *Molecular Biology of Aging.* New York, Plenum Pub. Corp., 1985, pp. 213-229.

Comfort, A. Youhotsky-Gore, I., and Pathmanathan, K.: Effect of ethoxyquin on the longevity of C3H mice. *Nature, 229*:254, 1971.

Conard, A., Lowrey, A., Eicher, M., Thompson, K., and Scott, W.A.: Aging studies in a Marshallese population exposed to radioactive fall-out in 1954. In Lindop, P., and Sacher, G.A. (Eds.): *Radiation and Aging*. London, Taylor & Francis, Ltd., 1966, pp. 345-360.

Conybeare, G.: Effect of quality and quantity of diet on survival and tumor incidence in outbred Swiss mice. *Fd Cosmet Toxicol, 18*:65, 1980.

Cooper, B., Weinblatt, F., and Gregerman, R.I.: Enhanced activity of hormone-sensitive adenylate cyclase during dietary restriction in the rat. Dependence on age and relation to cell size. *J Clin Invest, 59*:467, 1977.

Cooper, E.L.: Invertebrate defense systems, an overview. In Cohen, N., and Sigel, M.M. (Eds.): *Ontogeny and Phylogeny of the Reticuloendothelial System*. New York, Plenum Press, 1982, pp. 1-35.

Cooper, W.C., Good, R.A., and Mariani, T.: Effects of protein insufficiency on immune responsiveness. *Am J Clin Nutr, 27*:647, 1974.

Corbett, S.W., Stern, J.S., and Keesey, R.E.: Energy expenditure in rats with diet-induced obesity. *Am J Clin Nutr, 44*:173, 1986.

Corraze, G.R., Lacombe, C.R., and Nibbelink, M.M.: Dietary restriction amplifies the hypercholesterolemic effect of cholesterol feeding in the rat. *Nutr Res, 5*:781, 1985.

Corso, J.F.: Sensory processes and perception in ageing. In Viidik, A. (Ed.): *Lectures on Gerontology. Volume I: On Biology of Ageing*, Part B. New York, Academic Press, 1982, pp. 441-479.

Cosgrove, G.E., Satterfield, L.C., Bowles, N.D., and Klima, W.C.: Diseases of aging in untreated virgin female RFM and BALB/c mice. *J Gerontol, 33*:178, 1978.

Costa, P.T., Jr., and McCrae, R.R.: Functional age: a conceptual and empirical critique. In Haynes, S.G., and Feinleib, M. (Eds.): *Second Conference on the Epidemiology of Aging*. NIH Pub. No. 80-969, 1980a, pp. 23-46.

Costa, P.T., Jr., and McCrae, R.R.: Concepts of functional or biological age: a critical review. In Andres, R., Bierman, E.L., and Hazzard, W.R. (Eds.): *Principles of Geriatric Medicine*. New York, McGraw Hill, 1980b, pp. 30-37.

Cotzias, G.C., Miller, S.T., Tang, L.C., Papavasiliou, P.S., and Wang, Y.Y.: Levodopa, fertility and longevity. *Science, 196*:549, 1977.

Council for Agricultural Science and Technology, Diet and coronary disease. *Nutr Action, 21*:26, 1986.

Covelli, V., Marini, S., Di Majo, V., Bassani, B., Mancini, C., Adorini, L., and Doria, G.: Life-span, tumor incidence, and natural killer cell activity in mice selected for high or low antibody responsiveness. *JNCI, 72*:1127, 1984.

Cox, G.B., Hatch, L., Webb, D., Fimmel, A.L., Lin, Z.H., Senior, A.E., and Gibson, F.: Amino acid substitutions in the ϵ-subunit of the F_1-F_0-ATPase of *Escherichia coli*. *Biochim Biophys Acta, 890*:195, 1987.

Cox, M.D., Dalal, S.S., Heard, C.R.C., and Millward, D.J.: Metabolic rate and thyroid status in rats fed diets of different protein-energy value: the importance of free T_3. *J Nutr, 114*:1609, 1984.

Craig, B.W., Garthwaite, S.M., and Holloszy, J.O.: Adipocyte insulin resistance: effects of aging, obesity, exercise, and food restriction. *J Appl Physiol, 62*:95, 1987.

Crew, M.D., Spindler, S.R., Walford, R.L., and Koizumi, A.: Age-related decreases of growth hormone and prolactin mRNAs in pituitary glands of C57BL/6 mice. *Endocrinology, 121*:1251, 1987.

Cristofalo, V.J.: The destiny of cells: mechanisms and implications of senescence. *Gerontologist, 25*:577, 1983.

Csukas, S., and Green, K.: In vivo modification of catalase activity designed to mimic age-related changes in the rabbit eye. *Gerontologist, 27*:152A, 1987.

Curfman, G.D., O'Hara, D.S., Hopkins, B.E., Smith, T.W.: Suppression of myocardial protein degradation in the rat during fasting. Effects of insulin, glucose, and leucine. *Circ Res, 46*:581, 1980.

Curtis, H.J.: Biologic mechanisms underlying the aging process. *Science, 141*:688, 1963.

Cutler, R.G.: Evolution of human longevity and the genetic complexity governing aging rate. *Proc Natl Acad Sci USA, 72*:4664, 1975.

Cutler, R.G.: Nature of aging and life maintenance processes. In Cutler, R.G. (Ed.): *Interdiscip Top Gerontol*, Vol. 9. Basel, Karger, 1976, pp. 83-133.

Cutler, R.G.: Evolutionary biology of senescence. In Behnke, J.A., Finch, C.E., and Moment, G.B. (Eds.): *Biology of Aging*. New York, Plenum Press, 1978, pp. 311-360.

Cutler, R.G.: Lifespan extension. In McGaugh, J.L., and Kiesler, S.B. (Eds.): *Aging: Biology and Behavior*. New York, Academic Press, 1981, pp. 31-76.

Cutler, R.G.: Longevity is determined by specific genes: testing the hypothesis. In Adelman, R.C., and Roth, G.S. (Eds.): *Testing the Theories of Aging*. Boca Raton, CRC Press, 1982, pp. 25-114.

Cutler, R.G.: Antioxidants and longevity. In Armstrong, D., Sohal, R.S., Cutler, R.G., and Slater, T.F. (Eds.): *Free Radicals in Molecular Biology, Aging, and Disease*. New York, Raven Press, 1984a, pp. 235-266.

Cutler, R.G.: Urate and ascorbate: their possible roles as antioxidants in determining longevity of mammalian species. *Arch Gerontol Geriatr, 3*:321, 1984b.

Cutler, R.G.: Carotenoids and retinol: their possible importance in determining longevity of primate species. *Proc Natl Acad Sci USA, 81*:7627, 1984c.

Cutler, R.G.: Antioxidants and longevity of mammalian species. In Woodhead, A.D., Blackett, A.D., and Hollaender, A. (Eds.): *Molecular Biology of Aging*. New York, Plenum Press, 1985a, pp. 15-73.

Cutler, R.G.: Peroxide-producing potential of tissues: Inverse correlation with longevity of mammalian species. *Proc Natl Acad Sci USA, 82*:4798, 1985b.

Czaplicki, J., and Blonska, B.: Some cases of animal longevity following treatment with early fetal thymic extracts (Letter to the editor). *Thymus, 3*:185, 1981.

Dalderup, L.M., and Visser, W.: Influence of extra sucrose in the daily food on the life-span of Wistar albino rats. *Nature, 222*:1050, 1969.

Darby, W.J.: Diet and coronary atheroma. *JAMA, 182*:1328, 1962.

Dauncey, M.J.: Activity-induced thermogenesis in lean and genetically obese (ob/ob) mice. *Experientia, 42*:547, 1986.

David, J., Van Herrewege, J., and Fouillet, P.: Quantitative under-feeding of Drosophila: Effects on adult longevity and fecundity. *Exp Gerontol*, 6:249, 1971.

Davidson, J.K.: Controlling diabetes mellitus with diet therapy. *Postgrad Med*, 59:114, 1976.

Davis, T.A., Bales, C.W., and Beauchene, R.E.: Differential effects of dietary caloric and protein restriction in the aging rat. *Exp Gerontol*, 118:427, 1983.

De, A.K., Chipalkatti, S., and Aiyar, A.S.: Some biochemical parameters in relation to dietary protein. *Mech Ageing Dev*, 21:37, 1983.

Dean, W. Biological aging measurement: clinical applications. Aging Research Institute, El Toro, CA, 1986.

DeFronzo, R.A.: Glucose intolerance and aging. In Reff, M.E., and Schneider, E.L. (Eds.): *Biological Markers of Aging*. NIH Publication No. 82-2221, 1982, pp. 98-119.

DeFronzo, R.A., Ferrannini, E., Sato, Y., Felig, P., and Wahren, J.: Synergistic action between exercise and insulin on peripheral glucose uptake. *J Clin Invest*, 68:1468, 1981.

DeGroot, L.J., Coleoni, A.H., Rue, P.A., Seo, H., Martino, E., and Refetoff, S.: Reduced nuclear triiodothyronine receptors in starvation-induced hyperthyroidism. *Biochem Biophys Res Commun*, 79:173, 1977.

Dell'Orco, R.T., and Whittle, W.L.: Micrococcal nuclease and DNase I digestion of DNA from aging human diploid cells *Biochem Biophys Res Commun*, 107:117, 1982.

Denckla, W.D.: Role of the pituitary and thyroid glands in the decline of minimal O_2 consumption with age. *J Clin Invest*, 53:572, 1974.

Deneke, S.M., Lynch, B.A., and Fanburg, B.L.: Effects of low protein diets or feed restriction on rat lung glutathione and oxygen toxicity. *J Nutr*, 115:726, 1985.

Deshmukh, D.R., and Patel, M.S.: Age-dependent changes in pyruvate uptake by nonsynaptic and synaptic mitochondria from rat brain. *Mech Ageing Dev*, 20:343, 1982.

Dewasmes, G., Le Maho, Y., Cornet, A., and Groscolas, R.: Resting metabolic rate and cost of locomotion in long-term fasting emperor penguins. *J Appl Physiol*, 49:888, 1980.

Deyl, Z., Juricova, M., Rosmus, J., and Adam, M.: The effect of food deprivation on collagen accumulation. *Exp Gerontol*, 6:383, 1971.

DiGirolamo, M., Crandall, D., Fried, S.K., Nickel, M., and Hill, J.O.: Effects of chronic food restriction (CFR) and aging on rat adipocyte metabolic activities and hormonal responsiveness. In: *Proc VIIth Intl Congr Endocrinol* (Book of Abstracts). Amsterdam, Elsevier/North Holland, Excerpta Medica, 1984, p. 547.

Dilman, V.: Age-associated elevation of hypothalamic threshold to feedback control, and its role in development, ageing and disease. *Lancet*, i:1211, 1971.

Dilman, V.M.: The hypothalamic control of aging and age associated pathology: the elevation mechanism of aging. In Everitt, A.V., and Burgess, J.A. (Eds.): *Hypothalamus, Pituitary and Aging*. Springfield, Charles C Thomas, 1976, pp. 634-667.

Donato, K., and Hegsted, D.M.: Efficiency of utilization of various sources of energy for growth. *Proc Natl Acad Sci USA*, 82:4866, 1985.

Doorn, J.V., Van Der Heide, D., and Roelfsema, F.: The influence of partial food deprivation on the quantity and source of triiodothyronine in several tissues of athyreotic thyroxine-maintained rats. *Endocrinology*, 115:705, 1984.

Drori, D., and Folman, Y.: Environmental effects on longevity in the male rat: exercise, mating, castration and restricted feeding. *Exp Gerontol, 11*:25, 1976.

Duara, R., London, E.D., and Rapoport, S.I.: Changes in structure and energy metabolism of the aging brain. In Finch, C.E., and Schneider, E.L. (Eds.): *Handbook of the Biology of Aging.* New York, Van Nostrand Reinhold, 1985, pp. 595-616.

Dubos, R.: Nutritional adaptations. *Am J Clin Nutr, 32*:2623, 1979.

Dubuc, P.U., Wilden, N.J., and Carlisle, H.J.: Fed and fasting thermoregulation in ob/ob mice. *Ann Nutr Metab, 29*:358, 1985.

Duncan, K.H., Bacon, J.A., and Weinsier, R.L.: The effects of high and low energy density diets on satiety, energy intake, and eating time of obese and nonobese subjects. *Am J Clin Nutr, 37*:763, 1983.

Dunham, H.H.: Abundant feeding followed by restricted feeding and longevity in *Daphnia. Physl Zool, 11*:399, 1938.

Dunning, W.F., Curtis, M.R., and Maun, M.E.: The effect of dietary fat and carbohydrate on diethylstilbesterol-induced mammary cancer in rats. *Cancer Res, 9*:354, 1949.

Durand, A.M., Fisher, M., and Adams, M.: The influence of type of dietary carbohydrate. *Arch Pathol, 85*:318, 1968.

Durnin, J.V.G.A., Edholm, O.G., Miller, D.S., and Waterlow, J.C.: How much food does man require? *Nature, 242*:418, 1973.

Dutta, P., Smith, R.D., and Flynn, M.A.: Effects of medroxyprogesterone acetate and caloric restriction on the distribution of serum and liver lipids and proteins in female rats. *J Nutr, 111*:1380, 1981.

Edmundson, W.: Individual variations in work output per unit energy intake in East Java. *Ecol Food Nutr, 6*:147, 1977.

Edmundson, W.: Individual variations in basal metabolic rate and mechanical work efficiency in East Java. *Ecol Food Nutr, 8*:189, 1979.

Einhorn, D., Young, J.B., and Landsberg, L.: Hypotensive effect of fasting: possible involvement of the sympathetic nervous sytem and endogenous opiates. *Science, 217*:727, 1982.

Eisen, E.J., and Leatherwood, J.M.: Effect of postweaning feed restriction on adipose cellularity and body composition in polygenic obese mice. *J Nutr, 108*:1663, 1978.

Eklund, J., and Bradford, G.E.: Longevity and lifetime body weight in mice selected for rapid growth. *Nature, 265*:48, 1977.

El Haj, A.J., Lewis, S.E.M., Goldspink, D.F., Merry, B.J., and Holehan, A.M.: The effect of chronic and acute dietary restriction on the growth and protein turnover of fast and slow types of rat skeletal muscle. *Comp Biochem Physiol, 85A*:281, 1986.

Ellis, F.R., Holesh, S., and Ellis, J.W.: Incidence of osteoporosis in vegetarians and omnivores. *Am J Clin Nutr, 25*:555, 1972.

Else, P.L., and Hulbert, A.J.: Mammals: an allometric study of metabolism at tissue and mitochondrial level. *Am J Physiol, 248*:R415, 1985.

Enesco, H.E., and Kruk, P.: Dietary restriction reduces fluorescent age pigment accumulation in mice. *Exp Gerontol, 16*:357, 1981.

Engel, R.W., and Copeland, D.H.: Influence of diet on the relative incidence of eye, mammary, ear-duct, and liver tumors in rats fed 2-acetylaminofluorene. *Cancer Res, 11*:180, 1951.

Erickson, K.L., Gershwin, M.E., Canolty, N.L., and Eckels, D.D.: The influence of dietary protein concentration and energy intake on mitogen response and tumor growth in melanoma-bearing mice. *J Nutr, 109*:353, 1979a.

Erickson, K.L., Gershwin, M.E., McNeill, C.J., Ossmann, J.B., and Canolty, N.L.: Effects of low protein concentration and energy deprivation on lymphocyte transformation in melanoma-bearing mice. *J Nutr, 109*:1893, 1979b.

Erickson, K.L., Adams, D.A., and McNeill, C.J.: Dietary lipid modulation of immune responsiveness. *Lipids, 18*:468, 1983.

Ershler, W.B., Berman, E., and Moore, A.L.: Slower B16 melanoma growth but greater pulmonary colonization in calorie-restricted mice. *JNCI, 76*:81, 1986.

Evans, H.M., and Bishop, K.S.: On the relations between fertility and nutrition. II. The ovulation rhythm in the rat on inadequate nutritional regimes. *J Metab Res, 1*:335, 1922.

Everitt, A.V.: Food intake, growth and the ageing of collagen in rat tail tendon. *Gerontologia, 17*:98, 1971.

Everitt, A.V.: The hypothalamic-pituitary control of aging and age-related pathology. *Exp Gerontol, 8*:265, 1973.

Everitt, A.V.: Conclusion: Aging and its hypothalamic-pituitary control. In Everitt, A.V., and Burgess, J.A. (Eds.): *Hypothalamus, Pituitary and Aging.* Springfield, Charles C Thomas, 1976, pp. 676-701.

Everitt, A.V., and Webb, C.: The relation between body weight changes and life duration in male rats. *J Gerontol, 12*:128, 1957.

Everitt, A.V., and Cavanagh, L.M.: The ageing process in the hypophysectomized rat. *Gerontologia, 11*:198, 1965.

Everitt, A.V., and Porter, B.: Nutrition and aging. In Everitt, A.V., and Burgess, J.A. (Eds.): *Hypothalamus, Pituitary and Aging.* Springfield, Charles C Thomas, 1976, pp. 570-613.

Everitt, A.V., Seedsman, N.J., and Jones, F.: The effects of hypophysectomy and continuous food restriction, begun at ages 70 and 400 days, on collagen aging, proteinuria, incidence of pathology and longevity in the male rat. *Mech Ageing Dev, 12*:161, 1980.

Everitt, A.V., Porter, B.D., and Wyndham, J.R.: Effects of caloric intake and dietary composition on the development of proteinuria, age-associated renal disease and longevity in the male rat. *Gerontology, 28*:168, 1982.

Everitt, A.V., Wyndham, J.R., and Barnard, D.L.: The anti-aging action of hypophysectomy in hypothalamic obese rats: Effects on collagen aging, age-associated proteinuria development and renal histopathology. *Mech Ageing Dev, 22*:233, 1983.

Fabris, N.: Pathways of neuroendocrine-immune interactions and their impact with aging processes. In Facchini, A., Haaijman, J.J., and Labo, G. (Eds.): *Immunoregulation in Aging.* Rijswijk, Eurage, 1986, pp. 117-130.

Fabris, N., Mocchegiani, E., Muzzioli, M., and Imberte, R.: Thymus-neuroendocrine network. In Hadden, J., and Mitchison, N.A. (Eds.): *Immunoregulation.* New York, Plenum Press, 1983, pp. 341-362.

Failla, G.: The aging process and cancerogenesis. *Ann NY Acad Sci, 71*:1124, 1958.

Fanestil, D.D., and Barrows, C.H., Jr.: Aging in the rotifer. *J Gerontol, 20*:462, 1965.

Feinstein, R.N.: Acatalasemia in the mouse and other species. *Biochem Genet, 4*:135, 1970.

Feinstein, R.N., Fry, R.J.M., and Staffeldt, E.F.: Comparative effects of aminotriazole on normal and acatalasemic mice. *J Env Pathol Toxicol, 1*:779, 1978a.

Feinstein, R.N., Fry, R.J.M., and Staffeldt, E.F.: Carcinogenic and antitumor effects of aminotriazole on acatalasemic and normal mice. *J Natl Cancer Inst, 60*:1113, 1978b.

Feldman, D.B., McConnell, E.E., and Knapka, J.J.: Growth, kidney disease, and longevity of Syrian hamsters (*Mesocricetus auratus*) fed varying levels of protein. *Lab Anim Sci, 32*:613, 1982.

Feldman, J.D., and Woda, B.A.: Pathology and tumor incidence in aged Lewis and BN rats. *Clin Immunol Immunopathol, 15*:331, 1980.

Ferguson, S.J.: The ups and downs of P/O ratios (and the question of non-integral coupling stoichiometries for oxidative phosphorylation and related processes). In Hall, J. (Ed.): *TIBS*, Vol. 11. Amsterdam, Elsevier, 1986, p. 351-353.

Fernandes, G.: Nutritional factors: modulating effects on immune function and aging. *Pharmacol Rev, 36*:123S, 1984.

Fernandes, G.: Influence of nutrition on autoimmune disease. In Goidl, E.A. (Ed.): *Aging and the Immune Response*. New York, Dekker, 1987, pp. 225-242.

Fernandes, G., and Good, R.A.: Inhibition by restricted diet of lymphoproliferative disease and renal damage in MRL/lpr mice. *Proc Natl Acad Sci USA, 81*:6144, 1984.

Fernandes, G., Yunis, E.J., Jose, D.G., and Good, R.A.: Dietary influence on antinuclear antibodies and cell-mediated immunity in NZB mice. *Int Arch Allergy Appl Immunol, 44*:770, 1973.

Fernandes, G., Yunis, E.J., and Good, R.A.: Influence of protein restriction on immune functions in NZB mice. *J Immunol, 116*:782, 1976a.

Fernandes, G., Yunis, E.J., and Good, R.A.: Suppression of adenocarcinoma by the immunological consequences of calorie restriction. *Nature, 263*:504, 1976b.

Fernandes, G., Yunis, E.J., and Good, R.A.: Influence of diet on survival of mice. *Proc Natl Acad Sci USA, 73*:1279, 1976c.

Fernandes, G., Yunis, E.J., and Good, R.A.: Influence of dietary restriction on immunologic function and renal disease in (NZB × NZW)F_1 mice. *Proc Natl Acad Sci USA, 75*:1500, 1978a.

Fernandes, G., Yunis, E.J., Miranda, M., Smith, J., and Good, R.A.: Nutritional inhibition of genetically determined renal disease and autoimmunity with prolongation of life in kd/kd mice. *Proc Natl Acad Sci USA, 75*:2888, 1978b.

Fernandes, G., Alonso, D.R., Tanaka, T., Thaler, H.T., Yunis, E.J., and Good, R.A.: Influence of diet on vascular lesions in autoimmune-prone B/W mice. *Proc Natl Acad Sci USA, 80*:874, 1983.

Fernandes, G., Khare, A., Laganiere, S., Yu, B., Sandberg, L., and Friedrichs, B.: Effect of food restriction and aging on immune cell fatty acids, functions and oncogene expression in SPF Fischer 344 rats. *Fed Proc, 46*:567, 1987.

Finch, C.E.: The regulation of physiological changes during mammalian aging. *Q Rev Biol, 51*:49, 1976.

Finch, C.E.: Neuroendocrine mechanisms and aging. *Fed Proc, 38*:178, 1979.

Finch, C.E., and Mobbs, C.V.: Hormonal influences on hypothalamic sensitivity during aging in female rodents. In Meites, J. (Ed.): *Neuroendocrinology of Aging.* New York, Plenum Press, 1983, pp. 143-171.

Finch, C.E., and Landfield, P.W.: Neuroendocrine and autonomic functions in aging mammals. In Finch, C.E., and Schneider, E.L. (Eds.): *Handbook of the Biology of Aging,* 2nd Ed. New York, Van Nostrand Reinhold, 1985, pp. 567-594.

Finch, C.E., Felicio, L.S., Mobbs, C.V., and Nelson, J.F.: Ovarian and steroidal influences on neuroendocrine aging processes in female rodents. *Endocr Rev, 5*:467, 1984.

Fischer, W., Wictorin, K., Bjorlslund, A., Williams, L.R., Varon, S., and Gage, F.H.: Amelioration of cholinergic neuron atrophy and spatial memory impairment in aged rats by nerve growth factor. *Nature, 329*:65, 1987.

Fischer-Piette, E.: Sur la croissance et la longevite' de *Patella vulgata* L. en fonction du milieu. *J Conchyliologie, 83*:303, 1939.

Flatt, P.R., Bailey, C.J., Kwasowski, P., Swanston-Flatt, S.K., and Marks, V.: Glucoregulatory effects of cafeteria feeding and diet restriction in genetically obese hyperglycaemic (ob/ob) mice. *Nutr Rep Int, 32*:847, 1985.

Fleming, B.B.: The vitamin status and requirements of the elderly. In Moment, G.B. (Ed.): *Nutritional Approaches to Aging Research.* Boca Raton, CRC Press, 1982, pp. 84-117.

Fleming, J.E., Miquel, J., Cottrell, S.F., Yengoyan, L.S., and Economos, A.C.: Is cell aging caused by respiration-dependent injury to the mitochondrial genome? *Gerontology, 28*:44, 1982.

Flier, J.S., Cook, K.S., Usher, P., and Spiegelman, B.M.: Severely impaired adipsin expression in genetic and acquired obesity. *Science, 237*:405, 1987.

Flory, C.M., Furth, J., Saxton, J.A., Jr., and Reiner, L.: Chemotherapeutic studies on transmitted mouse leukemia. *Cancer Res, 3*:729, 1943.

Food and Nutrition Board, National Research Council: Toward Healthful Diets. *Natl Acad Sci,* Washington, D.C., 1980a.

Food and Nutrition Board, Committee on Dietary Allowances, National Research Council: Recommended Dietary Allowances. *Natl Acad Sci,* Washington, D.C., 1980b.

Forbes, E.B., Swift, R.W., Elliott, R.F., and James, W.H.: Relation of fat to economy of food utilization. *J Nutr, 31*:213, 1946.

Forsum, E., Hillman, P.E., and Nesheim, M.C.: Effect of energy restriction on total heat production, basal metabolic rate, and specific dynamic action of food in rats. *J Nutr, 111*:1691, 1981.

Foster, C., Jones, J.H., Henle, W., and Dorfman, F.: The effect of vitamin B_1 deficiency and of restricted food intake on the response of mice to the lansing strain of poliomyelitis virus. *J Exp Med, 79*:221, 1944a.

Foster, C., Jones, J.H., Henle, W., and Dorfman, F.: The comparative effects of vitamin B_1 deficiency and restriction of food intake on the response of mice to the lansing strain of poliomyelitis virus, as determined by the paired feeding technique. *J Exp Med, 80*:257, 1944b.

Franklin, A., Hinsull, S.M., and Bellamy, D.: The effect of dietary restriction on thymus autonomy. *Thymus, 5*:345, 1983.

French, C.E., Ingram, R.H., Uram, J.A., Barron, G.P., and Swift, R.W.: The influence of dietary fat and carbohydrate on growth and longevity in rats. *J Nutr, 51*:329, 1953.

Fridovich, I.: Biological effects of the superoxide radical. *Arch Biochem Biophys, 247*:1, 1986.

Friend, P.S., Fernandes, G., Good, R.A., Michael, A.F., and Yunis, E.J.: Dietary restrictions early and late: effects on the nephropathy of the NZB × NZW mouse. *Lab Invest, 38*:629, 1978.

Fries, J.F., and Crapo, L.M.: *Vitality and Aging.* San Francisco, Freeman, 1981.

Frisch, R.E.: Food intake, fatness, and reproductive ability. In Vigersby, R.A. (Ed.): *Anorexia Nervosa.* New York, Raven Press, 1977, pp. 149-161.

Frolkis, V.: The Hypothalamic Mechanisms of Aging. In Everitt, A.V., and Burgess, J.A. (Eds.): *Hypothalamus, Pituitary and Aging.* Springfield, Charles C Thomas, 1976, pp. 614-633.

Frolkis, V.V.: *Aging and Life-Prolonging Processes.* Vienna-New York, Springer-Verlag, 1982.

Fujita, Y., Ichikawa, M., Kurimoto, F., and Rikimaru, T.: Effects of feed restriction and switching the diet on proteinuria in male Wistar rats. *J Gerontol, 39*:531, 1984.

Fujita, Y., and Ichikawa, M.: Age-related changes in nitrogen balance and related variables in later life of aging male Wistar rats. *J Nutr Sci Vitaminol, 32*:381, 1986.

Fukami, M.H., and Flatmark, T.: Studies on catalase compartmentation in digitonin-treated rat hepatocytes. *Biochim et Biophys Acta, 889*:91, 1986.

Furukawa, T., Inoue, M., Kajiya, F., Inada, H., Takasuji, S., Fukui, S., Takeda, H., and Abe, H.: Assessment of biological age by multiple regression analysis. *J Gerontol, 30*:422, 1975.

Gabius, H., Engelhardt, R., Deerberg, F., and Cramer, F.: Age-related changes in different steps of protein synthesis of liver and kidney of rats. *FEBS Lett, 160*:115, 1983.

Gabrielsen, A.E., and Olsen, C.T.: Prolonged survival of hypertransfused NZB/NZW mice. *Immunology, 33*:449, 1977.

Gajjar, A., Kubo, C., Johnson, B.C., and Good, R.A.: Influence of extremes of protein and energy intake on survival of B/W mice. *J Nutr, 117*:1136, 1987.

Gallo, P.V., and Weinberg, J.: Corticosterone rhythmicity in the rat: Interactive effects for dietary restriction and schedule of feeding. *J Nutr, 111*:208, 1981.

Gansler, T.S., Muller, S., and Cleary, M.P.: Chronic administration of dehydroepiandrosterone reduces pancreatic β-cell hyperplasia and hyperinsulinemia in genetically obese Zucker rats. *Proc Soc Exp Biol Med, 180*:155, 1985.

Garrel, D.R., Todd, K.S., Pugeat, M.M., and Calloway, D.H.: Hormonal changes in normal men under marginally negative energy balance. *Am J Clin Nutr, 39*:930, 1984.

Garrow, J.S.: *Energy Balance and Obesity in Man,* 2nd ed. Amsterdam, Elsevier/North Holland Press, 1978.

Garrow, J.S.: Chronic effects of over- and under-nutrition on thermogenesis. *Int J Vitam Nutr Res, 56*:201, 1986.

Garthwaite, S.M., Cheng, H., Bryan, J.E., Craig, B.W., and Holloszy, J.O.: Ageing, exercise and food restriction: Effects on body composition. *Mech Age Develop, 36*:187, 1986.

Geissler, C.A., Muller, D.S., and Shah, M.: The daily metabolic rate of the post-obese and the lean. *Am J Clin Nutr, 45*:914, 1987.

Gellatly, J.B.M.: The natural history of hepatic parenchymal nodule formation in a colony of C57BL mice with reference to the effect of diet. In Butler, W.H., and Newberne, P.M. (Eds.): *Mouse Hepatic Neoplasia.* Amsterdam, Elsevier, 1975, pp. 77-109.

Genuth, S.M.: Perspective on very low calorie diets in the treatment of obesity. In Blackburn, G.L., and Bray, G.A. (Eds.): *Management of Obesity by Severe Caloric Restriction.* Littleton, Mass., PSG Publishing, 1985, pp. 21-32.

Gerbase-DeLima, M., Liu, R.K., Cheney, K.E., Mickey, R., and Walford, R.L.: Immune function and survival in a long-lived mouse strain subjected to undernutrition. *Gerontologia, 21*:184, 1975.

Gerstenblith, G.: Cardiovascular aging. In Reff, M.E., and Schneider, E.L. (Eds.): *Biological Markers of Aging.* NIH Publ. No. 82-2221, 1982, pp. 138-144.

Gibson, G.E., and Peterson, C.: Calcium and the aging nervous system. *Neurobiol Aging, 8*:329, 1987.

Gilbert, C., Gillman, J., Loustalot, P., and Lutz, W.: The modifying influence of diet and the physical environment on spontaneous tumor frequency in rats. *Br J Cancer, 12*:565, 1958.

Giles, J.S. and Everitt, A.V.: The role of the thyroid and food intake in the ageing of collagen fibers. I. In the young rat. *Gerontologia, 13*:65, 1967.

Giovanella, B.C., Shepard, R.C., Stehlin, J.S., Venditti, J.M., and Abbott, B.J.: Calorie restriction: Effect on growth of human tumors heterotransplanted in nude mice. *JNCI, 68*:249, 1982.

Giovannetti, P.M. and Strothers, S.C.: Influence of diet and age on ribonucleic acid, protein and free amino acid levels of rat skeletal muscle. *Growth, 39*:1, 1975.

Glass, A.R., and Swerdloff, R.S.: Nutritional influences on sexual maturation in the rat. *Fed Proc, 39*:2360, 1980.

Glass, A.R., Harrison, R. and Swerdloff, R.S.: Effect of undernutrition and amino acid deficiency on the timing of puberty in rats. *Pediatr Res, 10*:951, 1976.

Glass, A.R., Mellitt, R., Burman, K.D., Wartofsky, L., and Swerdloff, R.S.: Serum triiodothyronine in undernourished rats: Dependence on dietary composition rather than total calorie or protein intake. *Endocrinology, 102*:1925, 1978.

Gleeson, M., Brown, J.F., Waring, J.J., and Stock, M.J.: The effects of physical exercise on metabolic rate and dietary-induced thermogenesis. *Br J Nutr, 47*:173, 1982.

Goidl, E.A. (Ed.): *Aging and the Immune Response.* Immunology Series, Vol. 31, New York, Marcel Dekker, Inc., 1987.

Gold, A.J., and Costello, L.C.: Effects of semistarvation on rat liver, kidney, and heart mitochondrial function. *J Nutr, 105*:208, 1975.

Goldspink, D.F., and Merry, B.J.: Changes in protein turnover and growth of the rat lung in response to ageing and long term dietary restriction. *Mech Ageing Dev,* 1988 (in press).

Goldspink, D.F., Lewis, S.E.M., and Merry, B.J.: Effects of aging and long term dietary intervention on protein turnover and growth of ventricular muscle in the rat heart. *Cardiovasc Res, 20*:672, 1986.

Goldspink, D.F., El Haj, A.J., Lewis, S.E.M., Merry, B.J., and Holehan, A.M.: The influence of chronic dietary intervention on protein turnover and growth of the diaphragm and extensor digitorum longus muscles of the rat. *Exp Gerontol,* 22:67, 1987.

Goldstein, A.L., Low, T.L.K., Hall, N., Naylor, P.H., and Zatz, M.M.: Thymosin: can it retard aging by boosting immune capacity. In Regelson, W., Sinex, F.M. (Eds.): *Intervention in the Aging Process. Part A: Quantitation, Epidemiology, and Clinical Research.* New York, Alan R. Liss, Inc., 1983, pp. 169-198.

Golla, J.A., Larson, L.A., Anderson, C.F., Lucas, A.R., Wilson, W.R., and Tomasi, T.B., Jr.: An immunological assessment of patients with anorexia nervosa. *Am J Clin Nutr, 34*:2756, 1981.

Good, R.A., and Gajjar, A.J.: Diet, immunity, and longevity. In Hutchinson, M.L., and Munro, H.N. (Eds.): *Nutrition and Aging.* New York, Academic Press, 1986, pp. 235-249.

Good, R.A., Fernandes, G., Yunis, E.J., Cooper, W.C., Jose, D.C., Kramer, T.R., and Hansen, M.A.: Nutritional deficiency, immunologic function, and disease. *Am J Pathol, 84*:599, 1976.

Good, R.A., Jose, D.G., and Cooper, W.C.: The relation between nutritional deprivation and immunity. In Jankovic, B.D., and Isakovic, K. (Eds.): *Microenvironmental Aspects of Immunity.* New York, Plenum Press, 1981, pp. 321-326.

Good, R.A., Hanson, L.A., and Edelman, R.: Infections and undernutrition. *Nutr Rev, 40*:119, 1982.

Goodrick, C.L.: The effects of dietary protein upon growth of inbred and hybrid mice. *Growth, 37*:355, 1973.

Goodrick, C.L.: Body weight changes over the life span and longevity for C57BL/6J mice and mutations which differ in maximal body weight. *Gerontology, 23*:405, 1977.

Goodrick, C.L.: Body weight increment and length of life: the effect of genetic constitution and dietary protein. *J Gerontol, 33*:184, 1978.

Goodrick, C.L.: Effects of long-term voluntary wheel exercise on male and female Wistar rats. *Gerontology 26*:22, 1980.

Goodrick, C.L.: Effects of lifelong restricted feeding on complex maze performance in rats. *Age, 7*:1, 1984.

Goodrick, C.L., Ingram, D.K., Reynolds, M.A., Freeman, J.R., and Cider, N.L.: Effects of intermittent feeding upon growth and life span in rats. *Gerontology, 28*:233, 1982.

Goodrick, C.L., Ingram, D.K., Reynolds, M.A., Freeman, J.R., and Cider, N.L.: Effects of intermittent feeding upon growth, activity, and life span in rats allowed voluntary exercise. *Exp Aging Res, 9*:203, 1983a.

Goodrick, C.L., Ingram, D.K., Reynolds, M.A., Freeman, J.R., and Cider, N.L.: Differential effects of intermittent feeding and voluntary exercise on body weight and life span in adult rats. *J Gerontol, 38*:36, 1983b.

Goodrick, C.L., Ingram, D.K., Reynolds, M.A., Freeman, J.R., and Cider, N.L.: Differential effects of dietary restriction on growth and life span in genetically obese mice. *Age, 6*:145, 1983c.

Gori, G.B.: Dietary and nutritional implications in the multi-factorial etiology of certain prevalent human cancers. *Cancer, 43*:2151, 1979.

Gori, G.B., and Richter, B.I.: Macroeconomics of disease prevention in the United States. *Science, 200*:1124, 1978.

Gosnell, B.A.: Effects of dietary dehydroepiandrosterone on food intake and body weight in rats with medial hypothalamic knife cuts. *Physiol Behav, 39*:687, 1987.

Gottesman, S.R.S., and Walford, R.L.: Autoimmunity and aging. In Adelman, R.C. and Roth, G.S. (Eds.): *Testing the Theories of Aging,* Boca Raton, CRC Press, 1982, pp. 233-279.

Greenfield, H., and Briggs, G.M.: Nutritional methodology in metabolic research with rats. *Ann Rev Biochem, 40*:549, 1971.

Gregerman, R.I.: Mechanisms of age-related alterations of hormone secretion and action. An overview of 30 years of progress. *Exp Gerontol, 21*:345, 1986.

Grewal, T., Mickelsen, O. Haps, H.D.: Androgen secretion and spermatogenesis in rats following semistarvation. *Proc Soc Exp Biol Med, 138*:723, 1971.

Gross, J.: Studies on the formation on collagen. II. The influence of growth rate on neural salt extracts of guinea pig dermis. *J Exp Med, 107*:265, 1958.

Gross, L., and Dreyfuss, Y.: Reduction in the incidence of radiation-induced tumors in rats after restriction of food intake. *Proc Natl Acad Sci USA, 81*:7596, 1984.

Gross, L., and Dreyfuss, Y.: Inhibition in the development of radiation-induced leukemia in mice by reduction of food intake. *Proc Natl Acad Sci USA, 83*:7928, 1986.

Grossman, C.J.: Interactions between the gonadal steroids and the immune system. *Science, 227*:257, 1985.

Gundberg, C.M., Anderson, M., Dickson, I., and Gallop, P.M.: "Glycated" osteocalcin in human and bovine bone. *J Biol Chem, 261*:14557, 1986.

Gunter, T.E., and Jensen, B.D.: The efficiencies of the component steps of oxidative phosphorylation. I. A simple steady state theory. *Arch Biochem Biophys, 248*:289, 1986.

Haining, J.L., and Legan, J.S.: Catalase turnover in rat liver and kidney as a function of age. *Exp Gerontol, 8*:85, 1973.

Hall, K.Y., Hart, R.W., Benirschke, A.K., and Walford, R.L.: Correlation between ultraviolet-induced DNA repair in primate lymphocytes and fibroblasts and species maximum achievable lifespan. *Mech Ageing Dev, 24*:163, 1984.

Hallgren, H.M., Buckley, C.E., Gilbertson, V.A., and Yunis, E.J.: Lymphocytes phytohemagglutinin responsiveness, immunoglobulins and autoantibodies in aging humans. *J Immunol, 111*:1101, 1973.

Hallgren, H.M., and Yunis, E.J.: Immune function, immune regulation, and survival in an aging human population. In Segre, D., and Smith, L. (Eds.): *Immunological Aspects of Aging.* New York, Marcel Dekker, Inc., 1981, pp. 281-293.

Halliwell, B., and Grootveld, M.: The measurement of free radical reactions in humans. *FEBS Lett, 213*:9, 1987.

Hamilton, G.D., and Bronson, F.H.: Food restriction and reproductive development: male and female mice and male rats. *Am J Physiol, 250*:R370, 1986.

Hanawalt, P.: On the role of DNA damage and repair processes in aging: evidence for and against. In Warner, H.R., Butler, R.N., Sprott, R.L., and Schneider, E.L. (Eds.): *Modern Biological Theories of Aging,* Vol, 31. New York, Raven Press, 1987, pp. 183-198.

Hansen, P.J., Schillo, K.K., Hinshelwood, M.M., and Hauser, E.R.: Body composition at vaginal opening in mice as influenced by food intake and photoperiod: tests of critical body weight and composition hypothesis for puberty onset. *Biol Reprod, 29*:924, 1983.

Hansen-Smith, F.M., Maksud, M.G., and Van Horn, D.L.: Influence of chronic undernutrition on oxygen consumption of rats during exercise. *Growth, 41*:115, 1977a

Hansen-Smith, F.M., Maksud, M.G., and Van Horn, D.L.: Effect of dietary protein restriction or food restriction on oxygen consumption and mitochondrial distribution in cardiac and red and white skeletal muscle of rats. *J Nutr, 107*:525, 1977b.

Hansford, R.G.: Lipid oxidation by heart mitochondria from young adult and senescent rats. *Biochem J, 170*:285, 1978.

Hansford, R.G.: Bioenergetics in aging. *Biochim Biophys Acta, 726*:41, 1983.

Hansford, R.G., and Castro, F.: Age-linked changes in the activity of enzymes of the tricarboxylic acid cycle and lipid oxidation, and in carnitine content in muscles of the rat. *Mech Ageing Dev, 19*:191, 1982a

Hansford, R.G., and Castro, F.: Effect of senescence on Ca^{2+}-ion transport by heart mitochondria. *Mech Ageing Dev, 19*:5, 1982b.

Harden, K.K., and Robinson, J.L.: Hypocholesteremia induced by orotic acid; dietary effects and species specificity. *J Nutr, 114*:411, 1984.

Harman, D.: Aging: a theory based on free radical and radiation chemistry. *J Gerontol, 11*:298, 1956.

Harman, D.: Free radical theory of aging: effect of free radical reaction inhibitors on the mortality rate of male LAF_1 mice. *J Gerontol, 23*:476, 1968.

Harman, D.: The aging process. *Proc Natl Acad Sci USA, 78*:7124, 1981.

Harman, D.: Free radical theory of aging: consequences of mitochondrial aging. *Age, 6*:88, 1983.

Harman, D.: Free radical theory of aging: Role of free radicals in the origination and evolution of life, aging, and disease processes. In Johnson, J.E., Jr., Walford, R., Harman, D. and Miquel, J. (Eds.): *Free Radicals, Aging and Degenerative Diseases*. New York, Liss, 1986, pp. 3-49.

Harmon, H.J., Nank, S., and Floyd, R.A.: Age-dependent changes in rat brain mitochondria of synaptic and non-synaptic origins. *Mech Ageing Dev, 38*:167, 1987.

Harp, J.A., Tsuchida, C.B., Weissman, I.L., and Scofield, V.L.: Autoreactive blood cells and programmed cell death in growth and development of protochordates. *J Exp Zool*, 1988 (in press).

Harper, A.E.: Nutrition, aging, and longevity. *Am J Clin Nutr, 36*:737, 1982.

Harris, A.R.C., Fang, S.L., Azizi, F., Lipworth, L., Vagenakis, A.G., and Braverman, L.E.: Effect of starvation on hypothalamic-pituitary thyroid function in the rat. *Metabolism, 27*:1074, 1978.

Harris, P.M.: Changes in adipose tissue of the rat due to early undernutrition followed by rehabilitation. I. Body composition and adipose tissue cellularity. *Br J Nutr, 43*:15, 1980.

Harris, R.B.S., Kasser, T.R., and Martin, R.J.: Dynamics of recovery of body composition after overfeeding, food restriction or starvation of mature female rats. *J Nutr, 116*:2536, 1986.

Harrison, D.E.: Experience with developing assays of physiological age. In Reff, M.E., and Schneider, E.L. (Eds.): *Biological Markers of Aging*. NIH Pub. #82-2221, Washington, D.C., U.S. Dept. of Health and Human Services, 1982, pp. 2-12.

Harrison, D.E., and Archer, J.R.: Physiological assays for biological age in mice: relationship of collagen, renal function and longevity. *Exp Aging Res*, 9:245, 1984.

Harrison, D.E., and Archer, J.R.: Genetic differences in effects of food restriction on aging in mice. *J Nutr*, 117:376, 1987a.

Harrison, D.E., and Archer, J.R.: Biomarkers of aging: tissue markers, future research needs, strategies, directions and priorities. *Exp Gerontol*, 1987b (in press).

Harrison, D.E., Archer, J.R., and Astle, C.M.: Loss of proliferative capacity in immunohemopoietic stem cells caused by serial transplantation rather than aging. *J Exp Med*, 147:1526, 1978.

Harrison, D.E., Archer, J.R., and Astle, C.M.: The effect of hypophysectomy on thymic aging in mice. *J Immunol*, 129:2673, 1982.

Harrison, D.E., Archer, J.R., and Astle, C.M.: Effects of food restriction on aging: Separation of food intake and adiposity. *Proc Natl Acad Sci USA*, 81:1835, 1984.

Harrison, D., Astle, C., and Lerner, C.: A somatic tissue that does not age. *Gerontologist*, 27:144A, 1987.

Harrison, D.E., Ingram, D.K., and Archer, J.R.: Longevity prediction by 13 physiological, behavioral and growth parameters in 6 mouse strains. *J Gerontol*, 1988 (in press).

Hart, R.W., and Setlow, R.B.: Correlation between deoxyribonucleic acid excision-repair and life span in a number of mammalian species. *Proc Natl Acad Sci USA*, 71:2169, 1974.

Hart, R.W., and Turturro, A.: Theories of aging. In Rothstein, M. (Ed.): *Review of Biological Research in Aging*, Vol. 1. New York, Alan R. Liss, Inc., 1983, pp. 5-17.

Hart, R.W., and Turturro, A.: Review of recent biological research on theories of aging. In Rothstein, M. (Ed.): *Review of Biological Research in Aging*, Vol. 2. New York, Alan R. Liss, Inc., 1985, pp. 3-12.

Harvey, P.H., and Zammuto, R.M.: Patterns of mortality and age at first reproduction in natural populations of mammals. *Nature*, 315:319, 1985.

Hashmi, R.F., Siddiqui, A.M., Kachole, M.S., and Pawar, S.S.: Alterations in hepatic microsomal mixed-function oxidase system during different levels of food restriction in adult male and female rats. *J Nutr*, 116:682, 1986.

Hausman, P.B., and Weksler, M.E.: Changes in the immune response with age. In Finch, C.E., and Schneider, E.L. (Eds.): *Handbook of the Biology of Aging*. New York, Van Nostrand Reinhold, 1985, pp. 414-432.

Hawcroft, D.M., Jones, T.W., and Martin, P.A.: Studies on age related changes in cytochrome P-450, cytochrome b-5 and mixed function oxidase activity in mouse liver microsomes, in relation to their phospholipid composition. *Arch Gerontol Geriatr*, 1:55, 1982.

Hayashida, M., Yu, B.P., Masoro, E.J., Iwasaki, K., and Ikeda, T.: An electron microscope examination of age-related changes in the rat kidney: the influence of diet. *Exp Gerontol*, 21:535, 1986.

Hazelton, G.A., and Lang, C.A.: Glutathione contents of tissues in the aging mouse. *Biochem J, 188*:25, 1980.

Hegsted, D.M.: Nutrition: the changing scene. The 1985 W.O. Atwater Memorial Lecture. *Nutr Rev, 43*:357, 1985.

Heidrick, M.L., Hendricks, L.C., and Cook, D.E.: Effect of dietary 2-mercaptoethanol on the life span, immune system, tumor incidence and lipid peroxidation damage in spleen lymphocytes of aging BC3F$_1$ mice. *Mech Ageing Dev, 27*:341, 1984.

Heikkinen, E.: Assessment of functional aging. In Viidik, A. (Ed.): *Lectures on Gerontology. Vol. I: On Biology of Aging.* Part B, New York, Academic Press, 1982, pp. 481-516.

Helfman, P.M., and Bada, J.L.: Aspartic acid racemization in dentine as a measure of aging. *Nature, 262*:279, 1976.

Heller, T., Francisco, A., Washington, A., Richardson, A., and Holt, P.R.: Food restriction retards small intestinal aging changes in the Fischer rat. *Gerontologist, 27*:88A, 1987.

Hendrikx, A., Heyns, W., and DeMoor, P.: Influence of a low-calorie diet and fasting on the metabolism of dehydroepiandrosterone sulfate in adult obese subjects. *J Clin Endocrinol Metab, 28*:1525, 1968.

Henry, K.R.: Effects of dietary restriction on presbyacusis in the mouse. *Audiology, 25*:329, 1986.

Herbener, G.H.: A morphometric study of age-dependent changes in the mitochondrial populations of mouse liver and heart. *J Gerontol, 31*:8, 1976.

Heresi, G., and Chandra, R.K.: Effects of severe calorie restriction on thymic factor activity and lymphocyte stimulation response in rats. *J Nutr, 110*:1888, 1980.

Herlihy, J.T., and Yu, B.P.: Dietary manipulation of age-related decline in vascular smooth muscle function. *Am J Physiol, 238*:H652, 1980.

Hibbs, A.R., and Walford, R.L.: A systems analysis approach to multifactorial aging (submitted).

Hill, J.O., Latiff, A., and DiGirolamo, M.: Effects of variable caloric restriction on utilization of ingested energy in rats. *Am J Physiol, 248*:R549, 1985.

Hill, J.O., Talano, C.M., Nickel, M., and DiGirolamo, M.: Energy utilization in food-restricted female rats. *J Nutr, 116*:2000, 1986.

Himms-Hagen, J.: Very low energy diets and changes in metabolic rate: role of brown adipose tissue. In Blackburn, G.L., and Bray, G.A. (Eds.): *Management of Obesity by Severe Caloric Restriction.* Littleton, Mass., PSG Publishing, 1985a, pp. 143-154.

Himms-Hagen, J.: Food restriction increases torpor and improves brown adipose tissue thermogenesis in ob/ob mice. *Am J Physiol, 248*:E531, 1985b.

Hiramoto, R.N., Ghanta, U.K., and Soong, S.: Effect of thymic hormones in immunity and life span. In Goidl, E.A. (Ed.): *Aging and the Immune Response.* New York, Marcel Dekker, Inc., 1987, pp. 177-198.

Hirokawa, K.: Age-related changes of thymus: morphological and functional aspects. *Acta Pathol Jpn, 28*:843, 1978.

Hirokawa, K., and Makinodan, T.: Thymic involution: effect on T cell differentiation. *J Immunol, 114*:1659, 1975.

Hirokawa, K., Kuto, S., Utsuyama, M., Kurashima, C., Sado, T.: Age-related change in the potential of bone marrow cells to repopulate the thymus and splenic T cells in mice. *Cell Immunol, 100*:443, 1986.

Hochachka, P.W., and Guppy, M.: *Metabolic Arrest and the Control of Biological Time.* Cambridge, Harvard University Press, 1987.

Hochschild, R.: Effect of dimethylaminoethyl p-chlorophenoxyacetate on the life span of male Swiss Webster albino mice. *Exp Gerontol, 8*:177, 1973.

Hofecker, G., Skalicky, M., Kment, A., and Niedermueller, H.: Models of the biologic age of the rat. A factor model of age parameters. *Mech Ageing Dev, 14*:345, 1980.

Hoffman, H.A., and Grieshaber, C.K.: Genetic studies of murine catalase. *Biochem Genet, 14*:59, 1976.

Holehan, A.M.: The effect of aging and dietary restriction upon reproduction in the female Sprague-Dawley rat. Ph.D. Thesis, University of Hull, England, 1984.

Holehan, A.M., and Merry, B.J.: The control of puberty in the dietary restricted female rat. *Mech Ageing Dev, 32*:179, 1985a.

Holehan, A.M., and Merry, B.J.: Modification of the oestrous cycle hormonal profile by dietary restriction. *Mech Ageing Dev, 32*:63, 1985b.

Holehan, A.M., and Merry, B.J.: Follicular steroidogenesis in diet restricted rats with delayed reproductive ageing. *XIIIth Intl Congr Gerontol* (Book of Abstracts). 1985c, p. 135.

Holehan, A.M., and Merry, B.J.: Lifetime breeding studies in fully fed and dietary restricted female CFY Sprague-Dawley rats. I. Effect of age, housing conditions and diet on fecundity. *Mech Ageing Dev, 33*:19, 1985d.

Holehan, A.M., and Merry, B.J.: The experimental manipulation of ageing by diet. *Biol Rev, 61*:329, 1986.

Hollingsworth, J.W., Hashizume, A., and Jablon, S.: Correlation between tests of aging in Hiroshima subjects—an attempt to define "physiologic age." *Yale J Biol Med, 38*:11, 1965.

Hollander, D., Dadufalza, V., Weindruch, R., and Walford, R.L.: Influence of life-prolonging dietary restriction on intestinal vitamin A absorption in mice. *Age, 9*:57, 1986.

Holloszy, J.O., and Smith, E.K.: Aging of rats: the roles of food restriction and exercise. In Hutchinson, M.L., and Munro, H.N. (Eds.): *Nutrition and Aging.* New York, Academic Press, 1986, pp. 193-206.

Holloszy, J.O., Smith, E.K., Vining, M., and Adams, S.: Effect of voluntary exercise on longevity of rats. *J Appl Physiol, 59*:826, 1985.

Holmes, G.E., and Holmes, N.R.: Accumulation of DNA fragments in aging *Paramecium tetraurelia* in axenic and nonaxenic media. *Gerontologist, 27*:151A, 1987.

Hooper, A.C.B.: Muscle fibre length and bone length in adult mice during dietary restriction and refeeding. *Nutr Res, 6*:415, 1986.

Horn, P.L., Laver, J.L., Fogerty, A.C., and Johnson, A.R.: Effects of life span feeding of ruminant-derived human diets to rats. *J Nutr, 109*:1234, 1979.

Horst, K., Mendel, L.B., and Benedict, F.G.: The influence of previous diet, growth and age upon the basal metabolism of the rat. *J Nutr, 8*:139, 1934.

Horton, E.S.: Effects of low energy diets on work performance. *Am J Clin Nutr,* 35:1228, 1982.

Howard, A.N.: The development of a very low caloric diet: a historical perspective. In Blackburn, G.L., and Bray, G.A. (Eds.): *Management of Obesity by Severe Caloric Restriction.* Littleton, Mass., PSG Pub. Co., 1985, pp. 3-26.

Howard, G., Chitpativra, S.T., Feldhoff, R.C., and Geoghegan, T.E.: Effect of starvation on rat liver mRNA translation products. *Proc Soc Exp Biol Med, 181:*312, 1986.

Howarth, R.E., and Baldwin, R.L.: Concentrations of selected enzymes and metabolites in rat skeletal muscle: effects of food restriction. *J Nutr, 101:*485, 1971.

Howland, B.E.: The influence of feed restriction and subsequent re-feeding on gonadotrophin secretion and serum testosterone levels in male rats. *J Reprod Fertil,* 44:429, 1975.

Hruza, Z., and Hlavackova, V.: Effect of environmental temperature and undernutrition on collagen aging. *Exp Gerontol, 4:*169, 1969.

Hubert, H.B., Feinleib, M., McNamara, P.M., and Castelli, W.P.: Obesity as an independent risk factor for cardiovascular disease; a 26-year follow-up of participants in the Framingham heart study. *Circulation, 67:*968, 1983.

Hudson, J.W., and Scott, I.M.: Daily torpor in the laboratory mouse, Mus musculus var. albino. *Physl Zool, 52:*205, 1979.

Hughes, T.A., Gwynne, J.T., Swiitzer, B.P., Herbst, C., and White, G.: Effects of caloric restriction and weight loss on glycemic control, insulin release and resistance, and atherosclerotic risk in obese patients with type II diabetes mellitus. *Am J Med,* 77:7, 1984.

Huseby, R.A., Ball, Z.B., and Visscher, M.B. (Eds.): Further observations on the influence of simple caloric restriction on mammary cancer incidence and related phenomena in C3H mice. *Cancer Res,* 5:40, 1945.

Ichikawa, M., and Fujita, Y.: Effects of nitrogen and energy metabolism on body weight in later life of male Wistar rats consuming a constant amount of food. *J Nutr, 117:*1751, 1987.

Idrobo, F., Nandy, K., Mostofsky, D.I., Blatt, L., and Nandy, K.: Dietary restriction: effects on radial maze learning and lipofuscin pigment deposition in the hippocampus and frontal cortex. *Age,* 9:8, 1986.

Imre, S., and Juhasz, E.: The effect of oxidative stress on inbred mice of different ages. *Mech Ageing Dev, 38:*259, 1987.

Ingle, L., Wood, T.R., and Banta, A.M.: A study of longevity, growth, reproduction and heart rate in *Daphnia longispina* as influenced by limitations in quantity of food. *J Exp Zool, 76:*325, 1937.

Ingram, D.K.: Toward the behavioral assessment of biological aging in the laboratory mouse: concepts, terminology and objectives. *Exp Aging Res,* 9:225, 1984.

Ingram, D.K., and Reynolds, M.A.: Effects of protein, dietary restriction, and exercise on survival in adult rats: A re-analysis of McCay, Maynard, Sperling and Osgood (1941). *Exp Aging Res,* 9:41, 1983.

Ingram, D.K., and Reynolds, M.A.: The relationship of body weight to longevity within laboratory rodent species. In Woodhead, A.D., and Thompson, K.H. (Eds.): *Evolution of Longevity in Animals.* New York, Plenum Press, 1987.

Ingram, D.K., Reynolds, M.A., and Goodrick, C.L.: Relationship of sex, exercise, and growth rate to life span in the Wistar rat: a multivariate correlational approach. *Gerontology, 28*:23, 1982.

Ingram, D.K., Reynolds, M.A., and Les, E.P.: The relationship of genotype, sex, body weight, and growth parameters to life span in inbred and hybrid mice. *Mech Ageing Dev, 20*:253, 1983.

Ingram, D.K., Weindruch, R., Spangler, E.L., Freeman, J.R., and Walford, R.L.: Dietary restriction benefits learning and motor performance of aged mice. *J Gerontol, 42*:78, 1987.

Intersociety Commission for Heart Disease Resources: Primary prevention of the atherosclerotic diseases. *Circulation, 42*:A55, 1970.

Ip, C., and Sylvester, P.: Retardation of mammary cancer development by caloric restriction (CR) in rats fed a high fat (HF) diet. *Fed Proc, 46*:436, 1987.

Isaacs, J.T., and Binkley, F.: Cyclic AMP-dependent control of the rat hepatic glutathione disulfide-sulfhydryl ratio. *Biochim Biophys Acta, 498*:29, 1977.

Ismail, M.N., Dulloo, A.G., and Metler, D.S.: Genetic and dietary influences on the levels of diet-induced thermogenesis and energy balance in adult mice. *Ann Nutr Metab, 30*:189, 1986.

Itallie, T.B.V., and Hirsch, J.: Appraisal of excess calories as a factor in the causation of disease. *Am J Clin Nutr, 32*:2648, 1979.

Iwasaki, K., Gleiser, C.A., Masoro, E.J., McMahan, C.A., Seo, E., and Yu, B.P.: The influence of dietary protein source on longevity and age-related disease processes of Fischer rats. *J Gerontol, 43*:B5, 1988a.

Iwasaki, K., Gleiser, C.A., Masoro, E.J., McMahan, C.A., Seo, E., and Yu, B.P.: Influence of the restriction of individual dietary components on longevity and age-related disease of Fischer rats: the fat component and the mineral component. *J Gerontol, 43*:B13, 1988b.

Izui, S., Fernandes, G., Hara, I., McConahey, P.J., Jensen, F., Dixon, F.J., and Good, R.A.: Low-calorie diet selectively reduces expression of retroviral envelope glycoprotein gp70 in sera of NZB × NZW F_1 hybrid mice. *J Exp Med, 154*:1116, 1981.

Jacobson, D.: Diet for a long life. *The Hartford Courant, Health & Science,* Dec. 18, 1986.

Jalavisto, E.: The role of simple tests measuring speed of performance in the assessment of biological vigor: a factorial study in elderly women. In Welford, A.T., and Birren, J.E. (Eds.): *Behavior, Aging and the Nervous System.* Springfield, Charles C Thomas, 1965, pp. 353-360.

James, W.P.T., and Trayhurn, P.: Thermogenesis and obesity. *Br Med Bull, 37*:43, 1981.

Jensen, B.D., Gunter, K.K., and Gunter, T.E.: The efficiencies of the component steps of oxidative phosphorylation. II. Experimental determination of the efficiencies in mitochondria and examination of the equivalence of membrane potential and pH gradient in phosphorylation. *Arch Biochem Biophys, 248*:305, 1986.

Johnson, B.C.: Nutrition and aging: a current assessment (letter). *J Nutr, 116*:323, 1986.

Johnson, B.C., Gajjar, A., Kubo, C., and Good, R.A.: Calories versus protein in onset of renal disease in NZB × NZW mice. *Proc Natl Acad Sci USA, 83*:5659, 1986.

Johnson, J.E., Jr., and Barrows, C.H., Jr.: Effects of age and dietary restriction on the kidney glomeruli of mice: observations by scanning electron microscopy. *Anat Rec, 196*:145, 1980.

Johnson, J.E., Jr., Walford, R., Harman, D., and Miquel, J. (Eds.): *Free Radicals, Aging, and Degenerative Diseases.* New York, Alan R. Liss, 1986.

Johnson, T.E.: Analysis of the biological basis of aging in the nematode, with special emphasis on *Caenorhabditis elegans.* In Mitchell, D.H., and Johnson, T.E. (Eds.): *Selected Invertebrate Models in Aging Research.* Boca Raton, CRC Press, 1984, pp. 59-93.

Johnson, T.E., Mitchell, D.H., Kline, S., Kemal, R., and Foy, J.: Arresting development arrests aging in the nematode *Caenorhabditis elegans. Mech Ageing Dev, 28*:23, 1984.

Jose, D.G., and Good, R.A.: Absence of enhancing antibody in cell mediated immunity to tumor heterografts in protein deficient rats. *Nature, 231*:323, 1971.

Jose, D.G., and Good, R.A.: Quantitative effects of nutritional protein and calorie deficiency upon immune responses to tumors in mice. *Cancer Res, 33*:807, 1973a.

Jose, D.G., and Good, R.A.: Quantitative effects of nutritional essential amino acid deficiency upon immune responses to tumors in mice. *J Exp Med, 137*:1, 1973b.

Joseph, J.A., Whitaker, J., Roth, G.S., and Ingram, D.K.: Life-long dietary restriction affects striatally-mediated behavioral responses in aged rats. *Neurobiol Aging, 4*:191, 1983.

Jung, R.T., Shetty, P.S., and James, W.P.T.: Nutritional effects on thyroid and catecholamine metabolism. *Clin Sci, 58*:183, 1980.

Jung, L.K.L., Palladino, M.A., Calvano, S., Mark, D.A., Good, R.A., and Fernandes, G.: Effect of calorie restriction on the production and responsiveness to interleukin 2 in (NZB × NZW)F_1 mice. *Clin Immunol Immunopathol, 25*:295, 1982.

Kagawa, Y.: Impact of westernization on the nutrition of Japanese: changes in physique, cancer, longevity, and centenarians. *Prev Med, 7*:205, 1978.

Kahn, C.: A chilling solution. *Longevity Letter, 1*:49, 1987.

Kalu, D.N.: Comparison of the effects of DHEA and food restriction on serum calcitonin. *Exp Aging Res, 10*:3, 1984.

Kalu, D., Yu, B.P., and Norling, B.K.: Influence of aging and food restriction on senile osteopenia and hyperparathyroidism in F344 rats. *Age, 6*:141, 1983a.

Kalu, D.N., Cockerham, R., Yu, B.P., and Ross, B.A.: Lifelong dietary modulation of calcitonin levels in rats. *Endocrinology, 113*:2010, 1983b.

Kalu, D.N., Hardin, R.H., Cockerham, R., and Yu, B.P.: Aging and dietary modulation of rat skeleton and parathyroid hormone. *Endocrinology, 115*:1239, 1984a.

Kalu, D.N., Hardin, R.H., Cockerham, R., Yu, B.P., Norling, B.K., and Egan, J.W.: Lifelong food restriction prevents senile osteopenia and hyperparathyroidism in F344 rats. *Mech Ageing Dev, 26*:103, 1984b.

Kannel, W.B., and Hubert, H.: Vital capacity as a biomarker of aging. In Reff, M.E., and Schneider, E.L. (Eds.): *Biological Markers of Aging.* NIH Pub. No. 82-2221, 1982, pp. 145-160.

Kasiske, B.L., Cleary, M.P., O'Donnell, M.P., and Keane, W.F.: Effects of carbohydrate restriction on renal injury in the obese Zucker rat. *Am J Clin Nutr, 44*:56, 1986.

Katz, M.S., McNair, C.L., Hymer, T.K., and Boland, S.R.: Beta (β) adrenergic-responsive hepatic glucose output in male rats increases during postmaturational aging and is modulated by food restriction. *Fed Proc, 46*:567, 1987.

Kaufman, M.C., and Rao, M.V.N.: Alternative states of amoebae. Studies on nuclear RNA and DNA synthesis. *Gerontol, 26*:200, 1980.

Kaunitz, H., and Johnson, R.E.: Influence of dietary fats on disease and longevity. In Chavez, A., Bourges, H., and Basta, S. (Eds.): *Proc IXth Intl Congr Nutr,* Karger, 1975, pp. 362-373.

Kelley, K.W., Brief, S., Westly, H.J., Novakofski, J., Bechtel, P.J., Simon, J., and Walker, E.B.: GH_3 pituitary adenoma cells can reverse thymic aging in rats. *Proc Natl Acad Sci USA, 83*:5663, 1986.

Kellogg, V.L., and Bell, R.G.: Variations induced in larval, pupal and imaginal stages of Bombyx mori by controlled varying food supply. *Science, 18*:741, 1903.

Keys, A.: Overweight, obesity, coronary heart disease and mortality. *Nutr Rev, 38*:297, 1980.

Keys, A., Brozek, J., Henschel, A., Mickelson, O., and Taylor, H.L.: Cancer and other neoplasms. *The Biology of Human Starvation,* Vol. 2. Minneapolis, University of Minnesota Press, pp. 1051-1056, 1950.

Khan, M.A., and Bender, A.E.: Adaptation to restricted intake of protein and energy. *Nutr Metab, 23*:449, 1979.

Khare, A., Freidrichs, W., and Fernandes, G.: International Symposium on Nutritional Regulation of Immunity and Infection. Toronto, Canada, July 3-5, 1987 (cited by Fernandes).

Khilobock, I.Y., Mozzhukhina, J.G., Chabanny, V.N., and Kadura, S.N.: Some age-related structural peculiarities of fractionated chromatin. *Gerontology, 29*:9, 1983.

Kibler, H.H., and Johnson, H.D.: Temperature and longevity in male rats. *J Gerontol, 21*:52, 1966.

Kimmel, D.: Developing recommendations for reducing ageism in social science research. *Gerontologist, 27*:267A, 1987.

Kirkman, H.N., and Gaetani, G.F.: Catalase: a tetrameric enzyme with four tightly bound molecules of NADPH. *Proc Natl Acad Sci USA, 81*:4343, 1984.

Kirkman, H.N., Galiano, S., and Gaetani, G.F.: The function of catalase-bound NADPH. *J Biol Chem, 262*:660, 1987.

Klass, M.R.: Aging in the nematode *Caenorhabditis elegans:* major biological and environmental factors influencing life span. *Mech Ageing Dev, 6*:413, 1977.

Kleiber, W.: *The Fire of Life, An Introduction to Animal Energetics.* Huntington, New York, Robert E. Krieger, 1975.

Klevay, L.M., Reck, S.J., and Barcome, D.R.: Evidence of dietary copper and zinc deficiencies. *JAMA, 241*:1916, 1979.

Klug, G.A., Krause, J., Ostlund, A.K., Knoll, G., and Brdiczka, D.: Alterations in liver mitochondrial function as a result of fasting and exhaustive exercise. *Biochim Biophys Acta, 764*:272, 1984.

Klurfeld, D.M., Weber, M.M., and Kritchevsky, D.: Inhibition of chemically induced mammary and colon tumor promotion by caloric restriction in rats fed increased dietary fat. *Cancer Res, 47*:2759, 1987a.

Klurfeld, D.M., Lloyd, L.M., Buck, C.L., Davis, M.L., Tulp, O.L., and Kritchevsky, D.: Inhibition of mammary tumorigenesis by caloric restriction in LA/N-cp (corpulent) rats. *Fed Proc, 46*:436, 1987b.

Knuth, U.A., and Friesen, H.G.: Starvation induced anoestrus: effect of chronic food restriction on body weight, its influence on oestrous cycle and gonadotrophin secretion in rats. *Acta Endocrinol, 104*:402, 1983.

Koberle, S., and Spiegel, R.: A long-term study with codergocrine mesylate (Hydergine) in healthy pensioners. *Gerontology 30*:3, 1984.

Koga, A., and Kimura, S.: Influence of restricted diet on epithelial renewal and maturation in the mouse jejunum. *J Nutr Sci Vitaminol, 24*:323, 1978.

Koga, A., and Kimura, S.: Influence of restricted diet on the cell renewal of the mouse small intestine. *J Nutr Sci Vitaminol, 25*:265, 1979.

Koga, A., and Kimura, S.: Influence of restricted diet on the cell cycle in the crypt of mouse small intestine. *J Nutr Sci Vitaminol, 26*:33, 1980.

Kohn, R.R.: Effect of antioxidants on life span of C57BL mice. *J Gerontol, 26*:378, 1971.

Kohno, A., Yonezu, T., Matsushita, M., Irino, M., Higuchi, K., Takeshita, S., Hosokawa, M., and Takeda, T.: Chronic food restriction modulates the advance of senescence in the senescence accelerated mouse (SAM). *J Nutr, 115*:1259, 1985.

Koizumi, A., Walford, R.L., and Imamura, T.: Treatment with poly IC enhances lipid peroxidation and the activity of xanthine oxidase, and decreases hepatic p-450 content and activities in mice and rats. *Biochem Biophys Res Commun, 134*:632, 1986a.

Koizumi, A., Hasegawa, L., Walford, R.L., and Imamura, T.: H-2, *Ah*, and aging: the immune response and the inducibility of p-450 mediated monooxygenase activities, xanthine oxidase, and lipid peroxidation in H-2 congenic mice on C57BL/10, C_3H, and A strain backgrounds. *Mech Ageing Dev, 37*:119, 1986b.

Koizumi, A., Hasagawa, L., Rodgers, K.E., Ellefson, D., Walford, R.L., and Imamura, T.: Influence of H-2 haplotypes on poly IC induction of xanthine oxidase and poly IC induced decreases in p-450 mediated enzyme activities. *Biochem Biophys Res Commun, 138*:246, 1986c.

Koizumi, A., Hasegawa, L., Rodgers, K., Ali, B., Walford, R.L., and Imamura, T.: Influence of aging and H-2 haplotypes on poly IC induced depression of mixed function oxidase. In: *Liver and Aging*. Amsterdam, Elsevier/North Holland, 1986d, pp. 29-39.

Koizumi, A., Weindruch, R., and Walford, R.L.: Influences of dietary restriction and age on liver enzyme activities and lipid peroxidation in mice. *J Nutr, 117*:361, 1987a.

Koizumi, A., Walford, R.L., and Hasegawa, L.: Differences in H-2 recombinant mice in the β-naphthoflavone inducibility of the mixed function monooxygenase, p_1-450. *Immunogenetics, 26*:25, 1987b.

Kokkonen, G.C., and Barrows, C.H.: The effect of dietary vitamin, protein and intake levels on the life span of mice of different ages. *Age, 8*:13, 1985.

Kolata, G.: Diet fat-breast cancer link questioned. *Science, 235*:436, 1987.

Koletsky, S., and Puterman, D.I.: Reduction of atherosclerotic disease in genetically obese rats by low calorie diet. *Exp Mol Pathol, 26*:415, 1977.

Konoplya, E.F., Dubina, T.L., Zelezinskaya, G.A., Dyundikova, V.A., Pokrovskaya, R.V., Gulko, V.V., Mazhul, L.M., and Gatsko, G.G.: Vitamins and Periodic Fasting as possible factors of experimental prolongation of the life span. *Fiziol Zh* (Kiev), *30*:16, 1984.

Kopec, S.: Studies on the influence of inanition on the development and duration of life in insects. *Biol Bull, 46*:1, 1924.

Kotlikoff, L.J.: Some economic implications of life span extension. In March, J., McGaugh, J.L., and Kiesler, S.B. (Eds.): *Aging: Biology and Behavior.* New York, Academic Press, 1982, p. 97.

Kozubik, A., Pospisil, M., and Hosek, B.: Stimulatory effect of intermittent feeding on hemopoietic recovery in sublethally gamma-irradiated mice. *Acta Radiol [Oncol], 24*:199, 1985.

Krishnamachar, S. and Canolty, N.L.: Effects of energy restriction on diabetic rats. *Nutr Rep Int, 31*:777, 1985.

Kritchevsky, D., Weber, M.M., and Klurfeld, D.M.: Dietary fat versus caloric content in initiation and promotion of 7, 12-dimethylbenz (a) anthracene-induced mammary tumorigenesis in rats. *Cancer Res, 44*:3174, 1984.

Kritchevsky, D., Weber, M.M., Buck, C.L., and Klurfeld, D.M.: Calories, fat and cancer. *Lipids, 21*:272, 1986.

Kritchevsky, D., Buck, C.L., Weber, M.M., and Klurfeld, D.M.: Response of DMBA-induced mammary tumors to 25 percent caloric restriction at varying times during the promotion phase. *Fed Proc, 46*:436, 1987.

Kubo, C., Day, N.K., and Good, R.A.: Influence of early or late dietary restriction on life span and immunological parameters in MRL/Mp-lpr/lpr mice. *Proc Natl Acad Sci USA, 81*:5831, 1984a.

Kubo, C., Johnson, B.C., Day, N.K., and Good, R.A.: Caloric source, caloric restriction, immunity and aging of (NZB/NZW)F_1 mice. *J Nutr, 114*:1884, 1984b.

Kubo, C., Johnson, B.C., Gajjar, A., and Good, R.A.: Crucial dietary factors in maximizing life span and longevity in autoimmune-prone mice. *J Nutr, 117*:1129, 1987a.

Kubo, C., Johnson, B.C., Misra, H.P., Dao, M.L., and Good, R.A.: Nutrition, longevity and hepatic enzyme activities in mice. *Nutr Rep Int, 35*:1185, 1987b.

LaBella, F.S., and Vivian, S.: Effect of β-aminopropionitrile or prednisolone on survival of male LAF/J mice. *Exp Gerontol, 10*:185, 1975.

Laganiere, S. and Yu, B.P.: Anti-lipoperoxidation action of food restriction. *Age, 9*:117, 1986.

Laganiere, S., and Yu, B.P.: Anti-lipoperoxidation action of food restriction. *Biochem Biophys Res Commun, 45*:1185, 1987.

Laganiere, S., Yu, B.P., and Masoro, E.J.: Inhibition of membrane lipoperoxidation and modulation of the antioxidant status by food restriction. *Fed Proc, 46*:567, 1987.

Lambert, B., Ringborg, U., and Skoog, L.: Age-related decrease of ultraviolet light-induced DNA repair synthesis in human peripheral leukocytes. *Cancer Res, 39*:2792, 1979.

Lagopoulos, L., and Stalder, R.: The influence of food intake on the development of diethynitrosamine-induced liver tumours in mice. *Carcinogenesis, 8*:33, 1987.

Lammert, O., and Hansen, E.S.: Effects of excessive caloric restriction on body weight and energy expenditure at rest and light exercise. *Acta Physiol Scand, 114*:135, 1982.

Lammi-Keefe, C.J., Hegarty, P.V.J., and Swan, P.B.: Effect of starvation and refeeding on catalase and superoxide dismutase activities in skeletal and cardiac muscles from 12-month-old rats. *Experientia, 37*:25, 1981.

Lammi-Keefe, C.J., Swan, P.B., and Hegarty, P.V.J.: Effect of level of dietary protein and total or partial starvation on catalase and superoxide dismutase activity in cardiac and skeletal muscles in young rats. *J Nutr, 114*:2235, 1984.

Landsberg, L., and Young, J.B.: Diet-induced changes in sympathetic system activity. In Beers, R.F., Jr., and Bassett, E.G. (Eds.): *Nutritional Factors: Modulating Effects on Metabolic Processes*. New York, Raven Press, 1981, pp. 155-174.

Landsberg, L., and Young, J.B.: Changes in metabolic rate: role of cathecholamines and the autonomic nervous system. In Blackburn, G.L., and Bray, G.A. (Eds.): *Management of Obesity by Severe Caloric Restriction*. Littleton, Mass., PSG Publishing Co., 1985, pp. 129-141.

Landfield, P.W.: An endocrine hypothesis of brain aging and studies on brain-endocrine correlations and monosynaptic neurophysiology during aging. In Finch, C.E. (Ed.): *Parkinson's Disease, Vol. 2: Aging and Neuroendocrine Relationships*. New York, Plenum, 1978, pp. 179-199.

Lane, M.D., Pedersen, P.L., and Mildvan, A.S.: The mitochondrion updated. *Science, 234*:526, 1986.

Lane, P.W., and Dickie, M.M.: The effect of restricted food intake on the life span of genetically obese mice. *J Nutr, 64*:549, 1958.

Lapidus, L., Andersson, H., Bengtsson, C., and Bosaeus, I.: Dietary habits in relation to incidence of cardiovascular disease and death in women. *Am J Clin Nutr, 44*:444, 1986.

Larsen, C.D., and Heston, W.E.: Effects of cystine and calorie restriction on the incidence of spontaneous pulmonary tumors in strain A mice. *JNCI, 6*:31, 1945.

Ledvina, M. and Hodanova, M.: The effect of simultaneous administration of tocopherol and sunflower oil on the life span of female mice. *Exp Gerontol, 15*:67, 1980.

Lee, C.J., Panemangalore, M., and Wilson, K.: Effect of dietary restriction on bone mineral content of mature rats. *Nutr Res, 6*:51, 1986.

Lee, M., and Lucia, S.P.: Some relationships between caloric restriction and body weight in the rat. I. Body composition, liver lipids and organ weights. *J Nutr, 74*:243, 1961.

Lee, Y.C.P., King, J.T., and Visscher, M.B.: Calorie intake and fertility in C_3H-male mice. *Am J Physiol, 167*:375, 1951.

Lee, Y.C.P., Visscher, M.B., and King, J.T.: Life span and causes of death in inbred mice in relation to diet. *J Gerontol, 11*:364, 1956.

Leighton, B., Tagliaferro, A.R., and Newsholme, E.A.: The effect of dehydroepiandrosterone acetate on liver peroxisomal enzyme activities of male and female rats. *J Nutr, 117*:1287, 1987.

Lerner, S.P., Anderson, C.P., Walford, R.L., and Finch, C.E.: Genotype and reproductive aging of inbred female mice: effect of H-2 alleles. *Biol Reprod*, 1988 (in press).

Leslie, S.W., Chandler, L.J., Barr, E.M., and R.P. Farrar.: Reduced calcium uptake by rat brain mitochondria and synaptosomes in response to aging. *Brain Res, 329*:177, 1985.

Lesser, G.T., Deutsch, S., and Markofsky, J.: Aging in the rat: longitudinal and cross-sectional studies of body composition. *Am J Physiol, 225*:1472, 1973.

Leto, S., Kokkonen, G.C., and Barrows, C.H., Jr.: Dietary protein, life-span, and biochemical variables in female mice. *J Gerontol, 31*:144, 1976a.

Leto, S., Kokkonen, G.C., and Barrows, C.H., Jr.: Dietary protein, life-span, and physiological variables in female mice. *J Gerontol, 31*:149, 1976b.

Leveille, G.A.: the long-term effects of meal-eating on lipogenesis, enzyme activity, and longevity in the rat. *J Nutr, 102*:549, 1972.

Leveille, P.J., Weindruch, R.L., Walford, R.L., Bok, D., and Horwitz, J.: Dietary restriction retards age-related loss of gamma crystallins in the mouse lens. *Science, 224*:1247, 1984.

Levin, P., Janda, J.K., Joseph, J.A., Ingram, D.K., and Roth, G.S.: Dietary restriction retards the age-associated loss of rat striatal dopaminergic receptors. *Science, 214*:561, 1981.

Lewin, R.: Food fuels reproductive success. *Science, 217*:238, 1982.

Lewis, S.E.M., Goldspink, D.F., Phillips, J.G., Merry, B.J., and Holehan, A.M.: The effects of aging and chronic dietary restriction on whole body growth and protein turnover in the rat. *Exp Gerontol, 20*:253, 1985.

Licastro, F., and Walford, R.L.: Aging, proliferative potential and DNA repair capacity in short-lived and long-lived mice. *Mech Ageing Dev, 31*:171, 1985.

Licastro, F., and Walford, R.L.: Modulating effect of nicotinamide on unscheduled DNA synthesis in lymphocytes from young and old mice. *Mech Ageing Dev, 35*:123, 1986.

Licastro, F., Weindruch, R., and Walford, R.L.: Dietary restriction retards the age-related decline of DNA repair capacity in mouse splenocytes. In Facchini, A., Haaijman, J.J., and Labo, G. (Eds.): *Immunoregulation and Aging*. Rijswijk, Eurage, 1986, pp. 53-61.

Licastro, F., Weindruch, R., Davis, L.J., and Walford, R.L.: Effect of dietary restriction upon the age-associated decline of lymphocyte DNA repair activity in mice. *Age*, 1988 (in press).

Liepa, G.U., Masoro, E.J., Bertrand, H.A., and Yu, B.P.: Food restriction as a modulator of age-related changes in serum lipids. *Am J Physiol, 238*:E253, 1980.

Lindell, T.J.: Molecular aspects of dietary modulation of transcription and enhanced longevity. *Life Sci, 31*:625, 1982.

Lindstedt, S.L. and Calder, W.A.: Body size, physiological time, and longevity of homeothermic animals. *Q Rev Biol, 56*:1, 1981.

Lissner, L., Levitsky, D.A., Strupp, B.J., Kalkwarf, H.J., and Roe, D.A.: Dietary fat and the regulation of energy intake in human subjects. *Am J Clin Nutr, 46*:886, 1987.

Liu, R.K., and Walford, R.L.: Increased growth and lifespan with lowered ambient temperature in the annual fish, *Cynolebius adloffi*. *Nature, 212*:1277, 1966.

Liu, R.K., and Walford, R.L.: The effect of lowered body temperature on lifespan and immune and non-immune processes. *Gerontologia, 18*:363, 1972.

Liu, R.K., and Walford, R.L.: Mid-life temperature-transfer effects on life span of annual fish. *J Gerontol, 30*:129, 1975.

Liu, R.K., Leung, B.E., and Walford, R.L.: effect of temperature-transfer on growth of laboratory populations of a South American annual fish *Cynolebias bellottii*. *Growth, 39*:337, 1975.

Ljungren, H., Ikkos, D., and Luft, R.: Basal metabolism in women with obesity and anorexia nervosa. *Br J Nutr, 15*:21, 1961.

Lloyd, T.: Food restriction increases life span of hypertensive animals. *Life Sci, 34*:401, 1984.

Lockshin, R.A.: Symposia. Developmental biology of the post-mitotic cell. The regenerating neuron. The fate and death of cells. *Gerontologist, 27*:202A, 242A, 1987.

Loeb, J., and Northrop, J.H.: On the influence of food and temperature on the duration of life. *J Biol Chem, 32*:102, 1917.

London, E.D., Waller, S.B., Ellis, A.T., and Ingram, D.K.: Effects of intermittent feeding on neurochemical markers in aging rat brain. *Neurobiol Aging, 6*:199, 1985.

Loschen, G., Azzi, A., and Flohe, L.: Mitochondrial H_2O_2 formation: relationship with energy conservation. *FEBS Lett, 33*:84, 1973.

Loschen, G., Azzi, A., Richter, C., and Flohe, L.: Superoxide radicals as precursors of mitochondrial hydrogen peroxide. *FEBS Lett, 42*:68, 1974.

Lucas, J.A., Ahmed, S.A., Casey, M.L., and MacDonald, P.C.: Prevention of autoantibody formation and prolonged survival in New Zealand black/New Zealand white F_1 mice fed dehydroisoandrosterone. *J Clin Invest, 75*:2091, 1985.

Ludwig, F.C., and Elashoff, R.M.: Mortality in syngeneic rat parabionts of different chronological age. *Trans NY Acad Sci, 34*:582, 1972.

Ludwig, F.C., and Smoke, M.E.: Measurement of biological age. *Exp Aging Res, 6*:497, 1980.

Lyman, C.P., O'Brien, R.C., Greene, G.C., and Papafrangos, E.D.: Hibernationa and longevity in the Turkish hamster *Mesocricetus brandti*. *Science, 212*:668, 1981.

MacGregor, G.A.: Dietary sodium and potassium intake and blood pressure. *Lancet, 1*:750, 1983.

MacKay, I.R.: Aging and immunological function in man. *Gerontologia, 18*:285, 1972.

Maeda, H., Gleiser, C.A., Masoro, E.J., Murata, I., McMahan, C.A., and Yu, B.P.: Nutritional influences on aging of Fischer 344 rats: II. Pathology. *J Gerontol, 40*:671, 1985.

Makinodan, T., Lubinski, J., and Fong, T.C.: Cellular, biochemical, and molecular basis of T-cell senescence. *Arch Pathol Lab Med, 111*:910, 1987a.

Makinodan, T., Chang, M., Norman, D.C., and Li, S.: Vulnerability of the T-cell lineage to aging. In Goidl, E.A. (Ed.): *Aging and the Immune Response.* New York, Marcel Dekker, Inc., 1987b, pp. 27-44.

Makrides, S.C.: Protein synthesis and degradation during aging and sensecence. *Biol Rev, 58*:343, 1983.

Mammalian Models for Research on Aging. (Committee on Animal Models for Research on Aging). Washington, D.C., National Academy Press, 1981, pp. 62-71.

Mandelbrot, B.: *The Fractal Geometry of Nature.* San Francisco, W.H. Freeman, 1982.

Mann, D.M.A.: Nauronal loss in old people: the affects of ageing or disease. *Neurobiol Aging, 8:*550, 1987.

Mann, P.L.: The effect of various dietary restricted regimes on some immunological parameters of mice. *Growth, 42:*87, 1978.

Manson, J.E., Stampfer, M.J., Hennekens, C.H., and Willett, W.C.: Body weight and longevity. A reassessment. *JAMA, 257:*353, 1987.

Marcus, D.L., Ibrahim, N.G., and Freedman, M.L.: Age-related decline in the biosynthesis of mitochondrial inner membrane proteins. *Exp Gerontol, 17:*333, 1982a.

Marcus, D.L., Lew, G., Gruenspecht-Faham, N., and Freedman, M.L.: Effect of inhibitors and stimulators on isolated liver cell mitochondrial protein synthesis from young and old rats. *Exp Gerontol, 17:*429, 1982b.

Mareschi, J.P., Cousin, F., Villeon, B.D.L., and Brubacher, G.B.: Valeur calorique de l'alimentation et converture des apports nutritionnels conseilles en vitamins de l'homme adulte. *Ann Nutr Metab, 28:*11, 1984.

Mark, D.A., Alonso, D.R., Quimby, F., Thaler, H.T., Kim, Y.T., Fernandes, G., Good, R.A., and Weksler, M.E.: Effects of nutrition on disease and life span. I. Immune responses, cardiovascular pathology, and life span in MRL mice. *Am J Pathol, 117:*110, 1984a.

Mark, D.A., Alonso, D.R., Tack-Goldman, K., Thaler, H.T., Tremoli, E., Weksler, B.B., and Weksler, M.E.: Effects of nutrition on disease and life span. II. Vascular disease, serum cholesterol, serum thromboxane, and heart-produced prostacyclin in MRL mice. *Am J Pathol, 117:*125, 1984b.

Marmorston, J., Griffith, G.C., Geller, P.J., Fishman, E.L., Welsh, F., and Weiner, J.M.: Urinary steroids in the measurement of aging and of artherosclerosis. *J Am Geriatr Soc, 23:*481, 1975.

Marrale, J.C., Shepman, J.H., and Rhodes, M.L.: What some college students eat. *Nutr Today, 21:*16, 1986.

Marshall, E.: California's debate on carcinogens. *Science, 235:*1459, 1987.

Marshall, P.J., Warso, M.A., and Lands, W.E.M.: Selective microdetermination of lipid hydroperoxides. *Anal Biochem, 145:*192, 1985.

Martin, G.M.: Genetic syndromes in man with potential relevance to the pathobiology of aging. In Bergsma, D., and Harrison, D.E. (Eds.): *Genetic Effects on Aging.* New York, Alan R. Liss, Inc., 1978, pp. 5-39.

Martin, G.M.: Genotropic theories of aging: an overview. In Borek, C., Fenoglio, C.M., and King, D.W. (Eds.): *Aging, Cancer and Cell Membranes.* New York, Thieme-Stratton, 1980, pp. 5-20.

Maruyama, N., and Lindstrom, C.O.: H-2 linked regulation of serum gp 70 production in mice. *Immunogenetics, 17:*507, 1983.

Masoro, E.J.: Nutrition as a modulator of the aging process. *Physiologist, 27:*98, 1984.

Masoro, E.J.: Metabolism. In Finch, C.E., and Schneider, E.L. (Eds.): *Handbook of the Biology of Aging,* 2nd Ed. New York, Van Nostrand Reinhold, 1985a, pp. 540-566.

Masoro, E.J.: Nutrition and aging—a current assessment. *J Nutr, 115:*842, 1985b.

Masoro, E.J., Yu, B.P., and Bertrand, H.A.: Action of food restriction in delaying the aging process. *Proc Natl Acad Sci USA, 79*:4239, 1982.

Masoro, E.J., Compton, C., Yu, B.P., and Bertrand, H.: Temporal and compositional dietary restrictions modulate age-related changes in serum lipids. *J Nutr, 113*:880, 1983.

Masters, C., Pegg, M., and Crane, D.: On the multiplicity of the enzyme catalase in mammalian liver. *Mol Cell Biochem, 70*:113, 1986.

Matsubara, M., Nakagawa, K., and Akikawa, K.: Immunoreactive LHRH in chronic starved rats. *Horm Metabol Res, 18*:450, 1986.

Maurizo, A.: Lebendauer und Altern bei der Honibiene (*Apis mellifica L.*). *Gerontologia, 5*:110, 1961.

Mayer, J., and Goldberg, J.: Mild copper deficiency not uncommon in the United States. *Los Angeles Times,* Part VIII, p. 26, Sept. 22, 1983.

McCance, R.A., and Mount, L.E.: Severe undernutrition in growing and adult animals. Metabolic rate and body temperature in the pig. *Br J Nutr, 14*:509, 1960.

McCarron, D.A., Morris, C.D., and Cole, C.: Dietary calcium in human hypertension. *Science, 217*:267, 1982.

McCarter, R. and McGee, J.: Influence of nutrition and aging on the composition and function of rat skeletal muscle. *J Gerontol, 42*:432, 1987.

McCarter, R., Yu, B.P., and Radicke, D.: Effects of caloric restriction on contraction of skeletal muscle. *Nutr Rep Int, 17*:339, 1978.

McCarter, R.J.M., Masoro, E.J., and Yu, B.P.: Rat muscle structure and metabolism in relation to age and food intake. *Am J Physiol, 242*:R89, 1982.

McCarter, R., Yu, B.P., and Menefee, J.: Fast and slow muscle mechanics as a function of age and diet. *Gerontologist, 23*:80, 1983.

McCarter, R., Masoro, E.J., and Yu, B.P.: Does food restriction retard aging by reducing the metabolic rate? *Am J Physiol, 248*:E488, 1985.

McCay, C.M.: Chemical aspects of ageing and the effect of diet upon ageing. In Lansing, A.I. (Ed.): *Cowdry's Problems of Ageing.* Baltimore, Williams and Wilkins, 1952, pp. 139-202.

McCay, C.M., Crowell, M.F., and Maynard, L.A.: The effect of retarded growth upon the length of the life span and upon the ultimate body size. *J Nutr, 10*:63, 1935.

McCay, C.M., Maynard, L.A., Sperling, G., and Osgood, H.S.: Nutritional requirements during the latter half of life. *J Nutr, 21*:45, 1941.

McCay, C.M., Sperling, G., and Barnes, L.L.: Growth, ageing, chronic diseases and life span in rats. *Arch Biochem Biophys, 2*:469, 1943.

McGee, J., and McCarter, R.: Effect of short-term food restriction on 24-hour metabolic rate and spontaneous activity of Fischer 344 rats. *Fed Proc, 46*:435, 1987.

Meites, J., Goya, R., and Takahashi, S.: Why the neuroendocrine system is important in aging processes. Exp Gerontol, 22:1, 1987.

Meredith, P.J., and Walford, R.L.: Effect of age on response to T- and B-cell mitogens in mice congenic at the H-2 locus. *Immunogenetics, 5*:109, 1977.

Merimee, T.J., and Fineberg, E.S.: Starvation-induced alterations of circulating hormone concentrations in man. *Metabolism, 25*:79, 1976.

Merry, B.J.: Dietary manipulation of ageing: an animal model. In Bittles, A.H., and Collins, K.J. (Eds.): *The Biology of Human Ageing.* Cambridge, Cambridge University Press, 1986, pp. 233-242.

Merry, B.J., and Holehan, A.M.: Onset of puberty and duration of fertility in rats fed a restricted diet. *J Reprod Fertil, 57*:253, 1979.

Merry, B.J., and Holehan, A.M.: Serum profiles of LH, FSH, testosterone and 5-alpha-DHT from 21 to 1000 days of age in *ad libitum* fed and dietary restricted rats. *Exp Gerontol, 16*:431, 1981.

Merry, B.J., and Holehan, A.M.: The endocrine response to dietary restriction in the rat. In Woodhead, A.D., Blackett, A.D., and Holleander, A. (Eds.): *Molecular Biology of Aging.* New York, Plenum, 1985a, pp. 117-141.

Merry, B.J., and Holehan, A.M.: In vivo DNA synthesis in the dietary restricted long-lived rat. *Exp Gerontol, 20*:15, 185b.

Merry, B.J., Holehan, A.M., and Phillips, J.G.: Modification of reproductive decline and life span by dietary manipulation in CFY Sprague-Dawley rats. In Lofts, B., and Holmes, W.N. (Eds.): *Current Trends in Comparative Endocrinology.* Hong Kong, Hong Kong University Press, 1985, pp. 621-624.

Merry, B.J., Holehan, A.M., Lewis, S.E.M., and Goldspink, D.F. The effects of ageing and chronic dietary restriction on *in vivo* hepatic protein synthesis in the rat. *Mech Ageing Dev, 39*:189, 1987.

Mertz, W.: Trace minerals and atherosclerosis. *Fed Proc, 41*:2807, 1982.

Mervis, R.F., Moroi, S., London, E.D., and Ingram, D.K. Effect of dietary restriction on dendritic spines in aging rat neocortex. *Age 7*:144, 1984.

Miller, D.S., and Payne, P.R.: Longevity and protein intake. *Exp Gerontol, 3*:231, 1968.

Miller, R.A.: Calcium and the immune system. *Neurobiol Aging, 8*:368, 1987.

Miller, R.A., and Harrison, D.E.: Delayed reduction in T cell precursor frequencies accompanies diet-induced life span extension. *J Immunol, 134*:1426, 1985.

Milligan, L.P., and McBride, B.W.: Shifts in animal energy requirements across physiological and alimentational states. *J Nutr, 115*:1374, 1985.

Miquel, J., and Fleming, J.: Theoretical and experimental support for an "oxygen radical-mitochondrial injury" hypothesis of cell aging. In Johnson, J.E., Jr., Walford, R., Harman, D., and Miquel, J. (Eds.): *Free Radicals, Aging, and Degenerative Diseases.* New York, Alan R. Liss, 1986, pp. 51-74.

Mohan, P.F., and Rao, B.S.N.: Adaptation to underfeeding in growing rats. Effect of energy restriction at two dietary protein levels on growth, feed efficiency, basal metabolism and body composition. *J Nutr, 113*:79, 1983.

Mohan, P.F., and Rao, B.S.N.: Adaptation to underfeeding in adult rats. *Nutr Res, 5*:1419, 1985a.

Mohan, P.F., and Rao, B.S.N.: Adaptation to underfeeding in young growing rats. *Nutr Res, 5*:1409, 1985b.

Moment, G.B.: Editorial: Aging, arthritis and food allergies: A research opportunity revisited. *Growth, 44*:155, 1980.

Mondon, C.E., Sims, C., Dolkas, C.B., Reaven, E.P., and Reaven, G.M.: The effects of exercise training on insulin resistance in sedentary year old rats. *J Gerontol, 41*:605, 1986.

Monnier, V.M., Kohn, R.R., and Cerami, A.: Accelerated age-related browning of human collagen in diabetes mellitus. *Proc Natl Acad Sci USA, 81*:583, 1984.

Moore, M.A., Thamavit, W., Tsuda, H., Sato, K., Ichihara, A., and Ito, N.: Modifying influence of dehydroepiandrosterone on the development of dihydroxy-di-n-propylnitrosamine-initiated lesions in the thyroid, lung and liver of F344 rats. *Carcinogenesis, 7*:311, 1986.

Moreschi, C.: Beziehungen zwischen ernahrung und tumorwachstum. *Z Immunitatsforsch., 2*:651, 1909.

Morgan, R.F.: *The Adult Growth Examination.* CA, R. Morgan, 1986.

Morgan, R.W., Christman, M.F., Jacobson, F.S., Storz, G., and Ames, B.N.: Hydrogen peroxide-inducible proteins in *Salmonella typhimurium* overlap with heat shock and other stress proteins. *Proc Natl Acad Sci USA, 83*:8059, 1986.

Morin, R.J.: Longevity, hepatic lipid peroxidation and hepatic fatty acid composition of mice fed saturated or unsaturated fat-supplemented diets. *Experientia, 23*:1003, 1967.

Morrison, S.D.: Nutrition and longevity. *Nutr Rev, 41*:133, 1983.

Mos, J., and Hollander, C.F.: Analysis of survival data on aging rat cohorts: pitfalls and some practical considerations. *Mech Ageing Dev, 38*:89, 1987.

Muggleton, A., and Danielli, J.F.: Ageing of *Amoeba proteus* and *A. Discoides* cells. *Nature, 181*:1738, 1958.

Munro, H.N.: Nutrition and Aging. *Br Med Bull, 37*:83, 1981.

Myers, G.C., and Manton, K.G.: Compression of mortality: myth or reality? *Gerontologist, 24*:346, 1984.

Nadakavukaren, M.J., Fitch, K.L., and Richardson, A.: Dietary restriction retards the age-related decrease in cell population of rat corneal endothelium. *Proc Soc Exp Biol Med, 184*:98, 1987.

Nakagawa, I., Sasaki, A., Kajimoto, M., Fukuyama, T., Suzuki, T., and Yamada, E.: Effect of protein nutrition on growth, longevity and incidence of lesions in the rat. *J Nutr, 104*:1576, 1974.

Nandy, K.: Effects of caloric restriction on brain reactive antibodies in sera of old mice. *Age, 4*:117, 1981.

Nandy, K.: Effects of controlled dietary restriction on brain reactive antibodies in sera of aging mice. *Mech Ageing Dev, 18*:97, 1982.

National Research Council (NRC): Nutrient requirements of the mouse. In: *Nutrient Requirements of Laboratory Animals,* 3rd revised ed. Washington, D.C., National Academy of Sciences, 1978, pp. 38-53.

Nebert D.W., Brown, D.D., Towne, D.W., and Eisen, H.J.: Association of fertility, fitness and longevity with the murine Ah locus among (C57BL/6N) (C3H/HeN) recombinant inbred mice. *Biol Reprod, 30*:363, 1984.

Nelson, J.F., Gosden, R.G., and Felicio, L.: Effect of dietary restriction on estrous cyclicity and follicular reserves in aging C57BL/6J mice. *Biol Reprod, 32*:515, 1985.

Nelson, W., and Halberg, F.: Meal-timing, circadian rhythms and life span of mice. *J Nutr, 116*:2244, 1986.

Nesterenko, G.A., Nikitin, V.N., and Stavitskaya, L.I.: Prolongation of life with periodic growth-retarding diet and its effect on the age-bound changes in the hypothalamic-hypophysealadrenal system. *Fiziol Zh SSSR, 62*:73, 1977.

Nikitin, V.N.: Biochemism and the endocrine situation of the organism of laboratory animals when life is experimentally prolonged by nutrition with restrained growth. In: *Life Prolongation: Prognosis, Mechanisms, Control.* Kiev, Institute of Gerontology, 1979, pp. 27-34 (in Russian) (cited by Frolkis, 1982).

Nohl, H.: Influence of age on thermotropic kinetics of enzymes involved in mitochondrial energy metabolism. *Z Gerontol, 12*:9, 1979.

Nohl, H.: Age-dependent changes in the structure-function correlation of ADP/ATP-translocating mitochondrial membranes. *Gerontology, 28*:354, 1982.

Nohl, H.: Oxygen radical release in mitochondria: influence of age. In Johnson, J.E., Jr., Walford, R., Harman, D., and Miquel, J. (Eds.): *Free Radicals, Aging, and Degenerative Diseases.* New York, Alan R. Liss, 1986, pp. 77-97.

Nohl, H.: A novel superoxide radical generator in heart mitochondria. *FEBS Lett, 214*:269, 1987.

Nohl, H., and Hegner, D.: Do mitochondria produce oxygen radicals *in vivo*? *Eur J Biochem, 82*:563, 1978.

Nohl, H. and Hegner, D.: Responses of mitochondrial superoxide dismutase, catalase and glutathione peroxidase activities to aging. *Mech Ageing Dev, 11*:145, 1979.

Nohl, H., and Kramer, R.: Molecular basis of age-dependent changes in the activity of adenine nucleotide translocase. *Mech Ageing Dev, 14*:137, 1980.

Nohl, H., and Jordan, W.: The mitochondrial site of superoxide formation. *Biochem Biophys Res Commun, 138*:533, 1986.

Nolen, G.A.: Effect of various restricted dietary regimens on the growth, health and longevity of albino rats. *J Nutr, 102*:1477, 1972.

Northrop, J.H.: The effect of prolongation of the period of growth on the total duration of life. *J Biol Chem, 32*:123, 1917.

Novak, R., Bosze, Z., Matkovics, B. and Fachet, J.: Gene affecting superoxide dismutase activity linked to the histocompatibility complex in H-2 congenic mice. *Science, 207*:86, 1980.

Nutr Rev: (Anonymous) Role of liver in diet-induced thermogenesis. *43*:347, 1985.

Nyce, J.W., Magee, P.N., Hard, G.C., and Schwartz, A.: Inhibition of 1, 2-dimethylhydrazine-induced colon tumorigenesis in Balb/c mice by dehydroepiandrosterone. *Carcinogenesis, 5*:57, 1984.

O'Brian, J.T., Bybee, D.E., Burman, K.D., Osburne, R.C., Ksiazele, M.R., Watofsky, L., and Georges, L.P.: Thyroid hormone homeostasis in states of relative caloric deprivation. *Metabolism, 29*:721, 1980.

Odum, H.T.: *Systems Ecology: An Introduction.* New York, John Wiley & Sons, 1983.

Olewine, D.A., Barrows, C.H., and Shock, N.W.: Effect of reduced dietary intake on random and voluntary activity in male rats. *J Gerontol, 19*:229, 1964.

Oliver, C.N., Levine, R.L., and Stadtman, E.R.: A role of mixed-function oxidation reactions in the accumulation of altered enzyme forms during aging. *J Am Geriatr Soc, 35*:947, 1987.

Olsen, G.G., and Everitt, A.V.: Retardation of the ageing process in collagen fibres from the tail tendon of the old hypophysectomized rat. *Nature, 206*:307, 1965.

Ooka, H.: Changes in extrathyroidal conversion of thyroxine (T_4) to 3,3',5-triiodothyronine (T_3) *in vitro* during development and aging of the rat. *Mech Ageing Dev, 10*:151, 1979.

Ooka, H., Segall, P.E., and Timiras, P.S.: Neural and endocrine development after chronic trytophan deficiency in rats: II. Pituitary-thyroid axis. *Mech Ageing Dev,* 7:19, 1978.

Orentreich, N., Brind, J.L., Rizer, R.L., and Vogelman, J.: Age changes and sex differences in serum dehydroepiardrosterone sulfate concentrations throughout adulthood. *J Clin Endocrinol Metab, 59*:551, 1984.

Osborne, T.B., Mendel, L.B., and Ferry, E.L.: The effect of retardation of growth upon the breeding period and duration of life of rats. *Science, 45*:294, 1917.

Overall, J.E.: Estimating sample size for longitudinal studies of age-related cognitive decline. *J Gerontol,* 2:137, 1987.

Pahlavani, M.A., Cheung, H.T., and Richardson, A.: Influence of dietary restriction on the function of the immune system of rats. *Fed Proc, 46*:567, 1987.

Palmblad, J., Levi, L., Burger, A., Melander, A., Westgren, U., Schenck, H.V., and Skerde, G.: Effects of total energy withdrawal (fasting) on the levels of growth hormone, thyrotropin, cortisol, adrenaline, noradrenaline, T4, T3, and rT3 in healthy humans. *Acta Med Scand, 201*:15, 1977.

Panemangalore, M., Lee, C.J., and Wilson, K.: Comparative effects of dietary energy restriction in young adult and aged rats on body weight, adipose mass and lipid metabolism. *Nutr Res, 6*:981, 1986.

Papavasiliou, P.S., Miller, S.T., Thal, L.J., Nerder, L.J., Houlihan, G., Rao, S.N., and Stevens, J.M.: Age-related motor and catecholamine alterations in mice on levodopa supplemented diet. *Life Sci, 28*:2945, 1981.

Pariza, M.W.: Caloric restriction, *ad libitum* feeding, and cancer. *Proc Soc Exp Biol Med, 183*:293, 1986.

Pariza, M.W.: Dietary fat, caloric restriction, *ad libitum* feeding and cancer risk. *Nutr Rev, 45*:1, 1987.

Park, J.H.Y., Swan, P.B., and Hegarty, P.V.J.: Food restriction improves skeletal muscle maintenance during aging in rats. *Fed Proc, 41*:464, 1982.

Pashko, L.L., Hard, G.C., Rovito, R.J., Williams, J.R., Sobel, E.L., and Schwartz, A.G.: Inhibition of 7,12-dimethylbenz (a) anthracene-induced skin papillomas and carcinomas by dehydroepiandrosterone and 3-β-methylandrost-5-en-17-one in mice. *Cancer Res, 45*:164, 1985.

Payne, P.R.: Influence of energy intake on ageing and longevity. In Chavez, A., Bourges, H., and Basta, S. (Eds.): *Proc IXth Intl Congr Nutr.* Karger, Basel, 1975, pp. 353-361.

Pearl, R.: *The Rate of Living.* New York, Alfred Knopf, 1928.

Pedersen, P.L., and Carafoli, E.: Ion motive ATPases. II. Energy coupling and work output. *TIBS, 12*:186, 1987.

Pertshuk, M.J., Crosby, L.O., Earot, L., and Mullen, J.L.: Immunocompetency in anorexia nervosa. *Am J Clin Nutr, 35*:968, 1982.

Peters, A., Harriman, K.M., and West, C.D.: The effect of increased longevity, produced by dietary restriction, on the neuronal population of area 17 in rat cerebral cortex. *Neurobiol Aging, 8*:7, 1987.

Petros, T.V., Zehr, H.D., and Chabot, R.K.: Adult age differences in accessing and retrieving information from long-term memory. *J Gerontol, 38*:589, 1983.

Phillips, L.S., and Vassilopoulou-Sellin, R.: Nutritional regulation of somatomedin. *Am J Clin Nutr, 32*:1082, 1979.

Phinney, S.D.: The metabolic interaction between very low calorie diet and exercise. In Blackburn, G.L., and Bray, G.A. (Eds.): *Management of Obesity by Severe Caloric Restriction*. Littleton, Mass, PSG Pub. Co., 1985, pp. 99-105.

Piantanelli, L., Gentile, S., Fattoretti, P., and Viticchi, C.: Thymic regulation of brain cortex beta-adrenoceptors during development and aging. *Arch Gerontol Geriatr, 4*:179, 1985.

Pickering, R. and Pickering, C.E.: The effects of reduced dietary intake upon the body and organ weights, and some clinical chemistry and haematological variates of the young wistar rat. *Toxicol Lett, 21*:271, 1984.

Pierpaoli, W.: Changes of hormonal status in young mice by restricted caloric diet. Relation to life span extension. Preliminary results. *Experientia, 33*:1612, 1977.

Pinney, D.O., Stephens, D.F., and Pope, L.S.: Lifetime effects of winter supplemental feed level and age at first partuition on range beef cows. *J Anim Sci, 34*:1067, 1972.

Plesko, M.M., and Richardson, A.: Age-related changes in unscheduled DNA synthesis by rat hepatocytes. *Biochem Biophys Res Commun, 118*:730, 1984.

Pollard, M., and Luckert, P.H.: Tumorigenic effects of direct- and indirect-acting chemical carcinogens in rats on a restricted diet. *JNCI, 74*:1347, 1986.

Pollard, M., Luckert, P.H., and Pan, G.Y.: Inhibition of intestinal tumorigenesis in methylazoxymethanol-treated rats by dietary restriction. *Cancer Treat Rep, 68*:405, 1984.

Pomerantz, L., and Mulinos, M.G.: Pseudo-hypophysectomy produced by inanition. *Am J Physiol, 126*:601, 1939.

Poon, L.W.: Aging in the 1980's: Psychological issues. *American Psychological Association*, Washington, D.C., 1980.

Popper, H.: The liver in aging. In Warner, H.R., Butler, R.N., Sprott, R.L., and Schneider, E.L. (Eds.): *Modern Biological Theories of Aging*. New York, Raven Press, 1987, pp. 219-234.

Population Reference Bureau, Population Trends and Public Policy: In Scommegna, P.M. (Ed.): Death and taxes, the public policy impact of living longer, Washington, D.C., Sept. 1984, pp. 1-16.

Porta, E.A., Joun, N.S., and Nitta, R.T.: Effects of the type of dietary fat at two levels of vitamin E in Wistar male rats during development and aging. I. Life span, serum biochemical parameters and pathological changes. *Mech Ageing Dev, 13*:1, 1980.

Potvin, A.R., Sundulko, K., Tourtellotte, W.W., Lemmon, J.A., and Potvin, J.H.: Human neurologic function and the aging process. *J Am Geriatr Soc, 28*:1, 1980.

Prabhu, S.R., Squier, C.A., and Johnson, N.W.: The effect of ultra-violet radiation and restricted diet on rat labial mucosa. *J Oral Pathol, 7*:143, 1978.

Prasad, K.V.S., Madhavan Nair, K., and Sivakumar, B.: Effect of food restriction (undernutrition) on plasma sex hormone binding globulin (SHBG) capacity, liver drug metabolizing enzymes and uterine cytosol progesterone receptor levels in rabbits. *Contraception, 23*:563, 1981.

Priestly, G.C., and Robertson, M.S.M.: Protein and nucleic acid metabolism in organs from mice selected for large and smaller body size. *Genet Res, 22*:255, 1973.

Pryor, W.A.: The free-radical theory of aging revisited: a critique and a suggested disease-specific theory. In Warner, H.R., Butler, R.N., Sprott, R.L., and Schneider, E.L. (Eds.): *Modern Biological Theories of Aging.* New York, Raven Press, 1987.

Pullar, J.D., and Webster, A.J.F.: The energy cost of fat and protein deposition in the rat. *Br J Nutr, 37*:355, 1977.

Quigley, K., Goya, R., and Meites, J.: Rejuvenating effects of 10-week underfeeding period on estrous cycles in young and old rats. *Neurobiol Aging, 8*:225, 1987.

Rabbitt, P.: How can we tell whether human performance is related to chronologic age? In Samuel, D., Algeri, S., Gershon, S., and Grimm, V.E. (Eds.): *Aging of the Brain.* New York, Raven Press, 1983, pp. 9-18.

Reaven, E.P., and Reaven, G.M.: Structure and function changes in the endocrine pancreas of aging rats with reference to the modulating effects of exercise and caloric restriction. *J Clin Invest, 68*:75, 1981b.

Reaven, E., Wright, D., Mondon, C.E., Solomon, R., Ho, H., and Reaven, G.M.: Effect of age and diet on insulin secretion and insulin action in the rat. *Diabetes, 32*:175, 1983a.

Reaven, E., Curry, D., Moore, J., and Reaven, G.: Effect of age and environmental factors on insulin release from the perfused pancreas of the rat. *J Clin Invest, 71*:345, 1983b.

Reaven, G.M., and Reaven, E.P.: Prevention of age-related hypertriglyceridemia by caloric restriction and exercise training in the rat. *Metabolism, 30*:982, 1981a.

Reddy, B.S., Wang, C., and Maruyama, H.: Effect of restricted caloric intake on azoxymethane-induced colon tumor incidence in male F344 rats. *Cancer Res, 47*:1226, 1987.

Reff, M.E.: RNA and protein metabolism. In Finch, C.E., and Schneider, E.L. (Eds.): *Handbook of the Biology of Aging,* 2nd Ed. New York, Van Nostrand Reinhold, 1985, pp. 225-254.

Reff, M.E., and Schneider, E.L.: *Biological Markers of Aging.* Washington, D.C., U.S. Dept. of Health and Human Services (NIH Pub. #82-2221), 1982a.

Reff, M.E., and Schneider, E.L.: Introduction. In Reff, M.E., and Schneider, E.L. (Eds.): *Biological Markers of Aging.* Washington, D.C., U.S. Dept, of Health and Human Services (NIH Pub. #82-2221), 1982b, p. 1.

Regelson, W.: Biomarkers in Aging. In Regelson, W., and Sinex, F.M. (Eds.): *Intervention in the Aging Process, Part A: Quantitation, Epidemiology, and Clinical Research.* New York, Alan R. Liss, Inc., 1983, pp. 3-98.

Rehm, S., Dierksen, D., and Deerberg, F.: Spontaneous ovarian tumors in Han:NMRI mice: histologic classification, incidence, and influence of food restriction. *JNCI, 72*:1383, 1984.

Rehm, S., Rapp, K.G., and Deerberg, F.: Influence of food restriction and body fat on life span and tumour incidence in female outbred Han:NMRI mice and two sublines. *Z Versuchtierkd, 27*:249, 1985a.

Rehm, S., Nitsche, B., and Deerberg, F.: Non-neoplastic lesions of female virgin Han:NMRI mice, incidence and influence of food restriction throughout life span. I. Thyroid. *Lab Anim, 19*:214, 1985b.

Rehm, S., Wcislo, A., and Deerberg, F.: Non-neoplastic lesions of female virgin Han:NMRI mice, incidence and influence of food restriction throughout life span. II. Respiratory tract. *Lab Anim, 19*:224, 1985c.

Rehm, S., Sommer, R., and Deerberg, F.: Spontaneous nonneoplastic gastric lesions in female Han:NMRI mice, and influence of food restriction throughout life. *Vet Pathol, 24*:216, 1987.

Reigle, G.D.: Changes in hypothalamic control of ACTH and adrenal cortical functions during aging. In Meites, J. (Ed.): *Neuroendocrinology of Aging.* New York, Plenum Press, 1983, pp. 309-332.

Reimers, N.: A history of a stunted brook trout population in an alpine lake: A life span of 24 years. *California Fish and Game, 65*:196, 1979.

Reyman, K., and Schmidt, D.: Beeinflussung der herzfrequenz des kaninchens durch nahrungsentzug. *Acta Biol Med Ger, 38*:691, 1979.

Rhoads, G.G., and Kagan, A.: The relationship of coronary disease, stroke, and mortality to weight in youth and middle age. *Lancet, i*:492, 1983.

Richardson, A.: The effect of age and nutrition on protein synthesis by cells and tissues from mammals. In Watson, R.R. (Ed.): *Handbook of Nutrition in the Aged.* Boca Raton, CRC Press, 1985, pp. 31-48.

Richardson, A., and Cheung, H.T.: The relationship between age-related changes in gene expression, protein turnover, and the responsiveness of an organism to stimuli. *Life Sci, 31*:605, 1982.

Richardson, A., Birchenall-Sparks, M.C., and Staecker, J.L.: Aging and transcription. In Rothstein, M. (Ed.): *Review of Biological Research in Aging,* Vol. 1. New York, Alan R. Liss, 1983, *1*:275-294.

Richardson, A., Roberts, M.S., and Rutherford, M.S.: Aging and gene expression. In Rothstein, M. (Ed.): *Review of Biological Research in Aging,* Vol. 2. New York, Alan R. Liss, 1985, p. 395-419.

Richardson, A., Semsei, I., Rutherford, M.S., and Butler, J.A.: Effect of dietary restriction on the expression of specific genes. *Fed Proc, 46*:568, 1987a.

Richardson, A., Butler, J.A., Rutherford, M.S., Semsei, I., Gu, M., Fernandes, G., and Chiang, W.: Effect of age and dietary restriction on the expression of $\alpha_{2\mu}$-globulin. *J Biol Chem, 262*:12821, 1987b.

Ricketts, W.G., Birchenall-Sparks, M.C., Hardwick, J.P., and Richardson, A.: Effect of age and dietary restriction on protein synthesis by isolated kidney cells, *J Cell Physiol, 125*:492, 1985.

Ricotti, N.A., Nussbaum, S.R., Herzog, D.B., and Neer, R.M.: Osteoporosis in women with anorexia nervosa. *New Engl J Med, 311*:1601, 1984.

Ricquier, D., and Bouillaud, F.: The brown adipose tissue mitochondrial uncoupling protein. In Trayhurn, P., and Nicholls, D.G. (Eds.): *Brown Adipose Tissue.* London, Edward Arnold, 1986.

Riesen, W.H., Herbst, E.J., Walliker, C., and Elvehjem, C.A.: The effect of restricted caloric intake on the longevity of rats. *Am J Physiol, 148*:614, 1947.

Risley, J., Shao, R., Dao, M.L., Johnson, B.C., and Good, R.A.: Dietary regulation of gene expression, *Fed Proc, 46*:567, 1987.

Roberts-Thompson, I.C., Whittingham, S. Youngchaiyud, U., and Mackay, I.R.: Aging, immune response and mortality. *Lancet, ii*:368, 1974.

Robertson, T.B., and Ray, L.A.: Experimental studies on growth. XII. The influence of pituitary gland (anterior lobe) tissue, tethelin, egg lecithin, and cholesterol upon the duration of life of the white mouse. *J Biol Chem, 37*:427, 1919.

Robertson, T.B., and Ray, L.A.: Experimental studies on growth. XV. On the growth of relatively long-lived compared to short-lived animals. *J Biol Chem, 42*:71, 1920.

Robertson, T.B., Marston, H.R., and Walters, J.W.: The influence of intermittent starvation and of intermittent starvation plus nucleic acid on the growth and longevity of the white mouse. *Aust J Exp Biol Med Sci, 12*:33, 1934.

Romsos, D.R.: Efficiency of energy retention in genetically obese animals and in dietary-induced thermogenesis. *Fed Proc, 40*:2524, 1981.

Root, A.W., and Russ, R.D.: Short-term effects of castration and starvation upon pituitary and serum levels of luteinizing hormone and follicle stimulating hormone in male rats. *Acta Endocrinol, 70*:665, 1972.

Rosen, R.: Dynamical aspects of senescence. In Schimke, R.T. (Ed.): *Biochemical Mechanisms in Aging.* NIH Pub. No. 81-2194, 1981, pp. 108-195.

Rosenberg, B., Kemeny, G., Smith, L.G., Shurnick, I.D., and Bandurski, M.J.: The kinetics and thermodynamics of death in multicellular organisms. *Mech Ageing Dev, 2*:275, 1973.

Rosenthal, M., Doberne, L., Greenfield, M., Widstrom, A., and Reaven, G.M.: Effects of age on glucose tolerance, insulin secretion, and in vivo insulin action. *J Am Geriatr Soc, 30*:562, 1982.

Ross, M.H.: Proteins, calories and life expectancy. *Fed Proc, 18*:1190, 1959.

Ross, M.H.: Length of life and nutrition in the rat. *J Nutr, 75*:197, 1961.

Ross, M.H.: Life expectancy modification by change in dietary regimen of the mature rat. In Kuhnau, J. (Ed.): *Proc VIIth Intl Congr Nutr.* New York, Pergamon, Vol. 5, 1966, pp. 35-38.

Ross, M.H.: Aging, nutrition and hepatic enzyme activity patterns in the rat. *J Nutr, 97*:565, 1969.

Ross, M.H.: Length of life and caloric intake. *Am J Clin Nutr, 25*:834, 1972.

Ross, M.H.: Nutrition and longevity in experimental animals. In Winick, M. (Ed.): *Nutrition and Aging.* New York, Wiley, 1976, pp. 43-57.

Ross, M.H.: Nutritional regulation of longevity. In Behnke, J.A., Finch, C.E., and Moment, G.B. (Eds.): *The Biology of Aging.* New York, Plenum Press, 1978, pp. 173-189.

Ross, M.H., and Bras, G.: Tumor incidence patterns and nutrition in the rat. *J Nutr, 87*:245, 1965.

Ross, M.H., and Bras, G.: Lasting influence of early caloric restriction on prevalence of neoplasms in the rat. *JNCI, 47*:1095, 1971.

Ross, M.H., and Bras, G.: Influence of protein under- and overnutrition on spontaneous tumor prevalence in the rat. *J Nutr, 103*:944, 1973.

Ross, M.H., and Bras, G.: Dietary preference and diseases of age. *Nature, 250*:263, 1974.

Ross, M.H., and Bras, G.: Food preference and length of life. *Science, 190*:165, 1975.

Ross, M.H., Bras, G., and Ragbeer, M.S.: Influence of protein and caloric intake upon spontaneous tumor incidence of the anterior pituitary gland of the rat. *J Nutr, 100*:177, 1970.

Ross, M.H., Lustbader, E., and Bras, G.: Dietary practices and growth responses as predictors of longevity. *Nature*, 262:548, 1976.

Ross, M.H., Lustbader, E., and Bras, G.: Body weight, dietary practices, and tumor susceptibility in the rat. *JNCI*, 71:1041, 1983a.

Ross, M.H., Lustbader, E., and Bras, G.: Contribution of body weight and growth to risk of anterior pituitary gland tumors of the rat. *JNCI*, 70:1119, 1983b.

Ross, M.H., Lustbader, E.D., and Bras, G.: Dietary habits and the prediction of life span of rats: a prospective test. *Am J Clin Nutr*, 41:1332, 1985.

Roth, G.S., Ingram, D.K., and Joseph, J.A.: Delayed loss of striatal dopamine receptors during aging of dietarily restricted rats. *Brain Res*, 300:27, 1984.

Rothstein, M.: Biochemical studies of aging. *Chem Eng News*, Aug. 22, p. 26, 1986.

Rothstein, M.: Evidence for and against the error catastrophe hypothesis. In Warner, H.R., Butler, R.N., Sprott, R.L., and Schneider, E.L. (Eds.): *Modern Biological Theories of Aging*. New York, Raven Press, 1987, pp. 139-154.

Rothwell, N.J., and Stock, M.J.: Regulation of energy balance. *Annu Rev Nutr*, 1:235, 1981.

Rothwell, N.J., and Stock, M.J.: Effect of chronic food restriction on energy balance, thermogenic capacity, and brown—adipose-tissue activity in the rat. *Biosci Rep*, 2:543, 1982a.

Rothwell, N.J., and Stock, M.J.: Effects of early overnutrition and undernutrition in rats on the metabolic responses to overnutrition in later life. *J Nutr*, 112:426, 1982b.

Rothwell, N.J., and Stock, M.J.: Effects of age on diet induced thermogenesis and brown adipose tissue metabolism in the rat. *Int J Obes*, 7:583, 1983.

Rothwell, N.J., and Stock, M.J.: Stimulation of thermogenesis and brown fat activity in rats fed medium chain triglyceride. *Metabolism*, 36:128, 1987.

Rothwell, N.J., Saville, M.E., and Stock, M.J.: Sympathetic and thyroid influences on metabolic rate in fed, fasted, and refed rats. *Am J Physiol*, 243:R339, 1982a.

Rothwell, N.J., Stock, M.J., and Tyzbir, R.S.: Energy balance and mitochondrial function in liver and brown fat of rats fed "cafeteria" diets of varying protein content. *J Nutr*, 112:1663, 1982b.

Rotter, J.I., and Diamond, J.M.: What maintains the frequency of human genetic diseases? *Nature*, 329:289, 1987.

Rous, P.: The influence of diet on transplanted and spontaneous mouse tumors. *J Exp Med*, 20:433, 1914.

Rovner, S.: Breast cancer: more cases, more treatments, more decisions. In: *Health, A Weekly Journal of Medicine, Health, Science and Society*. The Washington Post, March 7, 1987, p. 12.

Rowe, J.W., Andres, R., Tobin, J.D., Norris, A.H., and Shock, N.W.: The effect of age on creatinine clearance in men: a cross-sectional and longitudinal study. *J Gerontol*, 31:155, 1976.

Rowe, J.W., Minaker, K.L., Pallotta, J.A., Flier, J.S.: Characterization of the insulin resistance of aging. *J Clin Invest*, 71:1581, 1983.

Rowlatt, C., Franks, L.M., and Sheriff, M.U.: Mammary tumour and hepatoma suppression by dietary restriction in C3H/A^{vy} mice. *Br J Cancer*, 28:83, 1973.

Rowlatt, C., Chesterman, F.C., and Sheriff, M.U.: Life span, age changes and tumour incidence in an ageing C57BL mouse colony. *Lab Anim*, 10:419, 1976.

Rozek, M., Pigg, M., and Fernandes, G.: Effect of food restriction and treadmill exercise on immune response of hypertensive SHR rats. *Fed Proc, 42*:1172, 1983.

Rubner, M. *Das Problem der Lebensdauer und Seine Beziehungen Zun Wachstum und Ernahrung.* Munich, Oldenbourg, 1908.

Rucker, R.: *Mind Tools. The Five Levels of Mathematical Reality.* Boston, Houghton Mifflin, 1987.

Rudzinska, M.A.: Overfeeding and life span in *Tokophyra infusionum. J Gerontol, 7*:544, 1952.

Rudzinska, M.A.: The use of a protozoan for studies on ageing. III. Similarities between young overfed and old normally fed *Tokophyra infusionum:* a light and electron microscope study. Gerontologia, 6:206, 1962.

Ruggerie, B.A., Klurfeld, D.M., and Kritchevsky, D.: Biochemical alterations in 7,12-dimethylbenz [a] anthracene-induced mammary tumors from rats subjected to caloric restriction. *Biochim Biophys Acta, 929*:239, 1987.

Rumsey, W.L., Kendrick, Z.V., and Starnes, J.W.: Bioenergetics in the aging Fischer 344 rat: effects of exercise and food restriction. *Exp Gerontol, 22*:271, 1987.

Rusch, H.P., Kline, B.E., and Baumann, C.A.: The influence of caloric restriction and of dietary fat on tumor formation with ultraviolet radiation. *Cancer Res, 5*:431, 1945a.

Rusch, H.P., Johnson, R.O., and Kline, M.S.: The relationship of caloric intake and of blood sugar to sarcogenesis in mice. *Cancer Res, 5*:705, 1945b.

Russell, R.L., and Jacobson, L.A.: Some aspects of aging can be studied easily in nematodes. In Finch, C.E., and Schneider, E.L. (Eds.): *Handbook of the Biology of Aging.* New York, Van Nostrand Reinhold, 1985, pp. 128-145.

Russell, J.C., and Amy, R.M.: Plasma lipids and other factors in the LA/N corpulent rat in the presence of chronic exercise and food restriction. *Can J Physiol Pharmacol, 64*:750, 1986.

Sachan, D.S.: Modulation of drug metabolism by food restriction in male rats. *Biochem Biophys Res Commun, 104*:984, 1982.

Sachan, D.S., and Das, S.K.: Alterations of NADPH-generating and drug-metabolizing enzymes by feed restriction in male rats. *J Nutr, 112*:2301, 1982.

Sacher, G.A.: Relation of life span to brain weight and body weight in mammals. In Wolstenholme, G.E.W., and O'Connor, M. (Eds.): *CIBA Foundation Colloquia on Ageing,* Vol. 5. London, Churchill, 1959, pp. 115-133.

Sacher, G.A.: Maturation and longevity in relation to cranial capacity in hominid evolution. In Tuttle, R. (Ed.): *Antecedents of Man and After. Primates: Functional Morphology and Evolution,* Vol. 1. The Hague, Mouton, 1975, pp. 417-441.

Sacher, G.A.: Evaluation of the entropy and information terms governing mammalian longevity. In Cutler, R.G. (Ed.): *Interdiscip Top Gerontol,* Vol. 9. Basel, Karger, 1976, pp. 69-82.

Sacher, G.A.: Life table modification and life prolongation. In Finch, C.E. and Hayflick, L. (Eds.): *Handbook of the Biology of Aging.* New York, Van Nostrand Reinhold, 1977, pp. 582-638.

Sacher, G.A.: Theories in gerontology, part 1. In Eisdorfer, C. (Ed.): *Annual Review of Gerontology and Geriatrics,* Vol. 1. New York, Springer, 1980, pp. 3-25.

Safai-Kutti, S., Fernandes, G., Wang, Y., Safai, B., Good, R.A., and Day, N.K.: Reduction of circulating immune complexes by calorie restriction in (NZB × NZW) F_1 mice. *Clin Immunol Immunopathol, 15*:293, 1980.

Salthouse, T.A.: Psychomotor indices of physiological age. In Reff, M.E., and Schneider, E.L. (Eds.): *Biological Markers of Aging.* NIH Publication 82-2221, 1982, pp. 202-209.

Sapolsky, R.M., Krey, L.C., and McEwen, B.S.: The neuroendocrinology of stress and aging: the glucocorticoid cascade hypothesis. *Endocr Rev, 7*:284, 1986.

Sarkar, N.H., Fernandes, G., Telang, N.T., Kourides, I.A., and Good, R.A.: Low calorie diet prevents the development of mammary tumors in C3H mice and reduces circulating prolactin level, murine mammary tumor virus expression, and proliferation of mammary alveolar cells. *Proc Natl Acad Sci USA, 79*:7758, 1982.

Satyanarayana, U. and Narasinga Rao, S.: Effect of diet restriction on some key enzymes of tryptophan-NAD pathway in rats. *J Nutr, 107*:2213, 1977.

Saudek, C.D., and Felig, P.: The metabolic events of starvation. *Am J Med, 60*:117, 1976.

Saul, R.L., Gee, P., and Ames, B.N.: Free radicals, DNA damage, and aging. In Warner, H., Butler, R.N., Sprott, R.L., and Schneider, E.L. (Eds.): *Modern Biological Theories of Aging.* New York, Raven Press, 1987, pp. 113-129.

Sawada, M., and Carlson, J.C.: Association between lipid peroxidation and life-modifying factors in rotifers. *J Gerontol, 42*:451, 1987.

Saxton, J.A., Jr.: Nutrition and growth and their influence on longevity in rats. In: *Biological Symposia,* Vol. 9. Lancaster, PA, Jacques Cattel Press, 1945, pp. 177-196.

Saxton, J.A., Jr., Boon, M.C., and Furth, J.: Observations on the inhibition of development of spontaneous leukemia in mice by underfeeding. *Cancer Res, 4*:401, 1944.

Scarpa, M., Rigo, A., Viglino, P., Stevanato, R., Bracco, F., and Battistin, L.: Age dependence of the level of the enzymes involved in the protection against active oxygen species in the rat brain. *Proc Soc Exp Biol Med, 185*:129, 1987.

Scarpace, P.J., and Yu, B.P.: Diet restriction retards the age-related loss of beta-adrenergic receptors and adenylate cyclase activity. *J Gerontol, 42*:442, 1987.

Schlesselman, J.J.: Planning a longitudinal study: I, sample size determination. II. Frequency of measurement and study duration. *J Chronic Dis, 26*:553, 1973.

Schmucker, D.L.: Subcellular and molecular mechanisms underlying the age-related decline in liver drug metabolizing. In Butler, R.N., and Bearn, A.G. (Eds.): *The Aging Process: Therapeutic Implications.* New York, Raven Press, 1985, pp. 117-136.

Schneeman, B.O., Lacy, D., Ney, D., Lefevre, M.L., Keen, C.L., Lonnerdal, B., and Hurley, L.S.: Similar effects of zinc deficiency and restricted feeding on plasma lipids and lipoproteins in rats. *J Nutr, 116*:1889, 1986.

Schneider, E.L. (Symposium moderator): A debate on obesity, dietary restrictions, and longevity. *Gerontologist, 25*:2, 1985.

Schneider, E.L., and Brody, J.A.: Aging, natural death, and the compression of morbidity: another view. *New Engl J Med, 309*:854, 1983.

Schneider, E.L., and Reed, J.D., Jr.: Life extension. *New Engl J Med, 312*:1159, 1985a.

Schneider, E.L., and Reed, J.D.: Modulations of aging processes. In Finch, C.E., and Schneider, E.L. (Eds.): *Handbook of the Biology of Aging,* 2nd Ed. New York, Van Nostrand Reinhold, 1985b, pp. 45-76.

Schneider, E.L., Reff, M.E., Finch, C.E., and Weksler, M.E.: Potential application of biological markers for assessing interventions of physiological aging. In Reff, M.E., and Schneider, E.L. (Eds.): *Biological Markers of Aging.* Washington, D.C., U.S. Dept. of Health and Human Services, NIH Pub. #82-2221, 1982, pp. 237-252.

Schroeder, H.A., and Mitchener, M.: Selenium and tellerium in rats: Effects on growth, survival and tumors. *J Nutr, 101*:1531, 1971.

Schussler, G.C., and Orlando, J.: Fasting decreases triiodothyronine receptor capacity. *Science, 199*:686, 1978.

Schwab, R., and Weksler, E.: Cell biology of the impaired proliferation of T-cells from elderly humans. In Goidl, E.A. (Ed.): *Aging and the Immune Response.* New York, Marcel Dekker, Inc., 1987, pp. 67-80.

Schwartz, A.G.: Correlation between species life span and capacity to activate 7,12-dimethylbenz (a) anthracene to a form mutagenic to a mammalian cell. *Exp Cell Res, 94*:445, 1975.

Schwartz, A.G.: Inhibition of spontaneous breast cancer formation in female C3H(A^{vy}/a) mice by long-term treatment with dehydroepiandrosterone. *Cancer Res, 39*:1129, 1979.

Schwartz, A.: The effects of dehydroepiandrosterone on the rate of development of cancer and autoimmune processes in laboratory rodents. *Basic Life Sci, 35*:181, 1985.

Schwerin, H.S., Stanton, J.L., Riley, A.M., Jr., Schaefer, A.E., Leveille, G.A., Elliott, J.G., Warwick, K.M., and Brett, B.E.: Food eating patterns and health: a reexamination of the ten-state and HANES 1 surveys. *Am J Clin Nutr, 34*:568, 1981.

Scott, M.D., Meshnick, S.R., and Eaton, J.W.: Superoxide dismutase-rich bacteria. Paradoxical increase in oxidant toxicity. *J Biol Chem, 262*:3640, 1987.

Segall, P.E.: Interrelations of dietary and hormonal effects in aging. *Mech Ageing Dev, 9*:515, 1979.

Segall, P.E., and Timiras, P.S.: Age-related changes in thermoregulatory capacity of tryptophan-deficient rats. *Fed Proc, 34*:83, 1975.

Segall, P.E., and Timiras, P.S.: Patho-physiologic findings after chronic tryptophan deficiency in rats: A model for delayed growth and aging. *Mech Ageing Dev, 5*:109. 1976.

Segall, P.E., and Timiras, P.S.: Low tryptophan diets delay reproductive aging. *Mech Ageing Dev, 23*:245, 1983.

Segall, P.E., Ooka, H., Rose, K., and Timiras, P.S.: Neural and endocrine development after chronic tryptophan deficiency in rats: I. Brain monoamine and pituitary responses. *Mech Ageing Dev, 7*:1, 1978.

Sekuler, R.: Vision as a source of simple and reliable markers of age. In Reff, M.E., and Schneider, E.L. (Eds.): *Biological Markers of Aging.* NIH Publication No. 82-2221, 1982, pp. 220-227.

Selwyn, M.J.: Holes in mitochondrial inner membranes. *Nature, 330*:424, 1987.

Shaffer, J.B., Sutton, R.B., and Bewley, G.C.: Isolation of a cDNA clone for a murine catalase and analysis of an acatalasemic mutant. *J Biol Chem, 262*:12908, 1987.

Shao, R., Risley, J., Dao, M.L., Johnson, B.C., and Good, R.A.: Regulation of intestinal alkaline phosphatase by dietary restriction. *Fed Proc, 46*:435, 1987.

Shatenstein, B., Srivastava, U., Tuchweber, B., and Nadeau, M.: Protein and nucleic acid metabolism in the liver of female rats during graded dietary restriction. *Nutr Rep Int, 32*:357, 1985.

Sherman, H.C., and Campbell, H.L.: Rate of growth and length of life. *Proc Natl Acad Sci USA, 21*:235, 1935.

Sherwin, R.S.: Influence of diet and carbohydrate on thyroid hormone metabolism. In Blackburn, G.L. and Bray, G.A. (Eds.): *Management of Obesity by Severe Caloric Restriction.* Littleton, M.A., PSG Publishing, 1985, pp. 155-163.

Shock, N.W.: The role of nutrition in aging. *J Am Coll Nutr, 1*:3, 1982.

Silberberg, R., Jarrett, S.R., and Silberberg, M.: Longevity of female mice kept on various dietary regimens during growth. *J Gerontol, 17*:239, 1962.

Simopoulos, A.P., and van Itallie, T.B.: Body weight, health, and longevity. *Ann Intern Med, 100*:285, 1984.

Sims, E.A.H., and Danforth, E., Jr.: Expenditure and storage of energy in man. *J Clin Invest, 79*:1019, 1987.

Sisk, C.L., and Bronson, F.H.: Effects of food restriction and restoration on gonadotropin and growth hormone secretion in immature male rats. *Biol Reprod, 35*:554, 1986.

Siskind, G.W.: Aging and the immune system. In Warner, H.R., Butler, R.N., Sprott, R.L., Schneider, E.L. (Eds.): *Modern Biological Theories of Aging.* New York, Raven Press, 1987, pp. 235-242.

Skalicky, M., Hofecker, G., Kment, A., and Niedermueller, H.: Models of the biological age of the rat. II. Multiple regression models in the study of influencing age. *Mech Aging Dev, 14*:361, 1980.

Skoldstam, L. and Lindstrom, F.D.: Effects of fasting and a lactovegetarian diet on rheumatoid arthritis. *Scand J Rheumatol, 8*:249, 1979.

Smith, E.L., Hill, R.L., Lehman, I.R., Lefkowitz, R.J., Handler, P., and White, A.: *Principles of Biochemistry: Mammalian Biochemistry.* New York, McGraw-Hill, 1983.

Smith, G.S., and Walford, R.L.: Influence of the main histocompatibility complex on aging in mice. *Nature, 270*, 727, 1977.

Smith, J.K., Sekaram, C., and Lifshitz, F.: Immune competence in anorexia nervosa. *Am J Clin Nutr, 31*:716, 1978.

Smith, K.C.: Chemical adducts to deoxyribonucleic acid: their importance to the genetic alteration theory of aging. *Interdisciplinary Topics in Gerontology, 9*:16, 1976.

Smith-Sonneborn, J.: How we age. In Oberlink, N., Butler, R.N., and Schechter, M. (Eds.): *The Promise of Productive Aging.* New York, Springer, 1988.

Snow, C.P.: *The Physicists.* Boston, Little, Brown, 1981.

Synder, D., and Pollard, M.: Life span and pathology of germfree and conventional rats fed ad libitum or restricted dietary intake. *Gerontologist, 27*:88A, 1987.

Snyder, D.L., and Wostmann, B.S.: Growth rate of male germfree Wistar rats fed *ad libitum* or restricted natural ingredient diet. *Lab Anim Sci, 37*:320, 1987.

Soboll, S., and Stucki, J.: Regulation of the degree of coupling of oxidative phosphorylation in intact rat liver. *Biochim Biophys Acta, 807*:245, 1985.

Sohal, R.S.: Metabolic rate, aging, and lipofuscin accumulation. In Sohal, R.S. (Ed.): *Age Pigments*. Amsterdam, Elsevier/North Holland, 1981, pp. 303-315.

Sohal, R.S., and Allen, R.G.: Relationship between metabolic rate, free radicals, differentiation and aging: a unified theory. In Woodhead, A.D., Blackett, A.D., and Hollaender, A. (Eds.): *Molecular Biology of Aging*. New York, Plenum Press, 1985, pp. 75-104.

Solomon, C., Tuchweber, B., Srivastava, U., and Nadeau, M.: Liver lysosomal enzymes in rats during long-term dietary restriction. I. Changes during the developmental period of life. *Mech Ageing Dev, 24*:9, 1984.

Sonntag, W.E., Forman, L.J., and Meites, J.: Changes in growth hormone secretion in aging rats and man, and possible relation to diminished physiological function. In Meites, J. (Ed.): *Neuroendocrinology of Aging*. New York, Plenum Press, 1983, pp. 275-308.

Sorrentino, S., Jr., Reiter, R.J., and Schalch, D.S.: Interactions of the pineal gland, blinding, and underfeeding on reproductive organ size and radioimmunoassayable growth hormone. *Neuroendocrinology, 7*:105, 1971.

Sparks, M.B., Ricketts, W.G., Rehwaldt, C.A., Cheung, H.T., and Richardson, A.: Effect of dietary restriction on gene expression. *Fed Proc, 42*:1307, 1983.

Spindler, S.R., Mellon, S.H., and Baxter, J.D.: Growth hormone gene transcription is regulated by thyroid and glucocorticoid hormones in cultures of rat pituitary tumor cells. *J Biol Chem, 257*:11627, 1982.

Spurgeon, H.A., Ingram, D.K., and Lakatta, E.G.: Long-term food restriction causes cardiac atrophy but does not alter rat cardiac muscle performance. *Fed Proc, 42*:466, 1983.

Srivastava, U. and Thakur, M.L.: Modulation of nucleic acid and protein metabolism in the liver of long-term graded dietary restricted rats. *Fed Proc, 46*:568, 1987.

Srivastava, U., Vu, M.L., Bhargava, S., and Goswami, T.: Metabolism of nucleic acids and protein in the liver, brain, and kidney of female rats subjected to dietary restriction during the period of gestation as well as the period of growth, gestation, and lactation. *Can J Physiol Pharmacol, 50*:832, 1972.

Srivastava, U., Ganguli, P.K., Brasseur, R. and Gyenes, L.: The metabolism of liver RNA in adult rats subjected to prolonged dietary restriction during the period of growth and development. *Nutr Rep Int, 17*:367, 1978.

Stallone, R.A.: Ishemic heart disease and lipids in blood and diet. *Ann Rev Nutr, 3*:155, 1983.

Stemmermann, G.N., Nomura, A.M.Y., and Heilbrun, L.K.: Dietary fat and the risk of colorectal cancer. *Cancer Res, 44*:4633, 1984.

Still, J.W.: The cybernetic theory of aging. *J Am Geriatr Soc, 17*:625, 1969.

Stocco, D.M., and Hutson, J.C.: Quantitation of mitochondrial DNA and protein in the liver of Fischer 344 rats during aging. *J Gerontol, 33*:802, 1978.

Stock, M., and Rothwell, N.: *Obesity and Leaness: Basic Aspects*. London, John Libbey, 1982.

Stoltzner, G.: Effects of life-long dietary protein restriction on mortality, growth, organ weights, blood counts, liver aldolase and kidney catalase in Balb/c mice. *Growth, 41*:337, 1977.

Stoltzner, G.H., and Dorsey, B.A.: Life-long dietary protein restriction and immune function: responses to mitogens and sheep erythrocytes in Balb/c mice. *Am J Clin Nutr, 33*:1264, 1980.

Storer, J.B.: Relation of life span to brain weight, body weight, and metabolic rate among inbred mouse strains. *Exp Gerontol, 2*:173, 1967.

Strong, R.: Neurochemistry of aging: 1982-1984. In Rothstein, M. (Ed.): *Review of Biological Research in Aging,* Vol. 2. New York, Alan R. Liss, 1985, p. 181-196.

Stuchlikova, E., Juricova-Horakova, M., and Deyl, Z.: New aspects of the dietary effect of life prolongation in rodents. What is the role of obesity in aging? *Exp Gerontol, 10*:141, 1975.

Stunkard, A.J.: Nutrition, aging and obesity. In Rockstein, M., and Sussman, M.L. (Eds.): *Nutrition, Longevity and Aging.* New York, Academic Press, 1976, pp. 253, 282.

Stunkard, A.J.: Anorectic agents lower a body weight set point. *Life Sci, 30*:2043, 1982.

Stunkard, A.J.: Nutrition, aging and obesity: A critical review of a complex relationship. *Int J Obes, 7*:201, 1983.

Sukhatme, P.V., and Margen, S.: Autoregulatory homeostatic nature of energy balance. *Am J Clin Nutr, 35*:355, 1982.

Sun, J., and Strobel, H.W.: Aging affects the drug metabolism systems of rat liver, kidney, colon and lung in a differential fashion. *Exp Gerontol, 21*:523, 1986.

Sun, J.Q., Lau, P.P., and Strobel, H.W.: Aging modifies the expression of hepatic microsomal cytochromes P-450 after pretreatment of rats with beta-naphthoflavone or phenobarbital. *Exp Gerontol, 21*:65, 1986.

Suominen, H., Heikkinen, E., Parkatti, T., Forsberg, S., and Kiiskinen, A.: Effects of "lifelong" physical training on functional aging in men. *Scand J Soc Med, 14*:225, 1980.

Surawicz, B.: Prognosis of ventricular arrhythmias in relation to sudden cardiac death: therapuetic implications. *J Am Coll Cardiol, 10*:435, 1987.

Suzuki, T., Makino, H., Kanatsuka, A., and Yoshida, S.: Effects of diet restriction on insulin-sensitive phosphodiesterase in rat fat cells. *Metabolism, 36*:43, 1987.

Svojtkova, E., Deyl, Z., Rosmus, J., and Adam, M.: Aging of connective tissue. The effect of diet and x-irradiation. *Exp Gerontol, 7*:157, 1972.

Swan, P.B.: Food consumption by individuals in the United States: Two major surveys. *Ann Rev Nutr, 3*:413, 1983.

Sylvester, P.W., Aylsworth, C.F., and Meites, J.: Relationship of hormones to inhibition of mammary tumor development by underfeeding during the "critical period" after carcinogen administration. *Cancer Res, 41*:1384, 1981.

Szilard, L.: On the nature of the aging process. *Proc Natl Acad Sci USA, 45*:30, 1959.

Szymura, J.M., Wabl, M.R., and Klein, J.: Mouse mitochondrial superoxide dismutase locus is on chromosome 17. *Immunogenetics, 14*:234, 1981.

Takahara, S. Progressive oral gangrene, probably due to lack of catalase in the blood. *Lancet, 2*:1101, 1952.

Takahashi, R., and Goto, S.: Influence of dietary restriction on accumulation of heat-labile enzyme molecules in the liver and brain of mice. *Arch Biochem Biophys, 257*:200, 1987.

Takata, H., Ishi, T., Suzuki, M., Sekiguchi, S., and Iri, H.: Influence of major histocompatibility complex region genes on human longevity among Okinawan-Japanese centenarians and nonagenarians. *Lancet,* Vol. II: 824, 1987.

Talan, M.I., and Ingram, D.K.: Effect of intermittent feeding on thermoregulatory abilities of young and aged C57BL/6J mice. *Arch Gerontol Geriatr, 4*:251, 1985.

Talmasoff, J.M., Ono, T., and Cutler, R.G.: Superoxide dismutase: correlation with life span and specific metabolic rate in primate species. *Proc Natl Acad Sci USA, 77*:2777, 1980.

Tam, C.F., and Walford, R.L.: Alterations in cyclic nucleotides and cyclase specific activities in T-lymphocytes of aging normal humans and patients with Down's Syndrome. *J Immunol, 125*:1665, 1980.

Tannenbaum, A.: The initiation and growth of tumors. Introduction. I. Effects of underfeeding. *Am J Cancer, 38*:335, 1940.

Tannenbaum, A.: The genesis and growth of tumors. II. Effects of caloric restriction per se. *Cancer Res, 2*:460, 1942.

Tannenbaum, A.: The dependence of the genesis of induced skin tumors on the caloric intake during different stages of carcinogenesis. *Cancer Res, 4*:673, 1944.

Tannenbaum, A.: The dependence of tumor formation on the degree of caloric restriction. *Cancer Res, 5*:609, 1945a.

Tannenbaum, A.: The dependence of tumor formation on the composition of the calorie-restricted diet as well as on the degree of restriction. *Cancer Res, 5*:616, 1945b.

Tannenbaum, A.: Effects of varying caloric intake upon tumor incidence and tumor growth. *Ann NY Acad Sci, 49*:5, 1947.

Tannenbaum, A., and Silverstone, H.: The influence of the degree of caloric restriction on the formation of skin tumors and hepatomas in mice. *Cancer Res, 9*:724, 1949.

Tannenbaum, A., and Silverstone, H.: Failure to inhibit the formation of mammary carcinoma in mice by intermittent fasting. *Cancer Res, 10*:577, 1950.

Tannenbaum, A., and Silverstone, H.: Nutrition in relation to cancer. In Greenstein, J.P., and Haddow, A. (Eds.): *Advances in Cancer Research,* Vol. 1. New York, Academic Press, Inc., 1953, pp. 451-501.

Tannenbaum, A., and Silverstone, H.: Nutrition and the genesis of tumors. In Raven, R.W. (Ed.): *Cancer,* Vol. 1. London, Butterworth, 1957, pp. 306-334.

Tannenbaum, G.S., Epelbaum, J., Cole, E., Brazeau, P., and Martin, J.B.: Antiserum to somatostatin reverses starvation-induced inhibition of growth hormone but not insulin secretion. *Endocrinology, 102*:1909, 1978.

Tannenbaum, G.S., Guyda, H.J., and Posner, B.I.: Insulin-like growth factors: A role in growth hormone negative feedback and body weight regulation via brain. *Science 220*:77, 1983.

Tappel, A.L., Fletcher, B., and Deamer, D.: Effects of antioxidants and nutrients on lipid peroxidation fluorescent products and aging parameters in the mouse. *J Gerontol, 28*:415, 1973.

Tas, S., and Walford, R.L.: Increased disulfide-mediated condensation of the nuclear DNA-protein complex in lymphocytes during postnatal development and aging. *Mech Ageing Dev, 19*:73, 1982a.

Tas, S., and Walford, R.L.: Influence of disulfide reducing agents on frantionation of the chromatin complex by endogenous nucleases and DNAse I in aging mice. *J Gerontol, 37*:673, 1982b.

Tas, S., Tam, C.F., and Walford, R.L.: Disulfide bonds and the structure of the chromatin complex in relation to aging. *Mech Ageing Dev, 12*:65, 1980.

Tauchi, H., and Sato, T.: Age changes in size and number of mitochondria of human hepatic cells. *J Gerontol, 23*:454, 1968.

Taylor, A.W., Cary, S., McNulty, M., Garrod, J., and Secord, D.C.: Effects of food restriction and exercise upon the deposition and mobilization of energy stores in the rat. *J Nutr, 104*:218, 1974.

Taylor, H.L., and Keys, A.: Adaptation to caloric restriction. *Science, 112*:215, 1950.

Thoman, M.L., and Weigle, W.O.: Age-associated changes in the synthesis and function of cytokines. In Goidl, E. (Ed.): *Aging and the Immune Response.* New York, Dekker, 1987, pp. 199-223.

Thomas, I.K., and Erickson, K.L.: Dietary fatty acid modulation of murine T-cell responses in vivo. *J Nutr, 115*:1528, 1985.

Thomson, T.J., Runcie, J., and Miller, U.: Treatment of obesity by total fasting up to 249 days. *Lancet, 2*:999, 1966.

Thompson, H.J., Meeker, L.D., Tagliaferro, A.R., and Roberts, J.S.: Effect of energy intake on the promotion of mammary carcinogenesis by dietary fat. *Nutr Cancer, 7*:37, 1985.

Tice, R.R., and Setlow, R.B.: DNA repair and replication in aging organisms and cells. In Finch, C.E., and Schneider, E.L. (Eds.): *Handbook of the Biology of Aging,* 2nd Ed. New York, Van Nostrand Reinhold, 1985, pp. 173-224.

Timiras, P.S.: Nueroendocrinology of aging. Retrospective, current and prospective views. In Meites, J. (Ed.): *Neuroendocrinology of Aging.* New York, Plenum Press, 1983, pp. 5-30.

Tollefsbol, T.O., and Cohen, H.J.: Expression of intracellular biochemical defects of lymphocytes in aging: proposal of a general aging mechanism which is not cell-specific. *Exp Gerontol, 21*:129, 1986.

Tollefsbol, T.O., Chapman, M.L., Zaun, R., Gracy, R.W.: Impaired glycolysis of human lymphocytes during aging. *Mech Ageing Dev, 17*:369, 1981.

Totter, J.R.: Food restriction, ionizing radiation, and natural selection. *Mech Ageing Dev, 30*:261, 1985.

Trayhurn, P., and James, W.P.T.: Thermoregulation and non-shivering thermogenesis in the genetically obese (ob/ob) mouse. *Pflugers Arch, 373*:189, 1978.

Treton, J.A., and Courtois, Y.: Correlation between DNA excision repair and mammalian life span in lens epithelial cells. *Cell Biol Int Rep, 6*:253, 1982.

Truswell, H.C.: Hypertension and salt. *Lancet, ii*:204, 1978.

Tuchweber, B., Perea, A., Ferland, G., and Yousef, I.M.: Dietary restriction influences bile formation in aging rats. *Life Sci, 41*:2091, 1987.

Tuck, M.L.: The effect of very low calorie diets on blood pressure control in obese subjects. In Blackburn, G.L., and Bray, G.A. (Eds.): Littleton, Mass., PSG Publishing Co., Inc., 1985, pp. 263-278.

Tucker, M.J.: The effect of long-term food restriction on tumours in rodents. *Int J Cancer, 23*:803, 1979.

Tucker, S.M., Mason, R.L., and Beauchene, R.E.: Influence of diet and feed restriction on kidney function of aging male rats. *J Gerontol, 31*:264, 1976.

Turnbull, G.J., Lee, P.N., and Roe, F.J.C.: Relationship of body-weight gain to longevity and to risk of development of nephropathy and neoplasia in Sprague-Dawley rats. *Fd Chem Toxic, 23*:355, 1985.

Tzagoloff, A.: *Mitochondria*. New York, Plenum, 1982.

Tzankoff, S.P., and Norris, A.H.: Longitudinal changes in basal metabolism in man. *J Appl Physiol, 45*:536, 1978.

Vagenakis, A.G.: Thyroid hormone metabolism in prolonged experimental starvation in man. In Vigersky, R.A. (Ed.): *Anorexia Nervosa*. New York, Raven Press, 1977, pp. 243-253.

Vallejo, E.A.: La dieta de hambre a dias alternos in la alimentacion de los viejos. *Rev Clin Exp, 63*:25, 1957.

Vander Tuig, J.G., Trostler, N., Romsos, D.R., and Leveille, G.A.: Heat production of lean and obese (ob/ob) mice in response to fasting, food restriction or thyroxine. *Proc Soc Exp Biol Med, 160*:266, 1979.

Vargas, R., and Castaneda, M.: Role of elongation factor 1 in the translational control of rodent brain protein synthesis. *J Neurochem, 37*:687, 1981.

Verzar, F.: Note on the influence of procaine (Novocain), para-aminobenzoic acid or dimethylethanolamine on the ageing of rats. *Gerontologia, 3*:351, 1959.

Vigersky, R.A., and Loriaux, D.L.: Anorexia nervosa as a model of hypothalamic dysfunction. In Vigersky, R.A. (Ed.): *Anorexia Nervosa*. New York, Raven Press, 1977, pp. 109-127.

Vigersky, R.A., Loriaux, D.L., Andersen, A.E., Meckelenburg, R.S., and Vaitukaitis, J.L.: Delayed pituitary hormone response to LRF and TRF in patients with anorexia nervosa and with secondary amenorhea associated with simple weight loss. *J Clin Endocrinol Metab, 43*:893, 1978.

Visscher, M.B., Ball, Z.B., Barnes, R.H., and Sivertsen, I.: The influence of caloric restriction upon the incidence of spontaneous mammary carcinoma in mice. *Surgery, 11*:48, 1942.

Vitorica, J., and Satrustegui, J.: Involvement of mitochondria in the age-dependent decrease in calcium uptake of rat brain synaptosomes. *Brain Res, 378*:36, 1986a.

Vitorica, J., and Satrustegui, J.: The influence of age on the calcium-efflux pathway and matrix calcium buffering power in brain mitochondria. *Biochim Biophys Acta, 851*:209, 1986b.

Vitorica, J., Machado, A., and Satrustegui, J.: Age-dependent variations in peroxide-utilizing enzymes from rat brain mitochondria and cytoplasm. *J Neurochem, 42*:351, 1984.

Vitorica, J., Clark, A., Machado, A., and Satrustegui, J.: Impairment of glutamate uptake and absence of alterations in energy-transducing ability of old rat brain mitochondria. *Mech Age Dev, 29*:255, 1985.

Voitenko, V.P., and Tokar, A.V.: The assessment of biological age and sex differences in human aging. *Exp Aging Res, 9*:239, 1984.

Volicer, L., West, C.D., Chase, A.R., and Greene, L.: Beta-adrenergic receptor sensitivity in cultured vascular smooth muscle cells: Effect of age and of dietary restriction. *Mech Ageing Dev, 21*:283, 1983.

Volicer, L., West, C., and Greene, L.: Effect of dietary restriction and stress on body temperature in rats. *J Gerontol, 39*:178, 1984.

Vorbeck, M.L., Martin, A.P., Park, J.K.J., and Townsend, J.F.: Aging-related decrease in hepatic cytochrome oxidase of the Fischer 344 rat. *Arch Biochem Biophys, 214*:67, 1982a.

Vorbeck, M.L., Martin, A.P., Long, J.W., Jr., Smith, J.M., and Orr, R.R., Jr.: Aging-dependent modification of lipid composition and lipid structural order parameter of hepatic mitochondria. *Arch Biochem Biophys, 217*:351, 1982b.

Voss, K.H., Masoro, E.J., and Anderson, W.: Modulation of age-related loss of glucagon-promoted lipolysis by food restriction. *Mech Ageing Dev, 18*:135, 1982.

Vruwink, K.G., Keen, C.L., Gershwin, M.E., and Hurley, L.S.: Studies of nutrition and autoimmunity. Failure of zinc deprivation to alter autoantibody production when initiated in disease-established mice. *J Nutr, 117*:177, 1987.

Walford, R.L.: Auto-immunity and aging. *J Gerontol, 17*:281 1962.

Walford, R.L.: *The Immunologic Theory of Aging.* Copenhagen, Munksgaard, 1969.

Walford, R.L.: The immunologic theory of aging: current status. *Fed Proc, 33*:2020, 1974.

Walford, R.L.: When is a mouse "old"? *J Immunol, 117*:352, 1976.

Walford, R.L.: A speculative proposal about the immemorial ancestry of the MHC. *AACHTion News, 5*:15, 1981.

Walford, R.L.: Studies in immunogerontology. *J Am Geriatr Soc, 30*:617, 1982.

Walford, R.L.: *Maximum Life Span.* New York, Norton, 1983.

Walford, R.L.: The extension of maximum life span. *Clin Geriatr Med, 1*:29, 1985.

Walford, R.L.: *The 120-Year Diet.* New York, Simon and Schuster, 1986a.

Walford, R.L.: Caloric restriction and aging in humans. *Chem Eng News, 64*:3, 1986b.

Walford, R.L.: MHC regulation of aging: an extension of the immunologic theory of aging. In Warner, H.R., Butler, R.N., Sprott, R.L., and Schneider, E.L. (Eds.): *Modern Biological Theories of Aging.* New York, Raven Press, 1987, pp. 243-260.

Walford, R.L., and Tam, C.F.: Lymphocyte biochemistry in relation to immune function in aging: cyclic nucleotides and purine salvage pathways. In Schimke, R.T., (Ed.): *Biochemical Mechanisms in Aging.* NIH Pub. No. 81-2194, National Institute on Aging, 1981, pp. 517-524.

Walford, R.L., and Tittor, W.: Einflusse des lymphatischen Systems auf den Alterungsvorgang. In: *Verhandlungen der Deutschen Gesellschaft f. Inner Medizin, 79*:137-153, 1973.

Walford, R.L., Liu, R.K., Gerbase-Delima, M., Mathies, M., and Smith, G.S.: Long-term dietary restriction and immune function in mice: Response to sheep red blood cells and to mitogenic agents. *Mech Ageing Dev, 2*:447, 1973/74.

Walford, R.L., Liu, R.K., Mathies, M., Lipps, L., and Konen, T.: Influence of caloric restriction on immune function: Relevance for an immunologic theory of aging. In Chavez, A., Bourges, H., and Basta, S. (Eds.): *Proc IXth Intl Congr Nutr.* Basel, S. Karger, 1975, pp. 374-381.

Walford, R.L., Meredith, P.J., and Cheney, K.E.: Immunoengineering: prospects for correction of age-related immunodeficiency status. In Makinodan, T., and

Yunis, E. (Eds.): *Immunology and Aging.* New York, Plenum Press, 1977, pp. 183-201.

Walford, R.L., Tam, C.F., and Weindruch, R.H.: Alterations in cyclic nucleotide metabolism in aging. *XIIth Intl Congr Gerontol* (Book of Abstracts). Hamburg, 1981a, p. 173.

Walford, R.L., Weindruch, R.H., Gottesmann, S.R.S., and Tam, C.F.: The immunopathology of aging. In Eisdorfer, C., Besdine, R.W., Cristofalo, V.J., Lawton, M.P., Maddox, G.L., and Starr, B.D. (Eds.): *Annual Review of Gerontology and Geriatrics.* Vol. 2, New York, Springer Publishing Co., 1981b, pp. 1-48.

Walford, R.L., Naeim, F., Hall, K.Y., Tam, C.F., Medici, M., and Gatti, R.: Accelerated aging in Down's Syndrome: the concept of hierarchical homeostasis in relation to local and global failure. In Fabris, N., Garaci, E., Hadden, J., and Mitchison, N.A. (Eds.): *Immunoregulation.* New York, Plenum Press, 1983, pp. 399-417.

Walford, R.L., Harris, S., and Weindruch, R.: Dietary restriction and aging: historical phases, mechanisms, current directions. *J Nutr, 117*:1650, 1987.

Walker, M.A., and Page, L.: Nutritive value of college meals. Proximate composition and vitamins. *J Am Diet Assoc, 66*:145, 1975.

Walker, R.F., McMahon, K.M., and Pivorun, E.B.: Pineal gland structure and respiration as affected by age and hypocaloric diet. *Exp Gerontol, 13*:91, 1978.

Ward, W.F.: Food restriction modulation of the age related decline in protein turnover. *Gerontologist, 26*:152A, 1986.

Ward, W.F.: Nutritional modulation of liver protein turnover in the aging Fischer 344 rat. *Fed Proc, 46*:567, 1987.

Warner, C.M., Briggs, C.J., Meyer, T.E., Spannaus, D.J., Yang, H.Y., Balinsky, D.: Lymphocyte aging in allophenic mice. *Exp Gerontol, 20*:35, 1985.

Warner, H.R., Butler, R.N., Sprott, R.L., and Schneider, E.L. (Eds.): *Modern Biological Theories of Aging.* New York, Raven Press, 1987.

Warren, M.J., Jewelewicz, R., Dyrenfurth, R.I., Ans, R., Kalef, S., and Wiele, R.L.V.D.: The significance of weight loss in the evaluation of pituitary response to LRF in women with secondary amenorrhea. *J Clin Endocrinol Metab, 40*:601, 1975.

Waterlow, J.C.: Metabolic adaptation to low intakes of energy and protein. *Annu Rev Nutr, 6*:495, 1986.

Webb, G.P., Jagot, S.A., Rogers, P.D., and Jakobson, M.E.: The effects of fasting on thermoregulation in normal and obese mice. *IRCS Med Sci, 8*:163, 1980.

Webb, G.P., Jagot, S.A., and Jakobson, M.E.: Fasting-induced torpor in *Mus musculus* and its implications in the use of murine models for human obesity studies. *Comp Biochem Physiol, 72A*:211, 1982.

Webster, G.C. and Webster, S.L.: Decline in synthesis of elongation factor one (EF-1) precedes the decreased synthesis of total protein in aging *Drosophila melanogaster. Mech Ageing Dev, 22*:121, 1983.

Webster, G.C., and Webster, S.L.: Specific disappearance of translatable messenger RNA for elongation factor one in aging *Drosophila melanogaster. Mech Ageing Dev, 24*:335, 1984.

Weinbach, E.C., and Garbus, J.: Oxidative phosphorylation in mitochondria from aged rats. *J Biol Chem, 234*:412, 1959.

Weindruch, R.: Dietary restriction and the aging process. In Armstrong, D., Sohal, R., Cutler, R., and Slater, T.F. (Eds.): *Free Radicals in Molecular Biology and Disease.* New York, Raven Press, 1984, pp. 181-202.

Weindruch, R., and Suffin, S.C.: Quantitative histologic effects on mouse thymus of controlled dietary restriction. *J Gerontol, 34*:525, 1980.

Weindruch, R., and Walford, R.L.: Dietary restriction in mice beginning at one year of age: Effects on life span and spontaneous cancer incidence. *Science, 215*:1415, 1982.

Weindruch, R.H., Kristie, J.A., Cheney, K.E., and Walford, R.L.: Influence of controlled dietary restriction on immunologic function and aging. *Fed Proc, 38*:2007, 1979.

Weindruch, R.H., Cheung, M.K., Verity, M.A., and Walford, R.L.: Modification of mitochondrial respiration by aging and dietary restriction. *Mech Aging Dev, 12*:375, 1980.

Weindruch, R., Gottesman, S.R.S., and Walford, R.L.: Modification of age-related immune decline in mice dietarily restricted from or after mid-adulthood. *Proc Natl Acad Sci USA, 79*:898, 1982a.

Weindruch, R., Chia, D., Barnett, E.V., and Walford, R.L.: Dietary restriction in mice beginning at one year of age: Effects on serum immune complex levels. *Age, 5*:111, 1982b.

Weindruch, R., Kristie, J.A., Naeim, F., Mullen, B., and Walford, R.L.: Influence of weaning-initiated dietary restriction on responses to T-cell mitogens and on splenic T-cell levels in a long-lived mouse hybrid. *Exp Gerontol, 17*:49, 1982c.

Weindruch, R., Devens, B.H., Raff, H.V., and Walford, R.L.: Influence of dietary restriction and aging on natural killer cell activity in mice. *J Immunol, 130*:993, 1983.

Weindruch, R., McFeeters, G. and Walford, R.L.: Food intake reduction and immunologic alterations in mice fed dehydroepiandrosterone. *Exp Gerontol, 19*:297, 1984.

Weindruch, R., Walford, R.L., Fligiel, S., and Guthrie, D.: The retardation of aging by dietary restriction: longevity, cancer, immunity and lifetime energy intake. *J Nutr, 116*:641, 1986.

Weindruch, R., Naylor, P.H., Goldstein, A.L., and Walford, R.L.: Influences of aging and dietary restriction on serum thymosin $\alpha 1$ levels in mice. *J Gerontol,* 1988 (in press).

Weinsier, R.L., Bacon, J.A., and Birch, R.: Time-calorie displacement for weight control: a prospective evaluation of its adequacy for maintaining normal nutrition status. In Blackburn, G.L., and Brody, G.A. (Eds.): *Management of Obesity by Severe Caloric Restriction.* Littleton, Mass., PSG Pub. Co., 1985, pp. 171-181.

Weksler, M.E.: The senescence of the immune system. *Hospital Practice, 16*:53, 1981.

Weksler, M.E.: A search for immunological markers of aging in man. In Reff, M., and Schneider, E.L. (Eds.): *Biological Markers of Aging.* NIH Pub. 82-2221, 1982, pp. 94-97.

Weksler, M.E., and Hutteroth, T.M.: Impaired lymphocyte function in aging humans. *J Clin Invest, 53*:99, 1974.

Weraarchakul, N., and Richardson, A.: Effect of age and dietary restriction on DNA repair. *Fed Proc,* 1988, (in press).

Whitaker, J., Roth, G.S., and Ingram, D.K.: Life-long dietary restriction affects striatally-mediated behavioral responses in aged rats. *Neurobiol Aging,* 4:191, 1983.

White, F., White, J., Mider, G.B., Kelly, M.G., and Heston, W.E.: Effect of caloric restriction on mammary-tumor formation in strain C3H mice and on the response of strain DBA to painting with methylcholanthrene. *JNCI,* 5:43, 1944.

White, J. and Andervont, H.J.: Effect of a diet relatively low in cystine on the production of spontaneous mammary-gland tumors in strain C3H female mice. *JNCI,* 3:449, 1943.

Widdowson, E.M., and Kennedy, G.C.: Rate of growth, mature weight and life span. *Proc R Soc Lond,* Series B, 156:96, 1962.

Will, L.C., and McCay, C.M.: Ageing, basal metabolism, and retarded growth. *Arch Biochem,* 2:481, 1943.

Willen, R., and Naftolin, F.: Pubertal food intake and body length, weight, and composition in the feed-restricted female rat: comparison with well fed animals. *Pediatr Res,* 12:263, 1978.

Williams, J.R., Spencer, P.S., Stahl, S.M., Borzelleca, J.F., Nichols, W., Pfitzer, E., Yunis, E.J., Carchman, R., Opishinski, J.W., and Walford, R.L.: Interaction of aging and environmental agents: the toxicological perspective. In Baker, S.R., and Rogul, M. (Eds.): *Environmental Toxicity and the Aging Process.* New York, Alan R. Liss, 1987, pp. 81-135.

Williams, V.J., and Senior, W.: The effects of coprophagy in the adult rat on rate of passage of digesta and on digestibility of food fed ad libitum and in restricted amounts. *J Nutr,* 115:1147, 1985.

Wilson, P.D.: Enzyme levels in animals of various ages. In Florini, J.R. (Ed.): *CRC Handbook of Biochemistry in Aging.* Boca Raton, CRC Press, 1981, pp. 163-194.

Wimpfheimer, C., Saville, E., Voirul, M.J., Danforth, E., Jr., and Burger, A.G.: Starvation-induced decreased sensitivity of resting metabolic rate to triiodothyronine. *Science,* 205:1272, 1979.

Wise, P.H.: Significance of anomalous thermoregulation in the pre-diabetic spiny mouse (*Acomys cahirinus*): oxygen consumption and temperature regulation. *Aust J Exp Biol Med Sci,* 55:463, 1977a.

Wise, P.H.: Significance of anomalous thermoregulation in the pre-diabetic spiny mouse (*Acomys cahirinus*): blood glucose and food consumption responses to environmental heat. *Aust J Exp Biol Med Sci,* 55:475, 1977b.

Wohaieb, S.A., and Godin, D.V.: Starvation-related alterations in free radical tissue defense mechanisms in rats. *Diabetes,* 36:169, 1987.

Wolin, M.S., and Burke, T.M.: Hydrogen peroxide elicits activation of bovine pulmonary arterial soluble guanylate cyclase by a mechanism associated with its metabolism by catalase. *Biochem Biophys Res Commun,* 143:20, 1987.

Woodhead, A.D., Merry, B.J., Cao, E., Holehan, A.M., Grist, E., and Carlson, C.: Levels of O^6-methylguanine acceptor protein in tissues of rats and their relationship to carcinogenicity and aging. *JNCI,* 75:1141, 1985.

Wostmann, B.S., Johnson, M., and Snyder, D.L.: The germfree rat in aging studies. *Gerontologist,* 26:154A, 1986.

Wright, B.E., and Davison, P.F.: Guest editorial: mechanisms of development and aging. *Mech Ageing Dev, 12*:213, 1980.

Wulf, J.H., and Cutler, R.G.: Altered protein hypothesis of mammalian ageing processes. I. Thermal stability of glucose-6-phosphate dehydrogenase in C57BL/6J mouse tissue. *Exp Gerontol, 10*:101, 1975.

Wyndham, J.R., Everitt, A.V., and Everitt, S.F.: Effects of isolation and food restriction begun at 50 days on the development of age-associated renal disease in the male Wistar rat. *Arch Gerontol Geriatr, 2*:317, 1983.

Yates, F.E.: *Self-Organizing Systems. The Emergence of Order.* New York, Plenum Press, 1987.

Yielding, K.L.: A model for aging based on differential repair of somatic mutational damage. *Perspect Biol Med, 17*:201, 1974.

Yonei, S., Yokota, R., and Sato, Y.: The distinct role of catalase and DNA repair systems in protection against hydrogen peroxide in *Esherichia coli. Biochem Biophys Res Commun, 143*:638, 1987.

Young, V.R.: Diet as a modulator of aging and longevity. *Fed Proc, 38*:1994, 1979.

Young, V.R., and Schrimshaw, W.S.: The physiology of starvation. *Sci Am, 225*:14, 1971.

Youngman, R.J.: Oxygen activation: is the hydroxyl radical always biologically relevant? In Hall, J. (Ed.): *TIBS,* Vol. 9. Amsterdam, Elsevier, 1984, p. 280-283.

Yu, B.P., Bertrand, H.A., and Masoro, E.J.: Nutrition-aging influence of catecholamine-promoted lipolysis. *Metabolism, 29*:438, 1980.

Yu, B.P., Masoro, E.J., Murata, I., Bertrand, H.A., and Lynd, F.T.: Life span study of SPF Fischer 344 male rats fed ad libitum or restricted diets: Longevity, growth, lean body mass and disease. *J Gerontol, 37*:130, 1982.

Yu, B.P., Wong, G., Lee, H., Bertrand, H., and Masoro, E.J.: Age changes in hepatic metabolic characteristics and their modulation by dietary manipulation. *Mech Ageing Dev, 24*:67, 1984a.

Yu, B.P., Maeda, H., Murata, I., and Masoro, E.J.: Nutritional modulation of longevity and age-related disease. *Fed Proc, 43*:858, 1984b.

Yu, B.P., Masoro, E.J., and McMahan, C.A.: Nutritional influences on aging of Fischer 344 rats: I. Physical, metabolic and longevity characteristics. *J Gerontol, 40*:657, 1985.

Yunis, E.J., Watson, A.L., Gelman, R.S., Sylia, S.J., Vronson, R., and Dorf, M.E.: Traits that influence longevity in mice. *Genetics, 108*:999, 1984.

Zamenhof, S., and van Marthens, E.: Effects of prenatal and chronic undernutrition on aging and survival in rats. *J Nutr, 112*:972, 1982.

Zammuto, R.M., and Millar, J.S.: Environmental predictability, variability, and *Spermophilus columbianus* life history over an elevational gradient. *ECOL, 66*:1784, 1985.

Zannie, E., Calloway, D.H., and Zezulka, A.Y.: Protein requirements of elderly men. *J Nutr, 109*:513, 1979.

Zglinicki, T. von: A mitochondrial membrane hypothesis of aging. *J Theor Biol, 127*:1987.

Zglinicki, T. von, and Bimmler, M.: Intracellular water and ionic shifts during growth and ageing of rats. *Mech Ageing Dev, 38*:179, 1987.

Zimmerman, J., Kaufmann, N., Fainaru, M., Eisenberg, S., Oschray, Y., Friedlander, Y., and Stein, Y.: Effect of weight loss in moderate obesity on plasma lipoproten and apolipoprotein levels and on high-density lipoprotein composition. *Arteriosclerosis, 4*:115, 1984.

Zoler, M.: Diet restriction: new clues to slow the aging process. *Geriatrics, 39*:130, 1984.

Zongza, V., and Mathias, A.P.: The variation with age of the structure of chromatin in three cell types from rat liver. *Biochem J, 179*:291, 1979.

Zuniga-Guajardo, S., Garfinkel, P.E., and Zinman, B.: Change in insulin sensitivity and clearance in anorexia nervosa. *Metabolism, 35*:1096, 1987.

ABBREVIATIONS

↑,	increased
↓,	decreased
<——>,	no change
ACTH,	Adrenocorticotropin Hormone
ADP,	Adenosine Diphosphate
ADR,	Adult-onset Dietary Restriction
AIN,	American Institute of Nutrition
ATP,	Adenosine Triphosphate
B6,	C57BL/6 mice
BMI,	Body Mass Index
BMR,	Basal Metabolic Rate
BW,	Body Weight
B/WF$_1$,	(NZB × NZW)F$_1$ mice
ConA,	Concanavalin A
CPM,	Counts Per Minute
CRF,	Corticotropin Releasing Factor
DHEA,	Dehydroepiandrosterone
DMBA,	7,12-dimethylbenz[a]anthracene
DNP,	Dinitrophenol
DR,	Dietary Restriction
EDR,	Early-onset Dietary Restriction
EF-1,	Elongation Factor-1
EOD,	Every-Other-Day (feeding regimen)
FASEB,	Federation of American Societies for Experimental Biology
FSH,	Follicle-Stimulating Hormone
GH,	Growth Hormone
GH-RF,	Growth Hormone Releasing Factor
Hx,	Hypophysectomy (Hxed, Hypophysectomized)

IL-2,	Interleukin 2
LEI,	Lifetime Energy Intake
LH,	Leutinizing Hormone
LHRH,	Leutinizing Hormone Releasing Hormone
LOMO,	Lateral Omohyoideus Muscle
LS,	Life Span (LSs, Life Spans)
MAM,	Methylazoxymethanol Acetate
MBW,	Metabolic Body Weight
MDA,	Malondialdehyde
MHC,	Major Histocompatibility Complex
MNU,	N-methylnitrosourea
NAD,	Nicotinamide Adenine Dinucleotide
NADPH,	Nicotinamide Adenine Dinucleotide Phosphate-reduced
NIA,	National Institute on Aging
NK,	Natural Killer cell
NPD,	Non-Purified Diet
NR,	Not Reported
O_2^-,	Superoxide radical
PD,	Purified Diet
PFC,	Plaque-Forming Cell
PHA,	Phytohemagglutinin
Poly I:C,	Polyinosinic:Polycytidylic acid
PTH,	Parathyroid Hormone
RCI,	Respiratory Control Index
RDA,	Recommended Dietary Allowance
RF,	Releasing Factor
RH,	Releasing Hormone
SOD,	Superoxide Dismutase
SRBC,	Sheep Red Blood Cells
T−,	Tryptophan-deficient
T+,	Not Tryptophan-deficient
T_3,	3,5,3'-Triiodothyronine
T_4,	3,5,3',5'-Tetraiodothyronine (thyroxine)
TRH,	Thyrotropin (TSH)-Releasing Hormone
TSH,	Thyroid-Stimulating Hormone (thyrotropin)
TBA,	Thiobarbituric Acid
UDS,	Unscheduled DNA Synthesis

AUTHOR INDEX

A

Abbott, B. J., 107, 356
Abe, H., 331, 355
Adam, M., 119, 350, 388
Adams, D. A., 196, 352
Adams, M., 9, 10, 351
Adams, S., 62, 67, 152, 214, 362
Adelman, R. C., 120, 264, 339, 340, 349, 358
Adorini, L., 19, 281, 348
Ahmed, S. A., 255, 371
Ainley, C. C., 308, 346
Aiyar, A. S., 122, 126, 176, 177, 347, 350
Akikawa, K., 143, 373
Aksoy, M., 109, 112, 343
Albanes, D., 76, 103, 305, 326, 328, 339
Alberts, B., 241, 339
Alfin-Slater, R., 341
Algeri, S., 379
Ali, B., 367
Allen, 232, 260
Allen, R. G., 340, 387
Alonso, D. R., 67, 89, 175, 284, 353, 372
Ames, B. N., 233, 258, 270, 375, 384
Amy, R. M., 84, 383
An, L. C., 246, 343
Andersen, A. E., 307, 391
Anderson, C. F., 304, 308, 357
Anderson, C. P., 282, 369
Anderson, M., 268, 358
Anderson, W., 150, 392
Anderson, W. R., 150, 343
Andersson, H., 327, 369
Andervont, H. J., 85, 86, 395
Andreou, K. K., 101, 286, 339
Andres, R., 306, 309, 310, 333, 334, 339, 348, 382

Ans, R., 307, 393
Aoki, T. T., 307, 313, 345
Apfelbaum, M., 312, 318, 321, 339
Appleton, Carol, ix
Arai, K., 268, 339
Archer, J. R., 7, 16, 17, 24, 29, 58, 59, 119, 181, 214, 226, 249, 274, 275, 276, 360
Armario, A., 146, 147, 148, 339
Armstrong, D., 349, 394
Armstrong-Major, J., 267, 346
Arshavsky, I. A., 263, 340
Ascaso, J., 304, 346
Aschheim, P., 274, 276, 277, 340
Asdell, S. A., 45, 224, 340
Assenmacher, I., 149, 344
Astle, C. M., 181, 274, 275, 276, 281, 310, 317, 360
Atkinson, R. L., 327, 340
Au, B., 181
Austad, S. N., 8, 14, 15, 39, 340
Ayers, J. W. T., 303, 307, 340
Aylsworth, C. F., 109, 112, 114, 388
Azizi, F., 359
Azzi, A., 245, 371

B

Bacon, J. A., 321, 323, 351, 394
Bada, J. L., 18, 361
Bafitis, H., 29, 340
Bailey, C. J., 107, 354
Bailey, P. J., 264, 340
Bailey, R., 340
Baird, M. B., 247, 256, 257, 340
Baker, P. Y., 5, 8, 9, 343
Baker, S. R., 395
Balazs, E. A., 118, 340
Baldwin, R. L., 137, 363

Bales, C. W., 52, 54, 62, 64, 66, 84, 221, 341, 342, 350
Balin, A. K., 4, 260, 340
Balinsky, D., 282, 393
Ball, S. S., ix, 24, 86, 173, 340
Ball, Z. B., 58, 85, 86, 137, 225, 278, 340, 363, 391
Bandurski, M. J., 209, 381
Banta, A. M., 8, 32, 37, 363
Barcome, D. R., 366
Barnard, D. L., 52, 273, 276, 352
Barnes, L. L., 52, 224, 373
Barnes, R. H., 58, 85, 86, 225, 278, 340, 391
Barnett, E. V., 4, 197, 341, 394
Barr, E. M., 242, 370
Barrett-Connor, E., 279, 334, 341
Barron, G. P., 5, 8, 9, 355
Barrows, C. H., 9, 10, 36, 62, 63, 161, 172, 228, 265, 269, 333, 334, 341, 367, 376
Barrows, C. H., Jr., 8, 43, 44, 58, 95, 123, 124, 125, 126, 211, 232, 246, 260, 261, 341, 353, 365, 370
Barrows, K., 307, 308, 313, 341
Basta, S., 366, 377, 392
Bassani, B., 19, 281, 348
Bassett, E. G., 369
Bates, P. C., 172, 345
Batory, G., 19, 341
Battistin, L., 247, 384
Baumann, C. A., 103, 383
Baxter, J. D., 147, 387
Beach, R. S., 97, 99, 107, 341
Bearn, A. G., 384
Beatty, W. W., 228, 341
Beauchene, R. E., 52, 54, 62, 64, 66, 84, 221, 226, 341, 342, 350, 391
Bechtel, P. J., 272, 366
Beers, R. F., Jr., 369
Behnke, J. A., 349, 381
Bell, R. G., 38, 182, 342, 366
Bellamy, D., 9, 180, 342, 354
Bender, A. E., 202, 366
Benedict, F. G., 202, 320, 321, 342, 362
Bengtsson, C., 327, 369
Benirschke, A. K., 358
Bennett, W., 311, 342
Berg, B. N., 33, 48, 52, 53, 77, 79, 224, 231, 342
Berger, M. R., 109, 112, 343
Bergsma, D., 372

Berke, L. K., 327, 340
Berkman, J. M., 308, 346
Berkowitz, E. M., 267, 342
Berman, E., 107, 352
Berry, M. N., 13, 250, 342
Berry, R. J., 13, 342
Bertrand, M. A., 16, 32, 33, 34, 35, 43, 52, 69, 70, 71, 77, 124, 150, 151, 152, 155, 174, 175, 198, 214, 216, 218, 219, 220, 231, 249, 342, 343, 370, 373, 396
Besdine, R. W., 393
Beth, M., 109, 112, 343
Beyer, R. E., 217, 246, 343
Bewley, G. C., 259, 385
Bhargava, S., 160, 161, 387
Bhuyan, D. K., 259, 343
Bhuyan, K. C., 259, 343
Bickel, H., 144, 147, 343
Bierley, R. A., 228, 341
Bierman, E. L., 348
Bilder, G. E., 274, 343
Bimmler, M., 242, 396
Binkley, F., 136, 364
Birch, R., 321, 394
Birchenall-Sparks, M. C., 171, 264, 343, 380
Birren, J. E., 364
Birt, D. F., 5, 8, 9, 343
Bischoff, F., 102, 343
Bishop, K. S., 45, 223, 352
Bittles, A. H., 344, 374
Bjorlslund, A., 272, 354
Blackburn, G. L., 340, 346, 356, 361, 363, 369, 378, 386, 390, 394
Blackett, A. D., 9, 10, 343, 347, 349, 374, 387
Blatt, L., 228, 363
Blank, J. L., 47, 343
Bliznakov, E. G., 246, 343
Blom, A. K., 144, 147, 343
Blonska, B., 48, 349
Blum, J. W., 144, 147, 343
Boersma, W. J. A., 185, 343
Bohr, Niels, 329
Boissonneault, G. A., 109, 110, 111, 112, 255, 326, 343
Bok, D., 170, 259, 370
Boland, S. R., 155, 366
Bolla, R. I., 344
Boon, M. C., 58, 86, 384
Borek, C., 339, 372

Borkan, G. A., 19, 29, 305, 310, 327, 333, 334, 344
Borzelleca, J. F., 14, 33, 35, 45, 89, 395
Bosaeus, I., 327, 369
Bostarron, J., 312, 339
Bosze, Z., 376
Bouillaud, F., 244, 380
Bouille, C., 149, 344
Bouliere, F., 334, 344
Bourges, H., 366, 377, 392
Boutwell, R. K., 103, 184, 344
Boveris, A., 245, 345
Bowers, T. K., 303, 304, 308, 344
Bowles, N. D., 10, 74, 75, 347, 348
Boyd, E. M., 44, 344
Boyle, P. C., 202, 254, 344
Bracco, F., 247, 384
Bradford, G. E., 70, 351
Bradish, Helga, ix
Bradley, P. J., 318, 344
Brafield, A. E., 249, 344
Bragg, C. S., 52, 62, 64, 66, 221, 342
Brand, M. D., 239, 253, 344
Bras, G., 23, 49, 52, 54, 55, 70, 77, 80, 81, 82, 84, 249, 290, 325, 381, 382
Brasseur, R., 160, 161, 387
Braverman, L. E., 359
Bray, D., 241, 339
Bray, G. A., 252, 266, 340, 344, 346, 356, 361, 363, 369, 378, 386, 390
Brazeau, P., 389
Brdiczka, D., 244, 366
Brennan, M. J., 228, 344
Brett, B. E., 324, 385
Brief, S., 272, 366
Briggs, C. J., 282, 393
Briggs, G. M., 40, 358
Brind, J. L., 334, 377
Brody, J. A., 5, 329, 344, 384, 394
Bronson, F. H., 46, 47, 141, 344, 358, 386
Brown, D. D., 285, 375
Brown, G. M., 307, 345
Brown, J. G., 172, 345, 356
Brownlee, M., 267, 268, 346
Brozek, J., 76, 209, 304, 308, 312, 313, 320, 321, 366
Brubacher, G. B., 322, 372
Bruce, R. A., 18, 333, 345
Bruice, T. W., ix
Brush, M. K., 103, 184, 344

Bryan, J. E., 214, 355
Buck, C. L., 104, 108, 109, 367, 368
Buckley, C. E., 358
Bullough, W. S., 287, 345
Burch, R. E., 43, 345
Burger, A. G., 307, 308, 377, 395
Burgess, J. A., 77, 342, 350, 352, 355
Burke, T. M., 259, 395
Burman, K. D., 145, 146, 307, 345, 356, 376
Burnet, F. M., 282, 345
Burnett, B., 246, 343
Burns, E. M., 242, 345
Buschmann, M. T., 345
Butler, J. A., 126, 166, 269, 270, 380
Butler, R. N., 21, 358, 378, 379, 382, 384, 386, 392, 393
Butler, W. H., 356
Bybee, D. E., 146, 307, 376

C

Cadenas, E., 245, 345
Cahill, G. F., 307, 313, 345
Calder, W. A., 251, 370
Calloway, D. H., 307, 319, 321, 345, 355, 396
Calvano, S., 187, 188, 365
Campbell, B. A., 228, 345
Campbell, G. A., 142, 146, 147, 275, 307, 345
Campbell, H. L., 68, 386
Cancilla, P. A., ix
Canolty, N. L., 114, 190, 327, 352, 368
Cantoni, O., 134, 286, 345
Cao, E., 395
Carafoli, E., 243, 250, 345, 377
Carchman, R., 14, 33, 35, 45, 395
Carlisle, H. J., 261, 351
Carlson, A. J., 52, 53, 68, 76, 77, 345
Carlson, C., 395
Carlson, H. E., 307, 346
Carlson, J. C., 37, 384
Carman, J. M., 328, 346
Carmena, R., 304, 346
Carr, C. J., 13, 346
Carryer, H. M., 308, 346
Cartwright, K. J., 246, 343
Cary, S., 175, 390
Casey, M. L., 255, 371
Cason, J., 308, 346

Casper, R. C., 303, 307, 308, 346
Castaneda, M., 391
Castelli, W. P., 309, 310, 346, 363
Casteneda, 266
Castro, C. E., 242, 267, 346
Castro, F., 359
Cavanaugh, L. M., 77, 273, 352
Cawthorne, M. A., 262, 318, 346
Cerami, A., 267, 268, 306, 346, 375
Cerutti, P. A., 246, 346
Chabanny, V. N., 267, 366
Chabot, R. K., 334, 377
Chandler, L. J., 242, 370
Chandra, R. K., 181, 346, 361
Chang, M., 272, 283, 371
Chapman, M. L., 284, 390
Chase, A. R., 155, 211, 212, 261, 391
Chavez, A., 366, 377, 392
Chebotarev, D. F., 308, 340, 346
Chen, J. C., 242, 346
Cheney, K. E., ix, 4, 8, 9, 35, 58, 64, 66, 90, 91, 92, 93, 97, 101, 132, 178, 180, 187, 188, 189, 190, 191, 211, 233, 261, 268, 308, 341, 356, 392, 394
Cheng, H., 214, 355
Cherkin, A., 12, 13, 346
Chernoff, R., 310, 346
Chesky, J., 295, 300, 336, 346
Chesterman, F. C., 74, 75, 382
Cheung, H. T., 171, 192, 197, 233, 264, 286, 347, 377, 380, 387
Cheung, M. K., ix, 122, 204, 205, 206, 207, 394
Chia, D., 4, 197, 341, 394
Chiang, W., 166, 269, 380
Chipalkatti, S., 122, 126, 176, 177, 347, 350
Chitpativra, S. T., 308, 363
Chiu, Y. I. D., 242, 347
Chopra, I. J., 307, 346
Chowers, I., 347
Christadoss, P., 196, 347
Christman, M. F., 286, 375
Chvapil, M., 118, 119, 347
Cider, N. L., 8, 43, 44, 52, 58, 59, 62, 67, 69, 228, 357
Clapp, N. K., 10, 347
Clark, A., 391
Clark, D. G., 250, 342
Clarke, J., 332, 347
Cleary, M. P., 86, 123, 124, 125, 153, 347, 355, 365
Clemens, M., 267, 347
Clouse, B. A., 228, 341
Cockerham, R., 156, 158, 215, 221, 222, 223, 226, 303, 325, 365
Cohen, H. J., 284, 390
Cohen, L. A., 109, 110, 281, 283, 284, 326, 347
Cohen, N., 348
Cohn, C., 153, 347
Cole, C., 373
Cole, E., 389
Cole, G. M., 159, 273, 347
Coleman, D. L., 255, 263, 347
Coleoni, A. H., 145, 350
Collins, K. J., 344, 374
Comerford, L. E., 345
Comfort, A., 8, 10, 32, 36, 39, 301, 314, 333, 347, 348
Comptom, C., 150, 151, 373
Compton, C., 373
Compton, R. E., III, 217, 343
Conard, A., 29, 332, 333, 348
Cook, D. E., 10, 361
Cook, K. S., 250, 354
Conybeare, G., 89, 348
Cooper, B., 150, 282, 348
Cooper, E. L., 348
Cooper, W. C., 188, 308, 348, 357
Copeland, D. H., 108, 352
Corbett, S. W., 4, 202, 348
Cornet, A., 48, 350
Corraze, G. R., 176, 348
Corso, J. F., 334, 348
Cosgrove, G. E., 74, 75, 348
Costa, P. T., Jr., 29, 331, 332, 348
Costello, L. C., 136, 209, 356
Cottrell, S. F., 242, 354
Cotzias, G. C., 9, 10, 348
Courtois, Y., 265, 390
Cousin, F., 322, 372
Covelli, V., 19, 281, 348
Cox, G. B., 244, 348
Cox, M. D., 146, 307, 348
Craig, B. W., 153, 214, 349, 355
Cramer, F., 264, 266, 355
Crandall, D., 152, 233, 350
Crane, D., 373
Crapo, L. M., 314, 355
Crew, M. D., 268, 269, 349

Cristofalo, V. J., 288, 349, 393
Crosby, L. O., 303, 304, 308, 377
Crowell, M. F., 8, 15, 45, 47, 52, 53, 224, 231, 340, 373
Csukas, S., 259, 349
Curfman, G. D., 308, 349
Curry, D., 154, 233, 268, 307, 379
Curtis, H. J., 264, 349
Curtis, M. R., 108, 351
Cutler, Richard G., 8, 13, 22, 23, 27, 137, 247, 248, 269, 270, 314, 349, 383, 389, 394, 396
Czaplicki, J., 48, 349

D

Dadufalza, V., 287, 362
Dalal, S. S., 146, 307, 348
Dalderup, L. M., 8, 9, 349
Danford, 249
Danforth, E., Jr., 308, 386, 395
Danielli, J. F., 36, 375
Dao, M. L., 121, 129, 166, 368, 380, 386
Darby, W. J., 296, 349
Das, S. K., 122, 123, 124, 125, 175, 178, 285, 383
Dauncey, M. J., 250, 349
David, J., 38, 350
Davidson, J. K., 327, 350
Davis, J., ix
Davis, J. M., 307, 346
Davis, L. J., 24, 26, 167, 270, 370
Davis, M. L., 367
Davis, T. A., 5, 52, 54, 62, 64, 66, 84, 221, 342, 350
Davison, P. F., 289, 290, 396
Day, N. K., 68, 99, 328, 368, 383
De, A. K., 122, 126, 176, 177, 347, 350
Deamer, D., 10, 389
Dean, W., 333, 350
Deerberg, F., 58, 59, 89, 90, 91, 264, 266, 355, 379, 380
DeFronzo, R. A., 334, 350
DeGroot, L. J., 145, 350
Dell'Orco, R. T., 267, 350
De Moor, P., 279, 361
Denckla, W. D., 273, 274, 343, 344, 350
Deneke, S. M., 136, 350
Deshmukh, D. R., 242, 350
Desjardins, C., 47, 343

Deutsch, S., 69, 214, 370
Devens, B. H., ix, 22, 187, 188, 194, 195, 286, 394
Dewasmes, G., 48, 350
Deyl, Z., 62, 64, 119, 350, 388
Diamond, J. M., 328, 382
Dickie, M. M., 59, 369
Dickson, I., 268, 358
Dierksen, D., 58, 59, 89, 90, 379
DiGirolamo, E., 202, 254, 361
DiGirolamo, M., 152, 233, 350
Dilman, V. M., 141, 272, 273, 350
Di Majo, V., 19, 281, 348
Dimond, R. C., 307, 345
Dixon, F. J., 88, 283, 364
Doberne, L., 306, 381
Dolkas, C. B., 154, 374
Donato, K., 255, 350
Doorn, J. V., 350
Dorf, M. E., 270, 396
Dorfman, F., 102, 354
Doria, G., 19, 281, 348
Dorsey, B. A., 189, 388
Drenick, E. J., 307, 346
Dreyfuss, Y., 107, 113, 358
Drori, D., 9, 52, 77, 82, 351
Duara, R., 272, 351
Dubina, T. L., 321, 368
Dubos, R., 318, 351
Dubuc, P. U., 261, 351
Dulloo, A. G., 323, 364
Duncan, K. H., 323, 351
Dunham, H. H., 38, 351
Dunning, W. F., 108, 351
Durand, A. M., 9, 10, 351
Durnin, J. V. G. A., 318, 351
Dutta, P., 170, 351
Dyrenfurth, R. I., 307, 393
Dyundikova, V. A., 321, 368

E

Earot, L., 303, 304, 308, 377
Eaton, J. W., 258, 385
Ebling, F. J., 287, 345
Eckels, D. D., 190, 352
Eckert, E., 303, 304, 308, 344
Economos, A. C., 242, 354
Edelman, R., 357
Edholm, O. G., 318, 351

Edington, D. W., 217, 246, 343
Edmundson, W., 318, 319, 320, 351
Effros, R. B., ix
Egan, J. W., 303, 325, 365
Ehrlich, Paul, 330
Eicher, M., 29, 332, 333, 348
Einat, R., 347
Einhorn, D., 308, 351
Einstein, Albert, 329
Eisdorfer, C., 383, 393
Eisen, E. J., 215, 351
Eisen, H. J., 285, 375
Eisenberg, S., 304, 397
Eklund, J., 70, 351
Elashoff, R. M., 9, 371
El Haj, A. J., 164, 166, 308, 351, 357
Ellefson, D., 285, 367
Elliott, J. G., 324, 385
Elliott, R. F., 110, 354
Ellis, A. T., 121, 122, 135, 157, 371
Ellis, F. R., 325, 351
Ellis, J. W., 325, 351
Else, P. L., 237, 238, 351
Elson, C. E., 109, 110, 111, 112, 255, 326, 343
Elvehjem, C. A., 52, 380
Enesco, H. E., 176, 351
Engel, R. W., 108, 352
Engelhardt, R., 264, 266, 355
Epelbaum, J., 389
Erickson, K. L., 190, 196, 352, 390
Ershler, W. B., 107, 352
Evans, H. M., 34, 223, 352
Everitt, A. V., 9, 16, 52, 54, 68, 77, 81, 82, 118, 119, 137, 226, 273, 275, 276, 288, 342, 350, 352, 355, 356, 376, 396
Everitt, S. F., 52, 77, 226, 396

F

Facchini, A., 370
Fachet, J., 376
Fabris, N., 280, 282, 352, 393
Failla, G., 264, 353
Fainaru, M., 304, 397
Falzon, M. J., 246, 343
Fanburg, B. L., 136, 350
Fanestil, D. D., 8, 36, 260, 341, 353
Fang, S. L., 359
Fattoretti, P., 282, 378

Farrar, R. P., 242, 370
Feinleib, M., 309, 363
Feinstein, R. N., 259, 353
Feldhoff, R. C., 308, 363
Feldman, D. B., 8, 9, 353
Feldman, J. D., 74, 75, 353
Feldman, S., 347
Felicio, L. S., 211, 235, 276, 354, 375
Felig, P., 307, 334, 350, 384
Feinleib, M., 348
Fenoglio, C. M., 339, 372
Ferguson, S. J., 244, 353
Ferland, G., 226, 390
Fernandes, Gabriel, 8, 16, 55, 58, 67, 78, 86, 87, 89, 99, 166, 179, 186, 187, 188, 196, 197, 233, 269, 270, 283, 284, 307, 317, 340, 347, 353, 355, 357, 364, 365, 366, 372, 380, 383, 384
Ferrannini, E., 334, 350
Ferry, E. L., 8, 49, 377
Fimmel, A. L., 244, 348
Finch, Caleb E., 18, 159, 225, 273, 276, 277, 278, 279, 280, 282, 333, 340, 349, 351, 353, 354, 360, 369, 372, 379, 381, 383, 384, 385, 390
Fineberg, E. S., 307, 373
Fischer, W., 33, 272, 354
Fischer-Piette, E., 39, 354
Fisher, M., 9, 10, 351
Fishman, E. L., 372
Fisler, J. S., 252, 266, 344
Fitch, K. L., 226, 288, 375
Flatmark, T., 256, 355
Flatt, P. R., 107, 354
Fleming, B. B., 324, 354
Fleming J. E., 242, 354, 374
Fletcher, B., 10, 389
Flier, J. S., 250, 306, 354, 382
Fligiel, S., ix, 10, 11, 12, 15, 23, 46, 60, 71, 179, 180, 187, 188, 191, 192, 199, 200, 201, 231, 233, 249, 287, 317, 394
Flohe, L., 245, 371
Flory, C. M., 102, 354
Floyd, R. A., 359
Flynn, M. A., 170, 351
Fogerty, A. C., 10, 362
Folman, Y., 9, 52, 77, 82, 351
Fong, T. C., 272, 283, 371
Forbes, E. B., 110, 354
Forman, L. J., 274, 280, 387

Forsberg, S., 18, 29, 333, 388
Forsum, E., 202, 354
Foster, C., 102, 354
Fouillet, P., 38, 350
Foy, J., 286, 365
Francisco, A., 287, 361
Franklin, A., 180, 354
Franks, L. M., 88, 382
Freedman, M. L., 242, 372
Freeman, J. R., 8, 43, 44, 52, 58, 59, 62, 67, 69, 228, 357, 364
Freidrichs, W., 270, 366
French, C. E., 5, 8, 9, 355
Fridovich, I., 246, 257, 355
Fried, S. K., 152, 233, 350
Friedlander, Y., 304, 397
Friedrichs, B., 197, 353
Friend, P. S., 67, 78, 99, 328, 355
Fries, J. F., 314, 355
Frisch, R. E., 325, 355
Friesen, H. G., 143, 367
Frohman, L. A., 344
Frolkis, V. V., 263, 273, 308, 346, 355
Fry, R. J. M., 259, 353
Fujita, Y., 84, 168, 169, 170, 202, 355, 363
Fukami, M. H., 256, 355
Fukui, S., 331, 355
Fukuyama, T., 5, 8, 9, 375
Furth, J., 58, 86, 102, 354, 384
Furukawa, T., 331, 355

G

Gabius, H., 264, 266, 355
Gaddy, J. R., 228, 345
Gaetani, G. F., 135, 257, 366
Gage, F. H., 272, 354
Gajjar, A., 8, 10, 16, 59, 232, 328, 355, 357, 364, 368
Galiano, S., 135, 257, 366
Gallo, P. V., 148, 355
Gallop, P. M., 268, 358
Ganguli, P. K., 160, 161, 387
Gansler, T. S., 355
Garaci, E., 393
Garbus, J., 242, 393
Garfinkel, P. E., 307, 345, 397
Garrel, D. R., 307, 355
Garrod, J., 175, 390
Garrow, J. S., 266, 308, 312, 355

Garthwaite, S. M., 153, 214, 349, 355
Garsko, G. G., 321, 368
Gatti, R., 257, 289, 290, 393
Gee, P., 233, 270, 384
Geissler, C. A., 312, 321, 356
Gellatly, J. B. M., 88, 356
Geller, P. J., 372
Gelman, R. S., 270, 396
Gentile, S., 282, 378
Genuth, S. M., 304, 308, 356
Georges, L. P., 146, 307, 376
Georghegan, T. E., 308, 363
Gerbase-Delima, Maria, ix, 16, 58, 132, 189, 190, 265, 356, 392
Gershon, S., 379
Gershwin, M. E., 87, 97, 99, 107, 190, 341, 352, 392
Gerstenblith, G., 333, 356
Ghanta, U. K., 26, 361
Gibson, F., 244, 348
Gibson, G. E., 279, 356
Gibwani, G. P., 303, 307, 340
Gilbert, C., 52, 77, 79, 356
Gilbertson, V. A., 358
Giles, J. S., 119, 356
Gillman, J., 52, 77, 79, 356
Giovanella, B. C., 107, 356
Giovannetti, P. M., 44, 356
Glass, A. R., 45, 47, 146, 307, 356
Gleeson, M., 356
Gleiser, C. A., 9, 10, 74, 75, 77, 95, 232, 364, 371
Godin, D. V., 136, 395
Goidl, E. A., 281, 353, 356, 361, 385, 390
Gold, A. J., 136, 209, 356
Goldberg, J., 324, 373
Goldspink, D. F., 164, 165, 166, 173, 265, 308, 351, 356, 357, 370, 374
Goldstein, Allan L., 26, 33, 35, 181, 182, 283, 334, 357, 394
Golla, J. A., 304, 308, 357
Gompertz, 33, 34, 35
Good, Robert A., 8, 10, 16, 55, 58, 59, 67, 68, 78, 86, 87, 88, 89, 97, 99, 121, 129, 166, 179, 186, 187, 188, 196, 232, 233, 282, 283, 284, 287, 307, 308, 316, 317, 328, 348, 353, 355, 364, 365, 368, 372, 380, 383, 384, 386
Goodrick, C. L., 8, 43, 44, 52, 58, 59, 62, 67, 69, 228, 357, 364

Gori, G. B., 297, 329, 357, 358
Gosden, R. G., 211, 235, 375
Gosnell, B. A., 255, 358
Goswami, T., 160, 161, 387
Goto, S., 173, 286, 388
Gottesman, S. R. S., ix, 26, 184, 187, 188, 358, 393, 394
Goya, R., 140, 235, 272, 273, 275, 276, 277, 278, 328, 383, 379
Gracy, R. W., 284, 390
Green, K., 259, 349
Greene, G. C., 371
Greene, L., 155, 211, 212, 261, 391, 392
Greenfield, H., 40, 358
Greenfield, M., 306, 381
Greenstein, J. P., 389
Gregerman, R. I., 150, 273, 275, 348, 358
Grewal, T., 140, 358
Grieshaber, C. K., 248, 362
Griffith, G. C., 372
Grigorov, Iu. G., 308, 346
Grimm, V. E., 379
Grist, E., 395
Grivell, A. R., 250, 342
Grootveld, M., 246, 358
Groscolas, R., 48, 350
Gross, J., 107, 113, 118, 358
Gross, L., 358
Gross, M., 303, 307, 340
Grossman, C. J., 235, 358
Gruenspecht-Faham, N., 242, 372
Gu, M., 166, 269, 380
Gulko, V. V., 321, 368
Gundberg, C. M., 268, 358
Gunter, K. K., 244, 364
Gunter T. E., 244, 245, 358, 364
Guppy, M., 238, 251, 252, 362
Guthrie, D., ix, 10, 11, 12, 15, 23, 46, 60, 90, 92, 94, 179, 180, 187, 188, 191, 192, 199, 200, 201, 231, 233, 249, 287, 317, 394
Guyda, H. J., 389
Gwynne, J. T., 304, 306, 307, 363
Gyenes, L., 160, 161, 387
Gyodi, E., 19, 341

H

Haaijman, J. J., 185, 343, 352, 370
Hadden, J., 352, 393

Haddow, A., 389
Hadley, Evan, ix
Hahn, H. K. J., 43, 345
Haining, J. L., 247, 257, 358
Halberg, F., 55, 58, 59, 211, 212, 261, 375
Hall, D. A., 343
Hall, K. Y., 9, 10, 257, 265, 289, 290, 358, 393
Hall, N., 334, 357
Halleman, Susan, ix
Hallgren, H. M., 334, 358
Halliwell, B., 358
Hamilton, G. D., 47, 358
Hanawalt, P., 265, 271, 358
Handler, P., 143, 144, 253, 386
Hansen, E. S., 369
Hansen, M. A., 188, 357
Hansen, P. J., 47, 320, 359
Hansen-Smith, F. M., 48, 218, 359
Hansford, R. G., 241, 242, 359
Hanson, L. A., 357
Haps, H. D., 140, 358
Hara, I., 88, 283, 364
Hard, G. C., 10, 255, 376, 377
Harden, K. K., 300, 359
Hardin, R. H., 156, 221, 222, 303, 325, 365
Hardwick, J. P., 171, 343, 380
Harman, D., 9, 10, 24, 232, 241, 242, 243, 246, 340, 341, 359, 365, 374, 376
Harmon, H. J., 242, 359
Harp, J. A., 282, 359
Harper, A. E., 202, 315, 344, 359
Harriman, K. M., 226, 288, 377
Harris, 35
Harris, A. R. C., 359
Harris, Mel, 78
Harris, P. M., 359
Harris, R. B. S., 215, 359
Harris, S., 231, 286, 307, 393
Harris, S. B., ix
Harris, Steve, ix, 49
Harrison, D. E., 7, 16, 17, 24, 29, 55, 58, 59, 118, 119, 181, 187, 188, 193, 214, 226, 249, 274, 275, 276, 281, 310, 317, 360, 372, 374
Harrison, R., 45, 47, 356
Hart, R. W., 21, 22, 261, 264, 358, 360
Harvey, P. H., 13, 360
Hasegawa, L., 282, 285, 367
Hashizume, A., 29, 333, 334, 362

Hashmi, R. F., 125, 360
Hatch, L., 244, 348
Hauser, E. R., 47, 359
Hausman, P. B., 281, 360
Hawcroft, D. M., 285, 360
Hawkins, S. T., 52, 62, 64, 66, 221, 342
Hayashida, M., 83, 360
Hayflick, L., 340, 383
Haynes, S. G., 348
Hazell, L. A., 38, 182, 342
Hazelton, G. A., 248, 361
Hazzard, W. R., 348
Heard, C. R. C., 146, 307, 348
Hegarty, P. V. J., 136, 216, 369, 377
Hegner, D., 242, 246, 258, 376
Hegsted, D. M., 255, 298, 350, 361
Heidrick, M. L., 10, 361
Heikkinen, E., 18, 29, 333, 361, 388
Helfman, P. M., 18, 361
Heilbrun, L. K., 305, 387
Heller, T., 287, 361
Helmholtz, 333
Hendricks, L. C., 10, 361
Hendrikx, A., 279, 361
Henle, W., 102, 354
Hendrix, M. J., 52, 62, 64, 66, 221, 342
Hennekens, C. H., 310, 372
Henry, K. E. R., 226, 361
Henschel, A., 76, 209, 304, 308, 312, 313, 320, 321, 366
Herbener, G. H., 242, 361
Herbst, C., 304, 306, 307, 363
Herbst, E. J., 52, 380
Heresi, G., 181, 346, 361
Herlihy, J. T., 218, 361
Herrera, M. G., 307, 345
Herschman, J. M., 307, 346
Herzog, D. B., 303, 380
Heston, W. E., 86, 87, 103, 369, 395
Heyns, W., 279, 361
Hibbs, A. R., 290, 291, 293
Higgenbotham, S. M., 5, 8, 9, 343
Higuchi, K., 16, 367
Hill, J. O., 152, 202, 233, 254, 350, 361
Hill, R. L., 143, 144, 253, 386
Hillman, P. E., 202, 354
Himms-Hagen, J., 250, 261, 361
Hinshelwood, M. M., 47, 359
Hinsull, S. M., 180, 354
Hiramoto, R. N., 26, 361

Hirokawa, K., 183, 281, 283, 361, 362
Hirsch, J., 327, 364
Hlavackova, 119
Ho, H., 154, 306, 307, 379
Hochachka, P. W., 238, 251, 252, 362
Hochschild, R., 9, 10, 362
Hodanova, M., 10, 369
Hoelzel, F., 52, 53, 68, 76, 77, 345
Hofecker, G., 332, 362, 386
Hoffman, 248, 362
Holeckova, E., 119, 347
Holehan, A. M., 8, 13, 16, 43, 46, 47, 49, 52, 53, 137, 138, 139, 140, 141, 144, 145, 147, 148, 149, 162, 163, 164, 165, 166, 224, 231, 265, 277, 278, 307, 308, 351, 357, 372, 370, 374, 395
Holesh, S., 325, 351
Hollaender, A., 347, 349, 374, 387
Hollander, C. F., 375
Hollander, D., ix, 32, 186, 226, 287, 362
Holliday, M. A., 172, 345
Hollingsworth, J. W., 29, 333, 334, 362
Holloszy, J. O., 9, 53, 62, 67, 152, 153, 214, 231, 349, 355, 362
Holmes, G. E., 38, 362
Holmes, N. R., 38, 362
Holmes, W. N., 374
Holt, P. R., 287, 361
Hooper, A. C. B., 218, 362
Hopkins, B. E., 308, 349
Horn, P. L., 10, 362
Horst, K., 202, 362
Horton, E. S., 314, 363
Horwitz, J., ix, 170, 259, 370
Hosek, B., 287, 368
Hosokawa, M., 16, 367
Houlihan, G., 10, 377
Howard, A. N., 363
Howard, G., 304, 308, 327, 363
Howarth, R. E., 137, 363
Hruza, D. S., 5, 8, 9, 343
Hruza, Z., 347
Hubert, H. B., 309, 334, 363, 365
Hudson, J. W., 209, 210, 363
Hughes, T. A., 304, 306, 307, 363
Hulbert, A. J., 237, 238, 351
Hurley, L., 5, 87, 97, 99, 107, 176, 341, 384, 392
Huseby, R. A., 137, 363
Hutchinson, M. L., 357, 362

Hutson, J. C., 242, 387
Hurrweorh, R. M., 334, 394
Hymer, T. K., 366

I

Ibrahim, N. G., 242, 372
Ichikawa, M., 84, 168, 169, 170, 202, 355, 363
Idrobo, F., 228, 363
Iizuka, S., 268, 339
Ikeda, T., 83, 360
Ikkos, D., 313, 371
Imamura, T., 285, 367
Imberte, R., 282, 352
Imre, S., 247, 257, 363
Inada, H., 331, 355
Ingle, L., 8, 32, 37, 363
Ingram, Don K., ix, 8, 17, 29, 43, 44, 52, 58, 59, 62, 63, 67, 69, 121, 122, 135, 153, 156, 157, 158, 211, 218, 226, 227, 228, 229, 273, 317, 350, 357, 363, 364, 365, 370, 371, 374, 382, 387, 389, 395
Ingram, R. H., 5, 8, 9, 355
Inoue, M., 331, 355
Ip, C., 107, 112, 364
Iredale, Kirsty, ix
Iri, H., 302, 389
Irino, M., 16, 367
Isaacs, J. T., 136, 364
Isakovic, K., 357
Ishi, T., 302, 389
Ismail, M. N., 323, 364
Itallie, T. B. V., 327, 364
Ito, N., 255, 375
Iwasaki, K., 9, 10, 83, 232, 360, 364
Izui, S., 88, 283, 364

J

Jablon, S., 29, 333, 334, 362
Jacobson, D., 37, 312, 364
Jacobson, F. S., 258, 375
Jacobson, L. A., 37, 383
Jagot, S. A., 209, 308, 393
Jakobson, M. E., 13, 209, 308, 342, 393
Jalavisto, E., 334, 364
James, W. H., 110, 354
James, W. P. T., 146, 250, 261, 263, 307, 313, 364, 365, 390
Janda, J. K., 156, 227, 370

Jankovic, B. D., 357
Jarrett, S. R., 58, 386
Jensen, B. D., 244, 245, 258, 264
Jensen, F., 88, 283, 384
Jeuniewie, N., 307, 345
Jewelewicz, R., 307, 393
Johnson, A. R., 10, 362
Johnson, B. C., 16, 59, 99, 121, 129, 166, 232, 287, 328, 355, 361, 368, 380, 386
Johnson, H. D., 9, 52, 262, 366
Johnson, J. E., 340
Johnson, J. E., Jr., 232, 246, 359, 365, 374, 376
Johnson, M., 178, 395
Johnson, N. W., 113, 378
Johnson, R. E., 9, 10, 366
Johnson, R. O., 103, 383
Johnson, T. E., 286, 365
Jolin, T., 146, 147, 148, 339
Jones, F., 9, 16, 52, 54, 273, 352
Jones, J. H., 102, 354
Jones, T. W., 285, 360
Jordan, W., 245, 376
Jose, D. C., 188, 357
Jose, D. G., 188, 308, 353, 357, 365
Joseph, D., 347
Joseph, J. A., 153, 157, 158, 227, 273, 376, 370, 382
Joun, N. S., 10, 378
Juhasz, E., 247, 257, 363
Jung, L. K. L., 187, 188, 365
Jung, R. T., 146, 307, 365
Juricova, M., 119, 350
Juricova-Horakova, M., 62, 64, 388

K

Kachole, M. S., 125, 360
Kadura, S. N., 267, 366
Kagan, A., 310, 380
Kagawa, Y., 301, 302, 365
Kahn, C., 261, 365
Kahn, Herman, 330
Kaiser, D. L., 327, 340
Kajimoto, M., 5, 8, 9, 375
Kajiya, F., 331, 355
Kalef, S., 393
Kalkwarf, H. J., 322, 370
Kalu, D. N., 156, 157, 158, 215, 221, 222, 223, 226, 303, 325, 365

Kanatsuka, A., 388
Kannel, W. B., 334, 365
Kasiske, B. L., 86, 365
Kasser, T. R., 215, 359
Katz, M. S., 366
Kaufman, M. C., 366
Kaufmann, N., 304, 397
Kaunitz, H., 366
Keane, W. F., 86, 365
Keen, C. L., 87, 176, 384, 392
Keesey, R. E., 202, 254, 344, 348
Kelley, K. W., 272, 366
Kellogg, V. L., 38, 366
Kelly, M. G., 103, 395
Kemal, R., 286, 365
Kemeny, G., 209, 381
Kendrick, Z. V., 123, 124, 126, 127, 135, 233, 383
Kennedy, G. C., 8, 395
Kesler, P., 345
Keys, A., 76, 209, 304, 306, 308, 310, 312, 313, 320, 321, 366, 390
Khan, M. A., 202, 366
Khare, A., 197, 270, 353, 366
Khaw, K., 279, 334, 341
Khilobock, I. Y., 267, 366
Kibler, H. H., 9, 52, 262, 366
Kiesler, S. B., 349, 368
Kiiskinen, A., 18, 29, 333, 388
Kim, Y. T., 67, 372
Kimmel, D., 300, 366
Kimura, S., 278, 367
King, D. W., 339, 372
King, J. T., 13, 47, 58, 88, 346, 369
Kipnis, D. M., 307, 345
Kirkman, H. N., 135, 257, 366
Klass, M. R., 37, 366
Kleiber, W., 7, 322, 366
Klein, J., 248, 388
Klevay, L. M., 366
Klima, W. C., 74, 75, 348
Kline, B. E., 103, 383
Kline, M. S., 103, 383
Kline, S., 286, 365
Klug, G. A., 244, 366
Klurfeld, D. M., 84, 104, 108, 109, 123, 366, 367, 368, 383
Kment, A., 332, 362, 386
Knapka, J. J., 8, 9, 353
Knoll, G., 244, 366

Knuth, U. A., 143, 367
Knutson, D., 4, 341
Koberle, S., 333, 367
Koga, A., 287, 367
Kohn, R. R., 9, 10, 306, 367, 375
Kohno, A., 16, 367
Koizumi, A., ix, 24, 26, 124, 126, 132, 133, 134, 177, 203, 247, 256, 266, 268, 269, 270, 282, 285, 249, 267
Kokkonen, G. C., 8, 9, 10, 36, 43, 44, 58, 62, 122, 123, 124, 125, 126, 127, 161, 172, 211, 261, 265, 341, 367, 370
Kolata, G., 305, 367
Koletsky, S., 96, 367
Konen, Ted, ix, 189, 392
Konoplya, E. F., 368, 321
Kopec, S., 39, 368
Kotlikoff, L. J., 329, 368
Kourides, I. A., 86, 87, 233, 307, 384
Kozubik, A., 287, 368
Kramer, R., 242, 376
Kramer, T. R., 188, 357
Krause, J., 244, 366
Kreitman, K. R., 246, 343
Krey, L. C., 384
Krishnamachar, S., 114, 327, 368
Kristie, James A., ix, 64, 179, 180, 184, 185, 187, 188, 191, 192, 193, 194, 195, 211, 261, 308, 394
Kritchevsky, D., 84, 104, 108, 109, 123, 366, 367, 368, 383
Kruckerberg, T. W., 345
Kruk, P., 176, 351
Ksiazele, M. R., 146, 307, 376
Kubo, C., 16, 59, 68, 99, 129, 232, 287, 328, 355, 364, 368
Kuhn, T. W., 246, 343
Kuhnau, J., 381
Kunz, P. L., 144, 147, 343
Kurashima, C., 281, 362
Kurcz, M., 142, 146, 147, 275, 307, 345
Kurimoto, F., 355
Kuto, S., 281, 362
Kwasman, M. A., 217, 343
Kwasowski, P. 107, 354

L

La Bella, F. S., 9, 352, 368
Labo, G., 370

Lacatis, D., 312, 339
Lacombe, C. R., 348
Lacy, D., 176, 384
Laganiere, S., 178, 197, 353, 368
Lagopoulos, L., 107, 108, 368
Lakatta, E. G., 218, 367
Lambert, B., 265, 368
Lammert, O., 320, 369
Lammi-Keefe, C. J., 136, 369
Landfield, P. W., 272, 276, 278, 279, 280, 354, 369
Lands, W. E. M., 173, 372
Landsberg, L., 155, 307, 308, 351, 369
Lane, M. D., 243, 369
Lane, P. W., 369
Lang, C. A., 248, 361
Lansing, A. I., 373
Lanza-Jacoby, S., 125, 153, 347
Lapidus, L., 327, 369
Larsen, C. D., 86, 87, 369
Larson, L. A., 304, 308, 357
Laver, J. L., 10, 362
Latiff, A., 202, 254, 361
Lau, P. P., 388
Lawton, M. P., 393
Leatherwood, J. M., 215, 351
Ledvina, M., 10, 369
Lee, C. J., 88, 122, 220, 369, 377
Lee, H., 124, 150, 174, 396
Lee, M., 253, 369
Lee, P. N., 70, 391
Lee, Y. C. P., 47, 58, 88, 369
Lefevre, M. L., 176, 384
Lefkowitz, R. J., 143, 144, 253, 386
Legan, J. S., 247, 257, 358
Lehman, I. R., 143, 144, 253, 386
Leighton, B., 256, 369
Leiter, E. H., 255, 347
Le Maho, Y., 48, 350
Lemmon, J. A., 334, 378
Lerner, C., 260, 281, 310, 317, 360
Lerner, S. P., 282, 369
Les, E. P., 364
Leslie, S. W., 242, 370
Lesser, G. T., 69, 214, 370
Leto, S., 43, 44, 58, 211, 261, 370
Leung, B. E., 371
Leung, R. E., 8, 35, 58, 66, 90, 91, 268, 346
Leveille, G. A., 52, 202, 324, 370, 385, 391
Leveille, P. J., ix, 170, 259, 370

Levi, L., 307, 377
Levin, P., 156, 227, 370
Levine, R. L., 134, 171, 285, 376
Levitsky, D. A., 322, 370
Levy, P. L., 307, 345
Lew, G., 242, 372
Lewin, R., 235, 370
Lewis, J., 241, 339
Lewis, S. E. M., 164, 165, 166, 173, 265, 308, 351, 356, 357, 370, 374
Li, S., 371
Licastro, F., ix, 24, 26, 167, 265, 270, 290, 370
Liepa, G. U., 174, 175, 370
Lin, Z. H., 244, 348
Lindell, T. J., 268, 370
Lindop, P., 348
Lindstedt, S. L., 251, 370
Lindstrom, C. O., 283, 372
Lindstrom, F. D., 305, 328, 386
Lindstrom, J., 196, 347
Lipps, L., 189, 392
Lipton, R. J., 217, 343
Lipworth, L., 359
Lissner, L., 322, 370
Liu, Robert K., ix, 4, 8, 16, 27, 35, 58, 66, 90, 91, 92, 93, 97, 101, 132, 187, 188, 189, 190, 209, 211, 233, 260, 261, 265, 268, 308, 346, 356, 370, 371, 392
Ljungren, H., 313, 371
Llewyllyn, M. J., 249, 344
Lloyd, L. M., 367
Lloyd, T., 16, 54, 84, 371
Lockshin, R. A., 272, 371
Loeb, J., 8, 38, 371
Lofts, B., 374
London, E. D., 121, 122, 135, 157, 226, 272, 351, 371, 374
Long, J. W., Jr., 242, 392
Long, M. L., 102, 343
Lonnerdal, B., 176, 384
Loriaux, D. L., 307, 308, 391
Loschen, G., 245, 371
Loustalot, P., 52, 77, 79, 356
Low, T. L. K., 334, 357
Lowrey, A., 29, 332, 333, 348
Lubinski, J., 272, 283, 371
Lucas, A. R., 304, 308, 357
Lucas, J. A., 255, 371
Lucia, S, P., 253, 369

Author Index

Luckert, P. H., 11, 53, 112, 113, 378
Ludwig, F. C., 9, 332, 371
Luft, R., 313, 371
Lukes, Y., 145, 345
Lustbader, E., 70, 84, 249, 382
Lutz, W., 52, 77, 79, 356
Lynd, F. T., 32, 33, 35, 43, 52, 69, 70, 71, 77, 214, 216, 219, 220, 231, 249, 342
Lyman, C. P., 252, 371
Lynch, B. A., 136, 350

M

MacDonald, P. C., 255, 371
Mac Gregor, G. A., 297, 299, 371
Machado, A., 391
MacKay, I. R., 334, 371, 380
MacLeod, R. M., 344
Madden, Sidney, ix
Maddox, G. L., 393
Madhavan Nair, K., 125, 378
Maeda, H., 74, 75, 77, 95, 219, 342, 371, 396
Magee, P. N., 10, 255, 376
Makino, H., 388
Makinodan, T., 272, 283, 361, 371, 392
Maksud, M. G., 48, 218, 359
Mancini, C., 19, 281, 348
Mandelbrot, B., 290, 372
Mann, D. M. A., 372
Mann, P. L., 187, 188, 194, 288, 372
Manson, J. E., 310, 372
Manton, K. G., 5, 6, 375
March, J., 368
Marcus, D. L., 242, 372
Mareschi, J. P., 322, 372
Margen, S., 320, 388
Mariani, T., 188, 348
Marini, S., 19, 281, 348
Mark, D. A., 67, 99, 175, 372
Mark, D. A., 187, 188, 365
Markofsky, J., 69, 214, 370
Marks, V., 107, 354
Marmorston, J., 331, 334, 32
Marrale, J. C., 324, 372
Marshall, S., 142, 146, 147, 275, 298, 307, 345
Marshall, E., 372
Marshall, P. J., 173, 372

Marston, H. R., 58, 381
Martin, A. P., 242, 392
Martino, E., 145, 350
Martin, G. M., 21, 25, 247, 269, 372
Martin, J. B., 389
Martin, P. A., 285, 360
Martin, R. J., 215, 359
Maruyama, H., 113, 379
Maruyama, N., 283, 372
Masen, H. L., 308, 346
Mason, R. L., 52, 62, 64, 66, 221, 226, 341, 342, 391
Masoro, E. J., 8, 9, 10, 15, 16, 22, 23, 32, 33, 35, 43, 52, 53, 66, 69, 70, 71, 74, 75, 77, 83, 95, 124, 149, 150, 151, 152, 155, 171, 174, 175, 198, 199, 202, 214, 215, 216, 217, 218, 219, 220, 226, 228, 231, 232, 233, 249, 252, 298, 308, 311, 312, 313, 342, 343, 360, 364, 368, 370, 371, 372, 373, 392, 396
Massie, H. R., 247, 340
Masters, C., 256, 373
Mathias, A. P., 267, 397
Mathies, Meg, ix, 16, 189, 265, 392
Matkovics, B., 376
Matsubara, M., 143, 373
Matsushita, M., 16, 367
Maun, M. E., 108, 351
Maurizo, A., 36, 373
Maxwell, L. C., 102, 343
May, Patrick, 159, 225
Mayer, J., 324, 373
Maynard, L. A., 8, 15, 47, 52, 53, 62, 63, 231, 363, 373
Mazhul, L. M., 321, 368
McBride, B. W., 250, 374
McCance, R. A., 209, 373
McCarron, D. A., 298, 373
McCarter, R. J. M., 201, 202, 215, 216, 217, 252, 288, 312, 373
McCay, C. M., 8, 15, 45, 47, 52, 53, 62, 63, 68, 76, 202, 224, 231, 301, 363, 373, 395
McConahey, P. J., 88, 283, 364
McConnell, E. E., 8, 9, 353
McCrae, R. R., 29, 331, 332, 348
McEwen, B. S., 384
McFeeters, Glenda, ix, 10, 12, 255, 394
McGaugh, J. L., 349, 368
McGee, J., 201, 216, 288, 373

McMahan, C. A., 9, 10, 15, 23, 66, 74, 75, 77, 95, 199, 215, 226, 228, 232, 233, 308, 364, 371, 396
Mahon, K. M., 226, 393
McNair, C. L., 155, 366
McNamara, P. M., 309, 363
McNeill, C. J., 190, 196, 352
McNulty, M., 175, 390
Meckelenburg, R. S., 307, 391
Medici, M., 357, 389, 390, 393
Meeker, L. D., 108, 110, 390
Meites, J., 109, 112, 114, 140, 141, 142, 146, 147, 235, 272, 273, 274, 275, 276, 277, 278, 280, 307, 328, 340, 345, 354, 373, 379, 380, 387, 388, 390
Melander, A., 307, 377
Mellitt, R., 45, 47, 146, 307, 356
Mellon, S. H., 147, 387
Mendel, L. B., 8, 49, 202, 362, 377
Menefee, J., 215, 373
Meredith, P. J., ix, 8, 9, 19, 20, 35, 58, 66, 90, 92, 93, 97, 101, 187, 188, 190, 211, 282, 308, 331, 346, 373
Merimee, T. J., 307, 373
Merry, B. J., 8, 13, 16, 43, 46, 47, 49, 52, 53, 137, 138, 139, 140, 141, 144, 145, 147, 148, 149, 162, 163, 164, 165, 166, 173, 224, 231, 265, 277, 278, 307, 308, 351, 356, 357, 362, 370, 395
Mertz, W., 324, 374
Mervis, R. F., 226, 374
Meshnick, S. R., 258, 385
Metler, D. S., 323, 364
Meyer, T. E., 282, 393
Meyn, R. E., 134, 286, 345
Michael, A. F., 67, 78, 99, 355
Mickelson, O., 76, 140, 209, 304, 308, 312, 313, 320, 321, 358, 366
Mickey, M. R., 8, 35, 58, 66, 90, 91, 92, 93, 97, 101, 187, 188, 190, 211, 233, 261, 268, 308, 346
Mickey, R., ix, 58, 132, 189, 190, 356
Mider, G. B., 103, 395
Mildvan, A. S., 243, 369
Miles, W. E., 320, 321, 342
Millar, J. S., 13, 396
Miller, D. S., 62, 63, 318, 351, 374
Miller, R. A., 187, 188, 193, 272, 279, 284, 374
Miller, S. T., 9, 10, 348, 377

Miller, U., 321, 390
Milligan, L. P., 250, 374
Millward, D. J., 146, 172, 307, 345, 348
Minaker, K. L., 306, 382
Miquel, J., 232, 242, 246, 340, 354, 359, 365, 374, 376
Miranda, M., 16, 86, 353
Misra, H. P., 59, 129, 368
Mitchell, D. H., 286, 365
Mitchener, M., 9, 48, 385
Mitchison, N. A., 352, 393
Mobbs, C. V., 276, 354
Mocchegiani, E., 282, 352
Mohan, P. F., 123, 124, 127, 202, 228, 253, 254, 374
Moldofsky, A., 307, 345
Moment, G. B., 328, 341, 349, 354, 374, 381
Mondon, C. E., 154, 306, 307, 374, 379
Monnier, V. M., 306, 375
Montero, J. L., 146, 147, 148, 339
Moore, A. L., 107, 352
Moore, J., 154, 233, 268, 307, 379
Moore, M. A., 255, 375
Moreschi, C., 73, 102, 375
Morgan, A. D., 307, 345
Morgan, P. R., 101, 339
Morgan, R. F., 375
Morgan, R. W., 258, 286, 333, 375
Morin, R. J., 10, 375
Moroi, S., 226, 374
Morris, C. D., 298, 373
Morrison, S. D., 14, 215, 323, 329, 375
Mos, J., 32, 375
Mostofsky, D. I., 228, 363
Mount, L. E., 209, 373
Mozzhukhina, J. G., 267, 366
Muggleton, A., 36, 375
Mulinos, M. G., 137, 378
Mullen, Beagle, ix, 184, 185, 187, 188, 192, 193, 194, 195, 308, 394
Mullen, J. L., 303, 304, 308, 377
Muller, D. S., 312, 356
Muller, E. E., 344
Muller, S., 125, 153, 347, 355
Munro, H. N., 314, 357, 362, 375
Murata, I., 32, 33, 35, 43, 52, 69, 70, 74, 75, 77, 95, 214, 216, 219, 232, 242, 271, 296
Murphy, M. P., 293, 253, 344
Murray, D., 134, 286, 345

Myers, G. C., 5, 6, 375
Muzzioli, M., 282, 352

N

Nadakavukaren, M. J., 226, 288, 375
Nadeau, M., 126, 160, 161, 386, 387
Naeim, F., 184, 185, 187, 188, 191, 192, 193, 194, 195, 257, 289, 290, 308, 393, 394
Naftolin, F., 46, 395
Nakagawa, I., 5, 8, 9, 375
Nakagawa, K., 143, 373
Nandy, K., 196, 228, 363, 375
Nank, S., 359
Narasinga Rao, S., 384
Naylor, P. H., 26, 33, 35, 181, 182, 283, 334, 357, 394
Nebert, D. W., 285, 375
Neer, R. M., 303, 380
Nelson, J. F., 225, 235, 276, 354, 375
Nelson, W., 55, 58, 59, 211, 212, 375
Nemeskeri, J., 19, 341
Nesheim, M. C., 202, 354
Nerder, L. J., 10, 377
Nesterenko, G. A., 148, 279, 375
Newberne, P. M., 356
Newsholme, E. A., 256, 369
Ney, D., 176, 384
Nibbelinks, M. M., 176, 348
Nicholls, D. G., 380
Nichols, W., 14, 33, 35, 45, 89, 395
Nickel, M., 152, 233, 254, 350, 361
Niedermueller, H., 332, 362, 386
Nikitin, V. N., 144, 148, 267, 279, 307, 375, 376
Nitsche, B., 89, 379
Nitta, R. T., 10, 378
Nohl, H., 242, 245, 246, 258, 376
Nolen, G. A., 62, 64, 174, 213, 221, 376
Nomura, A. M. Y., 305, 387
Norling, B. K., 303, 325, 365
Norman, D. C., 272, 283, 371
Norris, A. H., 235, 239, 333, 334, 344, 382, 391
Northrop, J. H., 8, 38, 371, 376
Norton, K. R., 308, 346
Novak, R., 376
Novakofski, J., 272, 366
Nussbaum, S. R., 303, 380
Nyce, J. W., 10, 255, 376

O

Oberlink, N., 386
O'Brian, J. T., 146, 307, 376
O'Brien, R. C., 371
O'Connor, M., 383
O'Donnell, M. P., 86, 365
Odum, H. T., 289, 376
O'Hara, D. S., 308, 349
Oikawa, K., 268, 339
Olewine, D. A., 228, 376
Oliver, C. N., 134, 171, 285, 376
Olsen, C. T., 355
Olsen, G. G., 273, 376
Olson, 26
Ono, T., 247, 389
Onody, C., 19, 341
Ooka, H., 146, 376, 377, 385
Opishinski, J. W., 14, 33, 35, 45, 89, 395
Orco, 267
Ordy, J. M., 341
Orentreich, N., 334, 377
Orlando, J., 307, 385
Orr, R. R., Jr., 242, 392
Osborne, T. B., 8, 49, 377
Osburne, R. C., 146, 223, 307, 345, 376
Oschray, Y., 397
Osgood, H. S., 62, 63, 363, 373
Ossmann, J. B., 190, 352
Ostlund, A. K., 244, 366
Overall, J. E., 332, 333, 377

P

Page, L., 324, 393
Pahlavani, M. A., 197, 377
Palladino, M. A., 187, 188, 365
Pallotta, J. A., 306, 382
Palmblad, J., 307, 377
Pan, G. Y., 11, 53, 112, 113, 378
Pandey, G. N., 307, 346
Panemangalore, M., 88, 122, 220, 369, 377
Papafrangos, E. D., 371
Papavasiliou, P. S., 9, 10, 348, 377
Pariza, M. W., 109, 110, 111, 112, 255, 305, 326, 343, 377
Park, J. H. Y., 216, 242, 377, 392
Parkatti, T., 18, 29, 333, 388
Parke, D. V., 339
Pashko, L. L., 255, 377

Pasteur, Louis, 299
Patel, M. S., 242, 350
Patil, K., 5, 8, 9, 343
Pathmanathan, K., 10, 32, 36, 39, 348
Pawar, S. S., 125, 360
Payne, P. R., 43, 62, 63, 374, 377
Pearl, R., 243, 377
Pedersen, P. L., 243, 369, 377
Pegg, M., 373
Penniston, J. T., 250, 345
Perea, A., 226, 390
Pertshuk, M. J., 303, 304, 308, 377
Peters, A., 226, 288, 377
Peterson, C., 279, 356
Petranyi, G. G., 19, 341
Petros, T. V., 334, 377
Pfitzer, E., 14, 33, 35, 45, 89, 395
Phillips, J. G., 164, 165, 265, 370, 374
Phillips, L. S., 147, 378
Phinney, S. D., 304, 378
Piantanelli, L., 282, 378
Pickering, C. E., 178, 378
Pickering, R., 178, 378
Pierpaoli, W., 141, 378
Pigg, M., 340, 383
Pinney, D. O., 40, 301, 378
Pivorun, E. B., 226, 393
Plesko, M. M., 265, 271, 378
Podos, S. M., 259, 343
Pohl, S. L., 327, 340
Pokrovskaya, R. V., 321, 368
Pollard M., 53, 112, 113, 307, 378, 386
Pomerantz, L., 137, 378
Poon, L. W., 330, 378
Pope, L. S., 40, 301, 378
Popper, H., 288, 378
Porta, E. A., 10, 378
Porter, B. D., 52, 275, 288, 352
Posner, B. I., 389
Pospisil, M., 287, 368
Potvin, A. R., 334, 378
Potvin, J. H., 334, 378
Pour, P., 5, 8, 9, 343
Prabhu, S. R., 113, 378
Peasad, K. V. S., 125, 378
Price, P., 38, 182, 342
Priestly, G. C., 266, 378
Pryor, W. A., 243, 379
Pugeat, M. M., 307, 355
Pullar, J. D., 255, 379

Puterman, D. I., 96, 367

Q

Quartermain, D., 228, 344
Quigley, K., 140, 235, 278, 328, 379
Quimby, F., 67, 372

R

Rabbitt, P., 334, 379
Radicke, D., 215, 373
Raff, H. V., ix, 22, 187, 188, 194, 195, 286, 394
Raff, M., 241, 339
Ragan, C. I., 245, 345
Ragbeer, M. S., 81, 381
Ramirez, M. E., 267, 346
Ramp, B. J., 246, 343
Randt, C. T., 228, 344
Rao, B. S. N., 374
Rao, M. V. N., 366
Rao, S. N., 10, 36, 123, 124, 202, 228, 253, 254, 377
Rapoport, S. I., 272, 351
Rapp, K. G., 58, 59, 89, 91, 379
Raven, R. W., 389
Ray, L. A., 9, 68, 381
Reaven, Eve P., 153, 154, 233, 268, 306, 307, 374, 379
Reaven, Gerald M., 153, 154, 233, 268, 306, 307, 374, 379, 381
Reck, S. J., 366
Reddy, B. S., 113, 379
Reed, J. D., 8, 10, 24, 384
Refetoff, S., 145, 350
Reff, M. E., 17, 18, 264, 333, 334, 350, 356, 360, 365, 379, 384, 385, 394
Regelson, W., 333, 344, 357, 379
Rehm, S., 58, 59, 89, 90, 91, 379, 380
Rehwaldt, C. A., 171, 233, 387
Reichard, G. A., Jr., 307, 345
Reigle, G. D., 279, 380
Reimers, N., 40, 73, 301, 314, 380
Reiner, L., 102, 354
Reiter, R. J., 147, 387
Reyman, K., 307, 380
Reynolds, M. A., 8, 43, 44, 52, 58, 59, 62, 63, 67, 69, 228, 229, 363, 364
Rhee, S. Y. S., 246, 343

Rhoads, G. G., 310, 380
Rhodes, M. L., 372
Richardson, A., 126, 129, 166, 167, 171, 172, 192, 197, 226, 231, 233, 242, 264, 265, 267, 268, 269, 270, 271, 286, 288, 308, 343, 347, 361, 375, 377, 378, 380, 387, 394
Richter, B. I., 329, 358
Richter, C., 245, 371
Ricketts, W. G., 171, 233, 380, 387
Ricotti, N. A., 303, 380
Ricquier, D., 244, 380
Riesen, W. H., 52, 380
Rigo, A., 247, 384
Rikimaru, T., 355
Riley, A. M., Jr., 324, 385
Ringborg, U., 265, 368
Risley, J., 121, 166, 380, 386
Rizer, R. L., 334, 377
Roberts, J. S., 108, 110, 390
Roberts, K., 241, 339
Roberts, M. S., 171, 264, 265, 267, 268, 269, 270, 343
Roberts-Thompson, I. C., 334, 380
Robertson, T. B., 9, 58, 68, 266, 381
Robertson, M. S. M., 378
Robinson, J. L., 300, 359
Rockstein, M., 388
Rodgers, K. E., 285, 367
Roe, D. A., 322, 370
Roe, F. J. C., 70, 391
Roeder, L. M., 62, 63, 123, 124, 125, 126, 341
Rogers, P. D., 209, 393
Rogul, M., 395
Romsos, D. R., 202, 381, 391
Root, A. W., 142, 381
Rose, K., 385
Roselfsema, F., 350
Rosen, R., 289, 381
Rosenberg, B., 209, 381
Rosenthal, M., 306, 381
Rosenwasser, M. J., 246, 343
Rosmus, J., 119, 250, 350, 388
Ross, B. A., 156, 158, 215, 223, 226, 325, 365
Ross, M. H., 8, 9, 15, 23, 33, 43, 49, 52, 54, 55, 62, 63, 70, 77, 80, 81, 82, 84, 124, 126, 129, 130, 131, 132, 133, 174, 191, 198, 247, 249, 290, 317, 318, 323, 325, 326, 381, 382
Roth, G. S., 153, 156, 157, 158, 227, 273, 340, 349, 358, 365, 370, 382, 395
Roth, P., 320, 321, 342
Rothstein, M., 134, 301, 310, 342, 360, 380, 382, 388
Rothwell, N. J., 202, 249, 266, 307, 308, 318, 319, 323, 382, 387
Rotter, J.I., 328, 382
Rous, P., 74, 102, 382
Rovito, R. J., 255, 377
Rovner, S., 299, 382
Rowe, J. W., 306, 333, 382
Rowlatt, C., 74, 75, 88, 382
Rozek, M., 383
Rubner, M., 243, 383
Rucker, R., 290, 383
Ruderman, N. B., 307, 313, 345
Rudzinska, M. A., 7, 32, 36, 383
Rue, P. A., 145, 350
Ruggeri, B. A., 123, 383
Rumsey, W. L., 123, 124, 126, 127, 135, 206, 208, 233, 383
Runcie, J., 321, 390
Rusch, H. P., 103, 184, 344, 383
Russ, R. D., 142, 381
Russell, J. C., 84, 383
Russell, R. L., 37, 383
Rutherford, M. S., 126, 166, 264, 265, 267, 268, 269, 270, 219, 280

S

Sachan, D. S., 122, 123, 125, 175, 178, 285, 383
Sacher, G. A., 8, 21, 22, 27, 33, 34, 35, 198, 235, 236, 237, 247, 253, 260, 269, 315, 348, 383
Sado, T., 281, 362
Safai, B., 196, 383
Safai-Kutti, S., 196, 383
Salthouse, T. A., 334, 384
Samis, H. V., 340
Samis, H. V., Jr., 247, 256, 257, 340
Samuel, D., 379
Samuels, S., 228, 344
Sanadi, D. R., 242, 346
Sanborn, A. C., 342
Sandberg, L., 197, 353
Sapolsky, R. M., 278, 279, 384

Sargent, F., 29, 340
Sarkar, N. H., 86, 87, 233, 307, 384
Sasaki, A., 5, 8, 9, 375
Sato, K., 255, 375
Sato, T., 390
Sato, Y., 242, 258, 334, 350, 396
Satrustegui, J., 242, 391
Satterfield, L. C., 10, 74, 75, 347, 348
Satyanarayana, U., 124, 384
Saudek, C. D., 307, 384
Saul, R. L., 233, 270, 384
Saville, E., 308, 395
Saville, M. E., 382
Sawada, M., 37, 384
Saxton, J. A., Jr., 58, 77, 86, 87, 102, 354, 384
Scarpa, M., 247, 384
Scarpace, P. J., 155, 233, 384
Schaefer, A. E., 324, 385
Schalch, D. S., 147, 387
Schechter, M., 386
Schenck, H. V., 307, 377
Schillo, K. K., 47, 359
Schimke, R. T., 381, 392
Schlesselman, J. J., 332, 384
Schmahl, D., 109, 112, 343
Schmidt, D., 307, 380
Schmidt, I. M. V., 303, 307, 340
Schmucker, D. L., 285, 384
Schneeman, B. O., 176, 384
Schneider, Ed L., 5, 8, 10, 17, 18, 21, 24, 295, 329, 333, 334, 344, 350, 351, 354, 356, 358, 360, 365, 372, 378, 379, 382, 383, 384, 385, 386, 390, 392, 393, 394
Schnyder, W., 144, 147
Schroeder, H. A., 9, 48, 385
Schurch, A., 144, 147, 343
Schussler, G. C., 307, 385
Schwab, R., 272, 283, 385
Schwartz, A., 10, 255, 376
Schwartz, A. G., 10, 255, 284, 285, 377, 385
Schwerin, H. S., 324, 385
Schwizer, R. W., 255, 347
Scofield, V. L., 359
Scommegna, P. J., 378
Scott, I. M., 209, 210, 363
Scott, M. D., 209, 210, 258, 385
Scott, W. A., 29, 332, 333, 348
Scrimshaw, 308, 316
Secord, D. C., 175, 390

Seedsman, N. J., 9, 16, 52, 54, 273, 352
Segall, P. E., 52, 54, 137, 141, 146, 159, 225, 274, 347, 377, 385
Segre, D., 341, 358
Sekaram, C., 307, 308, 386
Sekiguchi, S., 302, 389
Sekuler, R., 334, 338
Selwyn, M. J., 239, 385
Semsei, I., 126, 166, 269, 270, 380
Senior, A. E., 244, 348
Senior, W., 45, 395
Seo, E., 9, 10, 232, 364
Seo, H., 145, 350
Selow, R. B., 24, 264, 265, 360, 390
Sevall, 267
Shaffer, J. B., 259, 385
Shah, M., 312, 321, 356
Shao, R., 121, 166, 380, 386
Shatenstein, B., 160, 161, 386
Shepard, R. C., 107, 356
Shepman, J. H., 372
Sheriff, M. U., 74, 75, 88, 382
Sherman, H. C., 68, 386
Sherwin, R. S., 143, 144, 307, 308, 386
Shetty, P. S., 146, 307, 365
Shock, N. W., 228, 322, 333, 376, 382, 386
Shurnick, I. D., 209, 381
Siddiqui, A. M., 125, 360
Sigel, M. M., 348
Silberberg, M., 58, 386
Silberberg, R., 58, 386
Silverstone, H., 15, 76, 86, 88, 97, 103, 389
Simms, 33, 48, 52, 53, 77, 79, 224, 231, 342
Simon, J., 272, 366
Simopoulos, A. P., 310, 386
Sims, C., 154, 374
Sims, E. A. H., 249, 386
Sinex, F. M., 344, 357, 379
Sisk, C. L., 141, 386
Siskind, G. W., 281, 386
Sivakumar, B., 125, 378
Sivertsen, I., 85, 86
Skalicky, M., 332, 362, 386
Skerde, G., 307, 377
Skoldstam, L., 305, 328, 386
Skoog, K., 265, 368
Slater, T. F., 349, 294
Smallridge, R. C., 307, 345
Smith, 67
Smith, C. A., 52, 62, 64, 66, 341

Smith, E. K., 9, 53, 62, 67, 152, 214, 231, 362
Smith, E. L., 143, 144, 253, 386
Smith, George S., ix, 8, 16, 35, 58, 66, 90, 91, 92, 93, 97, 101, 187, 188, 189, 190, 211, 233, 261, 265, 268, 282, 308, 346, 386, 392
Smith, H. M., 320, 321, 342
Smith, J., 16, 86, 353
Smith, J. K., 307, 308, 386
Smith, J. M., 242, 392
Smith, K. C., 264, 286
Smith, L. G., 209, 381
Smith, R. D., 170, 351
Smith, T. W., 308, 349
Smith-Sonneborn, J., 386
Smoke, M. E., 332, 371
Snook, J. T., 307, 308, 313, 341
Snow, C. P., 386
Snyder, D. L., 53, 141, 149, 178, 307, 386, 395
Sobel, E. L., 255, 377
Sobell, S., 245, 386
Soeldner, J. D., 307, 345
Sohol, R. S., 4, 232, 260, 249, 387
Solomon, C., 126, 387
Solomon, R., 154, 306, 307, 379
Sommer, R., 89, 90, 380
Sonntag, W. E., 274, 280, 387
Soong, S., 26, 361
Soriano, J., 346
Sorrentino, S., Jr., 147, 387
Spangler, E. L., 364
Spannaus, D. J., 282, 393
Sparks, M. B., 171, 233, 387
Sparrow, D., 305, 310, 327, 344
Spencer, P. S., 14, 33, 35, 45, 89, 395
Sperling, G., 52, 62, 63, 224, 363, 373
Spiegel, R., 333, 367
Spiegelman, B. M., 250, 354
Spindler, S. R., 147, 268, 269, 349, 387
Sprott, R. L., 21, 358, 378, 379, 382, 384, 386, 392, 393
Spurgeon, H. A., 218, 387
Squier, C. A., 113, 378
Srivastava, U., 126, 160, 161, 386, 387
Stacer, H. C., 307, 345
Stacy, C., 219, 342
Stadler, 107, 108
Stadtman, Earl R., 134, 171, 285, 376

Staecker, J. L., 171, 264, 343, 380
Staffeldt, E. F., 259, 353
Stahl, S. M., 14, 33, 35, 45, 89, 395
Stalder, R., 368
Stallone, R. A., 297, 387
Stampfer, M. J., 310, 372
Stanton, J. L., 324, 385
Starnes, J. W., 123, 124, 126, 127, 135, 217, 233, 343, 383
Starr, B. D., 393
Stavitskaya, L. I., 148, 279, 375
Stehlin, J. S., 107, 356
Stein, M., 246, 343
Steinke, J., 307, 345
Steinmeier, F. A., 185, 343
Stemmermann, G. N., 305, 387
Stephens, D. F., 40, 301, 378
Stern, J. S., 202, 348
Stevanato, R., 384
Stein, Y., 304, 397
Stevens, J. M., 10, 377
Still, J. W., 289, 387
Stocco, D. M., 242, 387
Stock, M., 202, 249, 266, 307, 308, 318, 319, 323, 387
Stock, M. J., 202, 307, 323, 356, 382
Stolzner, G. H., 43, 44, 58, 189, 387, 388
Stoppani, A. O. M., 245, 345
Storer, J. B., 27, 388
Storlien, L. H., 202, 254, 344
Storz, G., 258, 375
Strobel, H. W., 285, 388
Strong, R., 273, 388
Strothers, S. C., 44, 356
Strupp, B. J., 322, 370
Stuchlikova, E., 62, 64, 388
Stucki, J., 245, 386
Stunkard, A. J., 232, 303, 309, 310, 318, 388
Suddin, S. C., 122, 124, 180, 204, 205, 206, 207, 283, 316, 394
Sukhatme, P. V., 320, 388
Sun, J., 285, 388
Suominen, H., 18, 29, 333, 388
Sundulko, K., 334, 378
Surawicz, B., 299, 388
Sussman, M. L., 388
Sutton, R. B., 259, 385
Suzuki, M., 302, 389
Suzuki, T., 5, 8, 9, 375, 388
Suojtkova, E., 119, 388

Swan, P. B., 136, 216, 324, 369, 377, 388
Swanston-Flatt, S. K., 107, 354
Swerdloff, R. S., 45, 47, 146, 307, 356
Swift, R. W., 5, 8, 9, 110, 354, 355
Swiitzer, B. P., 304, 306, 307, 363
Sylia, S. J., 270, 396
Sylvester, P., 109, 112, 114, 364, 388
Szilard, L., 264, 388
Szymura, J. M., 248, 388

T

Tack-Goldman, K., 175, 372
Tada, Y., 268, 339
Tagliaferro, A. R., 108, 110, 256, 369, 390
Takahara, S., 388
Takahashi, R., 173, 286, 388
Takahashi, S., 272, 273, 275, 276, 277, 373
Takasuji, S., 331, 355
Takata, H., 301, 331, 355, 389
Takeda, T., 16, 367
Takeshita, S., 16, 367
Talal, N., 196, 340, 347
Talan, M. I., 62, 211, 389
Talano, C. M., 254, 361
Talmasoff, J. M., 247, 389
Tam, C. E., 257, 284, 289, 290, 392, 393
Tam, C. F., 268, 284, 290, 389, 390
Tanaka, T., 89, 284, 353
Tang, L. C., 9, 10, 348
Taniguchi, N., 268, 339
Tannenbaum, A., 15, 76, 85, 86, 88, 97, 98, 101, 103, 104, 147, 148, 389
Tappel, A. L., 10, 389
Tas, S., 264, 267, 268, 389, 390
Tauchi, H., 242, 390
Tayag, Augusto, ix
Taylor, A. W., 175, 390
Taylor, H. L., 76, 309, 304, 308, 312, 313, 320, 321, 366, 390
Tebar, J., 304, 346
Telang, N. T., 86, 87, 233, 307, 384
Thakur, M. L., 161, 387
Thal, L. J., 10, 377
Thaler, H. T., 67, 89, 175, 284, 353, 372
Thamavit, W., 255, 375
Thomas, M. L., 193, 390
Thomas, I. K., 196, 390
Thompson, H. J., 108, 110, 390
Thompson, K., 29, 332, 333, 348

Thompson, K. H., 363
Thompson, R. P., 308, 346
Thomson, T. J., 321, 390
Tice, R. R., 24, 264, 265, 390
Timiras, P. S., 52, 54, 146, 159, 225, 272, 347, 377, 385, 390
Tittor, W., 16, 308, 392
Tobin, J. D., 333, 382
Todd, K. S., 307, 355
Toffler, Alvin, 330
Tokar, A. V., 331, 333, 391
Tollefsbol, T. O., 281, 283, 284, 390
Tomasi, T. B., Jr., 304, 308, 357
Totter, J. R., 14, 234, 235, 239, 360, 278, 301, 390
Tourtellotte, W. W., 334, 378
Towne, D. W., 285, 375
Townsend, J. F., 242, 392
Trayhurn, P., 250, 261, 263, 313, 364, 380
Tremoli, E., 175, 372
Treton, J. A., 390
Triggs, G. S., 13, 342
Trostler, N., 202, 391
Truswell, H. C., 318, 390
Tsuchida, C. B., 359
Tsuda, H., 255, 375
Tuchweber, B., 126, 160, 161, 226, 386, 387, 390
Tuck, M. L., 328, 390
Tucker, M. J., 58, 59, 390
Tucker, S. M., 52, 62, 64, 66, 84, 89, 90, 226, 341, 391
Tulp. O. L., 367
Turnbull, G. J., 70, 391
Turturro, A., 21, 22, 261, 360
Tuttle, R., 383
Twu, J. S., 286, 347
Tyzbir, R. S., 382
Tzagoloff, A., 203, 204, 235, 239, 391

U

Uram, J. A., 5, 8, 9, 355
Usher, P., 250, 354
Utsuyama, M., 281, 362

V

Vagenakis, A. G., 307, 359, 391
Vaitukaitis, J. L., 307, 391

Author Index

Vallejo, E. A., 303, 317, 391
Van Der Heide, D., 350
Vander Tuig, J. G., 202, 391
van Doorn, 144
Van Herrewege, J., 38, 350
van Horn, D. L., 48, 218, 359
van Itallie, T. B., 310, 386
Van Lancker, Julien L., ix, 4, 341
van Marthens, E., 52, 396
Vargas, R., 266, 391
Varon, S., 272, 354
Vassilopoulou-Sellin, R., 378
Vaughan, D. W., 342
Venditti, J. M., 107, 356
Verity, M. A., ix, 122, 124, 204, 205, 206, 207, 394
Vernadakis, A., 347
Verzar, F., 9, 391
Victorica, 242, 258
Vigersky, R. A., 307, 308, 345, 346, 391
Viglino, P., 247, 384
Viidik, A., 348, 361
Villeon, B. D. L., 322, 372
Vining, M., 62, 67, 152, 214, 362
Visscher, M. B., 13, 47, 58, 85, 86, 88, 137, 225, 278, 340, 346, 363, 369, 391
Visser, W., 8, 9, 349
Viticchi, C., 282, 378
Vitorica, J., 391
Vivian, S., 9, 368
Vlassara, H., 267, 268, 346
Vogelman, J., 334, 377
Voirul, M. J., 308, 395
Voitenko, V. P., 331, 333, 391
Vokonas, P. S., 305, 310, 327, 344
Volicer, L., 155, 211, 212, 261, 391, 392
von Zglinicki, 242
Vorbeck, M. L., 242, 392
Voss, K. H., 150, 392
Vronson, R., 270, 396
Vruwink, K. G., 87, 392
Vu, M. L., 160, 161, 387

W

Wabl, M. R., 248, 388
Wahren, J., 334, 350
Walford, R. L., 3, 4, 8, 9, 10, 11, 12, 14, 15, 16, 19, 20, 21, 23, 24, 25, 26, 28, 33, 35, 40, 45, 46, 49, 58, 60, 62, 64, 66, 71, 86, 89, 90, 92, 93, 94, 97, 100, 101, 122, 124, 126, 132, 133, 134, 167, 170, 173, 177, 179, 181, 182, 184, 187, 188, 189, 190, 191, 192, 193, 194, 195, 197, 200, 201, 203, 204, 205, 206, 207, 209, 211, 231, 232, 233, 246, 247, 248, 249, 255, 256, 257, 259, 260, 261, 264, 265, 266, 267, 268, 269, 270, 271, 281, 282, 283, 284, 285, 286, 287, 289, 290, 291, 293, 300, 301, 302, 306, 308, 311, 314, 316, 317, 322, 329, 330, 331, 336, 340, 341, 346, 349, 356, 358, 359, 362, 364, 365, 367, 369, 370, 371, 373, 374, 376, 386, 389, 390, 392, 393, 394, 395
Walker, E. B., 272, 366
Walker, M. A., 324, 393
Walker, R. F., 226, 393
Wallace, P. G., 250, 343
Waller, S. B., 121, 122, 135, 157, 371
Walliker, C., 52, 380
Walters, J. W., 58, 381
Wang, C., 113, 379
Wang, Y. Y., 9, 10, 196, 348, 383
Ward, W. F., 172, 393
Waring, J. J., 356
Warner, C. M., 282, 393
Warner, Huber R., ix, 21, 358, 378, 379, 382, 384, 386, 392, 393
Warren, M. J., 307, 393
Warshaw, J. B., 242, 346
Warso, M. A., 173, 372
Wartofsky, L., 145, 146, 307, 345, 356
Warwick, K. M., 324, 385
Washington, A., 287, 361
Waterlow, J. C., 198, 303, 305, 307, 308, 310, 313, 318, 351, 393
Watofsky, L., 146, 307, 376
Watson, A. L., 270, 396
Watson, J. D., 241, 339
Watson, R. R., 380
Wcislo, A., 89, 90, 380
Webb, C., 77, 352
Webb, D., 244, 348
Webb, G. P., 68, 209, 308, 393
Weber, Larry, ix
Weber, M. M., 84, 104, 108, 109, 366, 368
Webster, A. J. F., 379
Webster, G. C., 255, 264, 266, 270, 340, 393
Webster, S. L., 255, 264, 266, 270, 393

Weigle, W. O., 193, 390
Weinbach, E. C., 242, 393
Weinberg, J., 148, 355
Weinblatt, F., 150, 348
Weindruch, Robin H., ix, 4, 8, 10, 11, 12, 15, 16, 21, 22, 23, 24, 26, 33, 35, 46, 60, 62, 64, 71, 86, 90, 92, 94, 97, 100, 122, 124, 126, 132, 133, 134, 167, 170, 173, 177, 179 180, 181, 182, 184, 185, 187, 188, 191, 192, 193, 194, 195, 197, 199, 200, 201, 203, 204, 205, 206, 207, 211, 231, 233, 247, 249, 255, 256, 259, 261, 266, 270, 282, 283, 284, 285, 286, 287, 308, 316, 317, 340, 341, 362, 364, 367, 370, 393, 394
Weiner, J. M., 372
Weinsier, R. L., 321, 323, 351, 394
Weissman, I. L., 359
Weksler, B. B., 175, 372
Weksler, E., 272, 283, 385
Weksler, M. E., 18, 67, 175, 281, 282, 333, 334, 360, 372, 385, 394
Welford, A. T., 364
Wells, John, 184
Welsh, F., 372
Weraarchakul, N., 167, 270, 394
West, C. D., 155, 211, 212, 226, 261, 288, 377, 391, 392
Westgren, U., 377
Westly, H. J., 272, 366
Whitaker, J., 153, 227, 273, 365, 395
White, A., 143, 144, 253, 386
White, F., 85, 86, 103
White, G., 304, 306, 307, 363
White, J., 85, 86, 103
Whittingham, S., 334, 380
Whittle, W. L., 267, 350
Whorton, N. E., 307, 345
Wictorin, K., 272, 354
Widdowson, E. M., 8, 395
Widstrom, A., 306, 381
Wiele, R L V D, 307, 393
Wilden, N. J., 261, 351
Wilhelmi, Paula, ix
Will, L. C., 202, 395
Willen, R., 46, 395
Willett, W. C., 310, 372
Williams, J. R., 14, 33, 35, 45, 89, 255, 377, 395
Williams, L. R., 272, 354

Williams, V. J., 395
Wilson, K., 88, 122, 220, 369, 377
Wilson, P. D., 120, 395
Wilson, W. R., 304, 308, 357
Wimpfheimer, C., 308, 395
Winick, M., 381
Wise, P. H., 13, 249, 263, 313, 328, 395
Wisniewski, C., 305, 310, 327, 344
Woda, B. A., 74, 75, 353
Wohaieb, S. A., 136, 395
Wolf, A., 77, 79, 224, 342
Wolin, M. S., 259, 395
Wolstencroft, R. A., 308, 346
Wolstenholme, G. E. W., 383
Wong, G., 124, 150, 174, 396
Wood, T. R., 8, 32, 37, 363
Woodhead, A. D., 347, 349, 363, 374, 387, 395
Wostmann, B. S., 141, 145, 178, 307, 386, 395
Wright, B. E., 289, 290, 396
Wright, D., 154, 306, 307, 379
Wright, F. D., 145, 345
Wulf, J. H., 137, 396
Wyndham, J. R., 52, 77, 82, 226, 273, 276, 352, 396

Y

Yamada, E., 5, 8, 9, 375
Yang, H. Y., 282, 393
Yates, F. E., 289, 396
Yen, S. S. C., 279, 334, 341
Yengoyan, L. S., 242, 354
Yielding, K. L., 264, 396
Yokota, R., 258, 396
Yonei, S., 258, 396
Yonezu, T., 367
Yoshida, S., 388
Youhotsky-Gore, I, 10, 32, 36, 39, 348
Young, J. B., 308, 351, 369
Young, V. R., 23, 155, 307, 308, 316, 396
Youngchaiyud, U., 334, 380
Youngman, R. J., 246, 396
Yousef, I. M., 226, 390
Yu, B. P., 9, 10, 23, 32, 33, 34, 35, 43, 52, 66, 69, 70, 71, 74, 75, 77, 83, 95, 124, 150, 151, 152, 155, 156, 158, 174, 175, 178, 197, 198, 199, 202, 214, 215, 216, 217, 218, 219, 220, 221, 222, 223, 226,

228, 231, 232, 233, 249, 252, 303, 305,
308, 312, 325, 342, 343, 353, 360, 361,
364, 365, 368, 370, 371, 373, 384, 396
Yunis, Edmund J., 8, 14, 16, 33, 35, 45, 55,
58, 67, 78, 86, 87, 89, 99, 188, 196,
270, 284, 317, 334, 353, 355, 357, 358,
393, 395, 396

Z

Zakeri, Z., 295, 300, 336, 346
Zamenhof, S., 52, 396
Zammuto, R. M., 13, 360, 396
Zanni, E., 319, 321, 345, 396
Zatz, M. M., 334, 357

SUBJECT INDEX

A

Acatalasemia, in humans and mice, 259
ACTH (*see* Adrenocorticotropin hormone)
Adenocarcinoma
  in DR mice, 91
  influence DR on growth of, 74
Adenoma, effects DR on incidence in rats, 82
Adipose tissue
  effects of DR on, 218-220
    and aging, 219
    results of, 220
ADR (*see* Adult-onset dietary restriction)
Adrenal cortex tumor
  in rodents on DR, 75
    incidence, 82
    morbidity, 81
Adrenal cortical atrophy, in rodents, 75
Adrenocorticotropin hormone (ACTH)
  and corticosterone
    effects DR on, 148-149
    plasma corticosterone levels, graph, 149
Adult-onset dietary restrictions (ADR)
  ability of to modify LS in rats, 63
  benefit to mice with ongoing disease, 67-68
  body weights and survival curves, 65
  correlations body weight and life span, 70-71
    table, 71
  effects of
    on body weight, 70-71
    on growth rate, 68-70
    on life span, 68
  effects on survivorship, 31-72 (*see also* Survivorship)
  history of studies of, 63
  influence DR and/or exercise and, 67
  negative impact of, 63

  results study ADR effect on longevity, 66
  results survey studies of, 64-65
  summary studies, table, 61-62
Aging
  approaches to study of, 3
  as distinct from disease, 232
  as multi-rate-limiting-events-process, 290, 294
  biomarkers of (*see* Biomarkers of aging)
  definition, 247
  dietary restriction and (*see* Dietary restriction)
  General Adaptation Syndrome, 298
  genes and longevity, 247
  immunologic theory of, 281-282
  life span (*see* Life span)
  maximum human life, 295
  multifactorial aging in humans, 332
  prospects for retarding in humans by DR, 295-337 (*see also* Human aging retardation)
  rate of living theory, 298
  retardation in mammals, 232
  systems analysis of, 289-293 (*see also* Systems analysis)
  syndromes accelerating, 25-26
  ways to investigate biology of, 4
American Cancer Society, on diet and prevention of cancer, 296-297
American Heart Association, on diet and heart disease, 296
American Medical Association, Council on Foods and Nutrition, on diet and heart disease, 296
Amyloidosis, in rodents, 75
Anorexia nervosa patients
  diet of, 303
    body responses to, 303-304

comparison with other diets, table, 307-308
Anterior pituitary tumor, in rats on DR, 84
Arthritis, 73
  benefit of DR in humans, 328
Autoimmune nephropathy (*see* Nephropathy, autoimmune)
Autoimmunity, influences DR on, 196-197

B

Basal/induced activity hypothesis, 286-289
  aging and proliferative cell populations, 288-289
  influence DR, 286
    table, 287
  lymphopenia and DR, 287
  protein synthesis, 286
  study of holometabolous insects, 288
  WBC count and DR, 287
Biogerontology (*see also* Gerontology)
  goal of, 3
Bile duct hyperplasia, in rodents, 75
Biological parameters, effects dietary restriction on divisions of, 117
  immunologic, 178-197 (*see also* Immunologic parameters)
  molecular, 118-179 (*see also* Molecular parameters)
  physiologic, 197-227 (*see also* Physiologic parameters)
Biomarkers of aging, 16-20
  criteria for, 17
  definition, 16
  division of into sets, 19
  genetic complication to utility of, 19
  not influenced by DR, 20
  predictive value of, 16, 17
  rodents used, 17-18
  selection of, 17, 18
Body composition, 213-215
  correlation LS and lean body mass, 214
  effects DR on, 213
    table, 213
  organ weights and, 215
  muscle mass and aging, 214
Body temperature, 209-213
  day long patterns of, 212
  effects long-term DR on, 209-213
    table, 211
  homeotherms, 261-263
  in state of torpor, 209
    graph, 210
    O_2 consumption during, 210
    measurement of in rodents, 209
  poikilotherms, 260
Bone
  effects long-term DR on, 221-223
    bone mineral content, 223
    femur strength, 221
    graphs, 222
    results of, 221
    role calciton in, 221, 223
    skeletal growth and senescence, 221
Brain receptors, effects DR on, 156-157, 158
Breast cancer (*see* Mammary tumors)
B/WF$_1$ (NZB x NZW) F$_1$ mice, autoimmunity syndromes of, 25-26

C

Carcinoma, 73
  effects DR on tumor incidence in rats, 82
  environmental factors and, 297
Cardiomyopathy, in rats, 83
Cardiovascular diseases, 73
Catalase
  acatalasemia, 259
  age-related declines in, 257
  and NADPH, 257
  definition, 256
  importance activity of to organism, 258
  involvement in control physiologic processes, 259
  protective role of, 258
  review literature on, 257-258
  role in prevention lens cataracts, 259
  summary, 260
Cataracts, 73
Catecholamines, effect long-term DR on, 155-156
Cerebrovascular diseases, 73
Cholesteral seum levels (*see* Lipid content)
Collagen
  effects DR on, 118
    findings, table, 119
Colon cancer, effect DR on, 112-113
Coronary disease, and DR in humans, 327
Council for Agricultural Science and Technology, on diet and coronary disease, 296

Council on Foods and Nutrition, AMA, on heart disease prevention, 296

D

Death hormone, 273, 274
Dementia, 73
Diabetes mellitus
 accelerated aging of, 4
 and DR in humans, 327
 induced in DR mice, 106
 insulin-dependent, 25
Dietary restriction (DR)
 between species/within species comparisons, 26-27
 biomarkers of aging (see Biomarkers of aging)
 composition diets used, 11-12
  table, 11
 decreased susceptibility to diseases by, 295
 definition, 6
 disease incidence, 74-75
 early onset type (see Early onset dietary restriction)
 effects on biological parameters, 117-229 (see also Biological parameters)
 effects on disease, 73-115 (see also Diseases)
 effects on survivorship, 31-72 (see also Survivorship)
 historical phases of research, 6-7, 29
  disease incidence and, 15-16
  human application, 28
  life span extension, 7-15 (see also Life span extension)
  physiologic changes and, 16-20 (see also Biomarkers of aging)
  search for mechanisms, 21
 human application of studies, 28
 interest developed in, vii
 life span extension (see Life span extension)
 maximum LS characteristic of species by, 295
 mechanisms, 21-28
  of retardation aging by (see Mechanisms)
 National Institute on Aging study, vii
 overview summary, 29
 physiologic changes (see Biomarkers of aging)
 potential benefits of besides LS extension, 326-328
 health benefits of diet, 326-327
 prevention certain diseases, 327-328
 potential dangers/disadvantages of for humans, 323-326
  American diet as borderline, 324
  decline in fecunidity, 324-325
  need begin diet in childhood, 323
  risks in later life, 325
  tumor incidence with DR, 325-326
  weight loss dangerous, 323
 prospects for retarding human aging by, 295-337 (see also Human aging retardation)
 retardation aging in rodents using 8-11
  agruments and responses, 12-15
 spontaneous diseases and (see Spontaneous diseases)
 statistical treatment of data, 28-29
 study environmental temperature and, 7
 successful defined, 8, 10
 theories of aging and, 21-24
  classification of, table, 22
  life spans and SMR, 23
  multifactorial aging, 24, 25
  organic disease, 25-26
  segmental juvenescence, 26
  unifactoral aging, 24
Diets used in rodent studies
 composition of, table, 11, 42
 low protein, 43
 non-purified (see Non-purified)
 normal, 11
 open formula, 42
 purified, 42
Diseases
 as distinct from aging, 232
 disease incidences in rodents, 74-75
  table, 75
 effects dietary restriction on, 73-115
 incidences in rodents fed ad lib, 74-75
 induced (see Induced diseases)
 main causes of death, 73
 of aging and causes of death, 73, 74
 spontaneous (see Spontaneous diseases)
 summary study effects DR on, 114-115
DNA
 and aging, 264
 and chromatin, 267-268
  effects DR on, 267
  nonenzymatic glycosylation, 267-268

Down's syndrome, 25

E

Early-onset dietary restriction (EDR)
  effects fat and protein in diets, 59
  effects in rodents, 45-60
    on growth, 45
    on health, 47-48
    on longevity, 48-60
    on puberty onset, 45-47
  effects on mice predeterimined to fatal diseases, 55, 59
  effects on rodent longevity, 48-60
    hypotension, 54-55
    maximum life span, 59-60
    of hypophysectomy, 54
    of injected ETCE, 49
    of tryptophan deficiency, 54
    protein enriched diet, 59-60
    study results, table, 56-58
    stunted growth, 49
    summary results, table, 50-52
  spontaneous diseases and DR started, EDR, 76-95 (*see also* Spontaneous diseases) use of, 10-11
Endocrine tumor, effects DR on incidence in rats, 82
Energy metabolism, 237-260
  age changes in normal metabolism, 237-241
    metabolic rate, 237-239
    mitochondria, 239-241
  dietary restriction, 251-260
    catalase activity, 256-257 (*see also* Catalase)
    decreased free radical production by, 256
    energy intake and use and, table, 254
    increased free radical neutralization by, 256-260
    measuring energy utilization, 253-254
    metabolic effects of DHEA and, 256
    metabolic efficiency and energy intake, 253-256
    metabolic rate and DR, 252-253
    quality of diet and metabolic efficiency, 255
    theory, 251-252
    weight loss and decreasing metabolic rate, 252-253
  free radicals and aging, 241-248
    activities/levels of antioxidants, 247-248
    energy coupling in mitochondria, 243-245
    energy usuage during oxidative phosphorylation, diagram, 245
    free radical neutralization, 246-248
    free radical production in mitochondria, 245-246
    future studies mitochondrial ATP production, 243-245
    longevity determinant gene hypothesis, 247
  metabolic efficiency, 248-251
    efficiency of energy generation, 248
    efficiency of energy usuage, 248
    energy flow in the body, 250
    energy used to pump ions, 250
    factors in thrift of, 250
    predicted differences inefficient and, table, 251
  metabolic rate, 237-239
    relative O_2 consumption values, table, 238
  mitochondria, 239-241
    age related changes in mammals, table, 242
    overview of mitrochondrial ATP generation, diagram, 240
Enzymes and metabolites
  long-term DR studies, 120-135
    ATPase activity in liver homogenates, 132
    catalase activity in liver homogenates, 132, 133-134
    conclusions, 135
    effects on enzyme activities, 133-134
    influences on, table, 122-127
    influences on liver composition in rats, 130, 131, 132
    results studies, 120, 128-130
  short-term DR studies, 135-137
    active oxygen defenses, 136
    catalase activity changes, 136
    definition short-term DR, 135
    hyperoxic stress tolerance, 136
Epithelial tumor, effects DR on incidence in rats, 82

F

Fibroadenomas, effect DR on radiation induced, 113-114
Fibromas
  effects DR on incidents, 82

in rats, 80
Fibrosarcomas
  effects DR on incidence, 82
  in rats, 80

G

Gene expression
  aging and DR
    conclusions of author, 269-270
    measurement activities/levels MRNA and aging, 268-270
  DNA and chromatin, 267-268
  DNA repair
  importance in aging phenomena, 270-271
  results study of, graph, 271
Gerontological Society of America, debate on use of DR, 295
Gerontology
  approaches to study of aging (*see* Aging)
  goals of, 3
Glucocorticoid cascade, effects DR on, 278-279
Glomerulonephritis, in rats on DR, 75, 76, 79, 82
Gout, and DR in humans, 327
Growth hormone and somatomedins, effects DR on, 147-148

H

Heart disease, and DR in humans, 327
Hepatocarcinoma, induced in DR mice, 107
Hepatoma
  classification nodules, 88
  incidence and longevity in DR mice, 100
  inhibition by EDR in mice, 86, 88, 89
  tumor incidence in different diet groups, 92, 94
  use of term, 88
Hematopoietic cancer
  effects DR on in mice, 90
  in rats, 81
Homeotherms, 261-263
  and life span, 262
  conclusions, 263
  decreased internal body temperature and DR, 261
  diet and, 261
  food intake and, 262-263

Human aging retardation by dietary restriction, 295-337
  comparison physiologic changes and diet, table, 207-208
  current attitudes toward diet and prevention of disease, 296-297
  evidence and conjecture against proposition, 306-316
    actuarial analyses, 306, 309-311
    aging control mechanism different humans and mammals, 314
    conclusions, 310-311, 315-316
    "desirable weight" tables, 309
    effect smoking habits, 310
    "heavier is better" thesis, 310
    lack increased longevity in underdeveloped countries, 315
    Masoro's objections, 311-313
    relation obesity and subsequent death rates, 309
    rodent growth goes beyond sexual maturity, 315
    species studies all short-lived, 314
    studies not true retardation of aging, 314-315
  evidence and conjecture in favor of proposition, 300-306
    human studies, 301-306
    question of animal data translatable to humans, 300-301
  human studies on DR and LS, 301-306
    anorexia nervosa, 303-304 (*see also* Anorexia nervosa)
    comment on, 306
    fasting, 305
    long-term dietary studies, 304-305
    Okinawan population isolate, 301-302 (*see also* Okinawan population isolate)
    Vallejo's experiment, 303
    vital capacity and weight change, 305
  method of human study, 316-323 (*see also* Human study method)
  past views on health disease and aging, 298-29
  possible lag period diet and disease, 298
  potential benefits DR besides LS extension, 326-328
  potential dangers/disadvantages DR for humans, 323-326
  professional "ageism," 299-300

proof and probability in medical practice, 296-299
research needs and recommendations for human studies, 330-337 (see also Human study)
social effects of LS extension, 328-330
summary, 336-337
Human study
  biomarkers of in study human aging, 330-335
    advantages use of, 333
    influenced by physical fitness, 334
    index of aging approach, 330, 331
    levels of lethality, 331
    mathematical problems in, 331-332
    past studies, 333-334
    prediction mortality, 334
    sample size, 332-333
  energy requirements, 319-321
    for U. S. male, 319
    individual variations, 320
    results studies, 321
    semistarvation study, 320-321
    study Japanese peasant farmers, 319-320
  essential nutrients, 321-322
  level of restriction and methodology appropriate for, 316-323
  primate populations prior to, 335
  rapidity of weight loss, 317
  research needs and recommendations for, 330-337
    biomarkers of aging, 330-335
    primate populations, 335
    social planning, 336
    testing of human cohorts, 335-336
  social planning, 336
  summary of, 336-337
    dietary recommendations, 322-323
    testing of human cohorts, 335-336
  weight loss limits, 317-319
  where to begin, 316-317
Hypertension
  and DR in humans, 327, 328
  effects DR on in rats, 84
Hypothalamus-pituitary axis
  death hormone, 273, 274
  effects long-term DR following Hx, 274-275
  effects long-term Hx with hormonal replacement, 274
    table, 274

pituitary theory and DR mechanism, 275-276
role in aging, 273-276

I

Immune response capacities of mice, 186-196
  conclusions studies, 196
  diet used, 191
  effects DR on, table, 187
  immunosenescence in male mice, 194
  study PHA and ConA responses, 191-193
  natural killer cell activity in splenocytes, 194
    table, 195
  new disease model mice used, 189
  results authors' study, 189-190
  study immunologic aging in mice, 190
  use amino acid deficient diet, 188-189
  use low protein diets, 186, 188-189
Immunologic interpretation, 281-286
  aging, immune function, MHC-related functions, 281-282
  conclusion, 286
  dietary restriction, immune function and MHC, 282-283
  long-lived strain, aging and DR, 283-284
  MHC-influenced but non-immune phenomena, 285-286
  role immunosenescence, 281
  short-lived strain, aging and DR, 284
Immunologic parameters, 179-197
  autoimmunity, 196-197
  cellnumbers, proportions and subpopulations, 183-186
    changes in cell numbers, table, 184
    changes in subpopulations, table, 185
    effects DR on, 183
    splenic lymphocyte subsets in mice, 186
  immune response capacities, 186-196 (see also Immune response capacities)
  influence DR on, 179
  lymphoid biochemistry, 197
  thymus, 179-183 (see also Thymus)
Induced diseases, 101-114
  benzpyrene-induced skin tumors in DBA mice, 104
  effect quality of DR regimen on induction of, 105, 107-108
  experimental animals used to study, 101

effect DR on tumor induction, 104-105
effect DR on tumor initiation and/or promation, 104
  in recent study DR mice, 105, 107
    table, 106
  relationship severity DR, time of onset and, 102-103
  resistance DR rodents to, 101
  results studies in DR mice, 102-103
    table, 103
  studies with DR rats, 108-114
    inhibiting chemical tumorigenesis, 108-112
  studies with mice, 102
  use gamma irradiation before institution DR, 107
Insulin and glucagon
  caloric dilution DR use, 153, 154-155
  conclusion, 155
  effects long-term DR on, 149
  exploration pancreatic islets, 153, 154
  influence diet and age on, 150, 151
  lipolytic response, 150
  plasma levels in rats studied, 150
  rat adipocytes studies, 152-153
Intersociety Commission for Heart Disease Resources, on diet and heart disease, 296

L

Learning and behavioral parameters, 227-229
  effects DR on in, 227-228
    biochemical findings, 227-228
    maze performance, 228-229
    psycho/physical function, 228
Leukemia
  induced in DR mice, 103, 106
  in rodents on DR, 75
  inhibition by EDR in mice, 86, 87
Life span
  definition maximum LS, 5
  effects dietary restriction on (see Survivorship)
  extension of (see Life span extension)
  maximum in developed societies today, 5
  strategies for increasing, 4-5
    by dietary restriction, 4-5
    by lowering core body temperature, 4-5
    table, 5
  survival curves, 5, 6, 12
Life span extension (see also Survivorship)
  dietary restriction and (see Dietary restriction)
  in invertebrates, 7-8
  in poikilothermic vertebrates, 7-8
  in rodents, 8-15
    age-specific tumor incidence, 12
    diets used in studies, table, 11
    early studies of, 8, 10
    results argument and responses, 12-15
    results author's studies, 11-12
    strategies tested, table, 9
  social effects of, 328-330
  study dietary restriction and (see Dietary restriction)
Lipid content and peroxidation, 173-178
  cholesterol serum levels, 174
    composition, 176
    studies DR and aging changes in, 174-179
    table, 175
  effects long-term DR on prostaglandin metabolism, 175
  influence DR and aging, 173-178
  lipid content after long-term DR, 174
  lipid peroxidation and lipofuscin, 176-178
    effects long-term DR on, 716
    heart lipofuscin, 177
    quantitation of, 176
  peroxidative tone indicators, 173
  phospholipids serum levels
    studies DR and aging changes in, 174-179
    table, 175
  triglycerides serum levels, 174
    studies DR and aging changes, 174-179
    table, 175
Lipid peroxidation and lipofuscin, 176-178
Lipoma, effects DR on incidence in rats, 82
Longevity determinant gene hypothesis, 247
LS (see Life span)
Lung tumor (see Pulmonary tumor)
Lymphoid biochemistry, effects DR on, 197
Lymphoma
  in rodents on DR, 75, 80
  incidence and longevity in DR mice, 100
Lymphoreticular cancer
  effects DR on incidence, 82
  in rats, 81
Lymphosarcomas

diet and incidence tumor, 92-93
in DR mice, 91
in lungs of DA rats, 76

M

Mammary carcinoma
  fat intake and, 305
  in DR mice ADR, 97
  relationship to caloric intake in mice, 97, 99
Mammary tumor
  DMBA-induced in DR rats, 104-105
  in DR mice, 90, 91
  in DR rodents, 75, 76, 79, 84
  inhibition by EDR in mice, 85, 86, 87
  study of DMBA-induced, 109-110
  effects energy and fat intakes on, 111-112
Mechanisms of DR retardation of aging, 231-294
  age-sensitive but DR-resistant parameters, table, 233
  basal/induced activity hypothesis, 286
  body temperature, 260-263 (see also Body temperature)
  chromatin, 267-268
  conclusion and interpretation, 293
  DNA, 264, 267-268
  DNA repair, 270-271
  energy metabolism, 237-260 (see also Energy metabolism)
  evolutionary perspective, 234-236
    Sacher's equations, 235-236
    Totter's hypothesis, 234-235
  focus of future studies, 233-234
  gene expression, 268-270
  hypothesis, 293-294
  immunologic interpretation, 281-286 (see also Immunologic interpretation)
  neuroendocrine interpretation, 272-280 (see also Neuroendocrine interpretation)
  phylogenetic independence of effect, 232
  protein synthesis, 263-264, 265-267 (see also Protein synthesis)
  retardation aging in mammals, 232
  systems analysis, 289-293 (see also Systems analysis)
Melanoma, induced in DR mice, 106
Metabolic rate, 197-209
  effect DR on, 197-198
    table, 202

lifetime energy intake, 198-201
  calculations used, 198, 199
  evaluation DR's impact on, 198, 200-201
  studies of in mice, 198-199
mitochondria, 203-209
  brain mitochondrial respiration, 205
  effect DR on live mitochondrial respiration, 206
  effect DR on mitochondial recovery in mice, 205
  effects exercise on oxidative capacity, 206-208
  isolated liver mitochondrial fractions, micrographs, 207
  long-term DR's influences on, 203
  measurements of, 206
  mitochondrial recovery, 204-205
  O_2 utilization in rats, 208
  results studies, 208-209
  stimulation respiration by ADP, 203-204
  O_2 consumption and heat production, 201-203
  measurement of heat production, 201
  use short-term DR in studies, 202-203
Metabolism, energy (see Energy metabolism)
Molecular parameters, 118-179
  collagen, 118 (see also Collagen)
  enzymes and metabolites, 120-137 (see also Enzymes and metabolites)
  lipid content and peroxidation, 173-178
  neuroendocrine, 137-159 (see also Enuroendocrine)
  nucleic acid, 159-167 (see also Nucleic acid)
  protein, 167-173 (see also Protein)
Muscle
  in long-term DR animals, 215-218
  composition muscles, 216
  effects aging, 216, 217
  non-skeletal, 218
Musculoskeletal and soft tissue tumor, incidence in rats, 82
Myocardial degeneration
  in rats on DR, 75, 79
  incidence, 79
Myocardial fibrosis, in rats on DR, 76
Myocardial infarction, in rats on DR, 84

N

National Heart, Lung and Blood Institute,

Task Force on Arteriosclerosis, on diet, 296
National Institute on Aging
 daily requirements study, viii
 establishment of, 3
National Research Council Committee on Chemical Toxicity and Aging, viii
National Research Council Food and Nutrition Board, on diet and heart disease, 296
Neoplasia, in rats, 83
Neoplasms, in rodents on DR, 75
Nephropathy
 autoimmune
  effects zinc deficiency on, 99-100
  in mice, 85, 97
 chronic, in rats on DR, 82, 83
 mechanisms inhibition EDR in, 88-89
Nephrosis, incidence in rats, 79
Neuroendocrine, 137-159
 changes associated with long-term DR, 137-159
 non-reproductive aspects, 143-159
  ACTH and corticosterone, 148-149
  brain receptors, 156-159
  catecholamines, 155-156
  growth hormone and somatomedins, 147-148
  influences DR on, table, 159
  insulin and glucagon, 149-155
  parathyroid hormone and calcitonin, 156
  synopsis, 159
  thyroid axis, 143-147 (see also Thyroid axis)
 pseudohypophysectomy defined, 137
 reproductive aspects, 138-143
  EDR's impact on hormone level, 138, 140
  effects long-term DR on reproduction, 140-141
  impact brief DR on serum hormone levels, 141-143
  influences aging and DR on serum levels, 139
  sensitivity to DR, 138
  studies reports reviewed, 141
  study tryptophane in rats, 141
Neutoendocrine cascade, and aging, 278-279
Neuroendocrine interpretation, 272-280
 conclusion, 280
 glucocorticoid and neuroendocrine cascades, 278-279
 hypothalamus-pituitary axis, 273-276
 hypotheses of, representation, 280
 neuroendocrine-immune interactions, 279-280
 reproductive senescence and the hypothalamus, 276-278
 theory of role DR and, 272-273
Neuroendocrine-immune interactions, and aging, 279-280
Non-purified diet, composition of, 42
Nucleic acid, 159-167
 content, 160-166
  DNA synthesis, 163, 164
  effects aging and DR on, 165
  RNA, DNA, protein changes, 162
  studies effects DR on, 160-161
  synthesis proteins and, 162-166
 expression, 166
 influences Dr on, table, 161
 repair, effect DR on, 167

O

Okinawan population isolate
 diet of, 301-302
 HLA distribution, 302
 incidence centenarians, 302
 total energy consumed by school children, 302
Osteoporosis, 73
Ovarian carcinoma, in rodents on DR, 75
Ovarian tumor
 in mice on DR, 90
 in rodents, 75

P

Pancreas tumor, effects DR on incidence in rats, 82
Pancreatic islet cell tumors, in rats on DR, 80, 81
Papilloma, effects DR on incidence in rats, 82
Parathyroid, effects DR on incidence in rats, 82
Parathyroid hormone and calcitonin
 effect DR on, 156
 effects aging and diet on, 157, 158
Periarteritis
 in rats on DR, 79
 incidence, 79

Peroxidation (*see* Lipid content)
Phospholipids (*see* Lipid content)
Physiologic parameters 197-227
  adipose tissue, 218-220
  age-sensitive, 226
  body composition, 213-215 (*see also* Body composition)
  body temperature, 209-213
  bone, 221-223
  effects DR on in rodents, 226-227
    table, 226
  learning and behavioral, 227-229
  muscle, 215-218
  metabolic rate, 197-209 (*see also* Metabolic rate)
  reproductive senescence, 223-225
  results studies DR effects on, 197
  summary, 229
Pituitary chromophobe adenomas
  in mice on DR, 90
  in rats, on DR, 76, 79, 81
Pituitary tumor
  in rodents, 75, 84
    effects DR on incidence, 82
  in DR mice, table, 91
Pneumonia, chronic, with bronchiectasis, and DR in, 76
Polyarteritis nodosa, in rats on DR, 79
Poikilotherms, and life span, 260
Prostaglandin metabolism, effects long-term DR on, 175
Protein
  content, 168-171
    age-related changes in, 168-171
    effects aging and DR on, table, 165
    method of study, 168
    results studies, 167
  synthesis and turnover
    effects DR on, 171, 172
    results studies, 171-173
Protein synthesis and aging
  effects DR on, 264, 265-267
  increase of in DR animals, 266-267
  selective upregulation of, 266
Pulmonary adenomas
  in DR mice, 91, 97
  in rats, 80
Pulmonary disease, in rats, 76
Pulmonary lymphosarcomas, in rats on DR, 76

Pulmonary tumor
  in DR mice, 91
  in DR rodents, 75
  incidence and longevity in DR mice, 100
  inhibition by EDR in mice, 80, 86, 87, 88, 89, 90
Purified diet (PD), composition rodent diet, 42
Pseudohypophysectomy, definition, 137

R

Radiculoneuropathy, in rats on DR, 79
RCA tumor, in DR mice, 91
RCS, 91
  lung, effects DR on incidence in rats, 82
  lymph, effects DR on incidence in rats, 82
Renal disease
  effects DR on in rats, 84
  inhibition by EDR in mice, 86, 88
Reproductive senescence, 223-225
  cycling capacities on EDR, 223-224
  effects long-term DR on, 223
  tryptophan restriction, 225
Reproductive senescence and the hypothalamus
  effects age on hypothalamus, 276-277
  effects DR on, 277-278
  effects ovariectomy, 276
  interplay between, 278
  long-term effects early Hx, table, 277
  long-term effects early ovariectomy, table, 277
  reciprocal relationship between, 276
Reticulum cell sarcomas, in rats, 80
Rheumatoid arthritis, fasting and, 305

S

Sacher's equations, 235-236
Sarcoma
  induced in DR mice, 106
  inhibition due DR ARD, 104
Skeletal muscle degeneration
  in rats on DR, 79
  incidence, 79
Somatomedins (*see* Growth hormone)
Spontaneous diseases, 76-101
  dietary restriction started in adulthood, 95-101

studies with mice, 97-101
studies with rats, 95-97
incidence in rodents fed lib, 74-75
table, 75
retardation of in rodents, 73-74
studies DR mice ADR, 97-100
  collective results of, 101
  of effects on late-life diseases, 97
  phases of, 97
  results phrases of studies, 97-101
  results Tannenbaum's studies, 98
  retardation ongoing diseases, 99-100
  tumor incidence and longevity, 100
studies DR mice EDR, 84-95
  long-lived species, 89-95
  short-lived species, 85-89
studies DR rats ADR, 95-97
  diet regimen, 96
studies DR rats EDR, 76-84
  diet regimen used, 80-81
  incidence lesions, table, 79
  reports of summarized, table, 77-78
  selection of diets, 84
  tumor incidence patterns, table, 81
studies long-lived DR mice EDR, 89-95
  ages at death of tumor bearing mice, 93, 94
  delayed development of tumors, table, 91
  development of diseases, 90-91
  diet groups and tumor incidence, 92, 94-95
  effects DR on tumor patterns, 91
  improved LS with mild DR regimen, 90
  reports studied, 89-90
  tumor incidence and DR effects, 93
studies short-lived DR mice EDR, 85-89
  breast cancer in, 85
  disease inhibition in, 85, 86
  inhibition hepatoma, 86, 88
  inhibition leukemia, 86, 87
  inhibition lung tumor, 86
  inhibition mammary carcinoma, 85-87
  inhibition renal disease, 86
  results of, 88-89
trout study results, 73
Stomach lesions, in DR mice, 90
Survival curves
  for USA females, 5
  graph, 6
Survivorship, effects dietary restriction on, 31-72 (*see also* Life span)
  analysis of, 31-35

results studies of, 34-35
studies in rodents, 40-71
  adult-onset DR, 60-71
  early-onset DR, 45-60
  fasting, 44-45
  feeding strategies, 41-44
  low protein diet, 43
  restricted feeding of adequate diet, 42-43
  types diets use, 40-41
studies in invertebrates, 36-39
studies in vertebrates, 36-71
  non-rodent, 39-40
  rodent, 40-71
"toxic stress" plotted, 35
summary, 71, 72
ways to express longevity
  Comperz equation, 33-34
  doubling time, 34
  Gompertz mortality parameters, 34
  Gompertz plot, 33, 34
  survival curves, 12, 31-31
Systemic lupus erythematosus, accelerated aging of, 4
Systems analysis of aging, 289-293
  approach to, 289
  couple system
    connection to concepts about aging, 292-293
    coupling constants, 292
    decay constants, 292
    definition, 291
    equations used, 291-292
    recovery constants, 291-292
  future of, 293
  hierarchical homeostasis, 290
  species survival over individual survival, 290

T

Thymus
  aging in hypophysectomized B6 mice, 181-182
  conclusions, 183
  effect DR on mice weight, 179, 180
  effects early-onset DR on, 180-181
  effects low protein diets, 182-183
  histologic make-up, 180
  hormone levels, 181
  table, 182

thymic factor activities, 181
Thyroid axis, 143-147
  diet and T_3 levels, 146
  diets used in studies, 146
  plasma T_1 levels in DR, 145
  proteins and thyroxine, table, 144
  study mechanism of DR's action, 143-144
  summary, 147
Thyroid lesion, in DR mice, 90-91
Thyroid tumor
  effects DR on in mice, 90
  effects DR on incidence in rats, 82
  morbidity, 81
Totter's hypothesis, 234-235
Triglycerides (see Lipid content)
Tryplophan, effects diet deficient in, 54
Tumorigenesis
  diabetes, 114
  hormones and cancer, 114
  inhibiting chemical, 108-112
    diet groups used, 110-111
    dietary regimen, 109
    hypothesis tested, 109
    restriction dietary energy vs. fat, 108-112
  intestinal by chemicals, 112-113
  radiation-induced, 113-114

U

U. S. Senate, Select Committee on Nutrition and Human Needs, on diet and arteriosclerosis, 296

W

Wechsler Adult Intelligence Scale, use as biomarker, 332-333